Manual and Atlas
of Fine Needle
Aspiration Cytology

For Churchill Livingstone

Publisher: Timothy Horne
Editorial Co-ordination: Editorial Resources Unit
  Copy Editor: Leslie Smillie
  Indexer: Laurence Errington
Production Controller: Lesley Small
Design: Design Resources Unit
Sales Promotion Executive: Hilary Brown

Manual and Atlas of Fine Needle Aspiration Cytology

Svante R. Orell
ML FRCPA FIAC

Consultant Pathologist, Gribbles Pathology; Former
Associate Professor of Pathology and Director of Diagnostic
Cytology, Flinders Medical Centre, Adelaide, South Australia

Gregory F. Sterrett
MBBS FRCPA MIAC

Clinical Associate Professor and Cytopathologist, Hospital and
University Pathology Services, The Queen Elizabeth II
Medical Centre, Perth, Western Australia

Max N-I. Walters
MD FRACP FRCPath FRCPA

Professor of Pathology, University of Western Australia;
Director, Hospital and University Pathology Services, The
Queen Elizabeth II Medical Centre, Perth, Western Australia

Darrel Whitaker
PhD CFIAC FIMLS AAIMLS

Cytologist, Hospital and University Pathology Services, The
Queen Elizabeth II Medical Centre, Perth, Western Australia

With contributions by

Måns Åkerman
MD PhD FIAC

Associate Professor, University of Lund; Director, Department
of Clinical Cytology, University Hospital, Lund, Sweden

Suzanne Le P. Langlois
MBBS FRACR DDU

Director, Department of Radiology, Royal Adelaide Hospital,
Adelaide, South Australia

Karin Lindholm
MD FIAC

Director, Cytodiagnostic Department, Malmö General
Hospital, Malmö, Sweden

Foreword by

Nils G. Stormby
MD PhD FIAC

Associate Professor of Pathology, The University of Malmö,
Malmö, Sweden; Former President of the International
Academy of Cytology

CHURCHILL LIVINGSTONE

EDINBURGH LONDON MADRID MELBOURNE
NEW YORK AND TOKYO 1992

CHURCHILL LIVINGSTONE
Medical Division of Longman Group UK Limited

Distributed in the United States of America by Churchill
Livingstone Inc., 650 Avenue of the Americas, New York, N.Y. 10011, and
by associated companies, branches and representatives
throughout the world.

First edition 1986
Second edition 1992

ISBN 0-443-04239-X

British Library Cataloguing in Publication Data
CIP catalogue record to this book is available from the British Library

Library of Congress Cataloging in Publication Data
Manual and atlas of fine needle aspiration cytology / Svante R. Orell
    . . . [et al.]; with contributions by Måns Åkerman, Suzanne Le P.
Langlois, Karin Lindholm; foreword by Nils G. Stormby. — 2nd ed.
        p. cm.
    Includes bibliographical references and index.
    1. Diagnosis, Cytologic—Handbooks, manuals, etc. 2. Biopsy,
Needle—Handbooks, manuals, etc. 3. Pathology, Surgical—Handbooks,
manuals, etc.   I. Orell, Svante R.
    [DNLM: 1. Biopsy, Needle. 2. Cytodiagnosis. WB 379 M294]
RB43.M36 1992
616.07'582—dc20
DNLM/DLC
for Library of Congress   91–23111
                                                   CIP

Produced by Longman Group (F-E) Ltd
Printed in Hong Kong

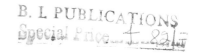
FOREWORD TO SECOND EDITION

The new edition of this Manual and Atlas of Fine Needle Aspiration Cytology is most welcome. Not because the first one was less than excellent or outdated – but simply because it was sold out. It has proved to be one of those work-mates not kept on the shelf but by necessity handily placed beside the microscope.

Cytological diagnosis means the interpretation of pictures and in daily work we refer to pictorial memories which constitute our experience. But, just as many of us store family and holiday photos unsorted in shoeboxes for years instead of providing them with text and storing them in an orderly way, so we are also less prone to approach a cytological problem logically and systematically.

This is the beauty of this book. It is not only an atlas but also a true manual with schematically presented criteria for diagnosis as well as for problems. The frustrated morphologist hunting to find an illustration which hopefully might resemble the actual diagnostic problem is common. In this book he or she is well served by the precise schematic approach to, and the encircling of the target, completed by an elaborate text where cytological features are solidly based on their histological base. Our profession has not only got a treasure for the innocent beginner but also an ample and crystal clear source for the experienced cytopathologist.

In a new edition you should of course expect an up-dating of the state of the science, new techniques and references, etc. The chapter on the cytology of breast lesions is now an example par excellence and the constructive and critical presentation of immunocytochemistry is very useful. The diagnostic edge from the first edition has been further sharpened. But Quintilianus is still right:

In omnibus fere minus valent praecepta quam experimenta.

Malmö, Sweden   Nils Stormby
April 1992

FOREWORD TO FIRST EDITION

Although the cradle of the technique can be found elsewhere, modern aspiration cytology is firmly rooted in Sweden, particularly in the sense that no other country has been such a fast and general acceptance of the method. This is due to two facts: first, two of the true pioneers, Dr Sixten Franzén – eventually heavily supported by the late Dr Joseph Zajicek – and Professor Nils Söderström, were both Swedish clinicians; secondly, the leading professors of surgical pathology were very quick to acknowledge both exfoliative and aspiration cytology as integrated aspects of morphology, thus also securing the histopathological base of cytology in the laboratory.

As a result of this, a cadre of young pathologists at different universities were encouraged to look into this new field. Influenced by the character of aspiration cytology as a bedside method, these doctors soon left their laboratories and went to see patients. They began to perform the technique after thorough clinical examination of the patients, or collaborated directly on the spot with roentgenologists or other visualising specialists. In this way a high diagnostic accuracy was obtained, to the delight of the clinicians.

The demand for laboratory services is set by clinicians and the complete success of aspiration cytology occurred when, particularly, ENT-doctors, oncologists and surgeons eventually found that this new method was indispensable to their clinical work. Since it was already established in tissue pathology and used by clinicians, disputes over the value of aspiration cytology were never heard in Sweden – to use modern phraseology, 'The market was there.'

It may seem unnecessary to give a lengthy description of the situation in Sweden in an Australian textbook; however, Dr Orell, who is the main author of this book, happens to be one of these exports from Sweden, who represents the second generation pioneers – a pathologist who in the early sixties became fascinated by the diagnostic possibilities mediated by a thin needle – parva sed apta!

This solid background of histopathology is, undoubtedly, the hallmark of all of the authors of this book and is strongly reflected in the strict and didactic presentation of diagnostic criteria as well as problems in differential diagnosis. Although 90% of interpretation is learned by microscopy and 10% by reading, the logical presentation of cytologic facts and features is of tremendous value to the beginner. Thus, there is a beneficial difference between this and a number of other publications that seem more to be collections of case reports than true textbooks.

The choice of staining method is a never-ending matter of discussion among cytopathologists. It is true that pathologists – including myself – from the beginning have been much more familiar and comfortable with wet-fixed smears stained with haematoxylin-eosin or according to Papanicolaou; however, it would be very unwise not to become familiar with the May-Grunwald-Giemsa (MGG) method also, since in a number of situations, particularly when it comes to cytoplasmic detail, it is superior to others and is actually often indispensable. In the procedure of wet fixation there is also a tendency for cells to shed off the glass slide. No wonder then, that MGG illustrations predominate here. Unfortunately, twin pictures with both MGG and Papanicolaou are not economically feasible.

In a specialty much dependent on visual impressions, illustrations obviously play an important role. Although economy also prevents the reproduction of all microphotographs in colour, the number of colour plates is uncommonly high and, moreover, the black and white reproductions are confined to histological sections where the illustration of cytological features is less dependent on colour. The stringent presentation of facts in the text supported by the pictures makes the reading both easy and enjoyable.

Indeed, this book should also be carefully studied by clinicians: one reason for this is that it gives the technical advice necessary to provide good smears – not all can or must be taken by the cytologist; another is the presentation of aspiration cytology as a diagnostic system with its possibilities as well as its limitations. Nobody can teach that better than the pathologist well experienced in cytology. Aspiration cytology is not a

substitute for histopathology but is one of the weapons
to be used to hit the diagnostic target. This book has a
sharp edge. Read and learn.

Malmö, Sweden   Nils Stormby
1986

ACKNOWLEDGEMENTS

Many people in both Adelaide and Perth have helped in the preparation of this book and we owe all of them our thanks; many have directly contributed; others have vigorously supported the introduction of fine needle aspiration cytology into medical practice in our respective hospitals, and thereby made this atlas possible. A major debt is owed to our teachers, particularly those from the Karolinska Hospital Cytology Department, for their help in guiding our initial steps in the discipline.

We would especially like to thank Professor Richard Whitehead, Head of the Department of Histopathology, Flinders Medical Centre, for his continuing support and stimulating interest in our work. All of the staff of the Department have given us generous assistance in the collection and follow-up of material; we are particularly grateful to Professor Douglas Henderson, Professor John Skinner and Dr Edward Chandraratnam for their contributions. We are greatly indebted to our clinical colleagues at the Flinders Medical Centre, especially to Dr Elizabeth McK. Cant, Professor V. Marshall and Dr R. R. Sanders for a critical review of the manuscript within their respective fields of expertise.

From The Queen Elizabeth II Medical Centre, all of the staff of the Pathology Department must be thanked, but in particular Professor Keith Shilkin and Professor John Papadimitriou; among the clinicians in the Hospital, Professor Harry Sheiner, and Drs John Glancy, Donald Gutteridge, and Ronald Yuen, have also been responsible for providing material. Their continuous interest and enthusiasm has been indispensable.

The members of the Cytology Department of both institutions have been surpassingly tolerant of the extra burdens imposed upon them in the collection and organisation of our material; we would like to thank Mrs Kay Dowling and Mr Barry Gormley in particular for their contributions.

The bulk of the secretarial assistance has come from Sandra Jones; Gillian Wilde, Lee Gardiner, Mrs E. Effinger, Catherine Bell and Beverley Corcoran have also been tireless and uncomplaining workers.

The Departments of Medical Illustration at both Flinders Medical Centre and The Queen Elizabeth II Medical Centre were heavily involved in the project and special thanks must go to Mr Peter Graaf and Mr Harry Upenieks for their talents and efforts on our behalf.

Many pathologists have contributed case material to the atlas. They include Dr N. Ferguson of Royal Newcastle Hospital, Dr Wendy Lew of the Queen Elizabeth Hospital, Adelaide, Dr Vincent Munro of St Vincent's Hospital, Sydney, Dr Dorothy Rosenthal of the UCLA School of Medicine, Los Angeles, Dr Terry Schultz of Wangaratta Base Hospital, Dr R. Seshadri of the Flinders Medical Centre, and in Perth, Dr John Armstrong, and Dr Elaine Waters from Royal Perth Hospital, Dr Ray Joyce of St John of God Hospital, Drs Trevor Kyle and David Knight of Kings Park Laboratories, and Dr Jim Carroll of Fremantle Laboratories. We are most grateful for their help.

In addition to the people mentioned above, a number of eminent colleagues in Australia and overseas have given us valuable advice and assistance in the preparation of the second edition of this book. Dr Antoine Zajdela of the Curie Institute, Paris, generously offered his time and unique experience to critically review the chapter of FNA of the breast. We are also greateful to Dr Melville Carter, Royal Adelaide Hospital, Adelaide, for updating the clinical/surgical aspects and implications of cytological diagnosis of breast lesions.

Additional case material has been made available to us by many pathologists in Australia: Dr Dennis Moir, Dr S. K. Tang, Dr B. H. Coombes; and overseas, Dr Karin Lindholm, Malmö, Sweden and Dr A. Kurniawan, University of Indonesia, Jakarta. Barry Greiger of the Department of Photography at Adelaide Children's Hospital and Frank Shilton of the Medical Illustration Department at The Queen Elizabeth II Medical Centre in Perth helped in preparing photographic material.

The publishers, Churchill Livingstone, deserve special praise for their perseverance with our undertaking; the project would undoubtedly not have reached fruition without their optimism, friendliness and encouragement.

CONTENTS

1

INTRODUCTION

1 *INTRODUCTION*

HISTORICAL PERSPECTIVE

For over 100 years the discipline of anatomical pathology has centred on diagnostic histopathology, and this, in turn, on the surgical biopsy. The pathologist sitting at his microscope, analysing the arrangement and tinctorial patterns of cells, frequently provides the definitive diagnosis by which therapy is determined.

For the last 50 years exfoliated and abraded samples of cells have also been collected from accessible anatomical surfaces, especially from the uterine cervix and the bronchus. Thus a diagnostic discipline has arisen in parallel with histopathology which subserves both a screening and a predictive function. Unfortunately, in many instances, these two streams in pathology developed as essentially separate disciplines so that the interchange of new ideas to the benefit of both did not occur as readily as it should have.

At about the same time as histopathologists and cytologists began their tentative initiatives, Leyden[18] and, three years later, Menetrier[23] employed needles to obtain cells and tissue fragments, the former to isolate pneumonic micro-organisms and the latter to diagnose pulmonary carcinoma. Few early pathologists were, however, involved in this pioneering work and the development of needle aspiration cytology along with exfoliative cytology was, to a large extent, performed by 'professional hybrids',[29] clinicians who used these simple techniques as aids to rapid diagnosis. For example, the wide acceptance of needling the bone marrow as an integral part of the investigation of haematological problems continued to serve as a reminder that almost every tissue could be sampled by an easily acquired technique requiring no anaesthesia nor the expensive intervention of surgeons.[10] In Great Britain in 1927, Dudgeon and Patrick[3] proposed the needling of tumours as a means of rapid microscopic diagnosis; similarly, Martin and Ellis[22] at the Memorial Hospital in the USA were also advocates of needle aspiration, although the pathologists working with them initially insisted on sectioning as well as smearing the samples, and would only make a confident diagnosis if cell-block preparations were obtained. Consequently, Martin and Ellis used needles of a thicker calibre (18 gauge) than those commonly in use today. The pathologists at Memorial continued to use the technique, but this hospital remained an oasis for 'aspiration biopsy' in America; limited interest was shown by other cancer centres.

It was in Europe and particularly Scandinavia, that 'fine-needle aspiration' (FNA) as the technique was usually called began to flourish in the 1950s and 1960s. Söderström[28] and Franzén[6] in Sweden, and also Lopes Cardozo[20] in Holland (all clinician/haemotologists by training) became major proponents, studying thousands of cases each year. Zajicek[36,37] among the first of pathologists to embrace FNA, in collaboration with Franzén at the Karolinska Hospital, applied the requisite scientific rigor to define precise diagnostic criteria and to determine diagnostic accuracy in a variety of conditions. Disciples of these pioneers have spread the gospel to Europe, the UK, the Americas, Japan and Australia, so that the technique should now be part of the service of all sophisticated departments of pathology.

It is interesting to note that in the last few years there has been a swing back to core needles, usually of a lesser calibre than those used in the pre-FNA era, and to histological sectioning of tissue fragments.[26] This may be the result of the increasing pressure on tissue pathologists, including those without sufficient training and experience in diagnostic cytology, to make definitive and specific diagnoses on needle biopsy material in all kinds of disease processes in all sites. The pressure on the pathologist is particularly strong in the investigation of disease processes in deep sites in which the only alternative to explorative laparotomy or thoracotomy is needle biopsy guided by ultrasonography or by computerised tomography. However, with reference to the older literature, one cannot help worrying that the use of core needles may carry a greater risk of complications than the simple fine needle of less than 21 gauge, without necessarily improving diagnostic accuracy.[27] We feel that core needle biopsy is an excellent tool in specific situations, but rather than using it routinely, one should make every effort to improve the fine needle cytology techniques.

ADVANTAGES AND LIMITATIONS

In the practice of FNA there are clear advantages to patients, to doctors, and to tax-payers. The technique is relatively painless, produces a speedy result, and is cheap.[5,11] Its accuracy in many situations, when applied by experienced and well-trained practitioners, can approach that of histopathology in providing an unequivocal diagnosis. We should stress, however, that aspiration cytology is not a substitute for conventional surgical histopathology; it should be regarded as an extremely valuable complement to it, and is itself becoming just as indispensable.

The method is applicable to lesions that are easily palpable; for example, superficial growths of the skin, subcutis and soft tissues, and organs such as the thyroid, breast, salivary glands, and superficial lymph nodes. New radiological techniques for internal imaging of organs and lesions in sites not easily accessible to surgical biopsy have opened vast opportunities for FNA of deeper structures. Aspirates may be taken from the lung, the prostate and the abdominal and retroperitoneal organs and tissues as the first step in laboratory investigation, and can quickly satisfy the avidity of clinicians for rapid diagnoses. Costly days in hospital can be saved, since a tissue diagnosis can be obtained within minutes rather than days.

FNA biopsy is less demanding technologically than surgical biopsy; in this respect it is eminently suitable for practice in countries with scant resources which are unable to fund teams of surgeons, anaesthetists, nurses, etc. The low risk of complications is an additional advantage which allows FNA biopsy to be performed as an office procedure, in out-patient departments, and in radiology theatres; it is also highly suitable in debilitated patients, is readily repeatable, and useful for multiple lesions. Instances of serious complications have been reported, such as major haemorrhage after FNA of lung, liver and kidney, septicaemia after prostatic aspiration, bile peritonitis following needling of the liver and acute pancreatitis resulting from pancreatic aspiration. However, such complications are extremely rare when compared to the many tens of thousands of uncomplicated FNA biopsies which have been performed in major centres where close follow-up of patients is the rule. The possibility of cancer cells being disseminated along the needle-track initially caused a great deal of concern, precipitated by occasional reports of tumour implants at the site of incisional biopsy or of core needle biopsy. The literature was recently reviewed by Roussel et al[27] who collected all reported cases of tumour implantation in the track after intraabdominal needle biopsy (see also Chs. 8, 9 and 10). They found 10 cases of seeding after the use of a fine needle (21 gauge or less). Multiple passes, larger needles and absence of normal parenchyma covering the lesion appear to increase the risk. The recent trend to return to larger cutting core needles therefore causes some concern. The rare severe complications do not diminish the clinical value and wide applications of FNA cytology but should serve as a reminder always to review the indications for any invasive procedure, however simple and traumatic.

Although FNA can be applied to practically every organ and tissue of the body, certain limitations do exist. In some areas experience is still rudimentary, and diagnostic cytological criteria are still being formulated. Even when routine smears can be supplemented by special investigations specific diagnostic conclusions may not be reached, although useful information indicating further lines of investigation may still be obtained. In some areas of diagnosis, such as soft tissue tumours, patients are best referred to major centres with specialised oncological expertise. Such centralisation is desirable so that the accumulated experience eventually allows the definition of diagnostic criteria for uncommon neoplasms and other diseases. On the other hand, because such cases will be seen initially in general surgical clinics, the hospital pathologist must be able to provide some indication of the nature of the condition as a basis for referral and must have a wide knowledge of the range of possible conditions in a particular site.

We should stress that FNA cytology as practised today is still a relatively new discipline and no single pathologist can lay claim to vast experience of its every facet. The numerous case reports of all kinds of rare and exotic tumours and other pathological processes diagnosed by FNA cytology found in the cytology journals give a strong impression that nothing is impossible for this technique. However, on second thought, one wonders just how confident was the pathologist of the specific diagnosis and how ready to accept full responsibility for major therapeutic decisions based on this diagnosis. Hajdu and Melamed 1984 issued a warning against overconfidence in FNAC diagnosis which led to a considerable debate in later issues of *Acta Cytologica*.[8] These thoughts were further developed and discussed at a recent symposium on the value and limitations of aspiration cytology in the diagnosis of primary tumours moderated by Hajdu and attended by a number of international experts.[9] We believe that such a debate is timely. Awareness of the limitations of any diagnostic procedure is most important and is the result of increasing experience and understanding of the use of the technique. The two fundamental requirements on which the success of FNA biopsy depends are representativeness of the sample and high quality of the preparation. If these prerequisites are not entirely fulfilled, definitive conclusions cannot possibly be drawn. It is true that the increasing use of electron microscopy (EM), fluorescent microscopy, immunocytochemistry, and morphometric analysis of FNA samples have significantly increased the potential to make precise, type-specific diagnoses, but the two prerequisites mentioned above will always remain a sine qua non, no matter how sophisticated the supplementary techniques. In addition, information obtained by FNA cytology must always be correlated with clinical judgment and with other investigations.

THE PRACTICE OF FNA

The debate over who should actually perform the procedure will continue regardless of the opinions expressed in this book. It is our belief that, in principle, the pathologist should be the protagonist; but, having made this claim, we concede that in many deeply sited lesions it is preferable for the radiologist who controls the various methods of tumour-imaging to direct the needle to the target. We cannot, however, believe that it is in the patient's best interest for the technique to be undertaken by every clinician in hospital or general medicine practice. No doubt every doctor may succeed in acquiring some material; but to achieve an ideal standard of proficiency, constant daily experience is essential. It has been our observation that material collected outside main centres of excellence is often unsatisfactory and impossible to interpret. When the radiologist or surgeon collects material it is of great value for the pathologist or a specially trained technologist to be present at the procedure to safeguard the quality of the preparations.

1 INTRODUCTION

Diagnosis by FNA cytology should only be attempted when the pathologist is cognisant of the details of the clinical history, physical examination, and the results of other laboratory tests. These will compensate for the shortcomings of the technique in demonstrating less of the architectural arrangement of tissues than do histological sections. Clinical data serves as a safeguard in the interpretation of the aspirate and should not bias the pathologist. In reporting his results, the pathologist must always make it quite clear if he is able to make a positive, definitive diagnosis, or if only indeterminate categories of diagnosis can be achieved which will require further needling or other confirmatory diagnostic procedures.

One should also realise that in FNA cytology it is extremely important to scrutinise the low-power, overall pattern of the smear, because it represents a direct sample which has been cut and withdrawn from the lesion and which contains microanatomical structures in addition to single cells and background material. Thus, the approach to the interpretation of the smear is closer to that used in histopathology than to exfoliative cytology. It is the pathologist who examines the entire slide, not the cyto-screener. If only a few abnormal cells can be found in a population of cells normal for the site, the aspirate in most cases should be regarded as unsatisfactory and the procedure repeated.

There has been a great deal of controversy regarding the advantages and disadvantages of using air-dried May-Grunwald-Giemsa (MGG)-stained smears as against wet-fixed Papanicolaou (Pap) and haematoxylin and eosin (H & E) preparations. We believe that the methods are complementary; both should be employed because certain features are particularly distinctive in each; familiarity with both stains is indispensable in specific situations (see Ch. 2). We emphasise that pathologists should keep an open mind concerning the benefits or otherwise of the two methods and make decisions on their worth from their own accumulating experience. The subject is elaborated further in the text in which we have tried to demonstrate the advantage of using both techniques.

NOMENCLATURE

The nomenclature applied to the discipline has been the subject of some discussion. Most Scandinavian and North American workers use the designation 'fine-needle aspiration biopsy' or 'aspiration biopsy cytology' for both the art as a whole and for the operative procedure. Thomson[31] prefers the term 'thin needle selective sampling' whereas Trott[32] makes a case for calling the products aspirates or samples. We believe that 'fine-needle aspiration cytology' is still an acceptable description of the whole of the art in spite of the fact that aspiration is not always used and that cytological preparation techniques are often supplemented by paraffin embedding. Like Trott we refer to the material expressed from the needle as samples, smears or aspirates. Since aspiration is often not applied and since the technique may involve also the collection of a fine core micro-biopsy, we prefer the terminology 'fine-needle biopsy' for the operative procedure.

THE AIMS OF THE ATLAS

We acknowledge the debt owed to clinicians in the development of FNA cytology, but the discipline now lies squarely in the realm of diagnostic pathology, along with surgical pathology and exfoliative cytology. It should be taught as an integral part of specialist training programmes in pathology. Until such training programmes evolve, however, there will be a need for self-education. Fresh surgical specimens provide an ideal source of material for smears, and, by using them, a reference set of slides can be accumulated as well as a feel for the operative technique gained.[11]

This book is therefore directed towards the practising diagnostic pathologist in whose hands we believe FNA cytology will flourish. The range of conditions which can be expected to constitute the main workload in a busy general hospital is treated in some depth, whereas rarer and more obscure lesions are described without too much detail. Some of our readers may find that certain areas have not been sufficiently covered; others may feel that too much space has been devoted to less important conditions. In this respect we have been guided by our own experience which may well differ from that of other centres.

In the time passed since the completion of the first edition, we have accumulated more experience which has allowed us to expand both the text and the illustrations, particularly in relation to less common conditions. Diagnostic criteria and differential diagnostic problems have been further clarified in many instances. The recent strong interest in mammographic screening and in stereotactically guided biopsy of non-palpable lesions in the breast has prompted an expansion of the chapter on FNA of the breast, particularly of the sections on benign proliferative lesions, in situ carcinoma, and well differentiated carcinoma. Dr Karin Lindholm, Malmö General Hospital, Sweden, who has a long and extensive experience in this area has made invaluable contributions to this chapter. We are also indebted to Dr M. Åkerman, University of Lund, Sweden, who reviewed and expanded the chapter on supporting tissues. Dr Åkerman has a special expertise in the cytology of soft tissue tumours — a notoriously difficult area in tissue pathology — the management of which is centralised to Lund Hospital from a large region in southern Sweden.

We have chosen to present FNA cytology within the

INTRODUCTION 1

framework of anatomical regions rather than on the basis of histopathological classifications; although this inevitably leads to some repetition, it conforms to the way problems present in clinical practice. Each of the descriptive chapters is subdivided into two parts; a text division in which indications, accuracy, techniques, and complications are discussed, and an atlas division in which the cytological patterns are described and illustrated. In this form we hope the book will fulfil the need for a practical atlas which will be kept close at hand beside the microscope. The text and illustrations are designed to be simple and to relate to daily diagnostic decisions. The magnifications used in the reproduction of microphotographs are simply recorded as low power (LP), intermediate power (IP), high power (HP), and high power using the oil immersion lens (HP Oil), which correspond approximately to × 100, × 250, × 400, and × 1000, respectively. Whenever possible, red blood cells or normal lymphocytes have been included in the field to provide a baseline for the appreciation of size.

One of the chapters is devoted to radiological aspects. Recent progress in organ imaging by computerised tomography and ultrasonography has made access to pulmonary and abdominal lesions almost routine. Because full consultation with radiologists is a fundamental requirement, we felt the viewpoint of the radiologist could best be expressed by one who had collaborated extensively with pathologists and we are grateful to Dr Suzanne Le P. Langlois for this contribution. Although the refinements of roentgenological techniques may appear foreign to some of our readers, the inclusion of this chapter emphasises our obligation to a sister discipline.

The demand of FNA cytology has grown in our own hospitals as a direct result of the demands of our surgeons and physicians. We are sure this experience is by no means unique. We have no doubt that as Koss[14] has said, 'thin-needle aspiration biopsy is a procedure whose time has come', and that pathologists not already versed in the technique will come under increasing and compelling pressure to provide it.

Like Ng[24] we believe that FNA cytology as part of the discipline of clinical cytology 'will be talked about and applied with equal competence and zeal as are other disciplines of anatomic pathology, such as surgical pathology, by all those who are involved in the study of disease, from medical students to clinicians, pathologists, cytotechnologists and researchers'. Our book, we hope, takes one step in this direction.

REFERENCES AND SUGGESTED FURTHER READING

1. Aspiration biopsy cytology. Editorial. Acta Cytol 28: 195–196, 1984.
2. Cohen M B, Miller T R, Gonzales J M, Sacks S T, Bottles K: Fine-needle aspiration biopsy. Perceptions of physicians at an academic medical center. Arch Pathol Lab Med 110: 813–817, 1986.
3. Dudgeon L S, Patrick C V: A new method for the rapid microscopical diagnosis of tumours. Br J Surg 15: 250–261, 1927.
4. Frable W J: Needle aspiration biopsy: past, present and future. Human Pathol 20: 504–517, 1989.
5. Frable W J: Thin-needle aspiration biopsy. Saunders, Philadelphia, 1983.
6. Franzen S, Giertz G, Zajicek J: Cytological diagnosis of prostatic tumours by transrectal aspiration biopsy: a preliminary report. Br J Urol 32: 193–196, 1960.
7. Grunze H, Spriggs A I: History of clinical cytology — A selection of documents. E.Giebeler, Darmstadt, 1980.
8. Hajdu S I, Melamed M R: Limitations of aspiration cytology in the diagnosis of primary neoplasms. Acta Cytol 28: 337–345, 1984, and 29: 487–492, 1985.
9. Hajdu S I, Ehya H, Frable W J et al: The value and limitations of aspiration cytology in the diagnosis of primary tumors. A symposium. Acta Cytol 33: 741–790, 1989.
10. Hirschfeldt H: Bericht über einige histologisch-mikroskopische und experimentelle Arbeiten bei den bösartigen Geschwulsten. Krebsforsch 16: 33, 1919.
11. Kaminsky D B: Aspiration biopsy for the community hospital. Masson, New York, 1981.
12. Kline T S: Fine-needle aspiration biopsy. Past, present and future (editorial). Arch Pathol Lab Med 104: 117, 1980.
13. Kline T S: Handbook of fine needle aspiration biopsy cytology. 2nd edn. Churchill Livingstone, New York, 1988.
14. Koss L G: Thin needle aspiration biopsy (editorial). Acta Cytol 24: 1–3, 1980.
15. Koss L G, Woyke S, Olszewski W: Aspiration biopsy; cytologic interpretation and histologic basis. Igaku-Shoin, New York, 1984.
16. Koss L G: Aspiration biopsy- a tool in surgical pathology. Am J Surg Pathol 12, suppl.1: 43–53, 1988.
17. Lever J V, Trott P A, Webb A J: Fine needle aspiration cytology. J Clin Pathol 38: 1–11, 1985.
18. Leyden O O: Ueber infectiöse Pneumonie. Dtsch Med Wschr 9: 52–54, 1883.
19. Linsk J A, Franzen S: Clinical aspiration cytology, 2nd edn. Lippincott, Philadelphia, 1989.
20. Lopes Cardozo P: Clinical cytology. Safleu, Leiden, 1954.
21. Lopes Cardozo P: Atlas of clinical cytology. Leiden, 1978.
22. Martin H E, Ellis E B: Aspiration biopsy. Surg Gynecol Obstet 59: 578–589, 1934.
23. Menetrier P: Cancer primitif du poumon. Bull Soc Anat (Paris) 11: 643, 1886.
24. Ng A B P: The future is coming — only you can decide where it is going (editorial). Acta Cytol 25: 593–598, 1981.
25. Orell S R: Fine needle aspiration biopsy in perspective (editorial). Pathology 14: 113–114, 1982.
26. Rode J: Fine needle cytology versus histology. Histopathology 15: 435–439, 1989.
27. Roussel F, Dalion J, Benozio M: The risk of tumoral

1 *INTRODUCTION*

seeding in needle biopsies. Acta Cytol 33: 936–939, 1989.

28. Söderström N: Fine needle aspiration biopsy. Almqvist & Wiksell, Stockholm, 1966.

29. Söderström N: Thin needle aspiration biopsy (letter). Acta Cytol 24: 468, 1980.

30. Tao L C, Sanders D E, McLoughlin M J, Weisbrod G L, Ho C S: Current concepts in fine needle aspiration biopsy cytology. Hum Pathol 11: 94–96, 1980.

31. Thomson P: Thin needle aspiration biopsy (letter). Acta Cytol 26: 262–263, 1982.

32. Trott P A: Needle aspiration terminology (letter). Acta Cytol 27: 83, 1983.

33. Utility of needle aspiration of tumours (editorial). Br Med J 1: 1507–1508, 1978.

34. Wakely P E, Kardos T F, Frable W J: Application of fine needle aspiration biopsy to pediatrics. Hum Pathol 19: 1383–1386, 1988.

35. Webb A J: Through a glass darkly (the development of needle aspiration biopsy). Bristol Med Chir J 89: 59–68, 1974.

36. Zajicek J: Aspiration biopsy cytology. Part 1. Cytology of supra-diaphragmatic organs. Monographs in clinical cytology, Vol. 4, Karger, Basel, 1974.

37. Zajicek J: Aspiration biopsy cytology. Part 2. Cytology of infra-diaphragmatic organs. Monographs in clinical cytology, Vol. 7. Karger, Basel, 1979.

2

THE TECHNIQUES OF FNA CYTOLOGY

2 THE TECHNIQUES OF FNA CYTOLOGY

PATIENT SELECTION

Indications for FNA biopsy of various organs and tissues will be explained in detail in the following chapters. Meanwhile, some general principles apply. To be suitable for FNA biopsy, the disease process must be localised and clearly defined by clinical examination or by any available radiological imaging technique. In this respect it is similar to any other biopsy method: core needle, endoscopic, incisional or excisional, and principally different to screening by exfoliative cytology. Occasionally, FNA biopsy can be of value in a diffuse process. For example, the causative agent can be demonstrated in an aspirate in some infectious processes such as pneumocystis pneumonia or miliary tuberculosis. If a diffuse abnormality is suspected to be neoplastic, FNA may be tried, but with the clear understanding that a negative result has no informative value at all. Although severe complications are very rare, the possible benefits and predicted specificity of a cytological diagnosis must always be weighed against the risk. For example: patients with coagulation disorders or with respiratory failure may not be suitable for biopsy of some sites; some highly malignant tumours such as melanomas, germ-cell tumours of the testis and ovarian cystadenocarcinomas are probably better managed without preoperative FNA if they appear to be localised.

Most FNA biopsies can safely be carried out as an office procedure. However, we prefer to do transpleural biopsies and biopsies of the spleen, sometimes also of the liver and some other deep sites, in hospital so that patients can be kept under observation for a few hours afterwards.

Whenever possible, the pathologist should be consulted before the biopsy is performed regarding the feasibility and the likely informative value of FNA in the case in question. He should have access to all relevant clinical and radiological data, without which a diagnosis should not be attempted.

PREPARATION FOR BIOPSY

Equipment

Needles (Fig. 2.1)

Standard disposable 25–22 gauge (less than 0.7 mm), 30–50 mm long needles are suitable for most superficial, palpable lesions. The finest (25 gauge) needles are recommended for children and for particularly sensitive areas such as the orbit and the eyelids. Although the yield with a 25 gauge needle is sparser than with 23–22 gauge, it is usually sufficient from any cellular and vascular tissue such as lymph nodes, thyroid and most cancers. Thicker needles on the whole offer no advantages. They are prone to cause more bleeding and can become blocked by a plug of tissue which may not

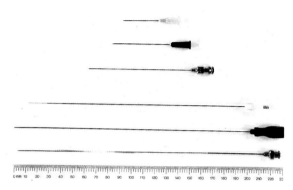

Fig. 2.1 Needles suitable for FNA
From top: standard disposable 23 gauge, 32 mm and 22 gauge 51 mm needles; disposable 22 gauge 90 mm lumbar puncture needle with trocar; disposable 22 gauge 205 mm Rotex II screw needle; 22 gauge 200 mm Chiba needle with trocar; Franzén needle for prostatic aspiration, 23 gauge 210 mm.

represent the process under investigation and which is difficult to smear. If the purpose of the biopsy is to obtain a core of tissue for paraffin embedding and sectioning, an 18 gauge needle is preferable, although cutting core needles as thin as 22 gauge are now available. With thick needles, the small but real risk of tumour implantation in the needle track must be considered, as well as the greater frequency of haemorrhage and other complications (see Ch. 1).[22] Anaesthesia and stricter sterility also become necessary. The 22 gauge, 90 mm disposable lumbar puncture needles with trocar are convenient for most deep biopsies. The needle is sufficiently rigid and the trocar prevents contamination during the passage of the needle through other tissues. If a needle of still greater length is required, a 22 gauge, 150 or 200 mm Chiba needle is used. Special long 23 gauge needles are supplied with the Franzén instrumentarium for biopsy of the prostate and other pelvic organs (Unimed, Lausanne, Switzerland). The choice of needles for bone biopsy is discussed in Chapter 11.[52] The Rotex II Screw Needle (Ursus Konsult AB, Stockholm, Sweden), which is available in 0.8 mm (21–22 gauge), 145 or 205 mm sizes, has been successfully used for deep biopsy of lung, liver, kidney, lymph nodes, etc.[40] We have found it particularly useful in fibrous lesions such as pulmonary hamartoma, lymphoma with sclerosis and various types of soft tissue tumours, and also in very vascular tumours in which conventional aspiration tends to yield mainly blood. It is also an excellent device for obtaining tissue fragments suitable for paraffin embedding and for EM. A wide range of specially designed small gauge cutting core needles are now commercially available.[25,26] However, standard needles are less expensive, easier to use, and give a satisfactory yield in the great majority of cases, provided the biopsy technique is correct.

THE TECHNIQUES OF FNA CYTOLOGY

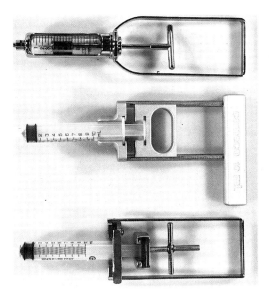

Fig. 2.2 Syringe holders
Top: Franzen stainless steel/glass aspiration syringe. Mid: Cameco syringe pistol with disposable 10 cc syringe. Bottom: simple home-made syringe holder for disposable 10 cc syringe.

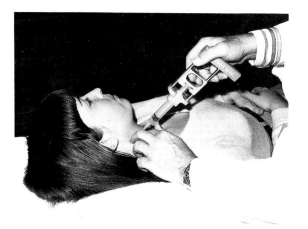

Fig. 2.3 FNA of thyroid
Needle and syringe are operated with one hand leaving the other free to feel and to fix the target lesion. Note the thumb supporting the syringe.

Syringes

Standard, disposable plastic syringes, 10–20 ml, are used. The syringe should be of good quality, of strong rigid material, and produce a good negative pressure.

Syringe holder (Fig. 2.2)

The use of a syringe holder is strongly recommended. Leaving one hand free to immobilise and to feel the target lesion allows for better precision in placing the needle exactly where desired (Fig. 2.3). We use the Cameco Syringe Pistol (Cameco AB, Taby, Sweden), made to fit either 10 or 20 ml plastic syringes. A similar, simpler device can be made to order by most hospital engineering workshops.

Slides

Glass slides must be thoroughly cleaned, dry and free of grease. Slides with frosted ends are convenient for immediate labelling. The aspirate can be smeared between two standard microscope slides. A 0.4 mm haemocytometer coverslip gives better control over the pressure used in smearing and a more even spread. Air-dried slides are best transported in a stainless steel slide carrier to avoid contamination and scratching.

Fixatives

For routine wet-fixation of smears, 70–90% ethanol, conveniently in Coplin jars, is preferable to spray fixatives. Carnoy's fixative has the advantage of lysing red blood cells. Glutaraldehyde and 10% buffered formalin should also be available if tissue fragments for EM or for paraffin embedding are obtained.

Sterile containers

Small sterile containers with tight lids containing physiological saline or Hank's balanced salt solution should be at hand if needles and syringe are to be rinsed to obtain material for culture or for preparation of a cell suspension. Special culture media may be required.

Other

Skin disinfectant (usually pre-injection swabs), sterile dressings, local anaesthetic, a watch glass, thrombin powder, a pencil, tongue depressors and sterile scalpel blades are other items which should be available at biopsy. We find it convenient to keep all this equipment in a light plastic box with suitable compartments, which is always at hand if the pathologist is called to do a biopsy.

Patient preparation

A clear explanation of the procedure will ensure the patient's consent and co-operation. Most patients, including children, readily accept FNA even when repeated. FNA is most conveniently carried out with the patient lying supine on an ordinary examination couch. A gynaecological examination couch with stirrups may be preferable for prostatic and pelvic biopsies, and a chair with a head rest for biopsy of lesions in the head and neck region.

Sterility

Simple skin disinfectant using pre-packed swabs as for

2 *THE TECHNIQUES OF FNA CYTOLOGY*

routine injections is adequate for superficial biopsies. For transpleural, transperitoneal, and bone biopsies we use a surgical skin disinfectant, a fenestrated sterile cloth, and sterile surgical gloves.

Anaesthesia

Pre-biopsy sedation is rarely justified, and then only in deep aspirations in very anxious or agitated patients. Atropine is recommended in preparation for transpleural biopsy to prevent the unlikely risk of vasovagal reflex. In some instances, FNA can be coordinated with other operative procedures which require general anaesthesia.

Local anaesthesia is hardly ever necessary when 22–25 gauge needles are used. Although it is probably as painful as the biopsy, we recommend the injection of a local anaesthetic in tranpleural, transperitoneal and transperiosteal biopsies. The reason is to prevent uncontrolled movements or jerks by the patient during the procedure; multiple passes also become more acceptable.

THE BIOPSY PROCEDURE

Insertion of the needle

When aspirating superficial lesions, better control of the needle is achieved by supporting the barrel of the syringe by the free hand (Fig. 2.3). Nearer vertical approaches tend to be less painful and allow better appreciation of depth.

The use of radiological imaging techniques to guide deep biopsies is described in detail in Chapter 3. Ultrasonography in particular, if readily available, is often helpful and time saving even if the lesion is palpable because it gives an exact measurement of the optimal depth. With practice and experience one will eventually develop a fingertip sensitivity projected to the point of the needle which, in most cases, allows accurate positioning without technical aids.

Aspiration

The aspiration technique is illustrated diagrammatically, step by step, in Figure 2.4. A few points need to be emphasised. The mechanism of FNA biopsy has been explained well by Thomson.[57] The function of the negative pressure is not to tear cells from the tissue but merely to hold the tissue against the sharp cutting edge of the needle. The softer tissue components protrude over the edge, are cut or scraped off, and accumulate in the lumen as the needle advances through the tissue. Aggregates of tumour cells as well as glandular and other epithelial structures are softer and more friable than the supporting stroma and are therefore selectively sampled, whereas the stroma is poorly represented in the aspirate. To obtain the greatest possible yield, the

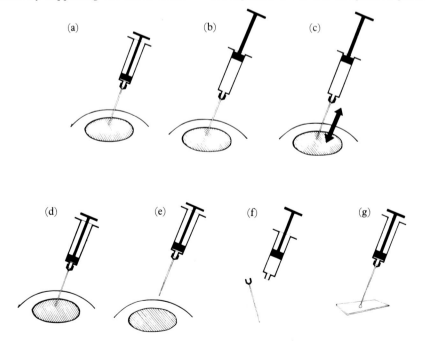

Fig. 2.4 Biopsy procedure
Diagrammatic stepwise illustration of biopsy procedure: (a) needle positioned within target tissue, (b) plunger pulled to apply negative pressure, (c) needle moved back and forth within target tissue, (d) negative pressure released while needle remains in target tissue, (e) needle withdrawn, (f) needle detached, air drawn into syringe, (g) aspirate blown onto slide.

THE TECHNIQUES OF FNA CYTOLOGY 2

needle should be moved back and forth within the lesion with the negative pressure maintained (Fig. 2.4c). This is important in the biopsy of fibrous tissues such as breast and soft tissues, and of fibrotic tumours with a low cell content. Many passes of the needle may be necessary to sample a satisfactory number of cells. In highly cellular and vascular tissues such as spleen, lymph nodes, liver and thyroid, one steady advance of the needle is usually sufficient, while multiple passes and a maintained negative pressure will only increase the amount of blood aspirated. The amount of blood also tends to be less if the needle is moved along the same track rather than in various directions. One should never wait to see material entering into the syringe except when evacuating a cyst or an abscess. Blood in the syringe usually means that the aspirate will be unsatisfactory. The ideal aspirate has a high cell content in a small amount of fluid, a creamy consistency, and remains within the lumen of the needle.

It is important to release the negative pressure (Fig. 2.4d) before the needle is withdrawn (Fig. 2.4e). A maintained negative pressure will draw the aspirate into the syringe which must then be rinsed with fluid to recover the specimen. In addition, the sample may be contaminated by material aspirated during withdrawal of the needle, e.g. rectal contents in biopsy of the prostate.

Needle biopsy without aspiration

As pointed out above, the negative pressure plays a relatively minor role compared to the scraping or cutting effect of the advancing sharp, oblique needle tip. Zajdela[64] recommended needle biopsy without aspiration based on the observation that the capillary pressure in a fine needle is sufficient to keep the scraped cells inside the lumen. In this technique, a 25–23 gauge needle is held directly with the fingertips, is inserted into the target lesion and is moved back and forth in various directions within the lesion to an extent that depends on the cellularity and the vascularity of the tissue (Fig. 2.5). The advantage of this technique over conventional aspiration is that the operator can feel the consistency of the tissues much better; this is a very valuable piece of diagnostic information and also improves precision, for example when sampling a tiny lymph node. Another important advantage is that admixture with blood is less than with aspiration, which makes the technique particularly suited for biopsy of the thyroid. The cell yield is somewhat less than with aspiration but not significantly so.[37] We have used this technique with 25 gauge needles increasingly during the last 5 years with such favourable results that it has become the routine for all superficial biopsies except for cystic lesions and for the more fibrous breast lumps and soft tissue tumours. The technique is an alternative also

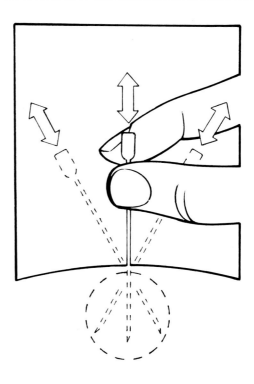

Fig. 2.5 Needle biopsy without aspiration
The needle is moved to and fro within the target tissue varying the angle to cover a larger area. Admixture with blood is less than with aspiration.

in deep biopsies (using the usual 22 gauge lumbar puncture needle) if traditional aspiration yields an excess of blood, for example in the liver and in renal cell tumours.

After biopsy of superficial lesions, pressure should be applied over the biopsy site to minimise bruising or to decrease the chance of haematoma formation, particularly in vascular tissues such as thyroid.

Failure to obtain a representative sample

The possible reasons for failure to obtain a representative sample are illustrated diagrammatically in Figure 2.6. If a tumour is narrowly missed and the needle passes it tangentially (Fig. 2.6b) only the adjacent inflammatory reaction is sampled and an erroneous diagnosis of an inflammatory process can easily be made. Central necrosis, haemorrhage, or cystic change is commonly seen in tumours and if the aspirate is taken from such areas no diagnostic cells may be found in the smears (Fig. 2.6c). Sometimes a small malignant neoplasm can be masked or hidden by a dominant benign tumour or cyst (Fig. 2.6d). This situation is not infrequently seen in the breast and in the thyroid and is one important cause of false negative diagnoses. In the breast, routine use of mammography can overcome this

2 *THE TECHNIQUES OF FNA CYTOLOGY*

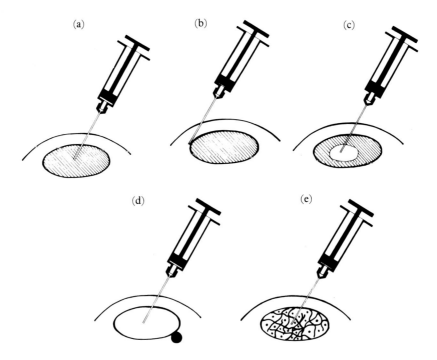

Fig. 2.6 Causes of unsatisfactory yield
(a) Needle well-positioned within target tissue should produce satisfactory yield, (b) needle has missed the lesion tangentially, (c) central cystic, necrotic or haemorrhagic area devoid of diagnostic cells, (d) small malignant lesion adjacent to dominant benign mass, (e) fibrosclerotic target tissue poor in cells.

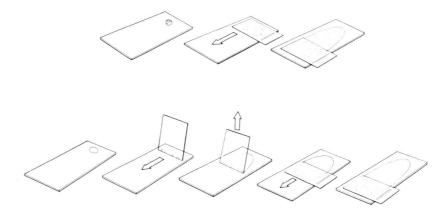

Fig. 2.7 Direct smearing
Upper: smearing technique suitable for a 'dry' aspirate. Lower: smearing technique suitable for a 'wet' aspirate. For details see text.

THE TECHNIQUES OF FNA CYTOLOGY

problem. Any palpable abnormality persisting after evacuation of a cyst must of course be biopsied again. Finally, it may be difficult to obtain a satisfactory sample from desmoplastic tumour tissue in which the cells are firmly held in a dense collagenous framework (Fig. 2.6e).

PREPARING THE ASPIRATE

Direct smearing (Figs 2.7–2.9)

In the following text an aspirate will be referred to as 'dry' if it consists of numerous cells suspended in a small amount of tissue fluid and has a creamy consistency. This represents the perfect sample obtainable from most highly cellular tissues. A 'wet' aspirate consists of a small number of cells suspended in fluid or blood. A 'dry' aspirate is best smeared with the flat of a 0.4 mm coverslip, exerting a light pressure to achieve a reasonably thin, even spread (Fig. 2.7). The flat of a standard microscopy slide can also be used. Too firm smearing pressure produces crush artefacts. It is there-

fore better to make the smear somewhat thicker than optimal than to make it too thin. Thin smears of a 'dry' aspirate dry almost instantaneously and drying artefacts are difficult to avoid when smears are wet-fixed. A 'wet' aspirate should be smeared in two steps as illustrated (Fig. 2.7). The first step is moving the coverslip or the smearing slide to the middle of the specimen slide, holding it at a blunt angle; this leaves most of the fluid behind while the cells follow the smearing slide like a buffy coat. The concentrated cells can then be smeared with the flat of the coverslip or slide as for a 'dry' aspirate. A correct technique is important, particularly in the preparation of air-dried smears. Good cell fixation depends on rapid drying: if drying is slow, artefacts appear which may render diagnosis impossible (Fig. 2.9). Optimal smearing is a fine balance between too thick and too thin, fixation artefacts and crush artefacts. If a large amount of blood is aspirated, this can be expressed on to and quickly spread over a watch glass before coagulation occurs. Minimal tissue particles or cell clumps, if present, become visible and can be picked up for direct smearing or be placed within a drop of blood to form a clot suitable for histological processing.

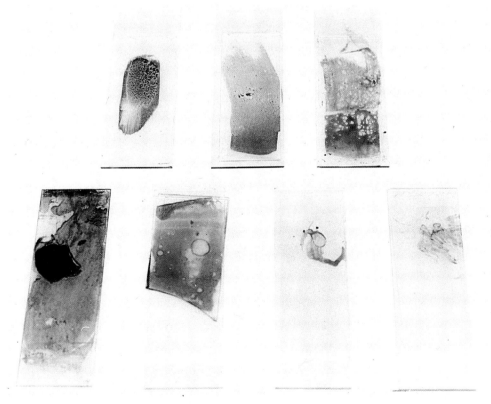

Fig. 2.8 Macro appearances of stained smears
Upper row from left to right: highly cellular aspirate; visible small particles evenly spread over slide; intermediate aspirate, some particles visible in thinner portion of smear; 'wet' aspirate spread with the two step technique; particles mainly at tail of smear.
Lower row (unsatisfactory smears referred from outside the hospital) from left to right: thick, bloody smear with clotting, poorly spread 'wet' smear on broken slide; thin and scanty smear unevenly spread.

2 *THE TECHNIQUES OF FNA CYTOLOGY*

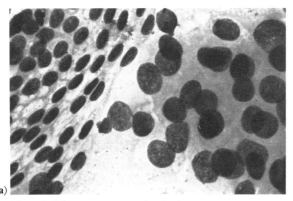
(a)

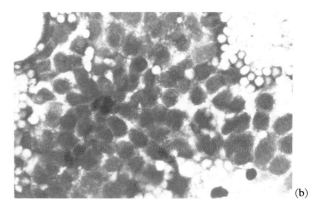
(b)

Fig. 2.9 Micro appearance of stained smears
(a) Optimal spread and fixation of 'dry' aspirate from carcinoma of prostate. (b) Slow drying of this thick and bloody smear of prostatic hyperplasia has resulted in artefacts which make a cytological diagnosis impossible in spite of good cell yield (MGG, HP).

If the sample is large enough, it should be divided up on to several slides, both air-dried and wet-fixed, so that special staining procedures can be carried out if required.

Indirect smearing

If thin fluid is aspirated, this is best processed by centrifugation on the cytocentrifuge.[54] Millipore or Nucleopore filtration is an alternative that we have found less satisfactory although it has been recommended by others.[11] In some laboratories the standard method of preparation of fine-needle aspirates is to rinse needles and syringes with saline or with a fixative which is then centrifuged or filtered onto slides.[8,45,55] This approach results in a significantly higher proportion of satisfactory specimens in a situation where the laboratory has no control over the biopsy procedure and the aspirates are

received from a number of outside sources. However, if the biopsy is correctly performed and direct smears are prepared by a trained and experienced person, results are at least as good, and there is no need for more complicated, expensive and time-consuming preparative procedures.

Standardised preparations with optimal preservation of cell and nuclear shapes are particularly important in the diagnosis of malignant lymphoma. For lymph node aspirates we therefore recommend that a cell suspension be prepared in addition to direct smears. Hank's balanced salt solution with the addition of 10–20% fetal calf serum is ideal for this purpose. The suspension is gently spun on the cytocentrifuge at 300 r.p.m. It may have to be diluted to achieve optimal dispersion of cells on the slide and to avoid clumping (Fig. 2.10). In most cases, a sufficient number of slides can be made from one aspirate to allow special stains or immunocytochemical studies.

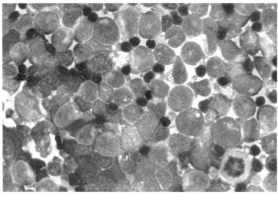
(a)

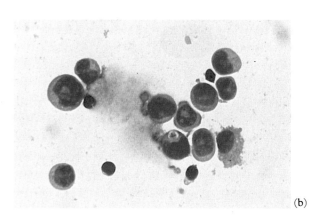
(b)

Fig. 2.10 Preparation of cell suspension
Suspension of lymphoid cells in Hank's balanced salt solution; smears prepared by cytocentrifugation. (a) Undiluted specimen shows clumping of cells with many smudged nuclei. (b) Optimal dilution (MGG, HP.)

THE TECHNIQUES OF FNA CYTOLOGY

2

Histological sections

Sometimes, a thin core of tissue or multiple visible tissue fragments are obtained with a 22 gauge standard needle, e.g. from the liver (Fig. 2.11). Multiple minimal fragments are easier to handle if assembled with a drop of blood and thrombin added to produce a clot. The tissue or clot is fixed in 5–10% buffered isotonic formalin and processed as for routine histology. Many laboratories recommend the routine preparation of cell blocks for paraffin embedding from FNA samples, by centrifugation or filtration.[5,28,31] Cell blocks are very helpful in selected cases as they give a better idea of tissue architecture and as they allow multiple sections for immunohistochemical studies but are time-consuming and expensive.

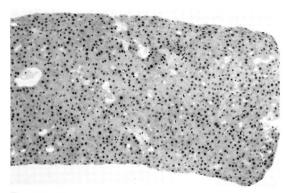

Fig. 2.11 Tissue core
Tissue section: core of tissue from a very well-differentiated hepatocellular carcinoma obtained with a standard 22 gauge lumbar puncture needle as shown in Figure 2.1 (H & E, LP)

Table 2.1 Electron microscopy and fine needle aspiration

Value	Tumour type
Unequivocal identification of cell type or differentiation (where available immune markers may not be specific enough for definitive diagnosis)	Melanoma
	Neuroendocrine differentiation
	Mesothelioma

	Small round cell tumours
	  Ewing's sarcoma
	  Rhabdomyosarcoma
	  Neuroblastoma
	  Primitive neuroectodermal tumour
	  Wilms' tumour

	Well differentiated spindle cell tumours
	  Schwann cell tumours
	  Smooth muscle tumours
	  Fibrohistiocytic tumours

Supports cytologic diagnosis or aids in subclassification (where immune marker studies are unlikely to be helpful)	Neuroendocrine malignancies
	  Carcinoid tumour
	  Well differentiated neuroendocrine carcinoma (atypical carcinoid)
	  Small cell carcinoma

	Adenocarcinoma subtyping
	  Acinic cell carcinoma
	  Hepatocellular carcinoma
	  Bronchiolo-alveolar carcinoma
	  Colonic carcinoma
	  Renal cell carcinoma
	  Adrenal carcinoma

Answers general questions of cell type (where immune markers have not been diagnostic or where material is insufficient for a panel of markers)	Small cell malignancies
	  Lymphoma
	  Small cell carcinoma

	Large cell malignancies
	  Lymphoma
	  Anaplastic carcinoma
	  Melanoma
	  Germ cell tumours

	Pleomorphic spindle cell tumours
	  Sarcoma
	  Sarcomatoid carcinoma
	  Melanoma

	Other tumours Thymoma/thymic carcinoma

2 *THE TECHNIQUES OF FNA CYTOLOGY*

Electron microscopy

The common applications of electron microscopy (EM) in FNA cytology have been discussed in many papers.[1,12,20,41,63] They are summarised in Table 2.1 based on our own experience. EM in tumour diagnosis is presented in several monographs such as the atlas by Henderson et al.[23]

Several methods have been described to process material from FNA biopsies for EM.[33,38,43] The most commonly used method is to eject the aspirate into a small test tube containing glutaraldehyde. The small pellet produced by centrifugation is then carefully removed and processed in the usual way. We have had better results with a simpler and gentler method developed in our laboratory (Figs 2.12–2.14). The aspirate is simply ejected as one or a few droplets directly onto a thoroughly cleaned glass slide. Without touching the droplets, the slide is immediately immersed in glutaraldehyde. After fixation, the droplet is processed on the slide.[46] This method is, of course, only suitable for good quality 'dry' aspirates. Some method of concentration must be applied to 'wet' aspirates, e.g. simple centrifugation, or more elaborate procedures. If we cannot obtain a satisfactory 'dry' aspirate, we prefer to use a Rotex II screw needle, or some other thin calibre core needle (see p. 8) to obtain a fragment of tissue which can be processed like any other tissue sample.

FIXATION AND STAINING

Two fundamentally different methods of fixation and staining are used in FNA cytology: air drying followed by staining with a haematological stain such as MGG, Jenner-Giemsa, Wright's stain, or Diff-Quik (Harleco, Philadelphia); and alcohol fixation and staining with Pap or H & E. Pathologists who had their basic training in gynaecological cytology find it natural to use alcohol fixation and Pap staining also in FNA cytology, whereas those with a background in haematology prefer air-dried Giemsa stained smears. Both methods have their advantages and deficiencies. We strongly recommend anyone practising FNA cytology to familiarise himself with both methods and to regard them as complementary. The effect produced on cells by air-drying and wet-fixation respectively, is easily understood if one compares the configuration of a fried egg with that of a poached or a boiled egg (Fig. 2.15). In air-drying, the cell, both cytoplasm and nucleus, is flattened on the glass surface and appears larger than a cell fixed in ethanol. Air-drying is therefore a helpful 'artefact' in cytological diagnosis as it exaggerates nuclear enlargment, one of the most important criteria of malignancy. For air-drying to be a successful method of fixation, smears must be carefully and expertly prepared and this requires the presence of cytology laboratory staff at the

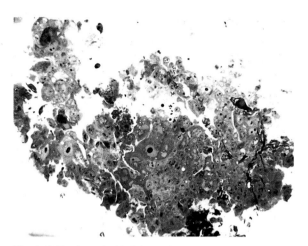

Fig. 2.12 Resin embedded tissue fragment for EM
Fragment of sarcoma obtained by a standard 22 gauge needle fixed in glutaraldehyde and processed on the slide: $1\mu m$ section (Toluidine blue, HP)

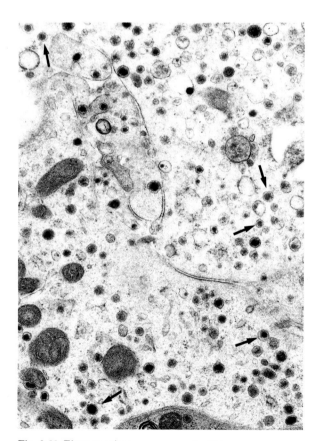

Fig. 2.13 Electron microscopy — carcinoid tumour
FNA biopsy of metastatic neoplasm in the liver. The cytoplasm of the tumour cells contains numerous rounded neurosecretory granules averaging 155 nm in diameter. In some, a submembranous lucent halo can be seen (arrows) EM × 13 650).

THE TECHNIQUES OF FNA CYTOLOGY 2

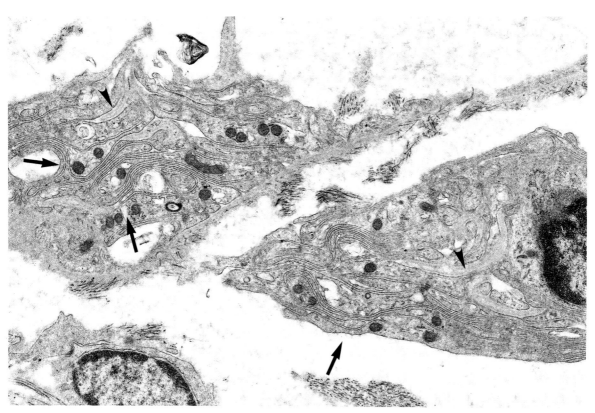

Fig. 2.14 Electron microscopy — Schwannoma
Fine-needle screw biopsy (Rotex II) of an atypical soft tissue tumour in the neck of a 20-year-old man. The complex intertwining cytoplasmic processes (arrows) and the associated external (basal) lamina (arrowheads) indicate Schwannian differentiation. The abundance of the lucent proteoglycan-containing extracellular matrix is in keeping with Antoni B tissue (EM × 9940).

biopsy procedure. Nuclear detail is poorly shown and confusing artefacts are common if smears are incorrectly made. However, difficulties can occur also with wet-fixation, in particular artefacts due to the extremely rapid drying of smears of a 'dry' aspirate as defined above.

Many pathologists are of the opinion that an evaluation of fine nuclear structure is not possible in air-dried Giemsa smears. However, haematologists have always relied entirely on this technique. Nuclear structure is important in haematological diagnosis, e.g. in megaloblastic anaemia, in typing of leukaemias, and in the recognition of metastatic malignancy in bone marrow aspirates. The fact is that nuclear chromatin patterns can also be studied in Giemsa smears, but the appearances are different to those of the Pap smear. It takes time for those who have not worked with blood films and bone marrow aspirates to become accustomed to air-dried smears, but it is time well spent since such smears are of great value in FNA cytology. The different properties of air-dried Giemsa smears and of

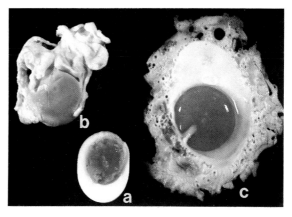

Fig. 2.15 Cell fixation
Three eggs of same weight illustrate the effects of different methods of fixation on individual cells: (a) the bisected boiled egg represents a cell as it appears in a tissue section; (b) the poached egg represents an alcohol fixed cell in a cytological preparation; (c) the fried egg illustrates the appearance of cells in an air dried smear.

2 *THE TECHNIQUES OF FNA CYTOLOGY*

alcohol-fixed Pap smears are listed in Tables 2.2 and 2.3. It is obvious from the tables that the two methods are complementary. Diff-Quik is a rapid haematology type stain (2–3 minutes) handy to use in theatre or in the radiology department, to check immediately during the biopsy procedure if a satisfactory specimen has been obtained. Rapid H & E, Pap and other stains are also available.[17,47,48]

To prevent cross infection, in cases in which there is a high level of suspicion of an infective process, we recommend that air-dried smears are sterilised by fixation in methanol soon after drying.

Table 2.2 Comparison of air-dried and wet-fixed smears – general properties

	Air-dried MGG	Wet-fixed Pap
Dependence on smearing technique	Strong	Moderate
The 'dry' smear	Good fixation	Drying artefacts common
The 'wet' smear	Artefacts common	Good fixation
Tissue fragments	Cells poorly seen due to heavily stained ground substance	Individual cells usually clearly seen
Cell and nuclear size	Exaggerated, differences enhanced	Comparable to tissue sections
Cytoplasmic detail	Well demonstrated	Poorly demonstrated
Nuclear detail	Pattern different to the familiar Pap stain	Excellently demonstrated
Nucleoli	Not always discernible	Well demonstrated
Stromal components	Well shown and often differentially stained	Poorly demonstrated
Partially necrotic tissue	Poor definition of cell details	Good definition of single intact cells

Table 2.3 Comparison of air-dried and wet-fixed smears – tissue specific properties

Tissue	Feature emphasized by MGG	Feature emphasised by Pap
Epithelial tissues	Mucin, intra- or extracellular Colloid (thyroid) Secretory granules (prostate) Lipofuscin granules (seminal vesicle) Lipid vacuoles Fire flares (thyroid) Bare bipolar nuclei (benign breast) Bile plugs Basement membrane globules (adenoid cystic carcinoma) Amyloid	Squamous differentiation/keratinisation Oncocytes (salivary gland tumours) Psammoma bodies
Lymphoid tissue	Cytoplasmic basophilia Lymphoid globules Haemopoietic cells Lipid vacuoles	Nuclear outline Nuclear chromatin pattern Nucleoli
Mesenchymal tissues	Fibromyxoid/chondromyxoid ground substance (pleomorphic adenoma, chondroid hamartoma, fibroadenoma, chondroid tissue, chordoma) Osteoid Basement membrane (vasoformative tumours) Amyloid Intracytoplasmic lipid vacuoles	Nuclear detail in solid tissue fragments
Neuroendocrine tissues	Cytoplasmic granularity (medullary carcinoma of thyroid, paraganglioma, carcinoid, islet cell tumours)	Speckled nuclear chromatin
Inflammatory tissue	Eosinophils	Macrophages (xanthogranulomatous pyelonephritis, old haematoma, fat necrosis)

THE TECHNIQUES OF FNA CYTOLOGY

2

Special stains

The common special stains in histopathology can also be used for cytological smears (air-dried or wet-fixed) without major modifications.[51] The most commonly used are PAS/diastase or Alcian blue for mucins, Prussian blue for iron, Masson-Fontana for melanin, Grimelius for argyrophilic granules, Congo Red for amyloid, Gram, PAS or Gomori's silver stain for micro-organisms and Ziehl-Neelsen for acid-fast bacilli. Special stains suitable for the demonstration of Pneumocystis, Nocardia and Actinomyces in smears have been described.[49,50] Glycogen can be demonstrated by PAS, and fat by oil-red-O or other fat stains in air-dried smears. Fouchet's reagent counterstained with Sirius red demonstrates bile pigment beautifully (Fig. 2.16). Formaldehyde-induced fluorescence is a simple rapid test for certain amines, particularly melanin precursors in amelanotic melanoma.

Cells containing certain aromatic amines show a granular yellow cytoplasmic autofluorescence after treatment with formaldehyde, e.g. melanocytes, argentaffin cells, chromaffin cells, mast cells, and thyroid C cells. The technique requires a fluorescence microscope with a BG 38, a UG 1 and a barrier filter and is carried out as follows:

1. Scan smear under UV light to exclude presence of autofluorescent lipofuscins.
2. Fix smear for at least 30 min in 30% formalin.
3. Rinse in water.
4. Dehydrate, clear, and mount in a fluorescence-free mounting medium.
5. Examine under UV light using filters as mentioned above.

Air-dried smears are suitable for enzyme histochemistry even if they have been kept for a couple of days at room temperature. The demonstration of acid phosphatase is helpful in the diagnosis of metastatic prostatic carcinoma (see p. 79), and naphthylamidase in hepa-

tocellular carcinoma.[15] Esterase and peroxidase can be significant in typing lymphoma and leukaemic infiltrates (see Fig. 11.4).[34]

The reader is referred to handbooks on histological techniques for descriptions of the staining methods mentioned here. Minor modifications to suit the variable quality of cytological material will, of course, be developed in the laboratory with experience.

Phase contrast microscopy

Phase contrast microscopy of unstained smears has been used by some authors in cytological diagnosis. We do not see it as a substitute for routine stains but it is a useful tool to check the quality and the representativity of smears to be used for immunoperoxidase staining or for EM, so that time and reagents are not wasted on unsatisfactory samples.[6]

Immunohistochemistry[10,13,14,19,24,39,42]

The increasing availability of monoclonal antisera to a variety of proteins and other cell products which are more or less specific to different cell lines is probably the most important recent development in diagnostic cytology. The demonstration and identification of such cell products by immunocytochemical methods (e.g. immunoperoxidase, immunoalkaline phosphatase) is of immense value as it offers a means of objectively recognising the line of differentiation shown by the cells.[56] In some situations, a confident specific diagnosis can be made on just a few cells, e.g. in medullary carcinoma of thyroid (Fig. 2.17), in several other endocrine tumours and in metastasis of prostatic carcinoma. Immune markers are extremely useful in the differentia-

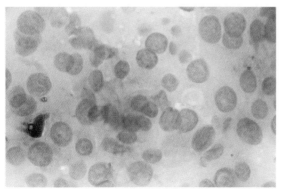

Fig. 2.16 Staining for bile pigment
Fouchet's reagent counterstained with Sirius red applied to smear from hepatocellular carcinoma (HP)

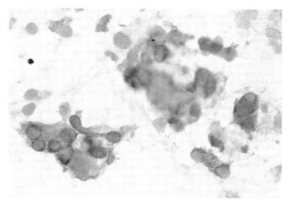

Fig. 2.17 Immunoperoxidase staining
Positive cytoplasmic staining for calcitonin in cells aspirated from a medullary carcinoma of thyroid (HP)

2 THE TECHNIQUES OF FNA CYTOLOGY

tion between anaplastic carcinoma, neuroendocrine tumours, malignant lymphoma and amelanotic melanoma (cytokeratin, EMA, chromogranin,[61] NSE, leucocyte common antigen, S100), and in the histogenetic typing of mesenchymal tumours (vimentin, desmin, factor VIII). Markers for B and T cells, immunoglobulins and light chains are used in the typing of lymphoma. Alpha-feto-protein and beta-human gonadotrophin may be of value in liver cell tumours and in germ cell tumours. Monoclonal antibodies to certain tumour antigens have been found to be useful in the distinction between malignant and benign epithelial cells.[27,35] A list of the most common immune markers used in aspiration cytology diagnosis is presented in Table 2.4.

Air-dried smears post-fixed in acetone, or sections of cell-blocks preferably fixed in mercury-based fixatives, are suitable for immunoperoxidase staining with a wide variety of markers. Cell-blocks have the great advantage of supplying a large number of sections sufficient for a panel of markers and for the indispensable negative controls. Some antigens are not well preserved in formalin fixed material, but are demonstrable in air-dried smears. If only smears are available, the number of tests possible can be increased by circling areas 3 mm apart on the same slide with a diamond pencil and wiping the smears between. It is possible to use previously Pap-stained smears if unstained smears are not available.[59]

The Avidin–Biotin complex method is the most commonly used with both monoclonal and polyclonal primary antibodies. Diaminobenzidine is used as the marker dye.[9,18,19,46] Immunoalkaline phosphatase staining appears to offer several advantages in cytological preparations.[58] Commercially produced kits have made immunohistochemistry a relatively simple method available to any cytology laboratory and an ever increasing number of antisera are being marketed in this form.

The interpretation of immunohistochemical stains is, however, more difficult in smears than in histological sections. The reason for this is that the cytoplasm of cells torn from their stroma is often fragile and diffusely dispersed in the background. In addition, there is often an admixture of blood, serum or secretory products, and this all combines to make it difficult to ascribe any positive staining to specific, identifiable cells. When examining smears, one should concentrate on tissue fragments in which the cytoplasm is left intact between the nuclei of the cells forming the fragments. Background staining is less of a problem in cytospin preparations of a cell suspension, particularly if the cells are washed, a technique particularly suitable for lymph node aspirates (Fig. 2.18, see also Ch. 5). The problem does not apply to paraffin-embedded cell blocks.

Table 2.4 Immunoperoxidase (IPOX) studies and fine needle aspiration

Tumour type or differential diagnosis	Useful tumour markers
Small cell malignancies	
Lymphoma	Leucocyte common antigen (LCA)
Small cell carcinoma	Keratins (AE1/AE3, CAM 5.2); neuroendocrine markers
Large cell malignancies	
Lymphoma	LCA
Anaplastic carcinoma	Keratins, carcino-embryonic antigen (CEA)
Melanoma	S-100; HMB.45
Germ cell tumours	Human chorionic gonadotrophin (HCG); Alpha-fetoprotein (AFP)
Pleomorphic spindle cell tumours	
Sarcoma	Vimentin, desmin (smooth muscle)
Sarcomatoid carcinoma	Keratins
Melanoma	S-100; HMB.45
Tubulo-glandular malignancies	
Mesothelioma	
Adenocarcinoma	CEA; Leu-1; 44–3A6
Lymphoma typing	LCA; pan-B, pan-T, kappa and lambda light chains Epithelial membrane antigen (EMA); BERH-2 (Ki-1 tumours)
Specific tumours	
Prostatic carcinoma	Prostate specific antigen (PSA); prostatic acid phosphatase (PAP)
Thyroid carcinoma	Thyroglobulin Calcitonin
Breast carcinoma	Breast cyst-fluid protein; lactalbumin
Neuroendocrine tumours (carcinoid; neuroendocrine carcinomas)	Neuron-specific enolase (NSE); synaptophysin; bombesin; chromogranin; ACTH; serotonin

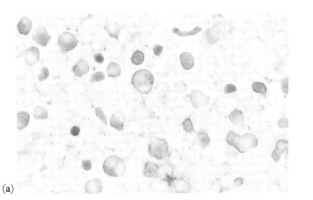
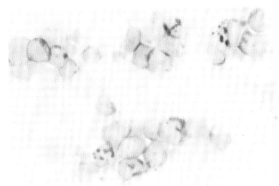

(a)   (b)

Fig. 2.18 Immunoperoxidase staining
Case of non-Hodgkin's lymphoma. a) Direct smear: difficult to interpret due to background staining. b) Cytospin preparation: positive staining distinctly related to individual cells (HP).

OTHER INVESTIGATIONS

Microbiology[32]

Providing material for microbiological culture is an important role of aspiration biopsy. However, there are difficulties in preserving small amounts of biopsy material and a flexible approach to this aspect of diagnosis is required. If an infective lesion is suspected in deep tissues, for example lung, prior to aspiration, optimal results are achieved if a microbiologist can be present at the biopsy to process material, particularly in the case of immunosuppressed patients where unusual infections are likely. Where the likelihood of infection is discovered only at the time of biopsy, either by the aspiration of macroscopically visible pus, or at preliminary microscopical examination, then several approaches are possible. Frank pus is best transported to the microbiology department in the aspirating needle and syringe, as rapidly as possible. Very small amounts of pus are best washed into a sterile container with a few mls of sterile normal saline, otherwise drying and dessication of organisms will occur. This may not provide for anaerobic or unusual organisms; however, dividing very small amounts of material into several types of media is singularly unprofitable. The use of needle washings, after most of the aspirate has been expelled onto slides, also seldom yields results. The single most important determinant of whether an organism can be cultured seems to be the amount of aspirated material and repeated biopsies, using all of the contents of the needle for culture, are most valuable.

Morphometry[4,21,36]

A number of morphometric techniques, for example planimetric methods including computer-assisted image analysis,[62] single cell microspectrophotometry[3] and flow cytometry,[30] have been applied to FNA preparations to a rapidly increasing extent. Morphometric analysis has mainly been used as an objective indicator of prognosis, particularly in carcinoma of the breast and of the prostate and in malignant lymphoma, but has also been found to be helpful in cytological diagnosis distinguishing benign from malignant processes, for example in the thyroid and in the breast.[2,7,29,60] A description of these techniques and a detailed review of their applications is beyond the scope of this book and the reader is referred to the excellent review by Frable,[16] the monograph by Baak[4], and to the numerous papers in this field published in *Analytical and Quantitative Cytology*.

2 THE TECHNIQUES OF FNA CYTOLOGY

REFERENCES AND SUGGESTED FURTHER READING

1. Akhtar M, Ali A, Owen E W: Application of electron microscopy in the interpretation of fine needle aspiration biopsies. Cancer 48: 2458–2463, 1981.
2. Auer G U, Casperson T O, Wallgren A S: DNA content and survival in mammary carcinoma. Anal Quant Cytol 2: 161–165, 1980.
3. Auer G, Askensten U, Ahrens O: Cytophotometry. Hum Pathol 20: 518–527, 1989.
4. Baak J P A, Oort J: A manual of morphometry in diagnostic pathology. Springer, Berlin, 1983.
5. Bell D A, Carr C P, Szyfelbeen W M: Fine needle aspiration cytology of focal liver lesions. Results obtained with examination of both cytologic and histologic preparations. Acta Cytol 30: 397–402, 1986.
6. Boccato P, Briani G, Bizzaro N et al: Cytology in 'black and white'. Acta Cytol 31: 643–645, 1987.
7. Boon M E, Löwhagen T, Willems J S: Planimetric studies of fine needle aspirations from follicular adenoma and follicular carcinoma of the thyroid. Acta Cytol 24: 145–148, 1980.
8. Boon M E, Lykles C: Imaginative approach to fine needle aspiration cytology. Lancet 2: 1031–1032, 1980.
9. Burns J: Background staining and sensitivity of the unlabelled antibody enzyme (PAP) method. Comparison with the peroxidase labelled antibody sandwich method using formalin fixed paraffin embedded material. Histochemistry 43: 291–294, 1975.
10. Chess Q, Hajdu S I: The role of immunoperoxidase staining in diagnostic cytology. Acta Cytol 30: 1–7, 1986.
11. Coleman D, Desai S, Dudley H, Hollowell S, Hulbert M: Needle aspiration of palpable breast lesions: A new application of the membrane filter technique and its results. Clin Oncol 1: 27–32, 1975.
12. Dabbs D J, Silverman J F: Selective use of electron microscopy in fine needle aspiration cytology. Acta Cytol 32: 880–884, 1988.
13. Domagala W, Lubinski J, Weber K, Osborn M: Intermediate filament typing of tumor cells in fine needle aspirates by means of monoclonal antibodies. Acta Cytol 30: 214–234, 1986.
14. Domagala W, Lubinski J, Lasola J et al.: Decisive role of intermediate filament typing of tumor cells in the differential diagnosis of difficult fine needle aspirates. Acta Cytol 31: 253–266, 1987.
15. Ekelund P, Wasastjerna C: Cytologic identification of primary hepatic carcinoma cells. Acta Med Scand 189: 373–375, 1971.
16. Frable W J: Thin-needle aspiration biopsy. Ch. 11. Research and special applications. W B Saunders, Philadelphia, 1983.
17. Godwin J T: Rapid cytologic diagnosis of surgical specimens. Acta Cytol 20: 111–115, 1976.
18. Gupta P K, Myers J D, Baylin S B, Mulshine J L, Cuttitta F, Gazdar A F: Improved antigen detection in ethanol-fixed cytologic specimens. A modified Avidin-Biotin-Peroxidase complex (ABC) method. Diagn Cytopathol 1: 133–136, 1985.
19. Gustafsson B, Manson J-C: Methodological aspects and application of the immunoperoxidase staining technique in diagnostic fine-needle aspiration cytology. Diagn Cytopathol 3: 68–73, 1987.
20. Hagelqvist E: Light and electron microscopic studies on material obtained by fine needle biopsy. Acta Otolaryngol (Suppl) 354: 1–75, 1978.
21. Hall T L, Fu Y S: Applications of quantitative microscopy in tumor pathology. Lab Invest 53: 5, 1985.
22. Hancke S: Hazards in percutaneous biopsy. In: Percutaneous biopsy and therapeutic vascular occlusion. Anacker H, Gulotta U, Rupp N (eds). Georg Thieme, Stuttgart, 1980.
23. Henderson D W, Papadimitriou J M, Coleman M: Ultrastructural appearances of tumors. A diagnostic atlas, 2nd edn. Churchill Livingstone, Edinburgh, 1986.
24. Heyderman E, Brown B M: Preparation of fine needle aspirates for immunocytochemical studies. Lancet 2: 520–521, 1986.
25. Isler R J, Ferrucci J T, Wittenberg J, Mueller P R, Simeone J F, van Sonnenberg E, Hall D A: Tissue core biopsy of abdominal tumors with a 22 gauge cutting needle. Am J Roentgenol 136: 725–728, 1981.
26. Jennings P E, Donald J J, Coral A, Rode J, Lees W R: Ultrasound-guided core biopsy. Lancet 1: 1369–1371, 1989.
27. Johnston W W, Szpak C A, Lottich S C, Thor A, Schlom J: Use of a monoclonal antibody (B72.3) as a novel immunohistochemical adjunct for the diagnosis of carcinoma in fine needle aspiration biopsy. Hum Pathol 17: 501–513, 1986.
28. Kern W H, Haber H: Fine needle aspiration microbiopsies. Acta Cytol 30: 403–408, 1986.
29. Klaus H, Roth K, Hufnagl P, Wildner G P: Automated image analysis in the cytological tumor diagnosis. Results in borderline cases of mammary tumors. Arch Geschwulstforsch 55: 253–258, 1985.
30. Koss L G, Czerniak B, Herz F, Wersto R P: Flow cytometric measurements of DNA and other cell components in human tumors: a critical appraisal. Hum Pathol 20: 528–548, 1989.
31. Krogerus L A, Andersson L C: A simple method for the preparation of paraffin-embedded cell blocks from fine needle aspirates, effusions and brushings. Acta Cytol 32: 585–587, 1988.
32. Layfield L J, Glasgow B J, DuPuis M H: Fine-needle aspiration of lymphadenopathy of suspected infectious etiology. Arch Pathol Lab Med 109: 810–812, 1985.
33. Lazaro A V: Technical note: Improved preparation of fine needle aspiration biopsies for transmission electron microscopy. Pathology 15: 399–402, 1983.
34. Lennert K: Histopathology of non-Hodgkin's lymphoma (based on the Kiel classification). Springer, Berlin, 1981.
35. Lundy J, Lozokowski M, Mishriki Y: Monoclonal antibody B72.3 as a diagnostic adjunct in fine needle aspirates of breast masses. Ann Surg 203: 399–402, 1986.
36. Machewsky A M, Gil J, Jeanty H: Computerized interactive morphometry in pathology. Current instrumentation and methods. Hum Pathol 18: 320–331, 1987.
37. Mair S, Dunbar F, Becker P J, DuPlessis W: Fine needle cytology — Is aspiration suction necessary? A study of 100 masses in various sites. Acta Cytol 33: 809–813, 1989.
38. Mather J, Stanbridge C M, Butler E B: Method for the removal of selected cells from cytological smear preparations for transmission electron microscopy. J Clin Pathol 34: 1355–1357, 1981.
39. Nadji M: The potential value of immunoperoxidase techniques in diagnostic cytology. Acta Cytol 24: 442–447, 1980.
40. Nordenstrom B: New instrument for biopsy. Radiology 117: 474, 1975.
41. Nordgren H, Åkerman M: Electron microscopy of fine needle aspiration biopsy from soft tissue tumors. Acta Cytol 26: 179–188, 1982.

THE TECHNIQUES OF FNA CYTOLOGY 2

42. Nordgren H, Nilsson S, Runn A C, Ponten J, Bergh J: Histopathological and immunohistochemical analysis of lung tumors: description of a convenient technique for use with fine needle biopsy. APMIS 97: 136–142, 1989.
43. Odselius R, Fält K, Sandell L: A simple method for processing cytologic samples obtained from body cavity fluids and by fine needle aspiration biopsy for ultrastructural studies. Acta Cytol 31: 194–198, 1987.
44. Oertel Y C, Galblum L I: Fine needle aspiration of the breast: diagnostic criteria. Pathol Annual 18: 375–407, 1983.
45. Olson N J, Gogel H K, Williams W L, Mettler F A: Processing of aspiration cytology samples. An alternative method. Acta Cytol 30: 409–412, 1986.
46. Orell S R, Skinner J: Fine needle aspiration cytology. In: Histochemistry in pathology, 2nd edn. Filipe M I, Lake B D (eds) Churchill Livingstone, Edinburgh, 1990.
47. Pak H Y, Yokota S, Teplitz R L, Shaw S L, Werner L J: Rapid staining techniques employed in fine needle aspiration of the lung. Acta Cytol 25: 178–184, 1981.
48. Pak H Y, Yokota S B, Teplitz R L: Rapid staining techniques employed in fine needle aspirations. Acta Cytol 27: 81–82, 1983.
49. Pintozzi R L, Blecka L J, Nanon S: The morphologic indentification of Pneumocystis Carinii. Acta Cytol 23: 35–39, 1979.
50. Pollock P G, Valicenti J F, Meyers D S, Frable W J, Durham J B: The used of fluorescent and special staining techniques in the aspiration of nocardiosis and actinomycosis. Acta Cytol 22: 575–579, 1978.
51. Sachdeva R, Kline T S: Aspiration biopsy cytology and special stains. Acta Cytol 25: 678–683, 1981.
52. Sanerkin N G, Jeffree G M: Cytology of bone tumors. John Wright & Sons, Bristol, 1980.
53. Sant'Agnese P A di, Mesy Jensen K L de, Bonfiglio T A, King D E, Patten S F Jr: Plastic-embedded semi-thin sections of fine needle aspiration biopsies with dibasic staining. Diagnostic and didactic applications. Acta Cytol 29: 477–483, 1985.
54. Sartorius J, Feldges A, Gysin R: Optimierung und Vereinfachung der klinischen Tumorzytodiagnostic mittels Zytozentrifugation. Schweiz Med Wschr 106: 761–764, 1976.
55. Smith M J, Kini S R, Watson E: Fine needle aspiration and endoscopic brush cytology. Comparison of direct smears and rinsings. Acta Cytol 24: 456–459, 1980.
56. Taylor C R: Immunomicroscopy: a diagnostic tool for the surgical pathologist. Vol. 19. Major Problems in Pathology. Saunders, Philadelphia, 1986.
57. Thompson P: Thin needle aspiration biopsy (letter). Acta Cytol 26: 262–263, 1982.
58. To A, Dearnley D P, Ormerod M G, Canti G, Coleman D V: Indirect immunoalkaline phosphatase staining of cytologic smears of serous effusions for tumor marker studies. Acta Cytol 27: 109–113, 1983.
59. Travis W D, Wold L E: Immunoperoxidase staining of fine needle aspiration specimens previously stained by the Papanicolaou technique. Acta Cytol 31: 517–520, 1987.
60. Tribukait B, Esposti P L, Ronstrom L: Tumor ploidy for characterization of prostatic carcinoma: flow-cytofluorometric DNA studies using aspiration biopsy material. Scand J Urol Nephrol (Suppl) 55: 59–64, 1980.
61. Watts A E, Said J W, Shintaker P, Lloyd R V: Chromogranin as a marker of neuroendocrine cells in cytologic material — an immunocytochemical study. Am J Clin Pathol 84: 273–277, 1985.
62. Wied G L, Bartels P H, Bibbo M, Dytch H E: Image analysis in quantitative cytopathology and histopathology. Hum Pathol 20: 549–571, 1989.
63. Wills E J, Carr S, Philips J: Electron microscopy in the diagnosis of percutaneous fine needle aspiration specimens. J Ultrastruct Pathol 11: 361–387, 1987.
64. Zajdela A, Zillhardt P, Voillemot N: Cytological diagnosis by fine needle sampling without aspiration. Cancer 59: 1201–1205, 1987.
65. Zajicek J: Aspiration biopsy cytology. Part 1. Cytology of supradiaphragmatic organs.Monographs in clinical cytology, Vol. 4. S Karger, Basel, 1974.

IMAGING METHODS FOR GUIDANCE OF ASPIRATION CYTOLOGY

Suzanne Le P. Langlois

3 GUIDANCE OF ASPIRATION CYTOLOGY

Percutaneous biopsy is the most frequent interventional radiographic procedure and is performed either as an in-patient or out-patient examination by most trained radiologists. There have been continuous improvements in needles, biopsy guides and mechanical biopsy devices, together with technological advances in the major imaging methods of computerised tomography (CT) and ultrasound, and more recently magnetic resonance imaging (MRI), plus development of stereotactic guidance, particularly for brain[1] and breast biopsies.[2] Previously inaccessible lesions can be safely sampled and many more areas of the body are now routinely biopsied under guidance. The technique has also allowed the development of more invasive procedures such as catheter drainage, villus biopsy and fetal blood and tissue sampling.[3,4]

FNA biopsy is now indicated in almost every mass detected where the aetiology is unclear. Close cooperation between the imaging and cytopathology departments provides maximum efficiency of machine and personnel time and ensures the most accurate diagnostic yield.

More than one imaging modality may be required, firstly to localise the lesion and then to obtain biopsy material. The discretion of the radiologist performing the procedure should determine the method used and will be influenced by availability of equipment, difficulty in scheduling, urgency of the procedure and operator preference and experience. Many prefer the speed of ultrasound guidance, while those in training are reassured by the greater resolution of CT.

All of the imaging techniques have advantages and disadvantages in various parts of the body (Table 3.1, Fig. 3.1). The single major advantage of ultrasound is mobility of the equipment. Modern portable realtime scanners can be transported to wards, intensive care units or operating theatres to assist biopsy or other more invasive procedures. While guidance by CT is easier for relatively unskilled operators (because the images are more easily interpreted) heavy utilisation of the equipment may result in delayed diagnosis; ultrasound departments often have a more flexible schedule, their procedures require shorter appointment times and they may acquire the major workload for biopsy guidance.[5] The problem of radiation exposure during fluoroscopically guided procedures, and to a lesser extent with CT, should also be considered. While this is not a significant factor for the patients, continued exposure to the operator may carry a risk.

The most critical factor in the success of guided needle aspiration biopsy is the presence of the pathologist during the procedure.[6] This will shorten the proce-

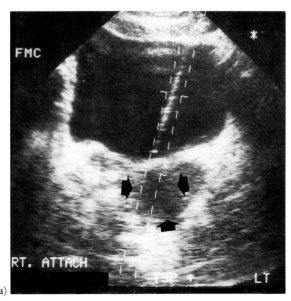

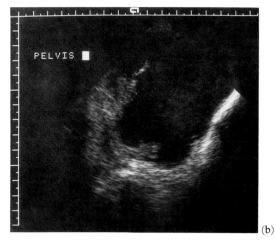

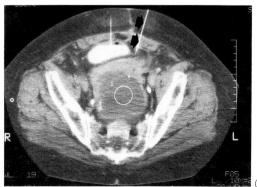

Fig. 3.1 Ultrasound guided biopsy of pelvic abscessess
(a) Transvesical needle aspiration for bacteriological diagnosis of an abscess (arrows) deep within the pelvis of a male patient following recent bowel resection. The echogenic fine needle can be seen within the bladder. (b) Transvaginal scan of an infected post-operative collection in a middle-aged woman. The central cystic or necrotic area is well demarcated from the peripheral solid walls of the collection. (c) CT-guided aspiration biopsy of the same collection as in (b), prior to insertion of a catheter for drainage. The needle (arrows) was obliquely placed to avoid the bladder.

GUIDANCE OF ASPIRATION CYTOLOGY

3

Table 3.1 Advantages and disadvantages of available imaging techniques

Method	Advantages	Disadvantages
Fluoroscopy	Rapid Flexible Mobile Readily available Needle easily visible Special areas, e.g. stereotaxis	Radiation exposure Difficult to visualise lesion Difficult to demonstrate depth
Ultrasound	Rapid Flexible Relatively inexpensive Mobile Real-time imaging	Poor needle visibility Limited by gas or bone Long learning curve
CT	Needle easily visible Precise localisation Suitable for deep/small lesions	More expensive Relatively slow Radiation exposure
MRI	Suitable for lesions not otherwise imaged	Very slow Most expensive Requires special needles

dure, as the number of aspirates is often reduced to one or two, and the pathologist may direct the radiologist to a different area of the lesion, for example to the viable periphery rather than the central necrotic area of a solid lesion, or request additional tissue for special stains, electron microscopy or culture.

The schedule of the imaging department should be modified if necessary to accomodate the pathologist. Optimal results can only be obtained by meticulous localisation before biopsy and this may occupy most of the procedural time; fortunately this can be performed prior to the arrival of the pathologist.

It matters little whether the radiologist or pathologist performs the actual aspiration. In many cases the radiologist is more skilled in interpreting the images and is better able to manipulate the needle in three dimensions while viewing a two-dimensional image. With ultrasound the image may be uninterpretable to all but the radiologist. Experience plays a part in obtaining adequate tissue[7] but some are more naturally skilled than others in this technique.[8]

FLUOROSCOPY

Fluoroscopy is the traditional method for guidance of biopsies to most parts of the body. With the advent of highly technical guidance methods such as CT and ultrasound it is used less and is often considered less accurate. However, it provides a quick alternative for those radiologists not experienced in ultrasound guidance and is most useful in guidance for small very

mobile lesions, such as focal lower zone lung lesions. In this instance, the real-time advantage of fluoroscopy may be the only method of accurately placing a needle tip within a small lesion. It is still the most rapid method for aspirating cortical bony lesions. It should always be considered as an alternative because of its low cost and general availability.

Fluoroscopy is most useful when bi-plane imaging is possible. If not, two-dimensional imaging can be used. Tube tilt can provide a stereotactic view to show the depth of the needle. When combined with other tissue or organ enhancement, however, its real-time features may permit biopsy of otherwise inaccessible areas such as lymph nodes or small vascular tumours when combined with lymphangiography, intra-abdominal selective angiography or endoscopic retrograde cholangiopancreatography.

ULTRASOUND

Ultrasound is the only real-time guidance which allows imaging in any plane and is the only suitable guidance for biopsy of fetal tissues. Its use is limited in certain areas as ultrasound is not transmitted through air or

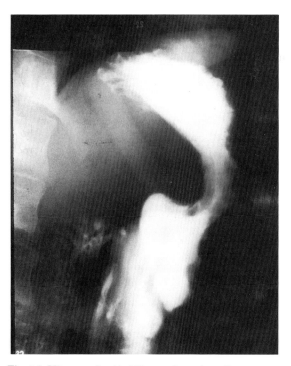

Fig. 3.2 Ultrasound-guided biopsy of gastric malignancy
A radiological diagnosis of 'linitis plastica' or infiltrating tumour on barium studies could not be confirmed by repeated endoscopic biopsies. After confirmation of the gastric distortion by fluoroscopy after Gastrografin ingestion, transabdominal ultrasound-guided biopsy of the stomach wall was performed, using a 22 G Rotex screw biopsy needle.

3 GUIDANCE OF ASPIRATION CYTOLOGY

bone. Some parts of the body, such as the chest and musculoskeletal system, though neglected in the past, are currently undergoing an increase in interest for both diagnostic and interventional studies (Fig. 3.2).[9] Recent developments such as operative probes and vaginal and rectal transducers combined with the portability of ultrasound equipment to intensive care areas and operating theatres have also increased the utility of ultrasound.

Real-time monitoring is a major advantage as the exact location of the needle tip can be seen during biopsy and adjustments to its position can be performed to increase the accuracy of sampling (Fig. 3.3). Visibility of needles can be a problem and needles should be tested for echogenicity prior to use. Needles such as the 'screw' type are popular because of their marked echogenicity (Fig. 3.3). Stilettes within needles, and particularly movement of the stilette within the needle, will improve visibility. The gauge of the needle does not necessarily relate to echogenicity and in many instances a fine needle will be more highly echogenic than a subsequent core-biopsy needle.

The choice of transducer and frequency is dictated by the area of the body to be biopsied. Sector scanners require less skin contact area than linear array transducers but many operators have greatest success with curvilinear probes. Intracavitary probes and future de-

velopments with intravascular and intraluminal transducers will allow biopsy and intervention into virtually every part of the body.

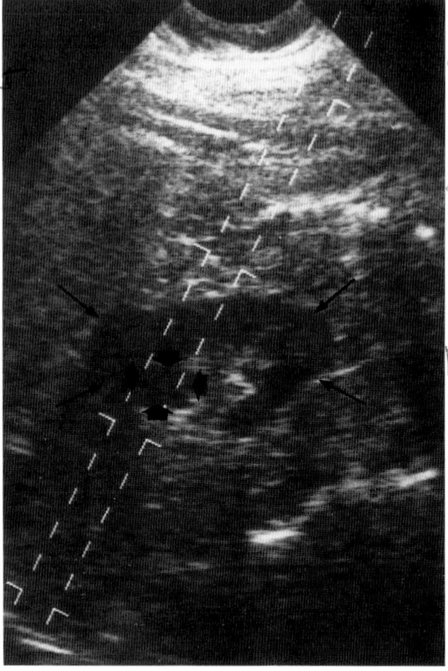

To reduce the risk of tearing of tissues there should be easy separation of the needle from the biopsy attachment, particularly in areas of the body where movement may occur, for example liver and kidney. The shortest puncture route is normally chosen, though with hepatic biopsies it is imperative that the needle traverses at least a rim of normal liver to reduce the risk of haemorrhage.

While sterile water can be used as a coupling medium, there appears to be no real risk of reaction from injection of sterile coupling medium. Sterilisation of the transducer and attachment is routine, including universal precautions against infection.

CT SCANNING

There are very few areas of the body which cannot be biopsied under CT control, and extremely small lesions can be sampled. Focal masses of a few millimetres within the lung can be biopsied and retroperitoneal biopsies are limited only by availability of needles long enough to traverse the abdomen of large patients. Interposed structures such as bowel are no longer considered a hazard with the use of fine needles (Fig. 3.4). The advantage of CT over ultrasound guidance is the ability of the needle to swing freely with respiratory or involuntary movement, whereas ultrasound guides produce a fixed system which may cause trauma to underlying tissues.

Localisation of the needle tip within a lesion is very accurate with CT. Unfortunately it is less readily available than other imaging techniques because of the high

Fig. 3.3 Renal cyst aspiration
A small mass lesion less than 1 cm in diameter (short arrows) was demonstrated in the para-pelvic region of a kidney (long arrows). Needle aspiration under real-time ultrasound control confirmed the position of the needle tip within the cyst and showed collapse of the cyst during aspiration of fluid.

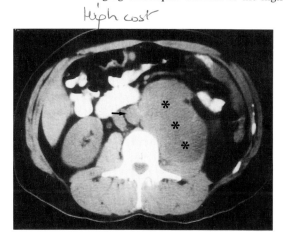

Fig. 3.4 Para-aortic lymphadenopathy
CT examination performed in a middle-aged man with a history of several months' of back pain reveals a large abnormal soft tissue mass (***) lying to the left of the aorta (arrow). Ultrasound-guided fine-needle aspiration confirmed metastatic disease from a testicular germ cell tumour, and testicular ultrasound then revealed a small mass in the left testis.

GUIDANCE OF ASPIRATION CYTOLOGY 3

clinical demand for the equipment and the prolonged time for examinations. However it provides detailed cross-sectional images of the body which are not limited by the same physical properties as are ultrasound images, such as interference from bowel gas and bone. The disadvantages are that the images are not produced in 'real-time' but require processing before display on the video-monitor. It is important that confirmation of the location of the needle-tip be obtained by scanning prior to each aspiration.

Disadvantages include changes in position of the needle and tissues with respiratory motion, and from scan to scan with time. The patient must be reasonably cooperative and it is advantageous to insert the needle in a plane vertical to the X-ray beam, so that the full length of the needle is demonstrated on one scan. This may also be obtained by gantry tilt.

The needle tip should be localised as accurately as possible to a position a few millimetres short of the lesion to be biopsied and the needle advanced the last few millimetres only during the biopsy. This prevents blood from accumulating around the needle tip and degrading the cytology specimen during the time required for scanning. Various techniques are available, including the use of guide or tandem needles,[10] or even stereotaxis.[11] Artefacts from metallic needles and respiratory movement are rarely significant, particularly with the latest generation of CT scanners.

MAGNETIC RESONANCE IMAGING (MRI)

One of the many predictions which were made during the development of magnetic resonance, and which were later proven wrong, was that MRI would never be suitable for guidance of biopsy and interventional procedures. However, the sensitivity of this new imaging technique is generally greater than that of other imaging methods and shows lesions which would not otherwise be detected. This is particularly evident in the brain and liver (Fig. 3.5). Needles with low ferromagnetic properties have therefore been developed to allow biopsy under MRI control. Fortunately the number of patients requiring this is small, as there are still logistic problems due to slow scanning times, which will probably be overcome by rapid-scan techniques, for example FLASH (Siemens), GRASS (General Electric) and further technological developments.

BREAST BIOPSY

The current enthusiasm for breast screening has brought added difficulties in biopsy and localisation of the small, clinically occult lesions detected by these programs. While many methods have been used, including ultrasound with and without a transducer

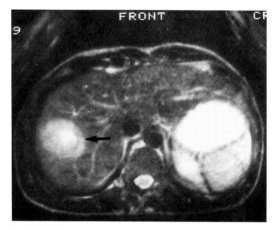

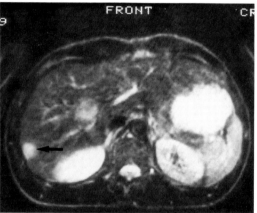

Fig. 3.5 Carcinoid metastases on MRI
T_2 weighted axial scans demonstrate two metastases (arrows) from the patient's known primary tumour. At least two more metastases were revealed by MRI than seen on CT scan.

attachment (Fig. 3.6), the most accurate method for localisation is the use of a stereotactic attachment for mammographic X-ray units (Fig. 3.7).[12,13] When combined with fine needle biopsy and localisation, either with a hookwire or preferably with carbon marking of the track, this technique efficiently provides maximal information for the clinician with the minimum of inconvenience to the patient.

USE OF GUIDE NEEDLES

A guide needle is a short 2–3 cm needle, through which a fine-gauge needle is passed in a co-axial method. The gauges of the needle combinations are usually 18/22 or 22/26. Use of these needles has been advocated during guided techniques for the following reasons:
1. Increase in needle stability.
2. Multiple passes can be made through the guide needle and the biopsy repeated several times in various

3 *GUIDANCE OF ASPIRATION CYTOLOGY*

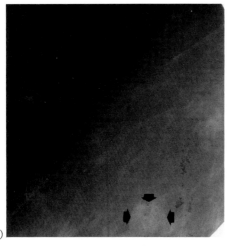

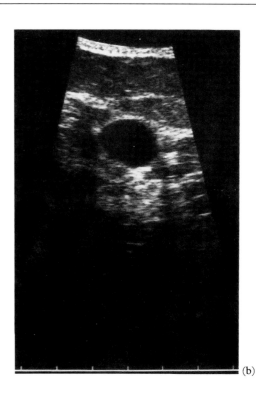

Fig. 3.6 Aspiration of breast cyst
(a) Mammography reveals a low-density well defined soft tissue mass (arrows) within a fat-replaced breast. (b) Ultrasound confirms the presence of a benign cyst, with acoustic enhancement posteriorly. (c) Real-time ultrasound-guided aspiration demonstrates the needle (arrows) within the cyst and gradual collapse of the walls as the cyst is emptied.

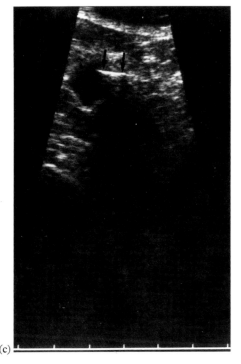

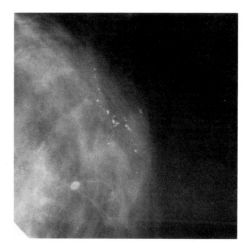

Fig. 3.7 Stereotactic biopsy of breast mass
Linear and irregular calcifications initially described as indeterminate to suspicious but which were subsequently proven to be histologically benign, are localised within a stereotactic device during carbon-marking prior to surgical excision. Fine-needle aspiration biopsy can be routinely performed during all stereotactic breast localisation procedures.

GUIDANCE OF ASPIRATION CYTOLOGY 3

directions and depths to obtain material from several areas of the lesion.

3. Any risk of spread of tumour or infection is minimised by reducing the path length of the contaminated biopsy needle.

4. Only one skin puncture is required thus lessening the discomfort of the procedure for the patient.

5. Deviation of the fine needle due to resistance to its passage through firm skin, subcutaneous tissues and muscle wall are avoided.

6. Microbubbles in local anaesthetic infiltrated into the tissues may obscure the scan field. This is prevented by using a focal area of anaesthesia for a single guide needle.

RISKS AND COMPLICATIONS

The overall mortality and morbidity related to fine needle biopsy has been estimated in many studies, and the risk of death is approximately 1:15 000.[14] This compares favourably with the more invasive studies which the technique replaces. Experience and the use of certain guidelines will reduce the risk of haemorrhage (Fig. 3.8) and spread of infection or tumour,[15] especially in liver biopsies.[16]

Ultrasound has considerable advantage in the upper abdomen because of the ability to guide biopsies in oblique planes (Fig. 3.9). While CT guidance is usually used in the axial plane to image the needle perpendicular to that plane, gantry tilt provides a practical and simple means of avoiding bone, pleura and other organs. It is particularly useful for spine and disc aspirates, and in the upper abdomen (Fig. 3.9).[17] The risk of puncturing lung, spleen and liver by a posterior percutaneous perpendicular approach has been calculated by examination of CT scans.[18] It is possible to demonstrate that the risk from a posterior intercostal approach between the 11th and 12th ribs for possible puncture of lung is 14–29%, while the risk from a posterior 10th to 11th intercostal approach is prohibitive.

Several techniques have been advocated for preventing development of pneumothorax,[19] a common complication of transpleural biopsy occuring in 10–40% of reported series. Usefulness of these techniques is not proven and where possible an extrapleural route for biopsy is recommended. There is also little data concerning the methods used to detect such a pneumothorax. In the authors' experience there is a 33% pneumothorax rate, with less than 1% requiring underwater seal drainage. However, this high incidence requires rigorous investigation, with radiographs taken 1 hour after the procedure and expiratory films if there is any doubt. Patients with chronic lung disease are at greater risk.[20]

The risk of late pneumothorax is probably extremely small. In the authors' experience the risk is negligible if no pneumothorax is detected at 1 hour. There is probably a similar risk of haemorrhage, and haemoptysis, if it occurs, usually manifests before the patient leaves the X-ray table. The procedure can be safely performed on out-patients, but there should be adequate counselling to return if pain, dyspnoea or haemoptysis occur.

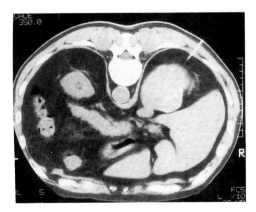

Fig. 3.8 Adrenal mass biopsy in a haemophiliac patient
The patient was a severe haemophiliac with only 2% of normal levels of Factor VIII. As he was experiencing discomfort in the right upper quadrant, a cytological diagnosis was sought for the mass within the right adrenal (arrow). Biopsy was performed during several days of infusion of Factor VIII. No complications occurred and the cytological diagnosis indicated old organising haemorrhage.

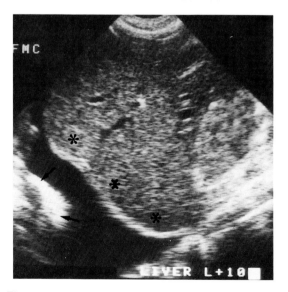

Fig. 3.9 Pleural effusion related to malignant mesothelioma
Free fluid is seen between the lung (arrows) and diaphragm and subjacent liver (***). With the increasing incidence of malignant mesothelioma it is becoming more important to diagnose the condition in the least invasive manner. Pleural biopsy under ultrasound control may provide sufficient tissue for diagnosis.

3 *GUIDANCE OF ASPIRATION CYTOLOGY*

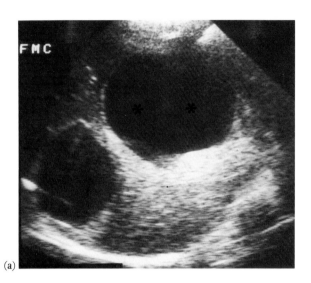

(a)

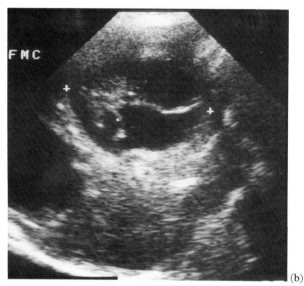

(b)

Fig. 3.10 Aspiration biopsy of hydatid disease without complication
(a) Two clearly defined anechoic cysts within the liver. The more anterior cyst (**) was completely aspirated (b) Five months later the patient was rescanned and multiple loculi within the cyst provided the diagnosis of hydatid disease. This was confirmed at surgery.

Various contraindications to fine needle biopsy have been given in the literature. These include the risk of biopsy of phaeochromocytomas,[21] hydatid cysts (Fig. 3.10) and haemangiomas, and of biopsy in the presence of ascites. The risks are considerably less than previously stated[16] and ascites does not affect the risk of biopsy.[22]

REFERENCES AND SUGGESTED FURTHER READING

1. Redmond M J, Saines N S, Coroneos M: The use of computed-tomographic-directed stereotaxis in the diagnosis of intracerebral lesions. Med J Aust 149: 468–472, 1988.
2. Azavedo E, Svane G, Auer G: Stereotactic fine-needle biopsy in 2594 mammographically detected non-palpable lesions. Lancet May 13, 1989.
3. Langlois S LeP, Henderson D W, Chen C, Sutherland G R: Antenatal diagnosis of lamellar ichthyosis by ultrasonically guided needle biopsy of foetal skin. In: Proceedings of 4th Meeting of the World Federation for Ultrasound in Medicine and Biology. Gill R W, Dadd M J (eds) Pergamon Press, Oxford, 1985, p. 305.
4. Kurjak A. Alfirevic Z, Jurkovic D: Ultrasonically guided fetal tissue biopsy. Acta Obstet Gynecol Scand 66: 523–527, 1987.
5. Pelaez J C, Hill M C, Dach J L et al: Abdominal aspiration biopsies — sonographic v computed tomographic guidance. JAMA 250: 2663–2666, 1983.
6. Givardi G, Fornari F, Cavanna L et al: Value of rapid staining and assessment of ultrasound-guided fine needle aspiration biopsies. Acta Cytol 32: 552–554, 1988
7. Lew W Y C, Lee W H: Fine-needle aspiration cytology: its role in the management of breast tumours. Aust NZ J Surg 58: 941–946, 1988.

8. Barrows G H, Anderson T J, Lamb J L, Dixon J M. Fine-needle aspiration of breast cancer — relationship of clinical factors to cytology results in 689 primary malignancies. Cancer 58: 1493–1498, 1986.
9. Christiansen R A, van Sonnenberg E, Casola G, Wittich G R: Interventional ultrasound in the musculoskeletal system. Radiol Clin N Am 26: 145–156, 1988.
10. van Sonnenberg E, Lin A S, Deutsch A L, Maltrey R F. Percutaneous biopsy of difficult mediastinal, hilar, and pulmonary lesions by computed tomographic guidance and a modified coaxial technique. Radiology 148(1): 300–302, 1983.
11. Onik G, Casman E R, Wells T H, Goldberg H I et al: CT-guided aspirations for the body: comparison of hand guidance with stereotaxis. Radiology 166: 389–394, 1988.
12. Evans W P, Cade S H: Needle localisation and fine-needle aspiration biopsy of non-palpable breast lesions with use of standard and stereotactic equipment. Radiology 173: 53–56, 1989.
13. Ciatto S, Del Turco M R, Bravetti P: Nonpalpable breast lesions: stereotaxic fine-needle aspiration cytology. Radiology 173: 57–59, 1989.
14. Holm H H, Torp-Pedersen S, Larsen T, Juul N: Percutaneous fine needle biopsy. Clin Gastroenterol 14(2): 423–448, 1985.

15. de Crespigny L Ch, Robinson H P, Davoren R A M, Fortune D W: Ultrasound-guided puncture for gynaecological and pelvic lesions. Aust NZ J Obstet Gynecol 25; 227–229, 1985.

16. Langlois S LeP: Fine-needle biopsy of hepatic hydatids and haemangiomas: an overstated hazard. Aust Radiol 33: 144–149, 1989.

17. Yueh N, Halvorsen A A, Letoureau J G, Grass J R: Gantry-tilt technique for CT-guided biopsy and drainage. J Comput Assist Tomog 13(1): 182–184, 1989.

18. Hopper K D, Yakes W F: The posterior intercostal approach for percutaneous renal procedures; risk of puncturing the lung, spleen and liver as determined by CT. Am J Roentgenol 154: 115–117, 1990.

19. Cassel D M, Birnberg F A: Preventing pneumothorax after lung biopsy: the roll-over technique. Radiology 1174: 282, 1990.

20. Fish G D, Stanley J H, Miller K S et al: Post-biopsy pneumothorax: estimating the risk by chest radiography and pulmonary function tests. Am J Roentgenol 150: 71–74, 1988.

21. Koenker R M, Mueller P R, van Sonnenberg E: Interventional radiology of the adrenal glands. Semin Roentgenol 22: 314–322, 1988.

22. Murphy F B, Barefield K P, Steinberg H V, Bernardino M E. CT- or sonography-guided biopsy of the liver in the presence of ascites: frequency of complications. Am J Roentgenol 151: 485–486, 1988.

4

HEAD AND NECK; SALIVARY GLANDS

HEAD AND NECK; SALIVARY GLANDS

CLINICAL ASPECTS

The proximity of tissues of various types and the wide range of primary and metastatic neoplasms are responsible for this site being among the most interesting in FNA diagnosis. Close co-operation with the clinician is necessary to be sure of the anatomical relations of the target lesion, the nature of any previous lesion or the details of prior therapy. The confirmation of metastatic spread to lymph nodes can be among the easiest of diagnoses but the variation in appearances of even common types of primary neoplasm of, for example, salivary glands, makes this a challenging and difficult area.

Incisional biopsy in this sensitive area may leave undesirable scars and can be difficult especially after radiotherapy. FNA can obviate the need for surgery if the lesion is shown to be non-neoplastic. If neoplastic, it may allow more rational preoperative planning of surgical treatment. This is important since curative surgery is often a delicate balance between radical excision and preservation of normal tissue and function. Finally, the psychological and economical advantages of an immediate diagnosis in the out-patient clinic are obvious.

HEAD AND NECK

The place of FNA in the investigative sequence

By far the most common and practically important indication for FNA biopsy in the region of the head and neck is the investigation of suspected local recurrence or nodal metastasis of previously diagnosed and treated cancer.[10] FNA is of great assistance in the management of patients with this type of problem since therapeutic decisions can be made earlier and without the need for further diagnostic surgery.[26] It is usually not difficult in non-irradiated tissue to distinguish between tumour recurrence on the one hand and inflammation, suture granuloma and scarring on the other; however, this can be quite a problem if the patient has had radiotherapy. Firstly, it is difficult to locate a small recurrence in an area of post-radiation oedema and fibrosis and therefore difficult to obtain a representative specimen. Secondly, the difficulties in distinguishing between radiation-induced cellular atypia and tumour recurrence are well known. Lymph node metastasis is easily distinguished from reactive lymphadenitis but a small metastatic deposit in an otherwise reactive node can be missed by the needle.

The most common primary tumour is a squamous cell carcinoma of the lip, tongue, oral cavity, larynx, etc. Adenoma, adenocarcinoma, lymphoma and sarcoma are also encountered in many different sites. Primary tumours involving the mucous membranes of the upper digestive and upper respiratory tracts are usually diagnosed by conventional surgical or endoscopic biopsy, sometimes preceded by a preliminary cytological diagnosis on scrape smears. FNA is mainly used for lesions which do not involve a mucous membrane. The majority of head and neck lesions are superficial and are easily accessible to needle biopsy. They may be located in the skin or subcutis of the scalp, eyelids, pinna of ear or nose, or in the salivary glands, lymph nodes, soft tissues or bone (for the latter two sites see Chapter 11). Lesions in the oral cavity, floor of mouth, tongue, palate, tonsils, posterior pharyngeal wall and orbit can also be needled directly under visual control.[22,32,33,36,39a] Branchial and thyroglossal cysts are eminently suitable to needling.[11] Carotid body and glomus jugulare tumours should not be needled as this can cause serious complications due to their vascularity.[9] Radiological investigation is preferable; however, as the correct diagnosis is not always suspected clinically and as paragangliomas occur in many other sites, one should be familiar with the cytological patterns of these tumours.

In deep lesions, needle biopsy is much facilitated if preceded by a CT scan which demonstrates the location, the extent and the anatomical relationships of the process. It is not often necessary to perform the biopsy with simultaneous CT guidance. A pituitary tumour can be needled through the nose guided by plain X-rays.[26] Intraocular tumours such as retinoblastoma and melanoma can be confirmed by FNA.[5,6]

Accuracy of diagnosis[15,16,26,31,34,37,39]

The diagnostic accuracy of FNA biopsy of tumours of the head and neck varies depending on the clinical situation; for example, it is higher for tumour recurrence in non-irradiated than in irradiated tissues. Patients who have received radiotherapy for cancer are closely followed and are frequently reviewed. The consequences of a false negative cytological report are, therefore, not too serious because the biopsy can easily be repeated if any abnormality persists or progresses; however there is some risk of false positive cytological diagnosis after radiotherapy. A positive diagnosis should not be made unless aspirates are entirely satisfactory both quantitatively and qualitatively and unless all criteria of malignancy are clearly present.

In primary diagnosis, diagnostic accuracy depends on the size and the site of the lesion, the tissue of origin and on the nature of the process. Meaningful figures based on large series of cases are not available for, for example, tonsillar, pharyngeal and paraganglionic tumours. The result is often non-diagnostic or imprecise, giving only a broad categorisation of the disease process or a short list of different diagnoses. This is still useful information as a guide to further investigations. Branchial cysts are, as a rule, easily diagnosed by FNA but metastasis of well differentiated squamous cell carcinoma undergoing liquefactive necrosis can occasionally present a difficult differential diagnostic problem.[11] The diagnostic accuracy of FNA of salivary gland tumours will be discussed in the following section.

HEAD AND NECK; SALIVARY GLANDS

4

Technical considerations

The biopsy technique is the same as for any superficial lesion. A 25 gauge needle without aspiration is recommended. It has the advantage of being minimally traumatic in this sensitive area and of lessening admixture with blood. In addition, it gives the operator a better fingertip sensitivity of the consistency of the tissues. The cell yield is perhaps less than with larger needles but the difference is not significant. To biopsy a target in the oral cavity or pharynx, the operating length given by a standard 23 gauge or a 90 mm 22 gauge needle on a 10 ml syringe mounted in a pistol grip is helpful. The use of a spray surface anaesthetic is recommended for intraoral and pharyngeal biopsies. When intraorbital or other deep masses are to be sampled a CT scan or ultrasonographic guidance helps to select the best approach and to decide the depth of the biopsy.[22,36] If possible, both air-dried and alcohol-fixed smears and a few spares for special stains, particularly immune markers, should be prepared. If there is any suspicion that the process may be of an inflammatory/infectious nature material should be obtained for microbiological investigation. Cell blocks can be useful in selected cases, or tissue fragments obtained with a 22 gauge core needle, but this inevitably renders the procedure more complicated and we do not feel that the routine preparation of cell blocks is justified.

SALIVARY GLANDS

Traditionally, salivary glands have not been subject to incisional or needle biopsy techniques because of the possible risks of fistula and, in the case of neoplasms, of tumor implantation. The tendency for benign neoplasms like pleomorphic adenomas, to recur after excision has added to this fear; however, there is no evidence that either of these complications occurs with FNA. Along with many other locations in the head and neck the glands are eminently accessible and material is usually obtained easily.

The place of FNA in the investigative sequence

In recent years a number of authors have advocated the use of FNAC as a substitute for frozen section diagnosis. We have observed an increasing acceptance of cytological diagnosis by ENT surgeons and a fall in the number of frozen sections from salivary gland tumours in which an unequivocal diagnosis was given by FNA. However, in experienced hands, tumour typing by frozen section is more accurate than by FNA cytology.[45] We therefore recommend histological examination (frozen section or paraffin) if there is doubt regarding the type or the malignant potential of a tumour and if important clinical decisions depend on exact typing.

FNA of salivary gland lesions is of clinical value for the following reasons:

1. It can provide a preoperative diagnosis of a benign versus a malignant neoplasm and in many cases also of the specific tumour type.

2. If the diagnosis is of a non-neoplastic lesion, there is no need for surgical intervention. In our practise, in nearly half of the cases referred for FNA biopsy the salivary gland enlargement was caused by a non-neoplastic condition.[66]

3. If the diagnosis is of a benign neoplasm, surgery can be avoided in the elderly or other patients who are poor surgical risks.

4. In case of high-grade malignancy or of recurrent cancer, a cytological diagnosis allows the administration of palliative treatment.

Accuracy of diagnosis

The Karolinska workers have provided the best guide to the level of diagnostic accuracy.[51–56,65,78,79] Even in the earliest years of their experience they were successful in recognising over 90% of neoplasms and, in particular, over 90% of pleomorphic adenomas were correctly typed and most malignant tumours were diagnosed. In later years an even greater accuracy has been achieved. This centre has a unique experience and for most pathologists salivary gland aspirations will be relatively uncommon. Using the criteria developed by Zajicek and his co-workers the diagnosis of pleomorphic adenoma and of Warthin's tumour is relatively easy in most cases. Most adenoid cystic and acinic cell carcinomas have distinctive features and can be recognised with a relative degree of certainty. The average accuracy reported in the literature in distinguishing benign and malignant lesions in the salivary glands is 93% while the average type-specific accuracy is 75%.[66]

However, there are limitations in the FNA diagnosis of salivary gland lesions due to sampling problems, particularly of cystic neoplasms, of small lesions, or of large lesions with considerable associated inflammation and fibrosis. Most false negative diagnoses relate to cystic tumours — Warthin's tumour, mucoepidermoid carcinoma and occasionally pleomorphic adenoma — in which the sample is only cyst contents. Mucoepidermoid and other carcinomas associated with focal inflammation and mucus retention may be misdiagnosed as sialadenitis. False positive diagnosis has mainly been related to the misinterpretation of squamous metaplasia and atypia associated with sialadenitis or Warthin's tumours, or of atypia and high cellularity in pleomorphic adenoma, as evidence of malignancy. Hyaline globules in monomorphic adenoma have been mistaken for the basement membrane globules of adenoid cystic carcinoma.[62] Also, the heterogenous structure of some pleomorphic adenomas may cause difficult diagnostic problems due to the selective

HEAD AND NECK; SALIVARY GLANDS

nature of the FNA sample.[68] A diagnosis of malignancy is easy in poorly differentiated adenocarcinoma and squamous carcinoma, but the distinction between and the subtyping of poorly differentiated primary or metastatic lesions are extremely difficult.

Complications

Needling of non-neoplastic lesions is often painful but not enough to prevent successful sampling. A little local bleeding may occur and may appear in the mouth but we have not caused severe haemorrhage. Tumour dissemination or implantation in a fine-needle track have not been reported; nor has damage to adjacent structures such as the facial nerve.

Technical considerations

Biopsy without aspiration using a 25-23G needle is recommended. A blood-stained sample is common in non-neoplastic lesions and smears may be suboptimal for this reason. In this event, two-step smearing is a helpful way of concentrating cells on one part of the slide (see Ch. 2). Cystic lesions provide special problems. Fluid obtained from cystic Warthin's tumours, muco-epidermoid tumours, or non-neoplastic cysts may be very similar cytologically and it is most important to sample diagnostic material from the walls of cysts. Most cystic lesions are multilocular so that complete emptying is not possible except in the rare simple cysts.

We strongly recommend the use of both MGG- and Pap-stained material, each method accentuates different features.

HEAD AND NECK; SALIVARY GLANDS 4

CYTOLOGICAL FINDINGS

HEAD AND NECK

Non-neoplastic lesions

Branchial cyst (Fig. 4.1)[11,15,39]

Criteria for diagnosis

1. Thick, yellow, pus-like fluid.
2. Anucleate, keratinising cells.
3. Squamous epithelial cells of variable maturity.
4. A background of amorphous debris.

A branchial cyst can develop relatively rapidly as a firm mass of significant size in the neck and may cause the patient considerable anxiety. It may become clinically apparent at any age. An instant diagnosis by FNA at the patient's first visit is therefore of clinical value.

The aspiration of fluid causes the mass to decrease in size but it rarely disappears completely. The macroscopic appearance of the aspirate is very much like pus even in non-inflamed cysts and may suggest suppurating lymphadenitis; however, the fluid is usually sterile. Smears sometimes show a large number of acute inflammatory cells. A component of multinucleate giant cells, representing a granulomatous reaction at the edge of the cyst, may be seen. Lymphoid tissue, although usually evident in tissue sections, is not often represented in smears.

Problems in diagnosis

1. Well differentiated squamous cell carcinoma.
2. Thyroglossal cyst.

A lymph node metastasis of highly differentiated squamous cell carcinoma undergoing liquefactive necrosis is an important and occasionally difficult differential diagnosis (Fig. 4.2). A careful search of the smears usually reveals some squamous epithelial cells with clearly malignant features such as nuclear hyperchromasia and chromatin clumping, or keratinised cells with bizarre shapes (see Fig. 4.5). Conversely, atypical cells in smears from an inflamed branchial cyst can occasionally cause concern.[38]

The aspirate from a thyroglossal cyst can be cytologically indistinguishable from that of a branchial cyst. The differential diagnosis is mainly based on the anatomical site of the lesion. Some thyroglossal cysts have a mucinous content and mucin-secreting columnar epithelial cells are found in the smears. Thyroid epithelial cells are rarely found (see p. 104).

Amyloid tumour (Fig. 4.3)

Criteria for diagnosis

1. Clumps of amorphous acellular material.
2. Apple-green birefringence with Congo red stain.

Solitary deposits of amyloid, so-called amyloid tumours, are occasionally found submucosally in the

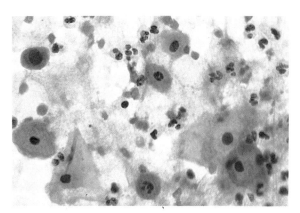

Fig. 4.1 Branchial cyst
Neutrophils, debris and mature squamous cells including degenerate forms (Pap, HP)

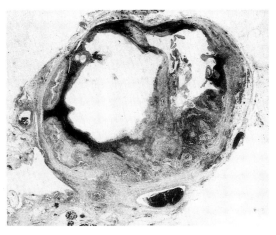

Fig. 4.2 Cystic metastasis of squamous carcinoma
Whole section of cervical lymph node containing cystically degenerated metastatic deposit of squamous carcinoma. Note similarity to branchial cyst (H & E)

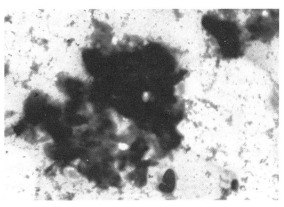

Fig. 4.3 Amyloid tumour
Clumps of amorphous acellular purple material (MGG, HP)

HEAD AND NECK; SALIVARY GLANDS

hypopharynx, the larynx and other parts of the upper respiratory tract. Amyloid has a fairly characteristic appearance in Giemsa-stained smears. It stains from pink to purple with a variable density; a finely fibrillar structure is discernible under high power. Its nature should be confirmed by special stains. Benign epithelial and/or mesenchymal cells from surrounding tissues may be included with the amyloid.

Others

The cytological diagnosis of *lymphadenitis* is discussed in Chapter 5. Special attention has been given to the diagnosis of *sarcoid* and of *tuberculous lymphadenitis* in the head and neck region.[13,14,24,25] We have seen examples of *actinomycosis* of the parotid region and of the pharynx which were clinically suspected of being neoplastic due to the induration of the tissues. Sulphur granules were not seen macroscopically, but microscopically a few small clumps of finely filamentous microorganisms surrounded by polymorphs suggested the correct diagnosis which was subsequently confirmed by culture of the aspirate (Fig. 4.4). *Pseudolymphoma* may occur, for example, as an orbital mass.[28] The differential diagnosis from malignant lymphoma is discussed in Chapter 5.

Myeloid metaplasia can give rise to an orbital mass in a patient with myelofibrosis. Erythroblasts, megakaryo-

cytes, and granulocytic precursors are found in the aspirate (see Fig. 9.76). *Mucocele* of the paranasal sinuses may sometimes be referred for FNA to exclude neoplasia or infection. The aspirated mucinous material may contain a small number of mucinophages and occasional columnar epithelial cells (goblet cells).

Neoplasms

Squamous cell carcinoma (Figs 4.2 and 4.5)

Squamous cell carcinoma is the commonest type of primary carcinoma of the head and neck. The criteria for diagnosis are listed in Chapter 8. One point of interest is the tendency for lymph node metastases of well differentiated squamous carcinoma to undergo liquefactive degeneration (Fig. 4.2). The aspirate may resemble pus. It is more often clear and yellow like fluid from a non-neoplastic cyst but with a characteristic mucoid, viscous consistency. Microscopically, intact tumour cells may be difficult to find; however, the appearances of the degenerate cells usually allow a very high order of suspicion of malignancy. Extremely dense, rounded, keratinised anucleate cells showing a varied staining reaction with Pap, together with irregular cell shapes are virtually diagnostic of malignancy (Fig. 4.5). A thorough search of the smears usually reveals occasional cells with cytologically malignant nuclear features (Fig. 4.5 inset).

Nasopharyngeal carcinoma (NPC)
(Figs 4.6 and 4.7)[3,4]

Criteria for diagnosis (undifferentiated)

1. Undifferentiated malignant cells, single and in compact aggregates.
2. Scanty but well defined eosinophilic cytoplasm.
3. Large vesicular nuclei with large central nucleoli.
4. Background of normal lymphoid cells.

Nasopharyngeal carcinoma usually presents to the cytologist as a lymph node metastasis in the neck without a known primary. It is important to recognise this cytological pattern since the primary is often clinically occult and difficult to detect.

A proportion of NPCs show squamous differentiation, usually without obvious keratinisation and with a basaloid pattern of relatively small cells, while the majority are undifferentiated. The dense clusters of malignant cells from an undifferentiated NPC resemble those of basal cell carcinoma and are characteristically mixed with lymphoid cells (Fig. 4.7). If the malignant cells are more dispersed, the differential diagnosis of Hodgkin's disease or large cell non-Hodgkin's lymphoma may pose a problem. In NPC, malignant cells form distinct aggregates and have a better defined, eosinophilic cytoplasm. In addition, the neoplastic cells contrast with the normal lymphoid cells in the background (Fig. 4.6). Immunocytochemical staining for keratin and with

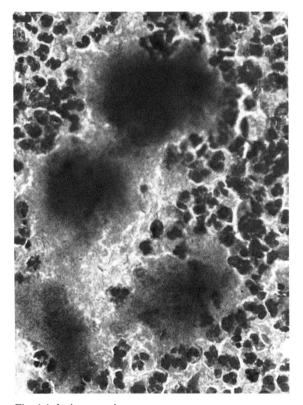

Fig. 4.4 Actinomycosis
Clumps of finely fibrillar organisms in a background of neutrophils (MGG, HP)

HEAD AND NECK; SALIVARY GLANDS

4

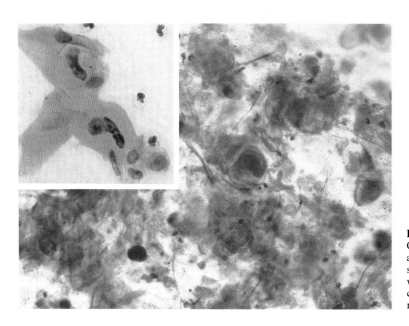

Fig. 4.5 2⁰ Well-differentiated SCC
Cystic change/necrosis; keratinised
anucleate squamous cells; irregular
shapes and staining reactions. Inset:
well-differentiated keratinising squamous
cells, some with nuclear features of
malignancy (Pap, HP).

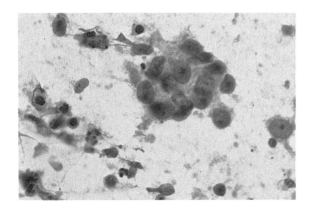

Fig. 4.6 Nasopharyngeal carcinoma
Cluster of undifferentiated epithelial cells, and a background of
lymphocytes. Note the eosinophilic cytoplasm and prominent
nucleoli in the tumour cells (H & E, HP).

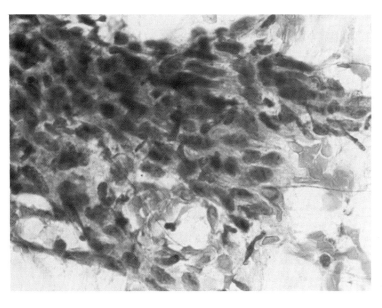

Fig. 4.7 Nasopharyngeal carcinoma
Cohesive cluster of small, poorly
differentiated, somewhat spindly
epithelial cells resembling basal cell
carcinoma; few scattered lymphocytes
(Pap, HP)

4 *HEAD AND NECK; SALIVARY GLANDS*

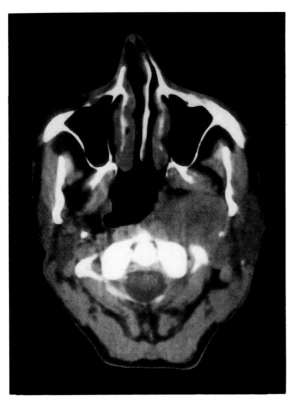

Fig. 4.8 Paraganglioma
CT scan showing large solid mass in left oropharynx; paraganglioma diagnosed by FNA

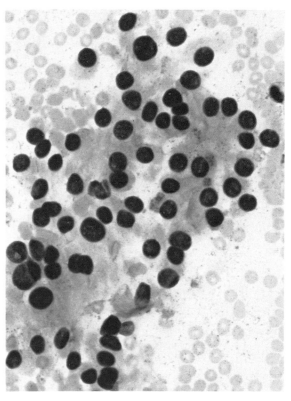

Fig. 4.9 Paraganglioma
Loose follicular arrangements of cells resembling thyroid epithelium. The very fine eosinophilic granules are visible only under the microscope and do not photograph well; the coarse blue granules are considered to be an artefact (MGG, HP)

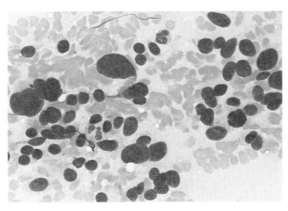

Fig. 4.10 Paraganglioma (atypical)
Striking nuclear pleomorphism but a uniformly bland chromatin pattern (MGG, HP)

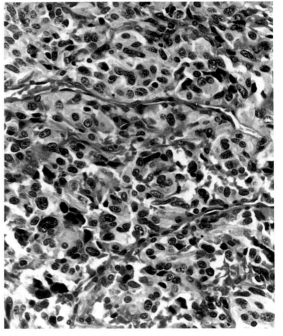

Fig. 4.11 Paraganglioma (atypical)
Tissue section of the case shown in Figure 4.7 (H & E, IP)

HEAD AND NECK; SALIVARY GLANDS

a panleucocyte marker is helpful in difficult cases. Epstein-Barr virus-associated nuclear antigen is demonstrable in undifferentiated tumours.[3] Other patterns of growth may occur and may cause diagnostic problems; for example, spindle cell forms may be difficult to identify as carcinoma.

If smears from a metastatic lymph node in the neck show larger malignant squamous cells with keratinisation, the primary is more likely to be found in the lung than in the nasopharynx.

Adenocarcinoma

Adenocarcinomas of the nasopharynx, nasal cavity and paranasal sinuses show no distinctive cytological features which allow their site of origin to be ascertained. Tumours arising from minor salivary glands of the upper respiratory and gastrointestinal tracts are described in the following section of this chapter.

Paraganglioma (carotid body and glomus jugulare tumours) (Figs 4.8–4.11)[7,9,17–19,21,29]

Criteria for diagnosis

1. Neoplastic cells single, in clusters, and in a loosely follicular arrangement.
2. Abundant but poorly defined, pale cytoplasm with fine red granularity (MGG).
3. Nuclei round to spindle with finely granular evenly distributed nuclear chromatin; moderate anisokaryosis.
4. Samples heavily admixed with fresh blood.

The cytological pattern is reminiscent of thyroid tissue and the main differential diagnosis is a thyroid neoplasm (Fig. 4.9). The follicular arrangement of the

tumour cells may suggest a follicular carcinoma, the fine red cytoplasmic granulation and the tendency for the cells to be spindle shaped, a medullary carcinoma. Furthermore, intranuclear vacuoles (cytoplasmic inclusions), common in papillary and sometimes found also in medullary carcinoma of the thyroid, may be seen in some paragangliomas.[19,23] In most cases, the anatomical site separate from the thyroid, in combination with the cytological pattern, allows a confident diagnosis. However, paragangliomas may occur in atypical locations. In one of our cases, the diagnosis was made on an aspirate from a mass in the tonsillar region thought clinically to be a deep parotid tumour (Fig. 4.8), in another case from a supraclavicular mass diagnosed clinically as lymphadenopathy. The FNAC diagnosis was later confirmed histologically in both cases. More prominent anisokaryosis and spindle cell patterns can cause diagnostic difficulties and occasionally nuclear pleomorphism may be severe enough to suggest malignancy (Figs 4.10 and 4.11).[9] However, mitotic rate and evidence of necrosis appear to be better related to clinical behaviour.[18] As these tumours are extremely vascular, the aspirate may consist predominantly of blood and tumour cells may be difficult to find.

Malignant lymphoma

Malignant lymphoma of Waldeyer's ring and of cervical lymph nodes have similar characteristics to lymphomas elsewhere (see Ch. 5). Differential diagnosis between malignant lymphoma of the orbit and pseudolymphoma may be particularly difficult.[28] A mixed population predominantly of small lymphocytes, together with a number of large transformed lymphoid cells, plasma cells and phagocytic histiocytes favours pseudolymphoma. The use of immunohistochemical techniques is of

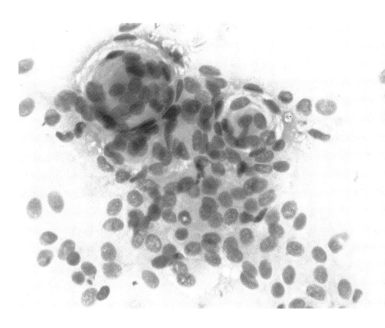

Fig. 4.12 Meningioma
Tight whorls of ovoid or spindle cells with a bland chromatin pattern (H & E, HP)

4 HEAD AND NECK; SALIVARY GLANDS

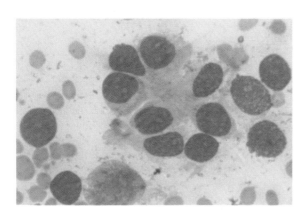

Fig. 4.13 Olfactory neuroblastoma
'Acinar' group of neoplastic cells with indistinct cytoplasm resembling adenocarcinoma (MGG, HP) (courtesy Dr A Kurniawan, University of Indonesia)

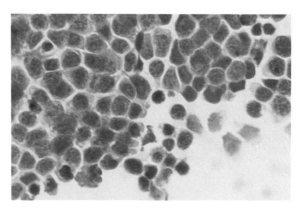

Fig. 4.14 Retinoblastoma
Cytological pattern of a malignant small round cell tumour without distinctive features (Pap, HP)

value in this situation. Demonstration of a monoclonal immunoglobulin product would confirm malignant lymphoma; a polyclonal pattern would help confirm pseudolymphoma, but does not exclude lymphoma.

Meningioma (Fig. 4.12)[35]

Criteria for diagnosis

1. Many fibroblast-like spindle cells in loose clusters, bundles and whorls.
2. Some small, tight whorls; occasional psammoma bodies.
3. Pale cytoplasm, indistinct cell borders.
4. Pale nuclei with finely granular, evenly distributed chromatin.

Extracranial meningiomas may occur in relation to the base of the skull, the scalp, the orbit, the nasal cavity, the paranasal sinuses and the middle ear. The exact anatomical site and the presence of characteristic whorls should allow differentiation from other mesenchymal tumours.

Olfactory neuroblastoma (Fig. 4.13)[12,20]
This rare tumour occurs in the upper nasal cavity and may cause nasal obstruction. Single cases diagnosed by FNA have been reported. The pseudorosettes formed by the tumour cells may be mistaken for the microacini of adenocarcinoma but the nuclear morphology is relatively bland.

Intra-ocular tumours (Fig. 4.14)[1,2]
Cells from a *retinoblastoma* may be found in fluid aspirated from the anterior chamber of the eye. The pattern is similar to other malignant, small, round cell tumours of undifferentiated cells.[5] In the only case we have seen, rosettes were not obvious (Fig. 4.14). *Malignant lymphoma* may rarely involve the uveal tract and can be diagnosed by cytological examination of fluid aspirated

from the vitreous.[27] FNA, performed in theatre, offers a means of distinguishing — in the exceptional case when this is a problem for clinical diagnosis and management — between a primary (*melanoma*) and a metastatic intraocular malignancy. The cells from uveal melanoma are often relatively bland, monomorphous spindle cells. Immunocytochemical staining provides a means of confirmation if melanin is not visible.[6]

Tumours of soft tissues and bone (see Ch. 11)
Rhabdomyosarcoma, usually of the embryonal type, is among the most common malignant head and neck tumours in children (see Fig. 11.34). Soft tissue tumours in general, such as *spindle cell lipoma, nerve sheath tumours and malignant fibrous histiocytoma* are not uncommon and may occur in sites where they are prone to be clinically mistaken for lymphadenopathy, salivary gland tumour etc. *Chordoma* may present as an orbital, nasal or posterior pharyngeal mass (p. 329). Of bone tumours affecting the skull, *eosinophilic granuloma* (p. 325), *multiple myeloma* (p. 324) and *metastatic carcinoma* led themselves to cytological diagnosis.

Metastatic tumours[10,30]
Metastatic tumours are of course common in this region. Guidelines for the indentification of the primary tumour are given on page 77.

SALIVARY GLANDS

Normal structures (Fig. 4.15)

1. Acinar cells (serous or mucinous).
2. Ductal epithelial cells.

Aspiration of normal or near normal glands usually yields scanty material, but occasionally a surprisingly large number of acinar cells are obtained which may raise a suspicion of neoplasia (acinic cell tumour). A

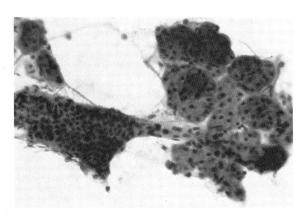

Fig. 4.15 Salivary acinar and ductal cells
Cohesive acinar and ductal cells in an arrangement similar to
that seen in histological sections (H & E, IP)

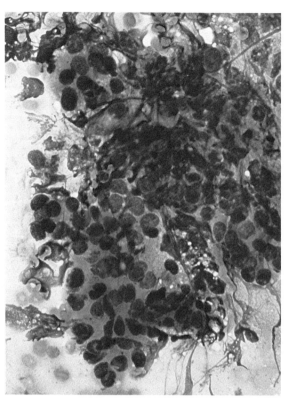

Fig. 4.16 Retention cyst
Debris and ductal epithelium showing degenerative and
regenerative atypia (MGG, HP)

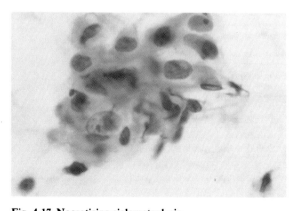

Fig. 4.17 Necrotising sialometaplasia
Cells resembling metaplastic squamous epithelial cells showing
mild atypia (Pap, HP)

heavy admixture with blood is frequent. Acinar cells
present as well-preserved acini and cohesive lobules,
sometimes with attached stromal and ductal tissue. Serous acinar cells have abundant, rather bubbly cytoplasm
and a small, central or slightly eccentric, rounded, dark
nucleus with a small nucleolus. Bare acinar cell nuclei
are commonly seen in the background of the smear and
should not be mistaken for lymphocytes. Ductal cells
are less plentiful and occur as small cohesive flat sheets
or tubules. These cells have denser, sometimes squamoid cytoplasm and may have oval nuclei. Other
findings include adipose and loose fibrous tissue. Lymphoid cells may sometimes be sampled from adjacent or
intraglandular lymph nodes.

Non-neoplastic lesions

Cysts[48]
We have seen several 'simple' parotid cysts; in one, a
completely cystic Warthin's tumour, the aspirated fluid
contained only cholesterol crystals and macrophages;
another contained debris and degenerate squamous cells
and was histologically designated a simple epidermoid
cyst. The findings in aspirates from *lymphoepithelial cysts*
have been described.[50] A *retention cyst* of the submandibular gland yielded abundant mucus, macrophages
and some ductal cells showing a moderate degree of
atypia (Fig. 4.16). Such atypia and sqamous metaplasia
of ductal epithelium in a cystic lesion may raise the
suspicion of mucoepidermoid tumour (see p. 56).

Sialadenitis[48]
Epithelial atypia and squamous metaplasia can be a
particularly difficult problem in cases of *necrotising
sialometaplasia* (Fig. 4.17). In a case of presumed *infective sialadenitis*, profuse purulent material was obtained
from a tender, swollen gland. There was a mixed cell
population of neutrophils, foamy cells and clumps of

endothelial cells. The lesion resolved after antibiotic
treatment. In cases clinically diagnosed as *chronic
sialadenitis* biopsy often yields only normal salivary
gland acini. In some cases, the diagnosis is supported by
a predominance of ductal cells and by the presence of
inflammatory cells and of fragments of fibrous tissue.
The bare nuclei of acinar epithelial cells commonly present in smears of salivary glands should not be mistaken

4 HEAD AND NECK; SALIVARY GLANDS

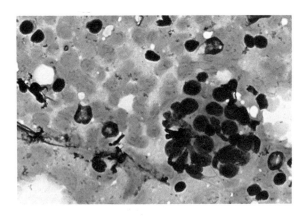

Fig. 4.18 Benign lymphoepithelial lesion
Lymphoid cells and an aggregate of mildly atypical ductal cells. Acinar cells absent (MGG, HP)

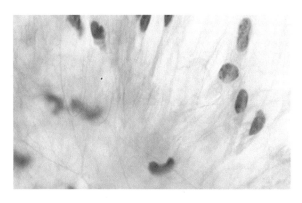

Fig. 4.19 Pleomorphic adenoma
Myxoid stromal tissue with a fine fibrillar structure and some spindle cells (Pap, HP)

for lymphocytes. In *sarcoidosis* affecting the parotid gland, epithelioid cells forming granulomatous clusters are prominent and multinucleated giant cells may be found. There is no evidence of necrosis and associated acute or chronic inflammatory cells are not present (see Fig. 5.17). Smears from a *'benign lymphoepithelial lesion'* were characterised by a pattern of monotonous, small lymphoid cells. Distinction from low grade lymphoma was not possible and, in fact, there was a circulating paraprotein, providing some evidence that transition to a low-grade lymphoma may have occurred. In another benign lymphoepithelial lesion, small clusters of ductal cells were seen with a background of lymphoid cells (Fig. 4.18).

Neoplasms

Pleomorphic adenoma (Figs 4.19–4.26)[54]

Criteria for diagnosis

1. Fibrillary chondromyxoid ground substance.
2. Epithelial cells single and in loose sheets.
3. Small ovoid nuclei with bland nuclear chromatin, well defined, dense cytoplasm.
4. Spindle shaped 'mesenchymal' cells seen mainly in stromal matrix.

With Pap staining the ground substance is grey/green to orange in colour and has a finely fibrillar structure (Fig. 4.19); with MGG staining it is intensely red to purple (Fig. 4.20). Spindle cells or rounded cells, either single or forming small clusters, are present within this myxoid stroma or lying free. Cells within tissue fragments may be difficult to visualise in MGG because of poor stain penetration through the connective tissue matrix; the matrix itself may be so intensely stained that it obscures the cellular content. For this reason, alcohol-fixed and air-dried smears should be done in parallel with all salivary gland aspirates. The epithelial cells are

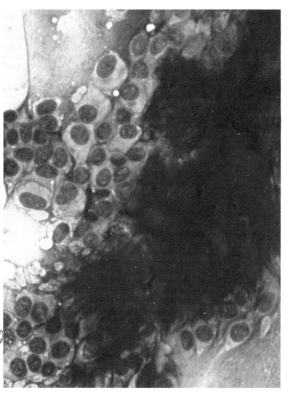

Fig. 4.20 Pleomorphic adenoma
Mixture of epithelial cells and myxoid stroma. Note the well-defined cytoplasm in the epithelial cells (MGG, HP).

relatively small, of uniform size and have round or oval, eccentric nuclei, a bland, granular chromatin, inconspicuous nucleoli and moderate amounts of densely staining cytoplasm with well-defined cell borders. They sometimes have a plasma-cell-like appearance (Fig. 4.21), and lie in moderately cohesive sheets as well as single.[72] Red-staining intercellular material (MGG) may be seen in some sheets. Tyrosine crystals have been noted in smears of pleomorphic adenoma.[43]

HEAD AND NECK; SALIVARY GLANDS

4

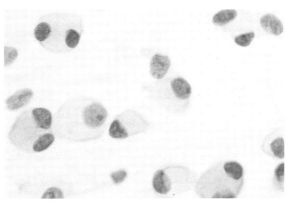

Fig. 4.21 Pleomorphic adenoma
Plasma cell like (hyaline-cell) pattern (Pap, HP) *Occur more often in tumours of minor of major saliv. gl.*

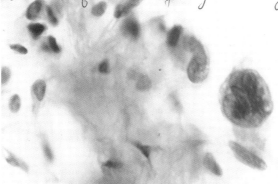

Fig. 4.23 Pleomorphic adenoma
Several pleomorphic bizarre epithelial cells among fragments of myxoid stroma; histology showed no evidence of malignancy (H & E, HP)

Cells melting away or c̄ a transition into chondromyxoid stroma.

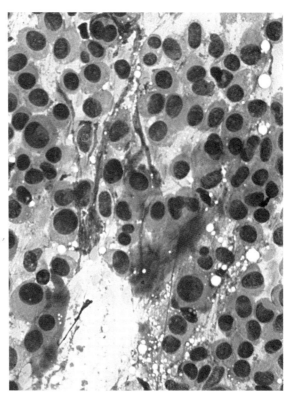

Fig. 4.22 Pleomorphic adenoma
Epithelial cell predominance; the degree of nuclear pleomorphism here should not suggest malignancy MGG, HP)

*Pitfalls
- Cystic
- DD from ACC
- Cellularity
- Atypia → may False +ve of CA
- Sq. metaplasia*

Problems in diagnosis

The cytological diagnosis of pleomorphic adenoma is obvious in typical cases. The focally striking variations in the histological pattern which is so characteristic of this tumour is rarely a problem in surgical pathology when the whole tumour can be examined, but can sometimes cause great difficulties in FNA cytology due to the limited sampling by needle biopsy. Thus, one particular feature may dominate the smears to the extent that the true nature of the tumour is not recognised. We have found the following problems to be the most important in the differential diagnosis:

1. Predominance of myxoid tissue in a particular tumour may result in only mucus-like material being sampled; confusion with epithelial mucus may occur if only Pap staining is used. Occasionally, the aspiration of mucoid fluid may suggest a cystic lesion and one may have to search carefully to find diagnostic tissue fragments.

2. Predominance of epithelial elements may lead to a diagnosis of monomorphic or basal cell adenoma.

3. The distinction of pleomorphic adenoma from well differentiated adenoid cystic carcinoma is not always easy. Myxoid stroma may be found in both and hyaline globules which appear identical to the globules of basement membrane material characteristic of adenoid cystic carcinoma can sometimes be seen in pleomorphic adenoma. One must look carefully at the epithelial cells; a well defined cytoplasm and a bland granular nuclear chromatin favours pleomorphic adenoma, scanty cytoplasm and nuclear hyperchromasia and coarseness favours adenoid cystic carcinoma. Sampling from several areas of the tumour will reduce the likelihood of error.

ACC - sharp borders betz cells ∧ stroma

4. Epithelial atypia in an otherwise typical mixed tumour (Figs 4.22 and 4.23) should not generally be interpreted as indicating malignancy. Enlarged, irregular, even bizarre nuclei are occasionally found in smears of histologically benign tumours. Unless clearly malignant cells are present in substantial numbers, epithelial atypia should be reported with caution and the assessment of malignancy should be deferred to histological examination. Malignant change in a pleomorphic adeno-

4 *HEAD AND NECK; SALIVARY GLANDS*

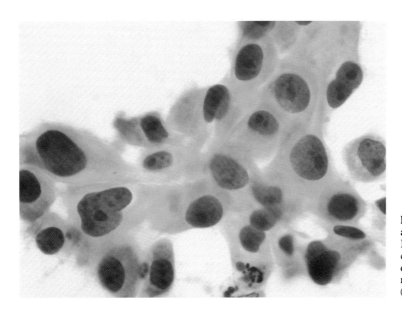

Fig. 4.24 Carcinoma in pleomorphic adenoma
Large, poorly-differentiated malignant cells. Histology showed poorly-differentiated carcinoma and small foci of residual typical pleomorphic adenoma (Pap, HP)

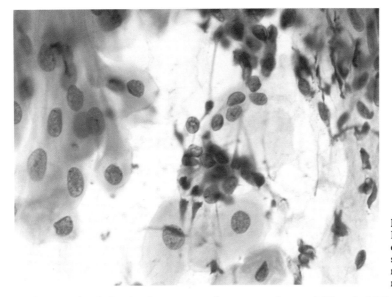

Fig. 4.25 Pleomorphic adenoma
Prominent component of squamous epithelial cells (left and centre); some small epithelial cells and fragments of myxoid stroma (upper right) reveal the nature of the lesion (Pap, HP)

ma is exceptional. In the few cases we have seen, the cytological findings were of a poorly-differentiated, large-cell carcinoma (Fig. 4.24). A specific diagnosis can only be made if poorly-differentiated malignant cells are present together with the usual components of pleomorphic adenoma.[78]

5. Mucin-secreting goblet cells are sometimes present in pleomorphic adenoma and may cause confusion with muco-epidermoid tumour, particularly if co-existing with squamous metaplasia. Sebaceous differentiation can also occur.

6. Squamous differentiation is not uncommon and can be a prominent feature. This is not a problem in histology but can be a difficult one in FNA cytology if the sample is mainly derived from such an area (Figs 4.25 and 4.26). The metaplastic squamous cells may appear atypical and may suggest a diagnosis of muco-epidermoid tumour.

7. We have encountered a few cases of nodular swellings in the submandibular gland which on histological examination were areas of acinar cell atrophy and ductal and ductular hyperplasia, mild atypia and a myxoid stromal background with a mild chronic inflammatory cell infiltration (Figs 4.27 and 4.28). These pseudotumours are of uncertain origin but may result from local obstruction. They closely mimic neoplasia clinically, and in smears the mixture of atypical ductal epithelium and myxoid stromal tissue may simulate pleomorphic adenoma. The presence of chronic inflammatory cells should induce caution in making this diagnosis.[41]

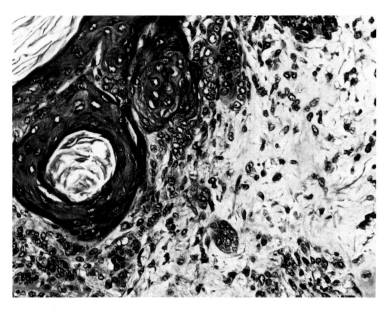

Fig. 4.26 Pleomorphic adenoma
Tissue section, same case as Figure 4.26.
Prominent squamous differentiation
(H & E, IP)

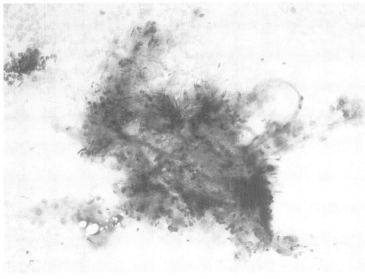

**Fig. 4.27 'Pseudotumour'
submandibular gland**
Myxoid stromal tissue containing darker
groups of ductal cells. One separate
aggregate of ductal cells (MGG IP).

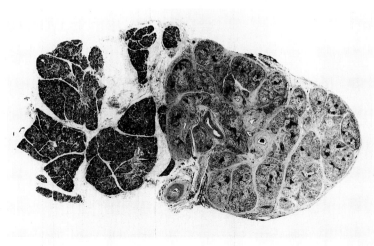

**Fig. 4.28 'Pseudotumour'
submandibular gland**
Tissue section, same case as Figure 4.27
(H & E, IP)

4 HEAD AND NECK; SALIVARY GLANDS

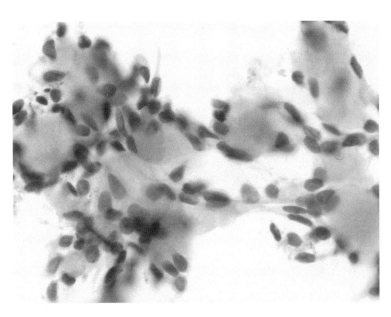

Fig. 4.29 Monomorphic adenoma trabecular variant
Many small hyaline globules of uniform size surrounded by small bland epithelial cells (Pap, HP)

The hallmark of pleomorphic adenoma is the combination of bland epithelial cells and fragments of fibromyxoid or chondromyxoid stroma with spindle cells (Fig. 4.19). In the presence of any such stromal fragments, pleomorphic adenoma should always be included in the differential diagnosis even if other features such as those mentioned above dominate the smears.[68] In difficult cases, immunoperoxidase staining for intermediate filaments may be helpful.[47]

Monomorphic adenoma (Figs 4.29–4.33)[51,59,62,68]

Criteria for diagnosis

1. Numerous cell clusters with few dissociated cells.
2. Regular round or oval nuclei and sparse cytoplasm.
3. Bland, granular nuclear chromatin.
4. Small amounts of homogenous stromal tissue.

Several distinctive subtypes of monomorphic adenoma have been described cytologically. Diagnosis of these uncommon lesions is difficult and a distinction from pleomorphic adenoma with epithelial cell predominance on the one hand and adenoid cystic carcinoma on the other may be a problem.[59] In particular, the trabecular variant of monomorphic adenoma can imitate adenoid cystic carcinoma closely; smears may show numerous hyaline globules and finger-like stromal structures similar to those of adenoid cystic carcinoma (Fig. 4.29).[62,68] However, the globules of monomorphic adenoma tend to be smaller, of more uniform size and of less hyaline appearance (Fig. 4.30). Close attention should also be paid to the appearance of the epithelial nuclei. These are bland with a finely granular chromatin and no or inconspicuous nucleoli in monomorphic adenoma, hyperchromatic and coarse in adenoid cystic carcinoma. The nuclear morphology is particularly important in the dis-

tinction of basal cell adenoma from poorly differentiated 'basaloid' adenoid cystic carcinoma with no hyaline globules. The stromal tissue in basal cell adenomas is generally homogenous and pale with the Pap stain and bright red in MGG staining. The fibrillar appearance seen in pleomorphic adenoma is not present.

We have seen two cases of the solid variant of monomorphic adenoma resembling cylindroma and called *membranous adenoma* or *dermal analogue tumour*. We believe the cytological diagnosis to be possible based on some distinctive features. Smears from both cases showed large cohesive masses of small basaloid neoplastic cells with a rim of basement membrane material which stained variably with Papanicolaou and MGG (Fig. 4.32). It was not particularly metachromatic with MGG in one case but was in the other. This pattern is unlike that seen in adenoid cystic carcinoma and in pleomorphic adenoma.

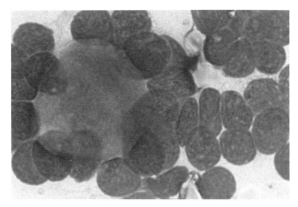

Fig. 4.30 Monomorphic adenoma trabecular variant
Small hyaline globules, small epithelial cells with bland granular chromatin (MGG, HP) (Courtesy Dr K. Lindholm, Malmö General Hospital)

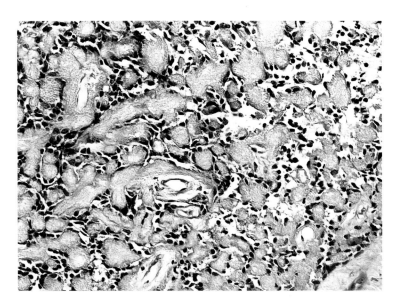

**Fig. 4.31 Monomorphic adenoma
trabecular variant**
Tissue section, same case as Figure 4.29
(H & E, IP)

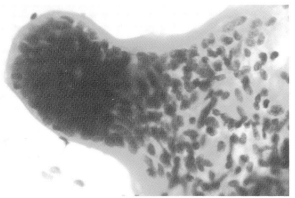

**Fig. 4.32 Monomorphic adenoma, dermal analogue type
(membranous adenoma)**
Cohesive sheets of small, uniform epithelial cells bordered by a
rim of hyaline basement membrane material (Pap, IP)

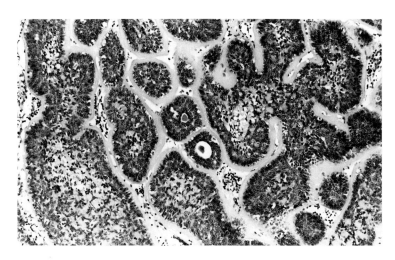

**Fig. 4.33 Monomorphic adenoma,
dermal analogue type (membranous
adenoma)**
Tissue section, same case as Figure 4.32,
jig-saw puzzle growth pattern: islands of
basaloid cells surrounded by eosinophilic
hyaline lamina, small eosinophilic
intercellular globules of hyaline material,
(H & E, IP)

4 HEAD AND NECK; SALIVARY GLANDS

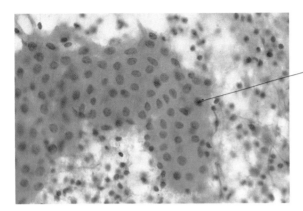

honeycomb.
Tightly packed large polyhedral
oncocytic cells c̄ abundant,
well demarcated granular cyto.

Fig. 4.34 Warthin's tumour
Monolayered sheet of uniform epithelial cells of oncocytic type;
background of lymphocytes and debris (Pap, HP).

Sheets have
irregular outlines.

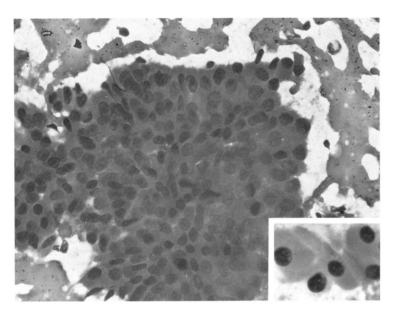

Fig. 4.35 Warthin's tumour
Monolayered sheet of oncocytes; note the
peripheral palisading (MGG, HP). Inset:
squamoid oncocytes with dense blue
cytoplasm (MGG, HP).

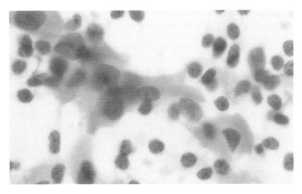

Fig. 4.36 Warthin's tumour
Note squamous metaplasia and mild epithelial atypia
(H & E, HP)

HEAD AND NECK; SALIVARY GLANDS 4

Warthin's tumour (Figs 4.34–4.36)[53]

Criteria for diagnosis

1. Aspirate of mucoid, murky fluid.
2. Background of amorphous and granular debris.
3. Oncocytic cells in cohesive, monolayered sheets.
4. Many lymphoid cells. *Honey comb arrangent*

The amorphous and granular debris representing cyst contents has a mucoid appearance and stains blue with MGG. The oncocytes present in flat, monolayered sheets with an irregular outline. These cells have plentiful cytoplasm and regular, small, round, central nuclei with a uniformly bland chromatin and inconspicuous nucleoli. With Pap staining their cytoplasm is dense and orangeophilic and may be granulated (Fig. 4.34); with MGG it is dense grey-blue and is more homogenous, though some granularity may be noted (Fig. 4.35). The cells are similar to oncocytes in other sites, for example Askanazy cells in the thyroid gland, although in Warthin's tumours the nuclei are uniformly small and bland. In MGG preparations, oncocytes may occasionally be confused with other types of cells, for example cells of acinic cell carcinoma. They are more easily identified in Pap preparations (see below).

Problems in diagnosis

1. Obtaining representative material may be difficult. Both oncocytic and lymphoid tissue may be sparse, absent or obscured by mucoid debris.

2. The mucoid material with flakes of homogenous and granular debris is rather characteristic but not specific, and similar material may be obtained from muco-epidermoid tumours or necrotic malignancies.

3. Degenerate oncocytic cells can resemble squamous epithelial cells and may look quite atypical. Confusion with metastatic or primary squamous cell carcinoma with central cystic liquefaction is possible. However, the glassy refractile nature of true keratinisation is absent in degenerate oncocytes. If only oncocytes are found in the smears, confusion with oncocytoma is likely, though the oncocytic cells in the latter should be in multilayered clumps rather than in flat sheets as in Warthin's tumour.

4. Distinction from muco-epidermoid tumour may be difficult, both tumours having a cystic component. If the smear pattern initially suggests Warthin's tumour but the cells show some atypia and lack a distinctly oxyphil cytoplasm, the alternative of a muco-epidermoid tumour should be considered.[64] A careful search may then reveal occasional cells with intracytoplasmic mucin vacuoles.

5. True squamous metaplasia is sometimes seen in Warthin's tumours (Fig. 4.36). The associated reactive/ inflammatory changes in the epithelium may simulate malignancy in FNA smears. This is among the most common causes of misdiagnosis of malignancy reported in the literature.

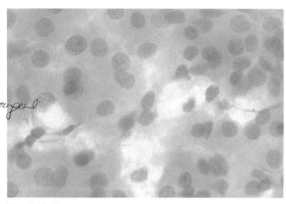

Fig. 4.37 Oncocytoma
Partly multilayered cohesive aggregate of oxyphil cells with bland nuclear morphology (Pap, HP)

Oncocytoma (Fig. 4.37)[53]

Criteria for diagnosis.

1. Cohesive, multilayered clumps of oncocytic cells with small, regular nuclei.
2. Absence of fluid, debris and lymphoid cells.

Problems in diagnosis

1. In some non-oncocytic tumours, cells with abundant cytoplasm may resemble oncocytes in MGG-stained preparations. The cells of acinic cell carcinoma, intermediate cells of muco-epidermoid tumours, and adenocarcinoma cells all have this appearance occasionally. In Pap-stained smears, acinic cell cytoplasm is pale and finely vacuolated or granular, contrasting with the dense staining of oncocytes. Acinic cell nuclei are generally larger and more variable in size than those of oncocytes; acinic cells are also more fragile and bare nuclei are more common in the background of smears from these tumours.

2. Oncocytomas may be cystic and their relationship to Warthin's tumours is then uncertain; however, in general, cyst fluid, debris and oncocytes would indicate a Warthin's tumour, especially if the oncocytes lie in flat sheets.

3. Malignant oncocytic neoplasms have been described.[53]

Acinic cell carcinoma (Figs 4.38–4.40)[52,69,76]

Criteria for diagnosis

1. Abundant cell material in a clean background.
2. Cohesive clusters of cells sometimes with central fibrovascular cores.
3. Abundant finely vacuolated or dense oncocyte-like cytoplasm.
4. Mildly pleomorphic medium-size nuclei, some nuclei bare, round, lymphocyte-like.

4 HEAD AND NECK; SALIVARY GLANDS

[handwritten margin notes: Uniform cells Monotonous Clear cyto. Eccentric nuc. Disintegrated cyto.]

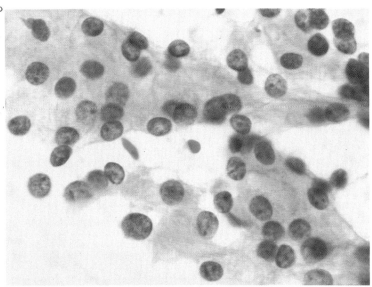

Fig. 4.38 Acinic cell carcinoma
Aggregate of fairly uniform epithelial cells with finely vacuolated cytoplasm (Pap, HP)

[handwritten note: Cyto - fine vacuolations oncocyte like or V. fragile but abundant]

Cells in smears from most acinic cell carcinomas are very well-differentiated, regular and cohesive. They may resemble normal acinar epithelial cells but acini are poorly formed, nuclei are larger and less evenly distributed and the nuclear/cytoplasmic ratio is higher. Most strikingly, the smears are far more cellular than one ever obtains from non-neoplastic salivary gland tissue. The adherence of the tumour cells to fibrovascular cores sometimes produce a papillary appearance. Although the cells always have plentiful cytoplasm, its density is variable from case to case; in MGG-stained material the cytoplasm may be either finely vacuolated, foamy or a dense gray colour resembling oncocytes (Fig. 4.39), in Pap-stained smears pale vacuolated or granular (Fig. 4.38).

Problems in diagnosis

1. The resemblance of acinic cells to oncocytes has been mentioned under oncocytoma. Infiltrates of lymphoid cells sometimes seen in acinic cell tumours may, when present in smears, contribute to confusion with Warthin's tumour.

2. Abundant cytoplasm may also be a feature of cells from muco-epidermoid tumour and adenocarcinoma. The variability in appearance in smears of muco-epidermoid tumours and the nuclear pleomorphism of adenocarcinomas should prevent error. It should be noted that intracellular mucus vacuoles are not found in acinic cell tumours. In difficult cases ultrastructural studies are helpful (Fig. 4.40).[58,76]

3. Acinic cell tumours are occasionally cystic and diagnostic epithelial cells may be difficult to find.

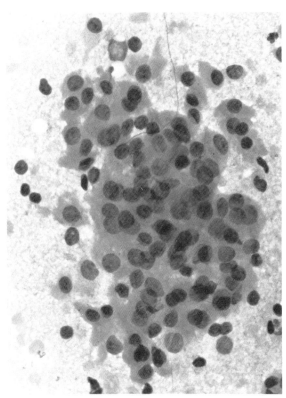

Fig. 4.39 Acinic cell carcinoma
Cells closely resembling oncocytes (MGG, HP)

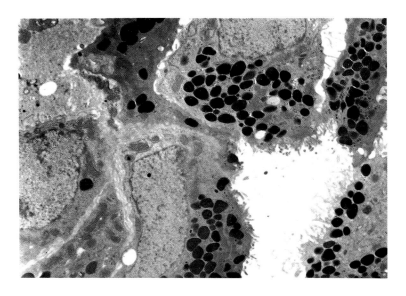

Fig. 4.40 Acinic cell carcinoma
Characteristic secretory granules in
aspirated tumour cells; same case as
Figure 4.38 (EM × 4650)

Adenoid cystic carcinoma (Figs 4.41–4.44)[40,55,74]

Criteria for diagnosis

1. Hyaline spherical globules of varying size (basement
   membrane material) surrounded by tumour cells.
2. Finger-like or rounded stromal structures between
   cell clusters.
3. Close-packed, cohesive cells with uniform round or
   oval nuclei and little cytoplasm.
4. Hyperchromatic nuclei, coarse nuclear chromatin,
   nucleoli.

The hyaline round basement membrane globules are
the most distinctive feature of this neoplasm. When
they are present in good numbers, and if the nuclear
morphology is typical, a confident diagnosis is possible.

The globules stain bright red or purple and appear very
dense with MGG (Fig. 4.41). With Pap or H & E staining they are pale, translucent and may be virtually invisible and therefore overlooked (Fig. 4.42). The finger-like
structures also represent stromal material (Fig. 4.43).
Although not diagnostic, they should raise the suspicion
of this neoplasm. The nuclei of adenoid cystic carcinoma cells are often quite uniform in size but are typically
hyperchromatic with a coarsely granular chromatin and
visible nucleoli. The malignant nuclear features are
more obvious in poorly differentiated tumours without
hyaline globules. Smears from tumours of this type
resemble basal cell carcinoma of skin; they contain
close-packed cohesive clusters or tissue fragments of
cells with hyperchromatic nuclei and a high nuclear/
cytoplasmic ratio (Fig. 4.44).

*darker
cells st
form grooves*

*- Tissue fragments c̄ a
lobulated pattern and c̄ a
c̄ spherical or 3D appearance
of small monotonous cancer cell
Central cores of hyaline material
- There may be large X layered ball
like structures of epithelial cells.
- Bg may show dispersed tumour
cells.
- Nucleoli easily seen.*

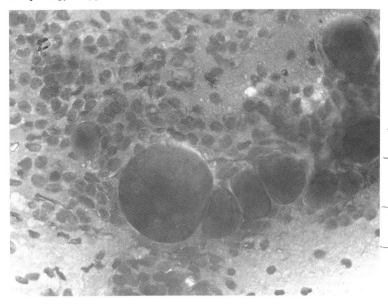

Fig. 4.41 Adenoid cystic carcinoma
Small uniform epithelial cells and
translucent hyaline globules (MGG, HP)

4 *HEAD AND NECK; SALIVARY GLANDS*

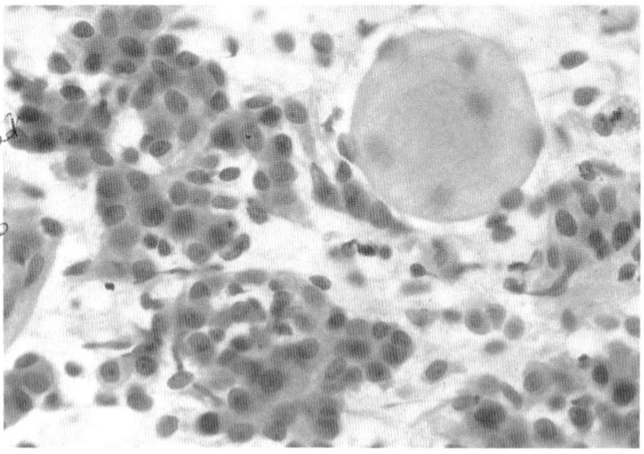

[handwritten margin notes: Monomorphic adenomas (trabecular variant); pleo. adenoma; derived usual gland tumours]

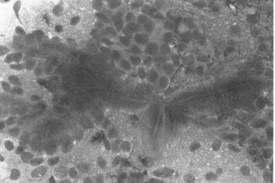

Fig. 4.42 Adenoid cystic carcinoma
Small uniform epithelial cells and a translucent hyaline globule (H & E, HP)

[handwritten margin notes: Sections here may st. show predominance of hyaline material. Cyts → shows a peculiar papillary arrangement č a tree branch effect →]

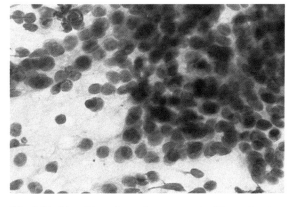

Fig. 4.43 Adenoid cystic carcinoma
Basement membrane material in finger-like structures (MGG, HP)

Fig. 4.44 Adenoid cystic carcinoma, poorly differentiated
Numerous small epithelial cells, single and in dense cluster; hyperchromatic nuclei with coarse chromatin, stromal elements absent (Pap, HP)

Problems in diagnosis

1. Distinction from monomorphic adenoma is a problem, particularly from the trabecular variant which also contains hyaline globules.[62,68] This problem has been discussed in the section on monomorphic adenoma. Very large basement membrane globules are not a feature of monomorphic adenoma and would seem to be the most reliable evidence of adenoid cystic carcinoma. The nuclear morphology must also be studied closely. The nuclei of adenoid cystic carcinoma may appear relatively bland although usually hyperchromatic in MGG-stained material. In Pap-stained smears, coarse chromatin granularity, or in some cases prominent irregular nucleoli and thickened nuclear membranes help to indicate a malignant lesion.

2. Anaplastic forms of adenoid cystic carcinoma may resemble anaplastic carcinoma from other sites; metastatic malignancy may therefore be difficult to exclude.

3. Pleomorphic adenoma may contain areas very similar to adenoid cystic carcinoma. If any fragments of myxoid mesenchymal tissue with spindle cells are found in a smear with globular bodies, the differential diagnosis of pleomorphic adenoma must be carefully considered.

4. Dermal sweat gland neoplasms may closely resemble adenoid cystic carcinoma in FNA smears.[42] We have seen a case of basal cell carcinoma arising in the skin invading the parotid gland deeply; the resemblance to adenoid cystic carcinoma in the FNA smear was striking.

Muco-epidermoid tumour (Figs 4.45–4.50)[79]

Criteria for diagnosis

1. A dirty background of mucus and debris.
2. Cohesive clumps and sheets of cells together with small streams of cells within mucus.
3. Variation in cell type — intermediate, squamous, mucin-secreting — most with abundant cytoplasm.
4. Rather regular nuclei, prominent nucleoli in some cells.

These criteria apply mainly to low-grade tumours; high-grade tumours are easily recognised as malignant but are difficult to type. The mucus and debris in the background of smears usually stains blue-violet with MGG and obscures the cellular component, producing an indistinct appearance similar to that sometimes seen in Warthin's tumour (Fig. 4.45). The cell detail is more evident in alcohol-fixed material. The variation in appearance of clumps of cells and of individual cells within the smear is a characteristic feature of muco-epidermoid tumours. Some cells appear to be more obviously squamoid or to have a clear cytoplasm, probably due to glycogen; others contain intracellular mucin vacuoles of varying size staining red in MGG preparations (Figs 4.46, 4.49 and 4.50). The 'intermediate' cells of this neoplasm presumably correspond to the 'meta- *[handwritten: Imp]*

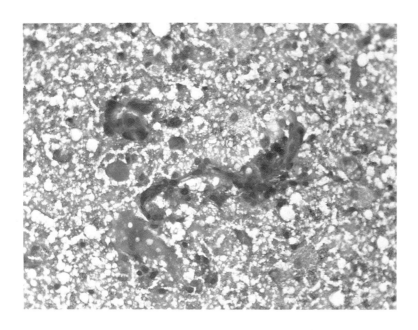

Fig. 4.45 Muco-epidermoid tumour
Degenerating squamoid cells partially obscured by background debris and mucus (MGG, IP)

Very variable appearance
Depends on differentiation.
Well diff —
Simultaneous presence of { mucus producing c̄ small dark nuc.
keratinizing cells
Clusters of intermed. c̄ perinuc. vacuoles
smaller cells and malig. nuclei

Poorly diff:-
Abundant clearcy malig. cells of epid. or keratin prod. Type.
Mucus prod. difficult to document

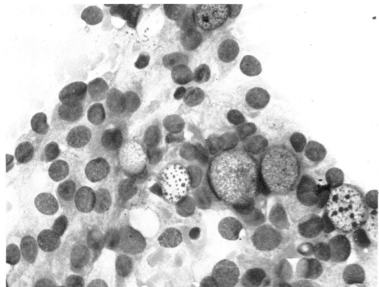

Fig. 4.46 Muco-epidermoid tumour *c̄ut sp. stains*
Intracytoplasmic mucin vacuoles (MGG, HP)

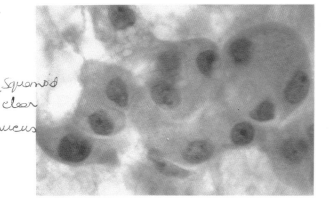

Squamoid
clear
mucus

Fig. 4.47 Muco-epidermoid tumour
Intermediate cells with some cytoplasmic vacuolation and mild nuclear atypia (H & E, HP Oil)

4 HEAD AND NECK; SALIVARY GLANDS

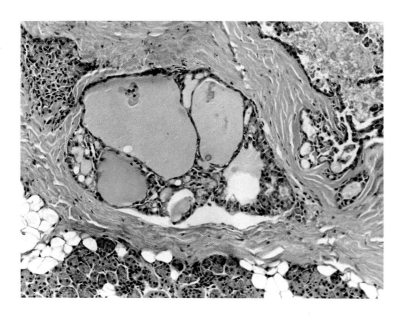

Fig. 4.48 Muco-epidermoid tumour
Tissue section; low-grade tumour; same
case as Figures 4.45 and 4.47 (H & E, IP)

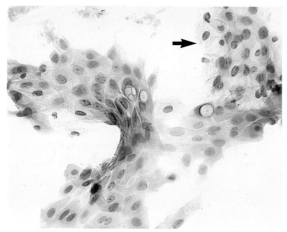

Fig. 4.49 Muco-epidermoid tumour
Moderately cohesive aggregate of atypical epithelial cells–
squamous, intermediate and with intracytoplasmic mucin
vacuoles; note cells with abundant foamy cytoplasm and small
nuclei resembling macrophages (arrow); intermediate grade
tumour (Pap, HP)

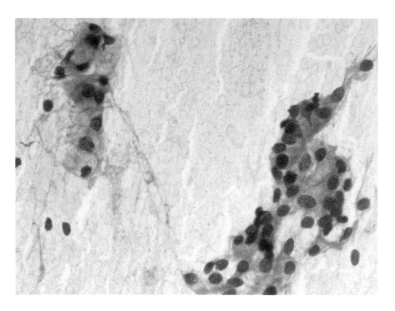

Fig. 4.50 Muco-epidermoid tumour
Thin fluid containing clusters of bland,
non-characteristic epithelial cells; a group
of mucin-containing goblet cells (left)
suggest the diagnosis (Pap, HP)

plastic' appearing cells in smears. At least some cells have prominent nucleoli, but may look otherwise bland in low-grade tumours (Figs 4.47 and 4.49). Cells with abundant, finely vacuolated cytoplasm and small nuclei closely resembling macrophages are commonly seen (Fig. 4.49). Lymphoid cells are present in some tumours.

A definitive diagnosis of muco-epidermoid tumour requires the co-existence in smears of cells showing squamous differentiation and of mucin-secreting cells. Unequivocal evidence of both may be difficult to prove, particularly in cystic tumours in which smears are poor in cells. In such cases, only a tentative diagnosis or a differential diagnosis can be offered.

Problems in diagnosis

1. This neoplasm is one of the most difficult to diagnose with confidence. Problems in distinguishing it from other squamous cell lesions, oncocytic tumours, acinic cell tumours and from other cystic tumours have been discussed.

2. Poorly differentiated forms are difficult to distinguish cytologically from other poorly differentiated primary or metastatic carcinomas.

3. Benign lesions such as retention cysts, or other simple cysts, as well as inflammatory processes, may yield mucus, debris, metaplastic squamous cells and glandular cells in a combination which simulates muco-epidermoid tumour.

4. Inflammatory cells may be prominent in smears of muco-epidermoid tumours, obscuring the neoplastic elements.

Adenocarcinoma

Criteria for diagnosis

1. Obvious nuclear features of malignancy.
2. Intracellular and/or extracellular mucus secretion.

There is a wide range in the types of primary adenocarcinoma encountered in the salivary glands. Adenocarcinoma may arise in pre-existing pleomorphic adenoma or de novo; there is a spectrum ranging from relatively well differentiated mucinous lesions (designated as 'adenopapillary' tumours by some authors)[78] to pleomorphic poorly differentiated carcinomas with minimal evidence of glandular differentiation. Separate subtypes have been defined histologically: salivary duct carcinoma, terminal duct (polymorphous low grade) adenocarcinoma, basaloid carcinoma and epithelial-myoepithelial carcinoma. The specific recognition of these subtypes depends to a great extent on architectural features which cannot be appreciated in FNA smears. The similarity to certain types of breast carcinoma can be striking, for example salivary duct carcinoma/

intraduct breast carcinoma of oxyphil type. The cytological appearances of some of these tumours have now been described.[57]

Problems in diagnosis

1. Metastatic adenocarcinoma.
2. Distinction of low grade tumours from pleomorphic adenoma and mucoepidermoid tumours.
3. Poorly differentiated muco-epidermoid carcinoma.
4. Other poorly differentiated carcinomas.

It will seldom be possible to completely exclude metastatic adenocarcinoma in aspirated material; histological confirmation will usually be necessary.

Squamous cell carcinoma
The criteria for diagnosis do not differ from those of other sites; distinction from poorly differentiated muco-epidermoid tumour, poorly differentiated adenocarcinoma and metastatic squamous cell carcinoma may be impossible.

Other neoplasms
Small cell anaplastic (neuroectodermal) carcinoma (Fig. 4.51) may occur as a primary lesion in the salivary glands. The diagnosis may need to be supported by ultrastructural examination. *Undifferentiated carcinoma* closely resembling nasopharyngeal carcinoma both histologically and cytologically may arise in the salivary glands.

Metastatic carcinoma[46] *melanoma* and *lymphoma* may involve either the salivary glands or lymph nodes adjacent to or within the gland; these possibilities, as well as certain *mesenchymal tumours* such as lipoma, neurinoma and some sarcomas, must be kept in mind when a smear from this site is examined.

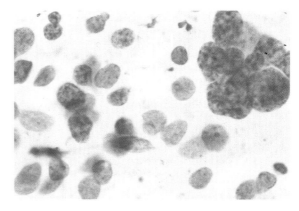

Fig. 4.51 Small cell carcinoma
This is an example of a high grade neuroendocrine carcinoma apparently primary in the parotid (Pap, HP)

4 HEAD AND NECK; SALIVARY GLANDS

REFERENCES AND SUGGESTED FURTHER READING

Head and neck

1. Augsburger J J, Shields J A: Fine needle aspiration biopsy of solid intraocular tumors: indications, instrumentation and techniques. Ophthalmic Surg 15: 34–40, 1984.
2. Augsburger J J, Shields J A, Folberg R, Lang W, O'Hara B J, Claricci J D: Fine needle aspiration biopsy in the diagnosis of intraocular cancer. Cytologic-histologic correlations. Ophthalmology 92: 39–49, 1985.
3. Chan M K, Huang D W, Ho Y H, Lee J C: Detection of Epstein-Barr virus-associated antigen in fine needle aspiration smears from cervical lymph nodes in the diagnosis of nasopharyngeal carcinoma. Acta Cytol 33: 351–354, 1989.
4. Chan M K, McGuire L J, Lee J C: Fine needle aspiration cytodiagnosis of nasopharyngeal carcinoma in cervical lymph nodes. A study of 40 cases. Acta Cytol 33: 344–350, 1989.
5. Chan D H, Miller T R, Descheues J: Fine needle biopsy of retinoblastoma. Am J Ophthalmol 97: 686–690, 1984.
6. Chan D H, Miller T R, Ljung B M, Hawes E L, Iboloff A: Fine needle aspiration biopsy in uveal melanoma. Acta Cytol 33: 599–605, 1989.
7. Chen L T, Hwang W-S: Fine needle aspiration of carotid body paraganglioma. Acta Cytol 33: 681–882, 1989.
8. Dekker A, Johnson B L, Kennerdell J S: Occurence of benign glandular tissue in orbital aspirates. Importance of recognizing its lacrimal gland origin. Acta Cytol 28: 171–174, 1984.
9. Engzell U, Franzen S, Zajicek J: Aspiration biopsy of tumours of the neck. II. Cytologic findings in 13 cases of carotid body tumour. Acta Cytol 15: 25–30, 1971.
10. Engzell U, Jakobsson P A, Sigurdson A, Zajicek J: Aspiration biopsy of metastatic carcinoma in lymph nodes of the neck: a review of 1101 consecutive cases. Acta Otolaryngol 72: 138–147, 1971.
11. Engzell U, Zajicek J: Aspiration biopsy of tumours of the neck. I. Aspiration biopsy and cytologic findings in 100 cases of congenital cysts. Acta Cytol 14: 51–57, 1970.
12. Ferris C A, Schnadig V J, Quinn F B, Des Jardins L: Olfactory neuroblastoma. Cytodiagnostic features in a case with ultrastructural and immunohistochemical correlation. Acta Cytol 32: 381–385, 1988.
13. Frable M A, Frable W J: Fine needle aspiration biopsy in the diagnosis of sarcoid of the head and neck. Acta Cytol 28: 175–177, 1984.
14. Frable M A, Frable W J: Fine-needle aspiration biopsy: efficacy in the diagnosis of head and neck sarcoidosis. Laryngoscope 94: 1281–1283, 1984.
15. Frable W J, Frable M A S: Thin-needle aspiration biopsy: the diagnosis of head and neck tumours revisited. Cancer 43: 1541–1548, 1979.
16. Gertner R, Podoshin L, Fradis M: Accuracy of fine needle aspiration biopsy in neck masses. Laryngoscope 94: 1370–1371, 1984.
17. Gonzales-Campora R, Otal-Salaversi C, Panea-Flores P, et al: Fine needle aspiration cytology of paraganglionic tumors. Acta Cytol 32: 386–390, 1988.
18. Hood I C, Qizilbash A H, Young J E M, Archibald S D: Fine needle aspiration cytology of paragangliomas. Cytologic, light microscopic and ultrastructural studies of three cases. Acta Cytol 27: 651–657, 1983.
19. Jacobs D M, Waisman J: Cervical paraganglioma with intranuclear vacuoles in a fine needle aspirate. Acta Cytol 31: 29–32, 1987.
20. Jelen M, Wozniak Z, Rak J: Cytologic appearance of esthesioneuroblastoma in a fine needle aspirate. Acta Cytol 32: 377–380, 1988.
21. Kapoor R, Saha M M, Das D K. Carotid body tumour initially diagnosed by fine needle aspiration cytology. Acta Cytol 33: 682–683, 1989.
22. Kennerdell J S, Dekker A, Johnson BL, Dubois PJ: Fine-needle aspiration biopsy: its use in orbital tumours. Arch Ophthalmol 97: 1315–1317, 1979.
23. Lack E E, Cubilla A L, Woodruff J M: Paragangliomas of the head and neck region. A pathologic study of tumours from 71 patients. Hum Pathol 10: 191–218, 1979.
24. Lau S K, Wei W I, Hsu C, Engzell U C: Efficacy of fine needle aspiration cytology in the diagnosis of tuberculous cervical lymphadenopathy. J Laryngol Otol 104: 24–27, 1990.
25. Lau S K, Wei W I, Hsu C, Engzell U C: Fine needle aspiration biopsy of tuberculous cervical lymphadenopathy. Aust NZ J Surg 58: 947–950, 1988.
26. Linsk A, Franzen S: Clinical aspiration cytology 2nd ed. Lippincott, Philadelphia, 1989.
27. Ljung B-M, Chan D, Miller T R, Deschenes J: Intraocular lymphoma. Cytologic diagnosis and the role of immunologic markers. Acta Cytol 32: 840–847, 1988.
28. Medeiros L J, Harris N L: Lymphoid infiltrates of the orbit and conjunctiva. A morphologic and immunophenotypic study of 99 cases. Am J Surg Pathol 13: 459–471, 1989.
29. Mincione G, Urso C: Fine needle aspiration cytologic findings in a case of carotid body paraganglioma (chemodectoma). Acta Cytol 33: 679–680, 1989.
30. Muraki A S, Mancuso A A, Harnsberger H R: Metastatic cervical adenopathy from tumors of unknown origin: the role of CT. Radiology 52: 749–753, 1984.
31. Qizilbach A H, Young J E M: Guides to Clinical Aspiration Biopsy. Head and Neck. Igaku-Shoin, New York, 1988.
32. Samuel P R: Aspiration biopsy: an aid in the diagnosis of paranasal tumours. J Laryngol Otol 90: 253–256, 1976.
33. Scholl A, Niemczyk H M: Cytological tumour diagnosis in maxillo-facial surgery. J Maxillofac Surg 8: 17–24, 1980.
34. Sismanis A, Merriam J, Yamaguchi K T, Shapshay S M, Strong M S: Diagnostic value of fine needle aspiration biopsy in neoplasms of the head and neck. Otolaryngol Head Neck Surg 89: 62–66, 1981.
35. Solares J, Lacruz C: Fine needle aspiration cytology diagnosis of an extracranial meningioma presenting as a cervical mass. Acta Cytol 31: 502–504, 1987.
36. Spoor T C, Kennerdell J S, Dekker A, Johnson B L, Rehkopf P: Orbital fine needle aspiration biopsy with B-scan guidance. Am J Ophthalmol 89: 274–277, 1980.
37. Thomsen J, Andreassen J C, Bangsbo C: Fine needle aspiration biopsy of tumours of head and neck. J Laryngol Otol 87: 1211–1216, 1973.
38. Warson F, Blommaert D, DeRoy G: Inflamed branchial cyst; a pitfall in aspiration cytology. Acta Cytol 30: 201–202, 1986.
39. Young J E, Archibald S D, Shier K J: Needle aspiration cytologic biopsy in head and neck masses. Am J Surg 142: 484–489, 1981.
39a. Zajdela A, Vielh P, Schlienger P, Haye C: Fine-needle cytology of 292 palpable orbital and eyelid tumors. Am J Clin Pathol 93: 100–104, 1990.

Salivary glands

40. Anderson R J, Johnston W W, Szpak C A: Fine needle aspiration of adenoid cystic carcinoma metastatic to the lung. Acta Cytol 29: 527–532, 1985.

HEAD AND NECK; SALIVARY GLANDS

4

41. Aufdemorte T B, Ramzy I, Holt G R, Thomas J R, Duncan D L: Focal adenomatoid hyperplasia of salivary glands. A differential diagnostic problem in fine needle aspiration biopsy. Acta Cytol 29: 23–28, 1985.
42. Bondeson L, Lindholm K, Thorstenson S: benign dermal eccrine cylindroma. A pitfall in the cytologic diagnosis of adenoid cystic carcinoma. Acta Cytol 27: 326–328, 1983.
43. Bottles K, Ferrell L D, Miller T R: Tyrosine crystals in fine needle aspirates of a pleomorphic adenoma of the parotid gland. Acta Cytol 28: 490–492, 1984.
44. Bottles K, Miller T, Cohen M, Ljung B. Fine needle aspiration biopsy cytology. Am J Med 81: 525–531, 1986.
45. Cross D L, Gansler T S, Morris R C: Fine needle aspiration and frozen section of salivary gland lesions. South Med J 83: 283–286, 1990.
46. Currens H S, Sajjad S M, Lukeman J M: Aspiration cytology of oat-cell carcinoma metastatic to the parotid gland. Acta Cytol 26: 566–567, 1982.
47. Domagala W, Halczy-Kowalik L, Welen K, Osborn M: Coexpression of glial fibrillary acid protein, keratin and vimentin. A unique feature useful in the diagnosis of pleomorphic adenoma in the salivary gland in fine needle aspiration biopsy smears. Acta Cytol 32: 403–408, 1988.
48. Droese M: cytological diagnosis of sialadenosis, sialadenitis and parotid cysts by fine needle aspiration. Adv Otorhinolaryngol 26: 49–96, 1981.
49. Droese M, Haubrick J, Tute M: Value of needle biopsy for the diagnosis of salivary gland tumours. Schweiz Med Wochenschr 108: 933–935, 1978.
50. Elliott J N, Oertel Y C: Lymphoepithelial cysts of the salivary glands. Histological and cytologic features. Am J Clin Pathol 93: 39–43, 1990.
51. Eneroth C M, Franzen S, Zajicek J: Cytologic diagnosis on aspirates from 1000 salivary gland tumours. Acta Otolaryngol Suppl 224: 168–171, 1967.
52. Eneroth C M, Jakobsson P, Zajicek J: Aspiration bipsy of salivary gland tumours. V. Morphologic investigations on smears and histologic sections of acinic cell carcinoma. Acta Radiol Suppl 310: 85–93, 1971.
53. Eneroth C M, Zajicek J: Aspiration biopsy of salivary gland tumours. II. Morphologic studies on smears and histologic sections from oncocytic tumours. Acta Cytol 9: 355–361, 1965.
54. Eneroth C M, Zajicek J: Aspiration biopsy of salivary gland tumours. III. Morphologic studies on smears and histologic sections from 368 mixed tumours. Acta Cytol 10: 440–454, 1966.
55. Eneroth C M, Zajicek J: Aspiration biopsy of salivary gland tumours. IV. Morphologic studies on smears and histologic sections from 45 cases of adenoid cystic carcinoma. Acta Cytol 13: 59–63, 1969.
56. Eneroth C M, Zetterberg A: A cytochemical method of grading the malignancy of salivary gland tumours preoperatively. Acta Otolaryngol 81: 489–495, 1976.
57. Frierson H F Jr, Covell J L, Mills S E: Fine-needle aspiration cytology of terminal duct carcinoma of minor salivary gland. Diagn Cytopathol 3: 159–162, 1987.
58. Hagelqvist E: Light and electron microscopic studies on material obtained by fine needle biopsy. A methodological study in aspirates from tumours of the head and neck with special emphasis on salivary gland tumours. Acta Otolaryngol (Suppl) 354: 1–75, 1978.
59. Hood I, Qizilbash A H, Salama S S, Alexopoulou I: Basal cell adenoma of parotid. Difficulty of differentiation from adenoid cystic carcinoma on aspiration biopsy. Acta Cytol 27: 515–520, 1983.
60. Kline T S, Merriam J M, Shapshay S M. Aspiration biopsy cytology of the salivary gland. Am J Clin Pathol 76: 263–269, 1981.
61. Lau T, Balle V H, Bretlau P. Fine-needle aspiration biopsy in salivary gland tumours. Clin Otolaryngol 11: 75–77, 1986.
62. Layfield L J: Fine needle aspiration cytology of a trabecular adenoma of the parotid gland. Acta Cytol 29: 999–1002, 1985.
63. Layfield L J, Tan P, Glasgow B J. Fine-needle aspiration of salivary gland lesions. Arch Pathol Lab Med 11: 346–353, 1987.
64. Lindberg L G, Åkerman M: Aspiration cytology of salivary gland tumours: diagnostic experience from six years of routine laboratory work. Laryngoscope 86: 584–589, 1976.
65. Mavec P, Eneroth C M, Franzen S, Moberger G, Zajicek J: Aspiration biopsy of salivary gland tumours. I. Correlation of cytologic reports from 652 aspiration biopsies with clinical and histological findings. Acta Otolaryngol 58: 472–484, 1964.
66. Nettle W J, Orell S R: Fine needle aspiration in the diagnosis of salivary gland lesions. Aust NZ J Surg 59: 47–51, 1989.
67. O'Dwyer P, Farrar W B, James A G, Finkelmeier W, McCabe D P:N needle aspiration biopsy of major salivary gland tumours; its value. Cancer 57: 554–557, 1986.
68. Orell S R, Nettle W J S: Fine-needle aspiration biopsy of salivary gland tumours. Problems and Pitfalls. Pathology 20: 332–337, 1988.
69. Palmer O, Torri A M, Christoforo J A, Fiaccavento S: Fine needle aspiration cytology in two cases of well-differentiated acinic-cell carcinoma of the parotid gland. Acta Cytol 29: 516–521, 1985.
70. Persson P S, Zettergren L: Cytologic diagnosis of salivary gland tumours by aspiration biopsy. Acta Cytol 17: 351–354, 1973.
71. Qizilbach A H, Sianos J, Young J E M, Archibald S D: Fine needle aspiration biopsy cytology of major salivary glands. Acta Cytol 29: 503–512, 1985.
72. Schultenover S J, McDonald E C, Ramzy I: Hyaline-cell pleomorphic adenoma diagnosed by fine needle aspiration biopsy. Acta Cytol 28: 593–597, 1984.
73. Sismanis A, Merriam J M, Kline T S, Davis R K, Shapshay S M, Strong M S: Diagnosis of salivary gland tumors by fine-needle aspiration biopsy. Head Neck Surg 3: 482–489, 1981.
74. Smith R C, Amy R W: Adenoid cystic carcinoma metastatic to the lung. Report of a case diagnosed by fine needle aspiration biopsy cytology. Acta Cytol 29: 533–534, 1985.
75. Webb A J: Cytologic diagnosis of salivary gland lesions in adult and pediatric surgical patients. Acta Cytol 17: 51–58, 1973.
76. Woyke S, Olsgewski W, Domagala W, Marzecki Z: Cytodiagnosis of acinic cell carcinoma. Ultrastructural study of material obtained by fine needle aspiration biopsy. Acta Cytol 19: 110–116, 1975.
77. Young J A: Fine needle aspiration cytology of salivary glands. Ear Nose Throat J 68: 120–129, 1989.
78. Zajicek J, Eneroth C M: Cytological diagnosis of salivary gland carcinomata from aspiration biopsy smears. Acta Otolaryng (Suppl) 263: 183–185, 1970.
79. Zajicek J, Eneroth C M, Jakobsson P: Aspiration biopsy of salivary gland tumours. VI. Morphologic studies on smears and histologic sections from mucoepidermoid carcinoma. Acta Cytol 20: 35–41, 1976.

5

LYMPH NODES

5 LYMPH NODES

CLINICAL ASPECTS

The commonest cause of peripheral lymphadenopathy is a reaction to some symptomatic or asymptomatic inflammatory process. Although surgical excision of a palpable peripheral node is relatively simple, it does require anesthesia, strict sterility and theatre time, and it may leave a scar; therefore patients are usually watched for some time unless the clinical suspicion of malignancy is strong. FNA biopsy offers the alternative of an immediate, preliminary, although not always specific diagnosis with little trauma and cost. FNA of lymph nodes has been practised in Central Europe and in Scandinavia for many years,[33,47,68,81,82] particularly by haematologists, in conjunction with aspiration of bone marrow and spleen, References to this method are less common in the Anglo-American literature. Martin and Ellis of the Memorial Hospital in New York[51] were pioneers in this field and their work was more recently followed up by Betsill and Hajdu.[7]

The emergence of the AIDS epidemic in recent years has presented lymph node cytology with formidable problems.[9,10,77] The exclusion or confirmation of malignant lymphoma and other malignant processes by FNA is of great practical importance in these patients, since it may obviate the need for surgical excision. So is the sampling of nodes for microbiological investigation when an opportunistic infection is suspected. However, the cytological evaluation and diagnosis of lymphadenopathy and the distinction between reactive and malignant change is particularly difficult in AIDS patients. There are also technical problems related to the safety precautions to be observed by staff involved with lymph node sampling.

The ever increasing number of commercially produced monoclonal antibodies to various antigens specific to different cell lines is proving very useful in lymph node cytology. In particular, it assists the pathologist in the identification of the source of tumour metastases to lymph nodes and in the distinction between undifferentiated carcinoma and malignant lymphoma. At the same time, experience accumulated over the years has rather emphasised the difficulty and limitations of FNA cytology in the exact diagnosis and subtyping of lymphoma. Conventional cell morphology is not sufficient and must be supplemented with a battery of immune markers. Although some workers have reported good results with immunohistological methods applied to cytocentrifuge preparations of lymph node aspirates,[2,46,63,67] most laboratories find that cytological preparations obtained in routine clinical work are often insufficient, both quantitatively and qualitatively. The amount of aspirated material may not allow the preparation of a sufficient number of slides for the required battery of antisera with appropriate controls, and the tendency for the cytoplasm of lymphoid cells to disperse in the background of smears introduces an element of uncertainty in the allocation of positive staining to individual cells. The role of cytology in the diagnosis of lymphoma has

subsequently become more clearly defined; it is to confirm a clinical suspicion of lymphoma, or to exclude it with the highest possible confidence. Confirmation is followed by open biopsy to provide tissue for histology and immune marker studies necessary for definitive diagnosis and subtyping, negative findings by clinical observation. Some of the new techniques developed in molecular biology may be applicable to FNA samples and may be of great value in this crucial distinction, such as gene re-arrangement studies and DNA monoclonality.[34,35,49]

The place of FNA in the investigative sequence

The primary purpose of FNA biopsy of an abnormal peripheral lymph node is to decide whether surgical excision for histological examination is indicated. The alternatives are to just observe the patient, to carry out further investigations or to try a course of conservative treatment for example with antibiotics. Obviously there are practical and psychological advantages if this decision can be made at the patient's first visit. Except in the rare event of significant haematoma and of post-aspiration infarction,[6,19] which we have not seen in our practice, preoperative FNA does not adversely affect subsequent histological examination of the node. Thus, any enlarged, abnormal lymph node in any site constitutes an indication for FNA biopsy.

As a rule, the cytological examination can decide whether the lymphadenopathy is due to reactive hyperplasia, to metastatic malignancy, or to malignant lymphoma.

In the case of reactive hyperplasia, surgical excision is not indicated, unless the subsequent course is atypical. Clinical follow up is justified in all cases in view of the small but significant rate of false negative cytological reports. Some specific diagnoses within this category can be made by FNA, but most often the aetiology remains obscure. Whenever possible, the biopsy material should therefore also be used for microbiological investigation.

Lymph nodes clinically suspected of metastatic malignancy constitute one of the commonest indications for FNA biopsy. In patients with known, histologically proven malignancy in whom enlarged nodes appear subsequently, a cytological diagnosis is usually easily obtained and further surgery merely to confirm metastasis can be avoided. In patients without a previous diagnosis, not only can metastatic malignancy be confirmed by FNA biopsy, but clues to the nature and the site of the primary are also given in most cases. The need for further investigations may therefore be reduced. Multiple smears which can be used for histochemical and immunohistochemical staining are of great value in this situation, or the FNA sample may be processed for electron microscopy, for example if a neuroendocrine tumour is suspected. Only when the primary cannot be found despite the evidence provided by FNA biopsy and supplementary investigations, and when this information is likely to be of therapeutic importance, is a diagnostic surgical excision of the node indicated. The primary tumours which are most important to confirm or exclude are obviously those in which an effective palliative treatment is available, mainly carcinoma of the prostate and of the breast, and also carcinoma of ovary and thyroid, germ cell tumour, and perhaps small cell anaplastic carcinoma. The distinction between anaplastic carcinoma and lymphoma is equally important.

If the cytological diagnosis is malignant lymphoma, or suspicious of lymphoma, this must be followed by surgical excision of the node. The exact diagnosis and classification necessary to select the appropriate treatment regimen can, in most cases, only be reached by histological and immunological examination of the whole node. Although FNA biopsy does not replace histological examination in the diagnosis of lymphoma, it is still of value in the management of these patients for the following reasons:

1. In a general practice situation, a cytological diagnosis suggests appropriate referral and further investigations without delay.

2. A representative node can be selected for surgical biopsy by FNA sampling of multiple nodes. The biggest or the most easily accessible node is not always the most suitable and may show only reactive change.

3. If a diagnosis or suspicion of lymphoma is known beforehand, steps can be taken to ensure that the node is sent fresh to the laboratory without fixation so that a complete immunological investigation can be carried out.

4. Other biopsies — bone marrow, liver, spleen — can be done at the same time as the node excision, saving time and additional anesthesia. In the case of Hodgkin's disease, lymph node excision can be deferred until the staging laparotomy.

5. In patients who have advanced intra-abdominal or mediastinal lymphoma without involvment of superficial nodes, cytological diagnosis and classification in combination with radiological and clinical evaluation of extent of disease may be sufficient basis for therapeutic decisions. It may be preferable to avoid a laparotomy only to obtain tissue for histological examination, particularly in elderly patients, since the procedure has a certain morbidity and can cause significant delay of treatment. In this situation, it may be advantageous to use a fine core needle for the biopsy to obtain sufficient tissue for immune marker studies.[79]

6. Suspected recurrent or residual disease in patients with previously confirmed lymphoma can in most cases be diagnosed by FNA alone without the need for a formal biopsy.[73] A change in the type of lymphoma will also usually be recognised. This is of clinical value as the recurrent tumour may be the only sign of disease by which the response to systemic therapy can be monitored and is therefore best left intact.

Accuracy of diagnosis

The accuracy of FNA of lymph nodes in the diagnosis of *metastatic malignancy* is influenced by many factors such as the size and the site of the node, fibrosis, previous irradiation and the number of punctures made. For example, small mobile nodes high up in the axilla are difficult to sample, while adequate material can easily be obtained from nodes only a couple of mm in diameter in a cervical or supraclavicular position.[81] Deep nodes are accessible to FNA only if they can be visualised by radiological methods.[83] Fibrosis in nodes sometimes makes it difficult to obtain sufficient material for diagnosis. This is commonly the case with reactive inguinal nodes and may also be a problem in nodular sclerosing Hodgkin's disease[28] and in some retroperitoneal non-Hodgkin's lymphomas.

If the biopsy material is adequate, diagnostic sensitivity is still limited by the fact that small metastatic deposits, metastases confined to the subcapsular sinus and single cell metastases can be missed even by multiple aspirations (Fig. 5.22). Although the diagnostic sensitivity reported in the literature varies, it is usually above 95% (metastatic and recurring malignancy).[7,12,23,39,40,43,47,50,61,65] Failure to obtain a representative sample is no doubt responsible for most false negative diagnoses. Interpretation of a representative aspirate can be a problem, but far more often so in lymphoma than in metastatic malignancy. For example, follicular lymphoma of mixed small and large cells can sometimes be mistaken for reactive follicular hyperplasia. Thus, although a negative cytological report makes malignancy unlikely, it cannot be taken as diagnostic on its own,[81] and if the lymphadenopathy does not show signs of regression within a few weeks of observation, FNA should be repeated or a node should be excised for histology.

Diagnostic specificity, on the other hand, is high. False positive diagnoses are rare[7,11,26,50] if particular caution is observed in the interpretation of smears from nodes in fields of previous irradiation and in the presence of necrosis. The existence of benign epithelial inclusions in lymph nodes (see p. 75) should be kept in mind. The main problem is in relation to lymphoma, particularly that of distinguishing between reactive follicular hyperplasia and follicular lymphoma of mixed cells. Most false positive diagnoses reported in the literature have been cases of reactive lymphadenopathy reported as suspicious of lymphoma.

Diagnostic accuracy not only depends on the representativity of the aspirate but also very much on the quality of the cytological preparations. This is particu-

5 LYMPH NODES

larly the case in the diagnosis of certain reactive lymphadenopathies and in the diagnosis and classification of lymphoma, which depends on the study of fine cytological detail and on an estimate of proportions of various cell types in the smear.[56,69] It is essential that the aspirates are handled and smears prepared by cytologically trained staff to achieve satisfactory results.

Conflicting opinions are expressed in the literature regarding the accuracy of cytological diagnosis and of typing of malignant lymphoma.[7,13,24,48,59,64] Diagnostic sensitivity has generally been found to be significantly lower for lymphoma than for metastatic malignancy.[50] For a diagnosis of lymphoma to be of clinical practical value, it must identify good and bad prognosis subgroups and therefore must include subtype according to one of the current classifications. Several of the reported studies in which the Kiel classification of non-Hodgkin's lymphoma[44] was applied to cytological preparations recorded an acceptable level of accuracy of both diagnosis and classification.[48,56,69,70] However, the material that can be obtained by FNA is not sufficient for a full immunohistological investigation, and interpretation of immune staining is often more difficult in cytological preparations than in sections. Although new markers with increasing specificity are being introduced, at the same time the number of defined subtypes of lymphoma is increasing. The definitive diagnosis must therefore still rely on the examination of tissue from an open biopsy, perhaps with the exception of some easily recognised high grade, large cell lymphomas. Other supplementary techniques, such as DNA analysis, morphometry and gene re-arrangement studies have been applied to cell samples obtained by FNA.[34,35,49]

Complications

Significant complications do not occur. Post-aspiration haematoma is rare. Septic complications or tumour implantation in the needle track have not been reported.

Contraindications

None.

Technical considerations

Both reactive nodes and nodes involved by metastatic malignancy or lymphoma are highly cellular and moderately vascular tissues. Sufficient material is therefore easily obtained using a 25 or a 23 gauge needle without aspiration, except in the presence of fibrosis. This technique, which we have used routinely for several years, has the advantage over the traditional aspiration of giving the operator a much better sensitivity projected to the tip of the needle. This is important when small or deep nodes are biopsied. Multiple passes of the needle in different directions within the node for wider sampling do not usually cause admixture with blood to the same extent as when aspiration is used. An abundance of blood in the sample adversely affects cell fixation and tends to distort the cells to some extent. If aspiration is used, the syringe should be mounted in a pistol grip so that one hand is free to hold the node firmly during puncture. Multiple rapid biopsies from different points of entry tend to give a better yield and less admixture with blood than several passes in various directions as recommended above for needle biopsy without aspiration.

Local anaesthetic is not used and simple skin disinfection as for an injection is adequate. Two to four samples are usually necessary to secure enough material for both routine smears and for special investigations, and to reduce sampling error in focal disease. The use of gloves and extreme care in handling used needles has become an important safety precaution. The techniques involved in the biopsy of deep nodes using radiological guidance are described in Chapter 3. If the standard technique does not yield sufficient material, for example due to fibrosis (nodular sclerosing Hodgkin's disease and some retroperitoneal non-Hodgkin's lymphomas), a 22 gauge cutting core needle or a Rotex screw needle may be tried.[79]

It is difficult to make perfect direct smears from samples of lymphoid tissue. An air-dried smear has to dry quickly for optimal fixation and therefore has to be made thin. The smearing pressure must be finely balanced to obtain a reasonably thin smear and at the same time avoid crush artefacts. A wet-fixed smear must be fixed immediately to minimise drying artefacts. Only those parts of the smears in which the cells are evenly dispersed, well-fixed and not distorted by the trauma of smearing should be chosen for diagnostic evaluation (Fig. 5.45). Areas in which cells show crush and/or drying artefacts, usually at the tail of the smear, should be ignored (Fig. 5.46).

While air-dried MGG-stained smears are essential for the evaluation of cytoplasm and background and for comparison with cells in blood and bone marrow, alcohol-fixation and staining with H & E or with Pap is helpful in assessing nucleoli and chromatin pattern. Whenever possible both air-dried and wet-fixed smears should be made. Extra smears to allow special stains are often of great value. Staining for micro-organisms (Ziehl-Neelsen, PAS, silver impregnation techniques, etc.), for mucin (PAS/D, Alcian blue), for melanin (Masson, formalin-induced fluorescence) and for acid phosphatase are those most commonly used.

Cell morphology is better preserved in a suspension made by gently dispersing a whole sample in Hank's balanced salt solution with 10–20% fetal calf serum, or by rinsing the needle with the fluid. The suspension is spun in the Cytocentrifuge at 300 r p m. for 3 minutes.

Processing should be done as soon as possible after biopsy since cell fragility increases rapidly with time. This method of preparation is a valuable complement to direct smears, especially in the diagnosis and classification of lymphoma (Figs 5.36 and 5.41b). It provides the best preparations for immunocytochemical staining. Background staining due to serum proteins and fragmented cells can be reduced by resuspending the cells in Hank's fluid after initial centrifugation. Direct smears are rarely suitable due to the dispersal of cytoplasm in the background (Fig. 2.18). Immunoperoxidase staining for demonstration of a variety of tissue-specific cell pro-

ducts is one of the most useful 'special stains' in diagnostic cytology. Immunocytochemistry is helpful in tracing the origin of metastatic malignancy (p. 79), in the differentiation of lymphoma from reactive processes and from anaplastic carcinoma (p. 87), and in the classification of lymphoma.[2,46,63,67]

If there is any suspicion of an infective process, the needle should be rinsed with sterile saline after the smears have been prepared or the biopsy should be repeated to provide material for culture for micro-organisms (p. 21).

5 *LYMPH NODES*

CYTOLOGICAL FINDINGS

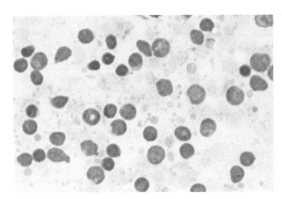

Fig. 5.1 Lymphoid globules
Spherical fragments of pale-blue cytoplasm of variable sizes dispersed between the lymphoid cells; absence of nuclear debris (MGG, HP)

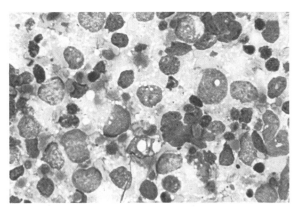

Fig. 5.2 Small cell carcinoma, intermediate type
Dispersed malignant cells with large pale nuclei, inconspicuous nucleoli and fragile cytoplasm; note irregular cytoplasmic and nuclear fragments in the background representing tumour necrosis (MGG, HP)

FNA samples of lymphoid tissue, nodal or extra-nodal, benign or malignant, are as a rule characterised by a very high cell content. This is obvious to the naked eye as the aspirate is smeared. It appears as a film of slimy material which becomes grey on drying. The cytoplasm of lymphoid cells is fragile. Many cells appear as naked nuclei and a variable number of rounded cytoplasmic fragments measuring up to 8 μm in diameter are seen in the background. Such cytoplasmic fragments (so called 'lymphoid globules' or 'lymphoglandular bodies'[68]) which stain an even pale-blue with Giemsa stains, are characteristic of lymphoid tissue, both neoplastic and non-neoplastic. They differ from necrotic debris by their regular round shape, their uniform staining, and by the absence of nuclear debris (compare Figs 5.1 and 5.2). The recognition of 'lymphoid globules' is of great diagnostic value, for example in the distinction of lymphoma from anaplastic carcinoma.

Most of the lymphoid cells in smears are seen as single cells but dense clumps or aggregates also occur. Cell detail is obscured in such clumps and they are of no diagnostic value as they can be found both in reactive and in malignant nodes. However, a characteristic aggregation of cells tends to occur in some follicle centre cell lymphomas.[68,82] Tissue fragments consisting of a vascular core of endothelial cells with adherent lymphoid cells and histiocytes are sometimes present in smears from reactive nodes (Fig. 5.3).

The reactive node (Figs 5.4–5.16)

Criteria for diagnosis

1. A mixed population of lymphoid cells.
2. A predominance of small lymphocytes.
3. Centroblasts, centrocytes, immunoblasts and plasma cells in variable but 'logical' proportions.
4. Dendritic reticulum cells associated with centroblasts and centrocytes (representing germinal centres).
5. Scattered histiocytes with intracytoplasmic nuclear debris (tingible body macrophages).
6. Pale histiocytes, endothelial cells, eosinophils, neutrophils (variable).

The reactive pattern is quite variable depending on the degree of stimulation, the number and size of germinal centres, and on whether the sample derives mainly from a germinal centre or from interfollicular or paracortical tissue (Fig. 5.4). A smear, which derives mainly from interfollicular tissue, consists predominantly of lymphocytes with a variable number of scattered immunoblasts, plasma cells, non-specific histiocytes and endothelial cells (Fig. 5.5). Material representing germinal centre tissue is characterised by poorly defined, loose tissue fragments of dendritic reticulum cells, to the syncytial cytoplasm (pale grey/violet in MGG) of

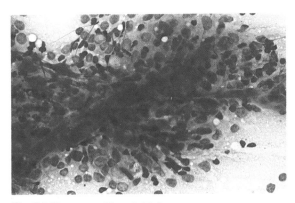

Fig. 5.3 Fragment of lymphoid tissue
Lymphoid cells and histiocytes adhering to a vascular core with prominent endothelial cells (MGG, IP)

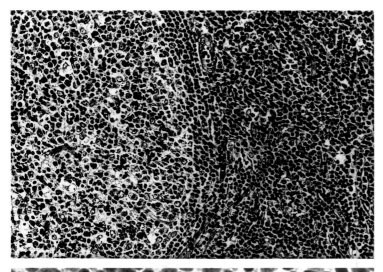

Fig. 5.4 Reactive lymphadenopathy
Tissue section showing germinal centre (left)
and paracortical tissue each of which may
be selectively sampled by FNA. The
corresponding cytological patterns are
shown in Figures 5.5 and 5.6 (H & E, IP)

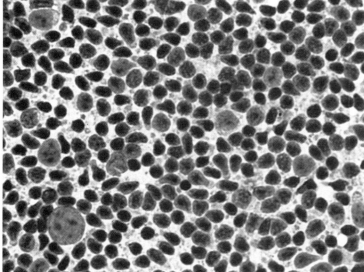

Fig. 5.5 Reactive lymphadenopathy
Smear derived from interfollicular tissue;
predominancy of lymphocytes with few
blasts (MGG, HP)

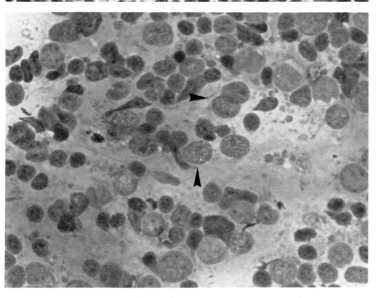

Fig. 5.6 Reactive lymphadenopathy
Smear derived from germinal centre;
loose tissue fragment of dendritic
reticulum cells (arrows), centroblasts,
centrocytes and some lymphocytes (MGG,
HP)

5 LYMPH NODES

which centroblasts, centrocytes and a smaller number of lymphocytes adhere (Fig. 5.6). Multiple biopsies diminish the bias caused by selective sampling. The most important features which distinguish a reactive process from lymphoma are: (1) a mixed population of lymphoid cells representing the whole range of lymphocyte transformation from small lymphocytes to immunoblasts and plasma cells; (2) a predominance of small, sometimes slightly larger 'stimulated' lymphocytes, which have small round nuclei and a characteristic chromatin pattern of large ill-defined condensations; and (3) centroblasts and centrocytes associated with dendritic reticulum cells derived from germinal centres as described above, and tingible body macrophages (Fig. 5.7).[54,71] FNA smears of truly normal lymphoid tissue are rarely seen as only clinically abnormal nodes are subjected to biopsy. However, axillary nodes undergoing fat involution are sometimes sampled as they may become quite large although of soft consistency. Smears of such nodes show fat droplets, fragments of adipose tissue, a number of small lymphocytes and a few blasts. Fibrotic but otherwise normal inguinal nodes also give a scanty yield.

Problems in diagnosis

1. Follicular hyperplasia with large germinal centres.
2. Follicular lymphoma.
3. Prominent immunoblastic and plasmacellular reaction.
4. Prominent histiocytic component.

Germinal centres may be very large in some cases of reactive follicular hyperplasia. If the aspirate derives from such a large germinal centre, the proportion of large cells (centroblasts, dendritic reticulum cells) and the number of mitoses may be impressive enough to suggest malignant lymphoma. However, the full range of lymphocyte transformation is still present, including small lymphocytes, and the various cell types occur in logical proportions. Small or slightly enlarged lymphocytes are still numerically predominant. A variable number of plasma cells can usually be found. The presence of macrophages with tingible bodies favours reactive hyperplasia but does not rule out lymphoma. The cytological pattern of reactive hyperplasia in which plasma cells are prominent but without other distinguishing features can be seen for example in cases of *secondary syphilis* and of *rheumatoid arthritis*.

The differential diagnosis between prominent follicular hyperplasia and follicular lymphoma of mixed cell type (centroblastic/centrocytic) can be very difficult in FNA smears. The characteristics of the former have been mentioned. In follicular lymphoma, the predominant cell type may appear small, but the nucleus is of intermediate size and has an irregular shape and a more granular chromatin similar to a centrocyte. Immunoblasts, plasma cells and tingible body macrophages are usually absent or few in numbers. The difficulty to distinguish the two conditions is largely due to the fact that dendritic reticulum cells associated with centroblasts and centrocytes are seen in both, and that interfollicular areas in lymphoma may contain large numbers of small lymphocytes. Immunological demonstration of poly- or monoclonality may be necessary to solve the problem.

A prominent immunoblastic and plasmacellular reaction is found in several conditions. In *viral lymphadenitis*, particularly in *infectious mononucleosis*,[36] immunoblasts, plasmacytoid cells, mature plasma cells and atypical lymphocytes can be numerous (Figs 5.8 and 5.9). The atypical lymphocytes have an abundant basophilic cytoplasm, an enlarged, often eccentric nucleus, and a paler nuclear chromatin than a normal lymphocyte. Atypical immunoblasts can cause differential diagnostic problems; the main differential diagnoses are T-immunoblastic lymphoma and Hodgkin's disease (atypical binucleate immunoblasts closely resembling Reed-Sternberg cells can occasionally be seen). In most cases, the diagnosis is already suggested by the clinical presentation, and can be confirmed by serological tests.

Prominent immunoblasts and sometimes Reed-

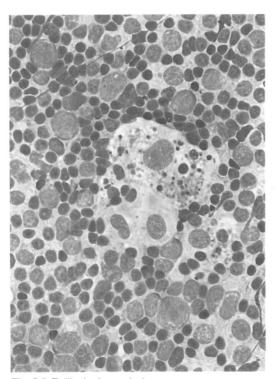

Fig. 5.7 Follicular hyperplasia
Tingible body macrophage; the full range of small and transformed lymphocytes (MGG, HP)

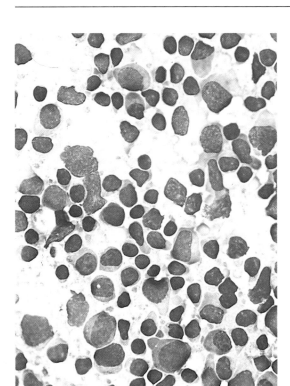

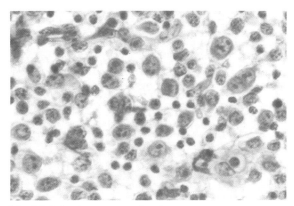

Fig. 5.9 Infectious mononucleosis
A similar pattern to Fig. 5.8 of a high proportion of transformed lymphocytes (Pap, HP)

Fig. 5.8 Infectious mononucleosis
Many transforming lymphocytes and immunoblasts (MGG, HP)

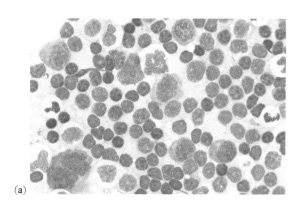

(a)

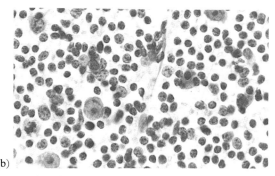

(b)

Fig. 5.10 Immunoblastic reaction
Several immunoblasts including a binucleate form; case of Dilantin lymphadenopathy (a. MGG, HP; b. H & E, HP)

Sternberg-like cells also occur in *post vaccinial lymphadenitis* and *Dilantin hypersensitivity lymphadenopathy* (Fig. 5.10). One is, of course, dependent on the clinical history in such cases. The cytological findings are at best only suggestive and unless the history is unequivocal, surgical excision for histological examination should usually follow. Immunoblastic reactions such as *angioimmunoblastic lymphadenopathy* (AILD) are difficult to distinguish from T-cell lymphoma and in some cases progress to lymphoma. In the absence of a clinical background such as the examples mentioned above, open biopsy is recommended. In AILD there may be a tendency to lymphocyte depletion. In the few cases we have seen, large pale cells which resembled histiocytes were also prominent and in fact, some form of histiocytosis was considered in the differential diagnosis. These cells may well represent swollen endothelial cells in keeping with the prominent vessels seen in histological sections (Fig. 5.11). In any case, the diagnosis can only be made by histological examination of the excised node. Malignant lymphoma of lymphoplasmacytoid type (immunocytoma, Waldenstrom's macroglobulinemia) must also be considered in the differential diagnosis in this group of conditions (p. 80).

Histiocytes, which have an abundant, pale or sometimes eosinophilic cytoplasm may be prominent in smears of lymph node aspirates. The histiocytes occur singly or in small groups. The cytoplasm is often vacuolated or granular and may contain phagocytosed debris or pigment. An increased number of histiocytes without specific features can be seen in smears from non-specific reactive nodes, perhaps indicating some de-

5 *LYMPH NODES*

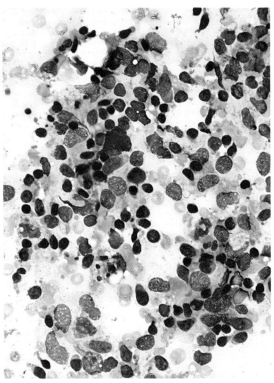

Fig. 5.11 Immunoblastic reaction
Case histologically diagnosed as angioimmunoblastic lymphadenopathy. Many histiocyte-like cells with large, elongated nuclei (possibly endothelial cells); lymphocyte depletion (MGG, HP)

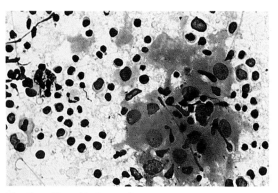

Fig. 5.12 Sinus histiocytosis
Loose cluster of histiocytes (non-epithelioid) with abundant eosinophilic cytoplasm (MGG, HP)

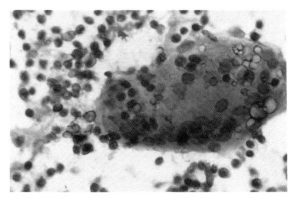

Fig. 5.13 Silicone adenopathy
Histiocytes and large multinucleated foreign-body-type giant cell with cytoplasmic vacuoles (Pap, IP)

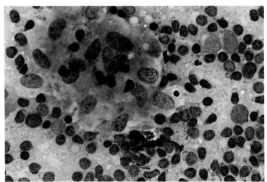

Fig. 5.14 Toxoplasmosis
Granuloma-like cluster of histiocytes without well-defined epithelioid features (MGG, HP)

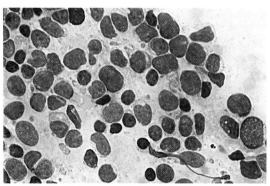

Fig. 5.15 Toxoplasmosis
Activated lymphoid cells including some monocytoid forms (MGG, HP)

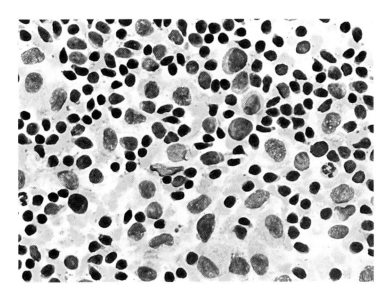

Fig. 5.16 Dermatopathic lymphadenopathy
Numerous pale histiocytes in a background of predominantly small lymphocytes. Intracytoplasmic pigment was sparse in this case (MGG, HP)

gree of sinus histiocytosis (Fig. 5.12). Histiocytes are particularly prominent in nodes sampled within a few days of *lymphangiographic examination*. Their cytoplasm contains lipid droplets, multinucleated histiocytic giant cells are common, and there is often a conspicuous number of eosinophils. Another condition with prominent histiocytes and multinucleated giant cells as a reaction to foreign material is *silicone lymphadenopathy* occasionally seen in axillary nodes of women with silicone breast prosthesis (Fig. 5.13).

Scattered small clusters of histiocytes which have ovoid, pale nuclei and resemble epithelioid cells, with a background of follicular hyperplasia, are suggestive of *toxoplasmosis* (Fig. 5.14). Atypical lymphoid cells with large, ovoid, pale nuclei may also be seen (Fig. 5.15). These cells probably correspond to the pale monocytoid cells observed in histological sections. Occasionally, the nuclei of these large cells may appear atypical enough to raise a suspicion of malignancy. The cytological pattern is not diagnostic in itself and needs to be confirmed by serological tests. Microcysts and organisms are hardly ever seen in smears.[3,15]

Numerous non-cohesive, pale, histiocyte-like cells (interdigitating reticulum cells) are present in *dermatopathic lymphadenopathy* (Fig. 5.16). Some of the histiocytes contain pigment — either haemosiderin or melanin. These have smaller and more consistently oval nuclei than dendritic reticulum cells and have a better defined cytoplasm. Some eosinophils are usually present. The background is predominantly of small lymphocytes which may appear slightly atypical (stimulated T-cells) and blast forms are less common.

For a description of *histiocytosis X* and of *malignant histiocytosis*, see pages 85, 325 (Fig. 11.46).[42] The nuclei of Langerhans' histiocytes of histiocytosis X are large and can have a very irregular shape: folded, convoluted,

lobulated and grooved. Mitotic activity may be seen and sometimes necrosis. Such cells seen in a lymph node aspirate, especially in the absence of eosinophils, may raise a suspicion of metastatic malignancy such as melanoma. However, the nuclear chromatin of Langerhans' histiocytes is bland and finely granular. If suspected, the diagnosis may be confirmed by immunocytochemistry and/or by EM.

The cytological presentation of *sinus histiocytosis* with *massive lymphadenopathy* in imprint preparations was detailed by Lampert and Lennert.[41] *Angiofollicular lymphoid hyperplasia* has been described in a case report by Hidvegi.[31]

Granulomatous lymphadenitis (Figs 5.17–5.20)[5,38,60,66]

Criteria for diagnosis

1. Histiocytes of epithelioid type forming cohesive clusters.
2. Multinucleated giant cells of Langhans' type.

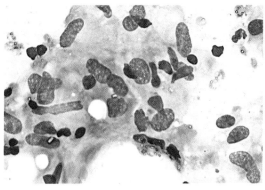

Fig. 5.17 Granulomatous lymphadentis (sarcoidosis)
Cluster of cohesive epithelioid histiocytes (MGG, HP)

5 LYMPH NODES

Epithelioid cells in smears from lymph nodes are quite characteristic. They have elongated nuclei, the shape of which can be described as resembling a footprint, or the sole of a shoe. The nuclear chromatin is very finely granular and pale and the cytoplasm is pale without distinct cell borders (Fig. 5.17). The epithelioid cells usually appear as cohesive clumps reminiscent of granulomas in tissue sections (Figs 8.5 and 8.6). Multinucleated Langhans' giant cells may be few in numbers or totally absent. Cohesive clusters of epithelioid cells in the absence of necrosis is suggestive but not diagnostic of *sarcoidosis*. However, *tuberculosis* has to be ruled out whether necrosis is present or not. Caseous material appears granular and eosinophilic in smears and usually lacks recognisable cell remnants (Figs 5.18 and 5.19). FNA smears of a tuberculous lymph node may sometimes show only polymorphs and necrotic de-

bris without histiocytes, particularly in immunocompromised patients. Acid-fast bacilli should, of course, be looked for both in direct smears and in culture from the aspirate. *Leprosy* in lymph nodes has also been diagnosed by FNAC.[14] If neutrophils are conspicuous in a smear showing epithelioid granulomas and necrosis, one should think of an *atypical mycobacterial infection* if the aspirate is from a cervical node in a child, of *cat scratch disease*[66] if from an axillary node, and of *lymphogranuloma venereum* if it is from an inguinal node (Fig. 5.20). Inclusions in histiocytes and giant cells such as birefringent particles, asteroid bodies, Schaumann bodies etc. are not particularly helpful in making a specific diagnosis. If no aetiological agent is found, one can only report the presence of granuloma with or without necrosis, and the aetiology must be pursued by other means.

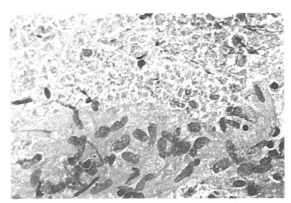

Fig. 5.18 Granulomatous lymphadenitis (tuberculosis)
Small epithelioid cell collection in a background of caseous necrosis (MGG, IP)

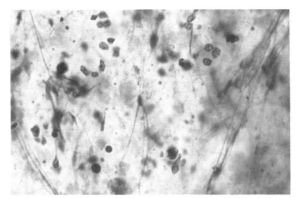

Fig. 5.19 Granulomatous lymphadenitis (tuberculosis)
Granular, acellular material of caseous necrosis. Note presence of polymorphs, a not uncommon feature particularly in AIDS patients (Pap, HP)

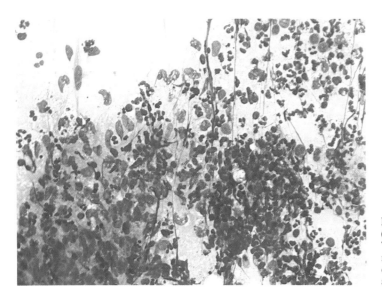

Fig. 5.20 Granulomatous lymphadenitis (lymphogranuloma venereum)
Tissue fragment of epithelioid histiocytes, neutrophils and debris, probably corresponding to the edge of a 'stellate abscess' (MGG, IP)

Problems in diagnosis

1. Tumour necrosis.
2. Other cell types resembling epithelioid cells (e.g. endothelial cells).
3. Granuloma in malignant lymphoma and in nodes regional to carcinoma.

If an aspirate consists entirely of necrotic material with no well-preserved cells, it may be difficult to decide whether it represents caseous necrosis or tumour necrosis (Fig. 8.7b). Re-aspiration, if possible from the periphery of the node, should be done if no bacilli, epithelioid cells or tumour cells are found on careful examination of the smears.

Sometimes only a few epithelioid cells are found in small groups, or as single cells, or the histiocytes may not quite have the typical appearance of epithelioid cells. The pattern then approaches that of non-specific, reactive lymphadenitis with prominent histiocytes. This may be the case in toxoplasma lymphadenitis and in early stages of sarcoidosis. Endothelial cells can sometimes also closely resemble epithelioid histiocytes (compare Fig. 5.3 with Fig. 5.20). Also, deposits of *Kaposi's sarcoma* in lymph nodes may be mistaken for granulomatous lymphadenitis, although the nuclei are more elongated spindly and the nuclear chromatin is darker and coarser than in epithelioid histiocytes (Fig. 5.21).[29,30]

Clusters of epithelioid cells are sometimes found in cases of malignant lymphoma, particularly in Hodgkin's disease and in Lennert's lymphoma (Fig. 5.56). They can also occur in lymph nodes regional to a carcinoma.

One must therefore look carefully for abnormal lymphoid cells and for metastatic cancer cells in smears containing epithelioid histiocytes. Full knowledge of the clinical presentation is obviously essential.

Metastatic malignancy

Criteria for diagnosis

1. Foreign cells amongst normal/reactive lymphoid cells.
2. Cytological criteria of malignancy.

Problems in diagnosis

1. Representative sampling — small metastatic deposits in a reactive lymph node.
2. Benign epithelial inclusions.
3. Necrosis or cystic change.
4. Malignant lymphoma.

Micrometastases, either in the subcapsular sinus (Fig. 5.22) or as scattered single cells, are unlikely to be sampled even by repeated aspirations and can sometimes be missed also by histological examination of an excised node. They are the main cause of false negative cytological reports. Benign epithelial inclusions of salivary gland or thyroid origin in cervical nodes and of Mullerian origin in pelvic nodes have been observed (Fig. 5.23). Such inclusions are usually very small. Although a rare occurrence, this possibility should be kept in mind when only a few epithelial cells without obvious malignant characteristics are found in lymph node aspirates in the appropriate context. Groups of

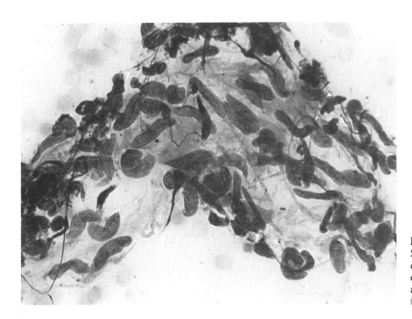

Fig. 5.21 Kaposi's sarcoma
Smear from involved lymph node showing cluster of spindle cells resembling epithelioid granuloma; however, nuclei are more irregular and hyperchromatic (MGG, HP)

5 LYMPH NODES

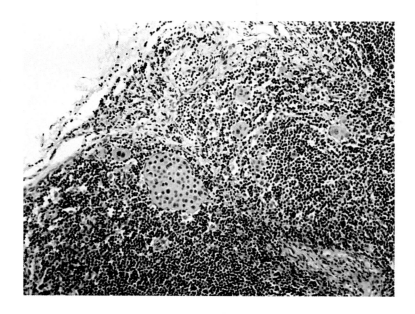

Fig. 5.22 Micrometastasis
Tissue section; minimal deposits of malignant melanoma cells in subcapsular sinus (H & E, LP)

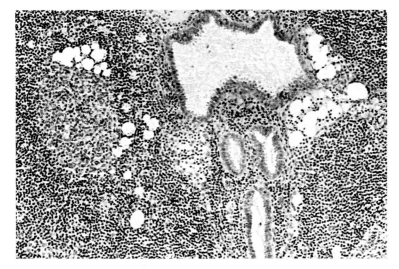

Fig. 5.23 Benign epithelial inclusions
Tissue section; glandular structures of benign Müllerian type in pelvic lymph node (H & E, MP)

glandular epithelial cells of apocrine type are not uncommonly found in FNA smears from axillary nodes. The presence of such cells could give rise to a suspicion of metastasis from breast cancer if the benign characteristics of the cells are not appreciated. In one case we had the opportunity to examine the excised node. No epithelial inclusions were found and we concluded that the apocrine epithelial cells were picked up accidentally by the needle from adjacent sweat glands (Fig. 5.24).

The uncommon problem of differentiating between necrotising lymphadenitis and necrotic tumour has already been mentioned (see also p. 90). Squamous cell carcinoma is particularly prone to undergo liquefactive necrosis. An aspirate from such a node consists of thin, mucoid, yellow fluid. Well-preserved neoplastic squamous cells may be few in numbers and may be very well-differentiated (see Fig. 4.5). There is therefore

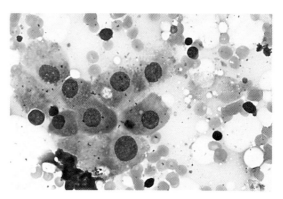

Fig. 5.24 Apocrine cells (axillary node)
Group of apocrine epithelial cells in an aspirate of an axillary lymph node; the anisokaryosis is characteristic of benign apocrine cells (MGG, HP)

a risk of mistaking a cystic metastasis of well-differentiated squamous carcinoma in a cervical gland for a branchial cyst (see p. 39).[82] Cystic nodes in the neck may also represent metastases of papillary carcinoma of the thyroid. This possibility should be remembered particularly in case of unexplained cervical lymphadenopathy in a young patient. The fluid from such nodes contains mainly cyst macrophages but a few groups of atypical epithelial cells found on careful examination of the smears may alert the observer to the possibility of thyroid cancer (Fig. 6.35).

Follicle centre cell lymphoma (centrocytic and mixed centroblastic/centrocytic) may resemble metastasis of small cell anaplastic carcinoma in FNA smears. This is because of the tendency for the centrocytes to form dense clusters of cells, often with nuclear moulding. The problem will be further discussed in the section on lymphoma. Also, large cell lymphoma (centroblastic, immunoblastic) can be difficult to distinguish from large cell anaplastic carcinoma without recourse to immunocytochemistry or electron microscopy.[21]

Indicators of the primary site
The cytological patterns seen in routinely stained smears often give clues to the site of the primary tumour. Columnar cells with elongated nuclei arranged in palisades, stringy mucus and necrosis suggest a primary in the *large bowel* (Fig. 9.62), while mucin-containing signet-ring cells suggest the *stomach* as the most likely primary site among several other possibilities. Glandular cells, moderately pleomorphic, arranged in a gland-in-gland or a cribriform pattern suggest *prostatic carcinoma* (Fig. 5.25a) whereas similar cells forming monolayered sheets are more in keeping with an origin from the *biliary tract*. Large cells with abundant pale, granular, or finely vacuolated cytoplasm and a low N/C ratio suggest a *renal cell carcinoma*. Very large central nucleoli are typical of less well differentiated forms of this tumour and are also seen in *large cell anaplastic carcinoma of lung* and in *hepatocellular carcinoma*. *Pulmonary* and *pancreatic adenocarcinoma* can have a variety of patterns. They usually show a moderate degree of glandular differentiation, prominent nuclear pleomorphism and obvious mucin secretion. As a rule the presence of intracytoplasmic mucin excludes renal, adrenal, hepatocellular and thyroid carcinoma. *Breast cancer* usually displays poor glandular differentiation while cell balls and single files of cells are more common. Some tumours form a monolayer of dispersed cells with intact cytoplasm. Nuclear pleomorphism is often relatively mild (Fig. 5.26).

The nuclei of a *small cell anaplastic carcinoma of lung* may appear large in air-dried smears but the amount of cytoplasm is minimal. Nucleoli are very small and indistinct in typical cases. The cells are closely packed together in aggregates or as single files with prominent nuclear moulding. Pyknotic nuclei and nuclear debris are commonly seen between preserved cells, in the abs-

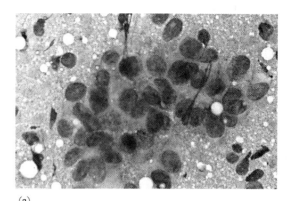
(a)

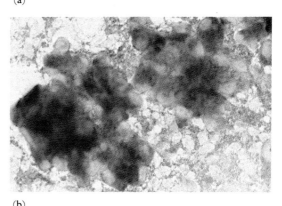
(b)

Fig. 5.25 2⁰ Prostatic carcinoma
(a) Supraclavicular node aspirate containing malignant cells from a metastatic adenocarcinoma (MGG, HP); (b) strongly positive staining for acid phosphatase (enzymatic method, HP)

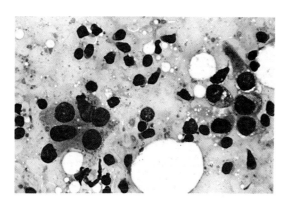

Fig. 5.26 2⁰ Breast carcinoma
Few aggregates of poorly differentiated carcinoma cells in a background of lymphocytes (MGG, HP)

ence of massive necrosis. 'Tear-drop' nuclear artefacts caused by smearing are characteristic (Figs 8.26–8.28). Smears of *malignant melanoma* show total dissociation of cells, well-defined cytoplasm, prominent anisokaryosis, a uniformly dense chromatin which does not vary much from nucleus to nucleus, large nucleoli, binucleate cells,

5 LYMPH NODES

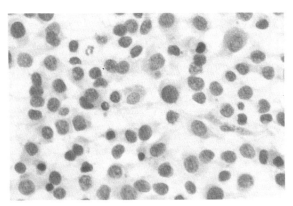

Fig. 5.27 Metastatic melanoma mimicking lymphoma
Dispersed malignant cells with eccentric nuclei and pale
cytoplasm; lymphoid globules absent (Pap, HP)

intranuclear vacuoles and, in most cases, some cells with
intracytoplasmic pigment (Figs 11.7–11.10). Malignant
melanoma can occasionally mimic lymphoma in FNA
smears (Fig. 5.27). Testicular tumours may be clinically

occult and present with metastases to pelvic, para-
aortic, or supraclavicular nodes. The cytological pattern
of *seminoma* is characteristic. The tumour cells are
mainly dissociated and are mixed with lymphocytes.
They have large, rounded, vesicular nuclei and an
evenly distributed nuclear chromatin. Nucleoli are
prominent but relatively small in wet-fixed smears. The
cytoplasm is pale and both cytoplasm and nuclei are
very fragile, the dispersed cytoplasm forming a 'tigroid'
background to the nuclei (Fig. 10.21).[32] Cells from a
transitional cell carcinoma are usually dispersed but may
form solid and sometimes papillary groups. The cells
have abundant, relatively dense cytoplasm with distinct
borders, and pleomorphic nuclei which are often eccentric (Fig. 9.54). A tendency to squamous differentiation
or a spindle cell pattern may be seen.

It is advisable to divide the cell sample on to multiple
slides so that spare slides are available for special stains.
Squamous differentiation is best seen in alcohol-fixed
Pap-stained smears. The histochemical demonstration of
intracytoplasmic mucin droplets is helpful in adeno-

Table 5.1 Entities of the Kiel classification and their equivalents in the Working Formulation (WF)

Kiel classification	WF equivalent
Low-grade malignant lymphomas	
Lymphocytic	
B-CLL	Small lymphocytic, consistent with CLL (A)
T-CLL	Small lymphocytic, consistent with CLL (A)
Hairy-cell leukaemia	Hairy cell leukaemia
Mycosis fungoides/Sézary's syndrome	Mycosis fungoides/Sézary's syndrome
T-zone lymphoma	Large cell, immunoblastic, polymorphous (H)
Lymphoplasmacytic/-cytoid	
lymphoplasmacytic	Small lymphocytic, plasmacytoid (A)
lymphoplasmacytoid	Small lymphocytic, plasmacytoid (A)
polymorphic	Diffused, mixed, small and large cell (F)
Plasmacytic	Extramedullary plasmacytoma
Centrocytic	Diffuse, small cleaved cell (E)
	Diffuse, large cell, cleaved cell (G)
Centroblastic-centrocytic	Follicular, predominantly small cleaved cell (B)
follicular	Follicular, mixed, small cleaved and large cell (C)
follicular and diffuse	Follicular, predominantly large cell (D)
diffuse	Diffuse, mixed, small and large cell (F)
	Diffuse, large cell, cleaved cell (F)
High-grade malignant lymphomas	
Centroblastic	Diffuse, large cell, non-cleaved cell (G)
Lymphoblastic	
B-lymphoblastic	Small non-cleaved cell (J)
Burkitt type	Small non-cleaved cell, Burkitt's (J)
T-lymphoblastic	Lymphoblastic, convoluted cell and non-convoluted cell (I)
convoluted-cell type	Lymphoblastic, convoluted cell (I)
unclassified	Lymphoblastic, non-convoluted cell (I)
Immunoblastic	Large cell, immunoblastic (H)

(Reproduced with permission from: Rilke F, Lennert K: A perspective of the Kiel Classification in relation to other recent
classification of non-Hodgkin's lymphoma, with special reference to the Working Formulation. In: Lennert K (ed.) *Histopathology
of non-Hodgkin's lymphoma*. Springer, New York, 1981.)

carcinoma. Strong positivity for acid phosphatase by the enzymatic method or positive immunocytochemical staining for prostatic acid phosphatase and/or prostate-specific antigen in an adenocarcinoma supports a prostatic origin (Fig. 5.25b).[1] This should be done in all metastatic adenocarcinomas of unknown origin in male patients in view of the effective palliative treatment available for disseminated prostatic carcinoma. Distant metastases, particularly to supraclavicular lymph nodes, are sometimes the first manifestation of prostatic cancer preceding any urinary symptoms. Formalin-induced fluorescence using an air-dried, unstained smear is a very simple test for melanin precursors in amelanotic melanoma (see p. 19, Figs 11.10–11.11). Other amines also react; the test is positive, for example, in carcinoid tumours. Immunoperoxidase staining for S100 or for more specific markers for melanoma is more reliable. Other useful tumour markers are NSE and chromogranin in neuroendocrine tumours, a variety of hormones and polypeptides in endocrine tumours, alphafetoprotein in hepatocellular carcinoma and certain germ cell tumours etc. (see Table 2.4). Electron micros-

copical examination of the aspirate can be most helpful, particularly in small round cell tumours and in some mesenchymal tumours (see Table 2.1).

Non-Hodgkin's lymphoma[8,25,27,40a,47,56,58,69,70]
Cytological subtyping of non-Hodgkin's lymphoma (NHL) in FNA smears is difficult and requires extensive experience. It can only be successful in centres with a team of oncology experts and with a regular flow of material. However, the diagnostic criteria of lymphoma in cytological preparations vary with the histological subtype. It is therefore necessary to describe the main subtypes in some detail. Of all current classifications of NHL, the Kiel classification can most readily be applied to cytological preparations and is, therefore, used in this presentation. Equivalent terms for the working formulation appear in Table 5.1. The Kiel and working formulation terms for the various lymphocyte subtypes are diagrammatically illustrated in Figure 5.28.[44,76] The classification of Lukes and Collins uses different terminology but is based on similar cytological criteria and is easily translated into the Kiel classification.[45]

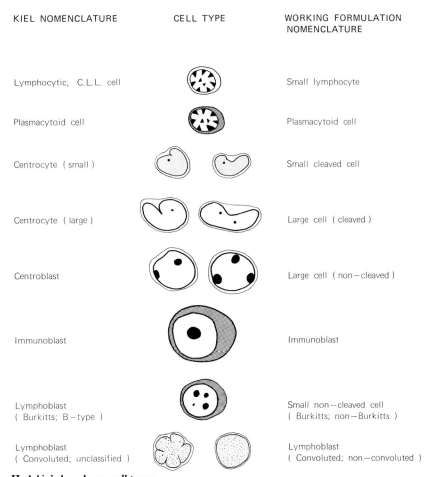

KIEL NOMENCLATURE	CELL TYPE	WORKING FORMULATION NOMENCLATURE
Lymphocytic, C.L.L. cell		Small lymphocyte
Plasmacytoid cell		Plasmacytoid cell
Centrocyte (small)		Small cleaved cell
Centrocyte (large)		Large cell (cleaved)
Centroblast		Large cell (non–cleaved)
Immunoblast		Immunoblast
Lymphoblast (Burkitts; B – type)		Small non–cleaved cell (Burkitts; non–Burkitts)
Lymphoblast (Convoluted; unclassified)		Lymphoblast (Convoluted; non–convoluted)

Fig. 5.28 Non-Hodgkin's lymphoma cell types
Diagrammatic representation of the various stages of lymphocyte transformation as seen mainly in alcohol-fixed material

5 *LYMPH NODES*

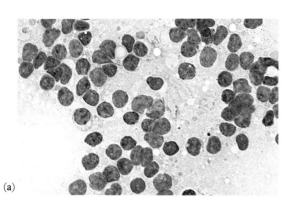

(a)

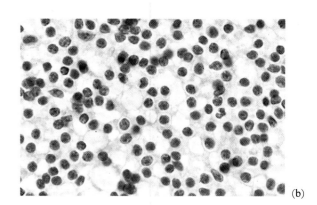

(b)

Fig. 5.29 ML lymphocytic (CLL)
Monotonous population of slightly enlarged lymphocytes with coarsely granular chromatin (a. MGG, HP; b. H & E, HP)

The various cell types and cytological patterns of non-Hodgkin's lymphomas as seen in imprint preparations of nodes have been beautifully illustrated by workers at the City of Hope National Medical Centre in California.[40a]

Criteria for diagnosis

Malignant lymphoma (ML) lymphocytic; CLL
(Figs 5.29 and 5.30)

1. A monotonous population of small lymphoid cells.
2. Mainly round nuclei slightly larger than those of normal small lymphocytes.
3. Nuclear chromatin paler and more granular than in normal lymphocytes; nucleoli absent.
4. Conspicuously few blast forms and histiocytes except in smears derived from proliferation centres.

Recognition of the subtle differences between small lymphocytes and the small cells of lymphocytic lymphoma requires optimal cytological preparations. The typical well differentiated lymphocytic lymphoma of CLL type is readily recognised by the monotonous population of cells resembling small lymphocytes (Fig. 5.29). Dif-

ficulties can arise if the process contains proliferation centres with many large and intermediate size cells — paraimmunoblasts and prolymphocytes (Fig. 5.30). If these are well represented in the smears, the characteristic monotony of the cell population is obviously lost. However, dendritic reticulum cells from germinal centres and tingible body macrophages are still absent and there are no centrocytes or centroblasts.

ML lymphoplasmacytoid; plasmacytic; myeloma
(Figs 5.31–5.33)

1. A mixed population of atypical lymphocytes, plasma cells and some blasts.
2. Many lymphocytes with plasmacytoid features.
3. Intracytoplasmic immunoglobulin globules in some lymphoid cells.
4. Plasmacytic subtype (plasmacytoma): predominance of differentiated plasma cells.
5. Cases with poorly differentiated immunoblast-like cells are difficult to distinguish from ML immunoblastic.

ML centroblastic/centrocytic (Figs 5.34–5.36)

1. Irregular, angular, comma-shaped, elongated or cleaved nuclei; moderately larger and paler and more variable in size than those of normal lymphocytes (centrocytes).
2. A tendency to form clusters of cells with some degree of nuclear moulding.
3. A variable proportion of centroblasts.

In centroblastic/centrocytic lymphoma the majority of cells are centrocytes. Intermingled with these is a variable number of centroblasts. Small lymphocytes are also present but they constitute a minority of the population (Fig. 5.34). The characteristic nuclear morphology of centrocytes is best demonstrated in cytocentrifuge preparations of cell suspensions (Fig. 5.36). The irregular nuclear shape is often less obvious in direct smears and

Fig. 5.30 ML lymphocytic (CLL)
Note the presence of many large cells (prolymphocytes) representing proliferation centre (MGG, HP)

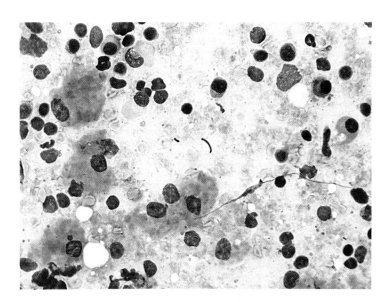

Fig. 5.31 ML lymphoplasmacytoid
Lymphoid cells distended with immunoglobulin (IgM by IPOX) and scattered plasmacytoid cells; clinically Waldenström's disease (MGG, HP)

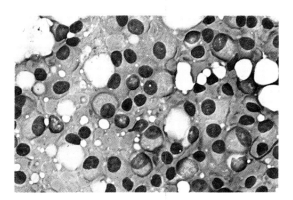

Fig. 5.32 ML plasmacytic
Pure population of well-differentiated plasma cells (MGG, HP)

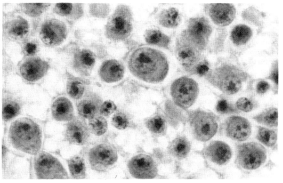

Fig. 5.33 Myeloma in lymph node
Poorly differentiated plasmacytoid cells. This patient had multiple myeloma (Pap, HP)

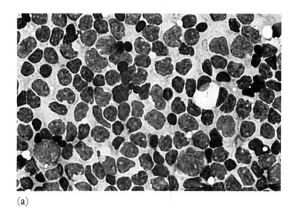

(a)

(b)

Fig. 5.34 ML centroblastic/centrocytic
Predominance of medium-sized cells with irregular sometimes cleaved nuclei; occasional centroblasts with multiple nucleoli (a. MGG, HP; b. H & E, HP)

5 LYMPH NODES

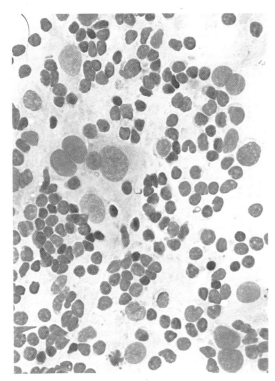

Fig. 5.35 ML centroblastic/centrocytic
Dendritic reticulum cells may be prominent, particularly in follicular lymphomas; note the predominance of centrocytes (MGG, HP)

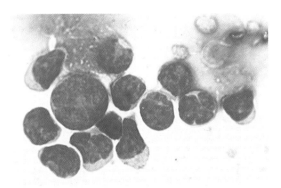

Fig. 5.36 ML centroblastic/centrocytic
Cytocentrifuge preparation; centrocytes showing cleaved nuclei; one centroblast (MGG, HP Oil)

centrocytes are then identified by the intermediate size of the nuclei and by the nuclear chromatin, paler and more granular than that of lymphocytes. Histiocytes, occasionally with tingible bodies, may be present, and dendritic reticulum cells are commonly seen (Fig. 5.35).

It is not possible in FNA smears to predict with a sufficient degree of confidence if a centroblastic/centrocytic lymphoma will be follicular or diffuse in histological sections. Cytological features which suggest a follicular lymphoma are a high proportion of lymphocytes and many dendritic reticulum cells. It is also difficult to assess the relative proportions of small and large centrocytes and of centroblasts, as these are influenced by sampling bias, and therefore to make a clear distinction between centroblastic/centrocytic and centroblastic lymphoma. For example, confluent areas of centroblasts which histologically define a lymphoma as centroblastic, may not be represented in the FNA sample. As a rule, we diagnose centroblastic lymphoma if 50% or more of the cell population, as assessed subjectively, are centroblasts, whereas the classification is uncertain in the range 25–50%.

ML centrocytic (Fig. 5.37)

1. A monotonous population of small or large centrocytes.
2. Only occasional centroblasts.

This is the type of lymphoma which is most easily confused with metastasis of small cell anaplastic carcinoma due to the tendency for centrocytes to adhere to each other in clumps with nuclear moulding. This problem is discussed on page 87. If more than a few centroblasts are present in the smears, the case is categorised as centroblastic/centrocytic.

ML centroblastic (Fig. 5.38)

1. A smear population of centroblasts and centrocytes; few lymphocytes or immunoblasts.
2. A high proportion of the cells are centroblasts.
3. Plasma cells, histiocytes, dendritic reticulum cells rare.

Centroblasts have large vesicular nuclei of moderately irregular shape. They have multiple nucleoli, characteristically present at the nuclear membrane. The cytoplasm is scanty, fragile (many nuclei are stripped), pale or basophilic. Some centrocytes are always present among the blasts. Nuclear pleomorphism can be very prominent in some cases including very large, multilobated nuclei which may resemble Reed-Sternberg cells, and nuclei with single central nucleoli (pleomorphic subtype).

ML lymphoblastic Burkitt's type (Figs 5.39 and 5.40)[17]

1. A relatively uniform cell population with a high mitotic rate.
2. Rounded nuclei of variable but predominantly intermediate size.
3. A granular or speckled chromatin pattern; multiple small but prominent nucleoli.
4. A thin rim of dense blue cytoplasm with small vacuoles (MGG).
5. 'Starry sky' histiocytes.

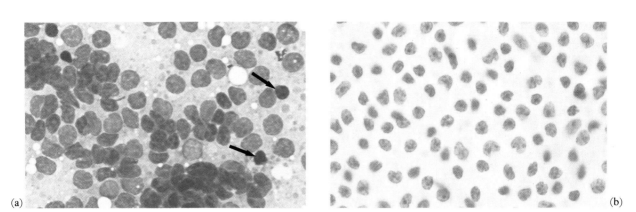

(a)

(b)

Fig. 5.37 ML centrocytic
Nuclei a little larger than those of lymphocytes, irregular shape, granular chromatin, tendency to clumping. A few normal lymphocytes (arrows) present. (a) MGG, HP. (b) Pap, HP

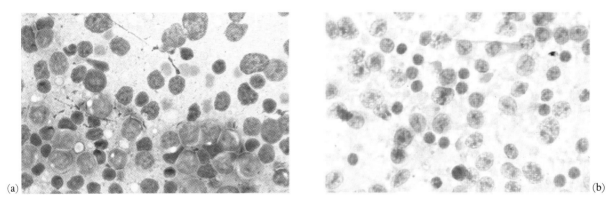

(a)

(b)

Fig. 5.38 ML centroblastic
Predominance of large lymphoid cells with pale nuclei, scanty cytoplasm and multiple, often peripheral nucleoli (a. MGG, HP; b. H & E, HP)

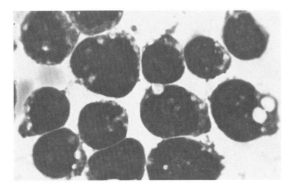

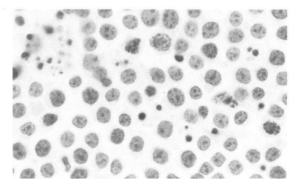

Fig. 5.39 ML lymphoblastic (Burkitt's)
Cytocentrifuge preparation; rounded lymphoid cells; some variation in nuclear size; granular chromatin; moderate amounts of dense blue cytoplasm and lipid vacuoles (MGG, HP oil)

Fig. 5.40 ML lymphoblastic (Burkitt's)
Lymphoblastic cells with round nuclei of varying size and small amount of cytoplasm; occasional 'starry sky' macrophages (Pap, HP)

5 LYMPH NODES

Lipid droplets can be demonstrated in the strongly basophilic cytoplasm of the neoplastic cells. Large histiocytes with intracytoplasmic debris ('starry sky' cells) are often prominent.

ML lymphoblastic convoluted type (Fig. 5.41)

1. A relatively uniform cell population with a high mitotic rate.
2. Intermediate size nuclei.
3. Some very complex — convoluted or cerebriform — nuclei.
4. Finely granular chromatin; inconspicuous nucleoli.
5. Scanty, pale, fragile cytoplasm.

In this type of lymphoblastic lymphoma some of the nuclei have a very complex shape. Their convoluted, lobulated or segmented (cerebriform) shape is most striking in cytocentrifuge preparations of cell suspensions. It seems to be related to the mode of preparation to some extent and appears to be exaggerated by centrifugation. Lymphoblasts with convoluted nuclei usually have markers for T cells, but in some cases the neoplastic cells have markers consistent with a B-cell origin. In

particular, we have noted a similar nuclear complexity in several B-cell lymphomas after treatment. The cytomorphology alone is thus insufficient to classify the lymphoma as of T-cell type. Also, the mere presence of convoluted nuclei does not establish a diagnosis of lymphoma since similar cells can be seen as a reactive component in B-cell lymphomas and in reactive processes.

ML lymphoblastic unclassified (acute lymphoblastic leukaemia) (Fig. 5.42)[22]

1. A homogenous population of cells of one type.
2. Round nuclei mainly of intermediate size but showing considerable variation in size.
3. Granular or 'speckled' nuclear chromatin; multiple small nucleoli.
4. Moderately basophilic, fragile cytoplasm.

A number of lymphoblastic lymphomas lack both B- and T-cell markers. This type of ML is mainly seen in children and the cytomorphology is similar to acute lymphoblastic leukaemia. B-lymphoblastic lymphomas of non-Burkitt type seen in adults, sometimes in extra-

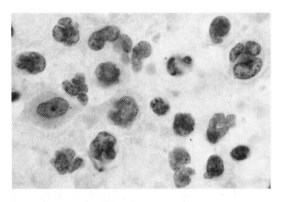

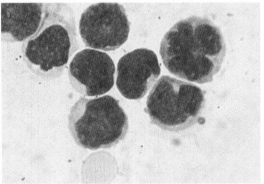

Fig. 5.41 ML lymphoblastic (convoluted)
Note the hyperlobulated appearance of the nuclei; the feature appears to be exaggerated in cytological preparations compared to histological section (a. H & E, HP Oil; b. cytocentrifuge preparation MGG, HP Oil)

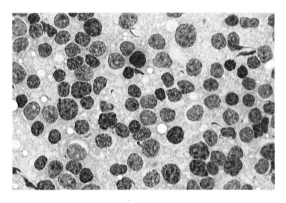

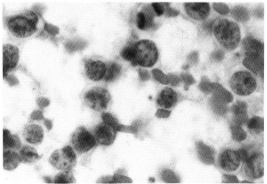

Fig. 5.42 ML lymphoblastic (unclassified)
Rounded nuclei of variable, mainly intermediate size; fragile cytoplasm; speckled nuclear chromatin. (a. MGG, HP; Pap, HP)

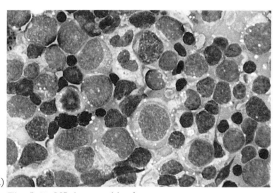
(a)

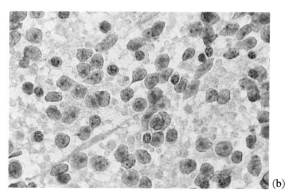
(b)

Fig. 5.43 ML immunoblastic
Predominantly large lymphoid cells with large vesicular nuclei, large central nucleoli (b) and abundant basophilic cytoplasm
(a. HGG, HP; b. H & E, HP)

nodal sites, have a similar cytomorphology, perhaps with a tendency to greater nuclear pleomorphism.

ML immunoblastic (Fig. 5.43)

1. A pleomorphic cell population dominated by large blasts; sometimes extreme pleomorphism and multinucleated cells (T-immunoblastic subtype).
2. Unevenly distributed nuclear chromatin; prominent, usually single central nucleoli; frequent mitoses.
3. A proportion of smaller, normal and abnormal lymphoid cells.
4. Abundant blue cytoplasm (MGG); eccentric nucleus and a perinuclear pale zone (plasmacytoid differentiation).

Tingible body macrophages may be seen in smears of immunoblastic lymphoma as in any lymphoma with a high mitotic rate. The distinction from pleomorphic centroblastic lymphoma with a proportion of immunoblasts can be subtle. T-immunoblastic lymphoma and Hodgkin's disease also present differential diagnostic problems.

True histiocytic lymphoma (Fig. 5.44)
It is difficult to recognise this rare type of lymphoma correctly in routine cytological smears. A very pleomorphic cell population with multilobed nuclei and multinucleated cells which may resemble Reed-Sternberg cells should make one think of this possibility. The differential diagnosis includes ML immunblastic, pleomorphic T-cell lymphoma, and Hodgkin's lymphoma. Immunocytochemistry and EM are required to confirm the diagnosis.

Problems in diagnosis of lymphoma

1. Suboptimal cytological preparations.
2. Variable pattern in one node.
3. Reactive lymphadenopathy.
4. ML with few neoplastic cells in a dominant population of reactive lymphoid cells.

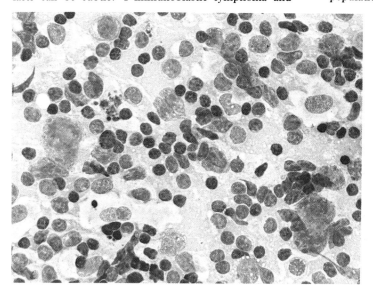

Fig. 5.44 ML true histiocytic
Many multinucleated large cells, somewhat resembling Reed–Sternberg cells; diagnosis confirmed by immunocytochemistry and EM (MGG. HP)

5 LYMPH NODES

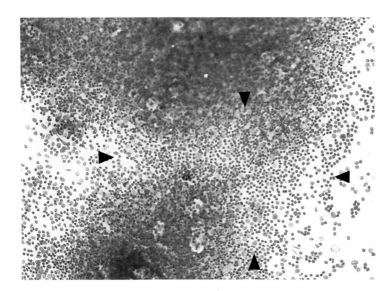

Fig. 5.45 Cellular smear
Only areas of optimal dispersal and fixation should be selected for evaluation in lymph node smears (arrowed) (MGG, LP)

5. Small cell anaplastic carcinoma and other small cell tumours, particularly versus ML centrocytic.
6. Large cell anaplastic carcinoma versus Ki-1 lymphoma.[75]
7. Effects of chemotherapy and radiotherapy.

Direct smears must be made expertly, since poor preparation makes accurate diagnosis impossible (Figs 5.45 and 5.46). In our experience, suboptimal smears are the commonest cause of diagnostic difficulties and misinterpretations. Both air-dried MGG-stained smears and alcohol-fixed smears stained by Pap or by H & E should be examined in parallel, as both provide complementary information (see Ch. 2). Smears of a cell suspension prepared in the cytocentrifuge, in addition to routine smears, are very helpful in the diagnosis and classification of NHL, and are better suited for immune marker studies (Figs 5.36, 5.41b and 2.18).

Sampling bias cannot always be avoided and may lead to an erroneous diagnosis. An aspirate from a node which is only partially involved by lymphoma may not be representative. In follicular lymphoma, the cell population of a sample mainly representing a nodule looks different compared to a sample derived from an interfollicular area. This can lead to errors in subclassification within the range ML centroblastic/centrocytic–centroblastic, which may have important prognostic implications.

The difference between normal lymphocytes and the neoplastic cells of ML lymphocytic (well-differentiated) is relatively subtle, and the most obvious diagnostic feature is the monotony of the cell population. However, a sample including proliferation centres does not appear monotonous since there can be many cells of intermediate and large size (prolymphocytes and paraimmunoblasts[44]) mixed with the typical cells of CLL type (Fig. 5.30). Such a case can be mistaken for

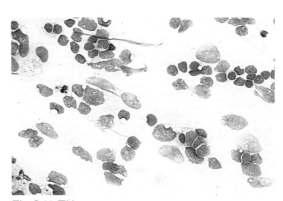

Fig. 5.46 Thin smear
Smudged nuclei, for example those in the tail of a smear, are impossible to evaluate (MGG, HP)

reactive lymphadenopathy unless close attention is paid to fine cytological detail of the lymphocytes. ML lymphoplasmacytoid can also be mistaken for reactive lymphadenopathy in view of the pleomorphic character of the smear population. Again, a close study of cell detail reveals atypical lymphoid cells with plasmacytoid features. Clinical and biochemical data must, of course, be taken into consideration. In ML centroblastic/centrocytic (follicular) there may be a high proportion of small lymphocytes to suggest a benign, reactive process, if the sample mainly derives from interfollicular areas. Also, the small cleaved cells of some follicular lymphomas can be difficult to distinguish from lymphocytes in a reactive process, particularly if smears are not technically optimal. Nuclei must be studied carefully in high power to appreciate the slightly larger size, irregular shape and granular chromatin. Follicular lymphoma with a predominance of small cleaved cells is the type of

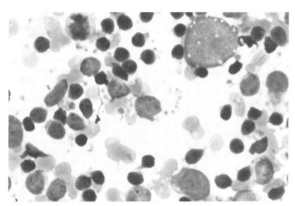

Fig. 5.47 Recurrent large cell lymphoma
A few neoplastic cells with very large nuclei scattered in dominant population of reactive cells (MGG, HP)

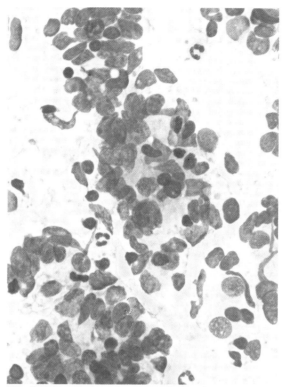

Fig. 5.48 Pseudoglandular clusters in lymphoma
Such clusters may simulate small cell anaplastic carcinoma or adenocarcinoma; this problem mainly occurs in follicular lymphomas (MGG, HP)

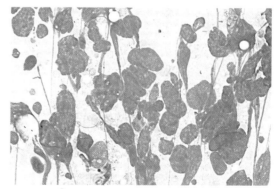

Fig. 5.49 2⁰ Melanoma
This cytological pattern, including cell clustering and nuclear moulding resembling that of a small cell carcinoma can be seen in lymphoma, particularly of follicular type; this case was in fact a metastatic melanoma; the main clue to a non-lymphoid origin here was the very large size of nuclei when compared to lymphoid cells in the smear; the pattern is very unusual for melanoma (MGG, IIP)

lymphoma which is most likely to be missed and misinterpreted as reactive lymphadenopathy by FNAC.

Occasionally, non-Hodgkin's lymphoma of large cell type may have relatively few neoplastic cells scattered in a background of reactive lymphoid cells (Fig. 5.47). Unless the neoplastic cells are very large and abnormal, such cases are impossible to diagnose correctly by FNA, especially since a few large, atypical-looking immunoblasts are sometimes seen in reactive lymphadenopathy.

In FNA smears, cleaved cells, particularly large cleaved cells, of ML centrocytic and ML centroblastic/centrocytic have a tendency to clump together into dense aggregates showing some moulding of the nuclei. Rows and palisades of closely apposed, ovoid nuclei which appear columnar through moulding may simulate small cell anaplastic carcinoma or even adenocarcinoma (Fig. 5.48). However, the proportion of isolated cells is usually larger in lymphoma and many of these have the typical appearance of lymphoid cells with a rim of basophilic cytoplasm and a nuclear chromatin pattern which is different from that of carcinoma cells. Importantly, nuclei of lymphoma cells of a similar size to those of small cell anaplastic carcinoma usually have prominent nucleoli. This is a helpful but not infallible feature: nuclei of large cleaved cells (centrocytes) and of small cell carcinoma of intermediate type may be very similar in size and may have similar nucleoli. Nuclear moulding and well formed single files of tumour cells are more obvious in small cell carcinoma and other metastatic small cell tumours (Fig. 5.49). The pale-blue, uniformly rounded cytoplasmic fragments characteristic of lymphoid tissue (lymphoid globules) are different from the cytoplasmic and nuclear fragments of tumour necrosis in smears of carcinomas (compare Figs 5.1 and 5.2). Immunoperoxidase staining for cytokeratin and a panleucocyte marker can usually solve the problem of distinguishing between lymphoma and small cell carcinoma in difficult cases.

Smears of large cell anaplastic carcinoma may show total dissociation of the tumour cells, nuclei may be large, vesicular and have prominent nucleoli, and the cells may have a rim of basophilic cytoplasm. This pattern can be indistinguishable from large cell lympho-

5 LYMPH NODES

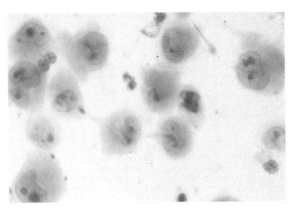

Fig. 5.50 ML large cell undifferentiated
Case of Richter's syndrome. Large, undifferentiated cells with vesicular nuclei and large nucleoli closely resembling large cell undifferentiated carcinoma (Pap, HP)

ma, particularly from Ki-1 lymphoma (Fig. 5.50). The presence of cytoplasmic fragments in lymphoma (lymphoid globules) is helpful. Well formed aggregates of tumour cells, not just clumping of cells, are not seen in lymphoma. Again, in difficult cases, immunological staining for cytokeratin and a panleucocyte marker is usually decisive. However, the commonly used immune markers may not solve the problem of distinguishing Ki-1 lymphoma from large cell carcinoma, and this may require electron microscopical examination.[75]

Chemotherapy and radiotherapy may cause changes to lymphoma cells which render typing more difficult. In particular, treatment seems to cause an increased irregularity of nuclear shapes. However, if a recurrence is of higher grade than the original process, for example a follicular mixed cell lymphoma recurring as large cell lymphoma, the change in cytological pattern is usually obvious.

Hodgkin's lymphoma (Figs 5.51–5.56)[20,28,37]

Criteria for diagnosis

1. Reed-Sternberg cells.
2. Atypical mononuclear cells.
3. A variable number of eosinophils, plasma cells and histiocytes.
4. A background population of lymphocytes.

A confident diagnosis of Hodgkin's disease can only be made in the presence of typical Reed-Sternberg cells with a background of lymphocytes and reactive cells as listed above. Reed-Sternberg cells have large, lobulated nuclei which may appear symmetrically double (mirror nuclei), or complex and multiple. The nuclear chromatin is coarse and is irregularly distributed in a reticular fashion with clear areas in between which give the nucleus an overall pale appearance. Nucleoli are large, often huge, eosinophilic in H & E preparations, pale grey-blue in MGG-stained smears. The cytoplasm is abundant, but is pale and fragile so that the nucleus often appears to be surrounded by an empty space (Figs 5.51–5.53). Sometimes the characteristic nucleoli are not well demonstrated and in some cases only mononuclear cells which have a nuclear structure similar to the typical Reed-Sternberg cells (mononuclear Hodgkin's cells, Fig. 5.54) are present. In such cases the definitive diagnosis must await histological examination, except in recurrent disease when classical Reed-Sternberg cells are not essential for diagnosis.

Histological examination is also necessary to distinguish confidently the four subtypes of Hodgkin's disease: lymphocyte predominance, nodular sclerosis, mixed cellularity, and lymphocyte depletion. The two extremes, lymphocyte predominance and lymphocyte depletion are, of course, reflected in the smears by the number of lymphocytes relative to the number of Reed-

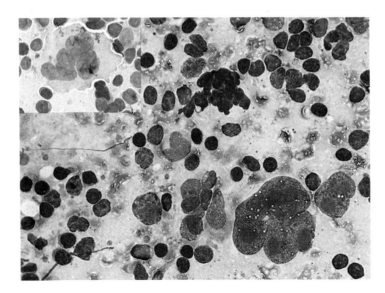

Fig. 5.51 Hodgkin's lymphoma
Reed–Sternberg cell with multiple nuclei, and large nucleoli. Inset: lacunar cell, with an irregular multilobulated nucleus and inconspicuous nucleoli (MGG, HP)

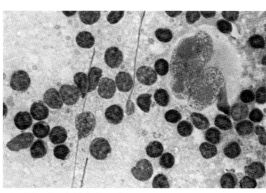

Fig. 5.52 Hodgkin's lymphoma
Reed–Sternberg cell; note the well-defined, but rather pale cytoplasm. (a. MGG, HP; b. Pap, HP)

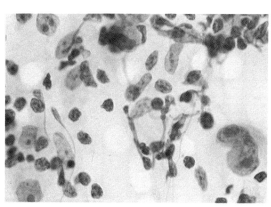

Fig. 5.53 Hodgkin's lymphoma
Reed–Sternberg cell with bilobed nucleus and large nucleoli (Pap, HP)

Sternberg and mononuclear Hodgkin's cells. The lacunar type of Reed-Sternberg cell recognised in histological sections of nodular sclerosis Hodgkin's disease can not often be distinguished as a specific variant in FNA smears (Fig. 5.51, inset). The tough consistency of the node felt with the needle, a scanty aspirate, and the presence of fibroblasts and collagen fragments in the smear are features suggestive of the nodular sclerosis type. In the mixed cellularity type, typical Reed-Sternberg cells are usually easy to find and there are many plasma cells and eosinophils as well as histiocytes in the background cell population.[53]

Problems in diagnosis

1. Poor biopsy yield.
2. Reed-Sternberg look-alike cells in other conditions.
3. T-immunoblastic and true histiocytic lymphoma.
4. Epithelioid histiocytes suggestive of granulomatous lymphadenitis.

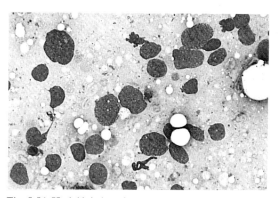

Fig. 5.54 Hodgkin's lymphoma
Recurrent lymphoma; atypical mononuclear cell forms only (MGG, HP)

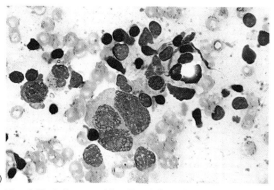

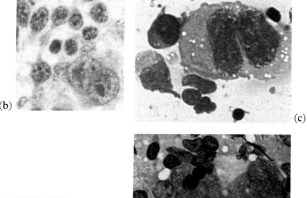

Fig. 5.55 Cells resembling Reed–Sternberg cells
(a) Large binucleate cell in case of immunoblastic lymphadenopathy (MGG, HP).
(b) Reed–Sternberg-like binucleate cell in case of infectious mononucleosis (Pap, HP).
(c) Large binucleate cell in large cell lymphoma (ML IB) (MGG, HP). (d) Very large binucleate cell in metastatic squamous cell carcinoma (MGG, HP)

5 LYMPH NODES

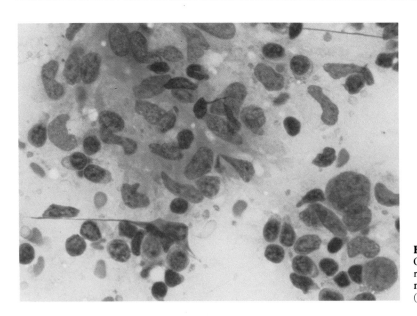

Fig. 5.56 Hodgkin's lymphoma
Clusters of epithelioid histiocytes resembling granulomatous lymphadenitis; note large abnormal cells lower right (MGG, HP)

Poor biopsy yield is a problem mainly in the nodular sclerosis subtype. Not infrequently, smears show only a few lymphocytes, fibroblasts and fragments of collagen suggestive of a chronic inflammatory process. Multiple biopsies or the use of a Rotex screw needle may be necessary to obtain sufficient material.

Large, multilobated nuclei resembling Reed-Sternberg cells can be seen in a variety of conditions (Fig. 5.55a–d). Atypical immunoblasts in non-neoplastic reactive lymphadenopathy, for example in mononucleosis, and in angioimmunoblastic lymphadenopathy, may have nuclei of this type. They usually differ from the typical Reed-Sternberg cells by having smaller and darker nucleoli, a denser chromatin and a basophilic cytoplasm. Cells of large cell non-Hodgkin's lymphoma (centroblastic, immunoblastic, T-immunoblastic, true histiocytic) can also have large nuclei similar but not identical to those of Reed-Sternberg cells.[72] Such cases are unlikely to be mistaken for Hodgkin's disease since the majority of the smear population consists of clearly abnormal lymphoid cells. The most difficult differential diagnosis is T-immunoblastic lymphoma in which both the giant cells and the background of predominantly small T cells may be very similar to Hodgkin's disease. Immunological studies may be necessary to solve the problem. Finally, we have seen an occasional example of large malignant cells with multilobated nuclei in a background of reactive lymphoid cells, representing single malignant cells of metastatic carcinoma (Fig. 5.55d), which were misdiagnosed as Hodgkin's lymphoma.

Clusters of epithelioid histiocytes are sometimes seen in smears of Hodgkin's lymphoma — as in some non-Hodgkin's lymphomas — and could suggest granulomatous lymphadenitis (Fig. 5.56). The lymphoid cells must therefore always be carefully scrutinised in lymph node smears containing epithelioid cells.

Lymph node necrosis (Fig. 5.57)[16,78]
Extensive or total necrosis/infarction of lymph nodes occurs in some inflammatory processes, in metastatic malignancy, in malignant lymphoma and rarely in relation to vasculitis and to trauma. If necrosis is extensive,

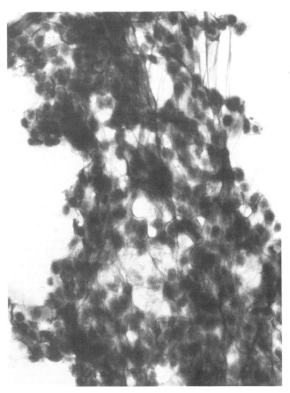

Fig. 5.57 Lymph node necrosis
Amorphous debris and necrotic single cells, reminiscent of ischaemic necrosis, or tumour necrosis; subsequent lymph node excision showed non-Hodgkin's lymphoma (MGG, HP)

LYMPH NODES 5

FNA smears may not include any well-preserved cells necessary for diagnosis.

Completely amorphous, granular material without identifiable cell remnants suggests caseous necrosis and smears should be searched for acid fast bacilli and other micro-organisms. In acute inflammatory necrosis, the aspirate and smears have a purulent character. Necrotising lymphadenitis (Kikuchi) is a condition seen mainly in young women in which there is focal necrosis in cervical lymph nodes.[78] The presence of large mononuclear cells in such nodes may cause a suspicion of malignant lymphoma. We have not yet seen an example of this disease in FNA smears. Necrosis in lymph nodes may also occur in systemic lupus.

Smears of infarcted nodes show numerous cell shadows, some with preserved but pyknotic nuclei. Unless there is a clear history of trauma, such findings suggest either metastatic carcinoma or malignant lymphoma. Nodal metastases of small cell anaplastic carcinoma of lung, melanoma and breast carcinoma are prone to necrosis and the necrotic cells with pyknotic nuclei can be indistinguishable from necrotic lymphoid cells. Extensive necrosis/infarction is not uncommon in malignant lymphoma, both non-Hodgkin's and Hodgkin's. Total infarction of a lymph node can sometimes precede manifest lymphoma.[16] FNA biopsy should be repeated, if possible from other abnormal nodes, and if a diagnosis can still not be made, surgical excision is indicated.

REFERENCES AND SUGGESTED FURTHER READING

1. Allhoff E P, Proppe K H, Chapman C M, Lin C-W, Prout G R Jr: Evaluation of prostatic specific acid phosphatase and prostatic specific antigen in identification of prostatic cancer. J Urol 129: 315–318, 1983.
2. Aratake Y, Tamura K, Kotani T, Ohtaki S: Application of the Avidin–Biotin complex method for the light microscopic analysis of lymphocyte subsets with monoclonal antibodies on air-dried smears. Acta Cytol 32: 117–122, 1988.
3. Argyle J C, Schumann G B, Kjeldsberg C R, Anthens J W: Identification of a toxoplasma cyst by fine needle aspiration. Am J Clin Pathol 80: 256–258, 1983.
4. Baatenburg de Jong R J, Rongen R J, Lameris J S, Harthoorn M, Verwoerd C D, Knegt P: Metastatic neck disease. Palpation vs ultrasound examination. Arch Otolaryngol Head Neck Surg 115: 689–690, 1989.
5. Bailey T M, Akhtar M, Ali M A: Fine needle aspiration biopsy in the diagnosis of tuberculosis. Acta Cytol 29: 732–736, 1985.
6. Behm F G, O'Dowd C J, Frable W J: Fine needle aspiration effects on benign lymph node histology. Am J Clin Pathol 82: 195–198, 1984.
7. Betsill W L, Hajdu S I: Percutaneous aspiration biopsy of lymph nodes. Am J Clin Pathol 73: 471–479, 1980.
8. Bizjak-Schwarzbartl M: Cytomorphologic characteristics of non-Hodgkin's lymphoma. Acta Cytol 32: 216–220, 1988.
9. Bottles K, Cohen M B, Brodie H, Jeffrey R B, Nyberg D A, Abrams D I: Fine needle aspiration cytology of lymphadenopathy in homosexual males. Diagn Cytopathol 2: 31–35, 1986.
10. Bottles K, McPhaul L W, Volberding P: Fine needle aspiration biopsy of patients with acquired immunodeficiency syndrome (AIDS): experience in outpatient clinic. Ann Intern Med 108: 42–45, 1988.
11. Cafferty L L, Katz R L, Ordonez N G, Carrasco C H, Cabanillas F R: Fine needle aspiration diagnosis of intraabdominal and retroperitoneal lymphomas by a morphologic and immunocytochemical approach. Cancer 65: 72–77, 1990.
12. Cardillo M R: Fine needle aspiration cytology of superficial lymph nodes. Diagn Cytopathol 5: 166–173, 1989.
13. Carter T R, Feldman P S, Innes D J Jr, Frierson H F Jr,

Frigy A F: The role of fine needle aspiration cytology in the diagnosis of lymphoma. Acta Cytol 32: 848–853, 1988.
14. Cavett J R, III, McAfee R, Ramzy I: Hansen's disease (leprosy). Diagnosis by aspiration biopsy of lymph nodes. Acta Cytol 30: 189–193, 1986.
15. Christ M L, Feltes-Kennedy M: Fine needle aspiration cytology of toxoplasmic lymphadenitis. Acta Cytol 26: 425–428, 1982.
16. Cleary K R, Osborne B M, Butler J J: Lymph node infarction foreshadowing malignant lymphoma. Am J Surg Pathol 6: 435–442, 1982.
17. Das D K, Gupta S K, Pathak I C, Sharma S C, Datta B N: Burkitt-type lymphoma. Diagnosis by fine needle aspiration cytology. Acta Cytol 31: 1–7, 1987.
18. David J F, Marques B, de Graeve P, Combes P F: Etude comparative de la cytoponction et de la ponction-biopsie dans le diagnostic des adenopathies suspectes de malignité. Arch Anat Cytol Pathol 27: 239–243, 1979.
19. Davies J D, Webb A J: Segmental lymph-node infarction after fine-needle aspiration. J Clin Pathol 35: 855–857, 1982.
20. Dmitrovsky E, Martin S E, Krudy A G, Chu E W, Jaffe E S, Longo D L, Young R C: Lymph node aspiration in the management of Hodgkin's disease. J Clin Oncol 4: 306–310, 1986.
21. Domagala W, Weber K, Osborn M: Differential diagnosis of lymph node aspirates by intermediate filament typing of tumor cells. Acta Cytol 30: 225–234, 1986.
22. Dunphy C H, Katz R L, Fanning C V, Dalton W T Jr: Leukemic lymphadenopathy: diagnosis by fine needle aspiration. Hematol Pathol 3: 35–44, 1989.
23. Engzell U, Jakobsson P A, Sigurdson A, Zajicek J: Aspiration biopsy of metastatic carcinoma in lymph nodes of the neck: a review of 1101 consecutive cases. Acta Otolaryngol 72: 138–147, 1971.
24. Erwin B C, Brynes B K, Chan W C, Keller J W, Phillips V M, Gedgaudas-McClees R K, Torres W E, Bernardino M E: Percutaneous needle biopsy in the diagnosis and classification of lymphoma. Cancer 57: 1074–1078, 1986.
25. Feinberg M R, Bhaskar A G, Bourne P: Differential diagnosis of malignant lymphomas by imprint cytology. Acta Cytol 24: 16–25, 1980.

5 *LYMPH NODES*

26. Frable W: Fine needle aspiration biopsy. Saunders, Philadelphia 1983.
27. Frable W J, Kardos T F: Fine needle aspiration biopsy. Applications in the diagnosis of lymphoproliferative diseases. Am J Surg Pathol 12 (Suppl 1): 62–72, 1988.
28. Friedman M, Kim U, Shimaoka K, Panahon A, Han T, Stutzman L: Appraisal of aspiration cytology in management of Hodgkin's disease. Cancer 45: 1653–1663, 1980.
29. Gagliano E F: Fine needle aspiration cytology of Kaposi's sarcoma in lymph nodes. A case report. Acta Cytol 31: 25–28, 1987.
30. Hales M, Bottles K, Miller T, Donegan E, Ljung B M: Diagnosis of Kaposi's sarcoma by fine needle aspiration biopsy. Am J Clin Pathol 88: 20–25, 1987.
31. Hidvegi D F, Sorensen K, Lawrence J B, Nieman H L, Isoe C: Castleman's disease. Cytomorphologic and cytochemical features of a case. Acta Cytol 26: 243–246, 1982.
32. Highman W J, Oliver R T: Diagnosis of metastases from testicular germ cell tumours using fine needle aspiration cytology. J Clin Pathol 40: 1324–1333, 1987.
33. Hirschfeld H: Bericht über einige histologisch-mikroskopische und experimentelle Arbeiten bei den bösartigen Geschwulsten. Z. Krebsforsch 16: 33, 1919.
34. Hu E, Horning S, Flynn S, Brown S, Warnke R, Sklar J: Diagnosis of B cell lymphoma by analysis of immunoglobulin gene rearrangements in biopsy specimens obtained by fine needle aspiration. J Clin Oncol 4: 278–283, 1986.
35. Joensuu H, Klemi P J, Eerola E: Flow cytometric DNA analysis combined with fine needle aspiration biopsy in the diagnosis of palpable metastases. Anal Quant Cytol Histol 10: 256–260, 1988.
36. Kardos T F, Kornstein M J, Frable W J: Cytology and immunocytology of infectious mononucleosis in fine needle aspirates of lymph nodes. Acta Cytol 32: 722–726, 1988.
37. Kardos T F, Vinson J H, Behm F G, Frable W J, O'Dowd G J: Hodgkin's disease: diagnosis by fine needle aspiration biopsy. Analysis of cytologic criteria from a selected series. Am J Clin Pathol 86: 286–291, 1986.
38. Klemi P J, Elo J J, Joensuu H: Fine needle aspiration biopsy of granulomatous disorders. Sarcoidosis 4: 38–41, 1987.
39. Kline T S, Kannan V, Kline I K: Lymphadenopathy and aspiration biopsy cytology. Review of 376 superficial nodes. Cancer 54: 1076–1081,1984.
40. Kline T S, Neal H S: Needle aspiration biopsy: A critical appraisal. Eight years and 3,267 specimens later, JAMA 239: 36–39, 1978.
40a. Koo C H, Rappaport H, Sheibani K, Pangalis G A, Nathwani B N, Winberg C D: Imprint cytology of non-Hodgkin's lymphomas. Based on a study of 212 immunologically characterized cases. Human Pathol 20, suppl.1: 1–137, 1989.
41. Lampert F, Lennert K: Sinus histiocytosis with massive lymphadenopathy. Fifteen new cases. Cancer 37: 783–789, 1976.
42. Layfield L J, Bhuta S: Fine needle aspiration cytology of histiocytosis X: a case report. Diagn Cytopathol 4: 140–143, 1988.
43. Lee R E, Valaitis J, Kalis O, Sophian A, Schultz E: Lymph node examination by fine needle aspiration in patients with known or suspected malignancy. Acta Cytol 31: 563–572, 1987.
44. Lennert K: Histopathology of non-Hodgkin's lymphomas (based on the Kiel classification). Springer, Berlin, 1981.
45. Lennert K, Collins R D, Lukes R J: Concordance of the Kiel and Lukes-Collins classification of non-Hodgkin's lymphomas. Histopathology 7: 544–559, 1983.
46. Levitt S, Cheng L, DuPuis M H, Layfield L J: Fine needle aspiration diagnosis of malignant lymphoma with confirmation by immunoperoxidase staining. Acta Cytol 29: 895–902, 1985.
47. Lopes Cardozo P: The cytologic diagnosis of lymph node punctures. Acta Cytol 8: 194–205, 1964.
48. Lopes Cardozo P: The significance of fine needle aspiration cytology for the diagnosis and treatment of malignant lymphomas. Folia Haematol (Leipzig) 107: 601–620, 1980.
49. Lubinski J, Chosia M, Kotanska K, Huebner K: Genotypic analysis of DNA isolated from fine needle aspiration biopsies. Anal Quant Cytol Histol 10: 383–390, 1988.
50. Martelli G, Pilotti S, Lepera P, Piromalli D, Bono A, Di Pietro S, Galante E. Fine needle aspiration cytology in superficial lymph nodes: an analysis of 266 cases. Eur J Surg Oncol 15: 13–16, 1989.
51. Martin H E, Ellis E B: Aspiration biopsy. Surg Gynaecol Obstet 59: 578–589, 1934.
52. Meatheringham R E, Ackerman L V: Aspiration biopsy of lymph nodes: a critical review of the results of 300 aspirations. Surg Gynaecol Obstet 84: 1071–1076, 1947.
53. Moriarty A T, Banks E R, Bloch T: Cytologic criteria for subclassification of Hodgkin's disease using fine-needle aspiration. Diagn Cytopathol 5: 122–125, 1989.
54. O'Dowd G J, Frable W J, Behm F G: Fine needle aspiration cytology of benign lymph node hyperplasias. Diagnostic significance of lymphohistiocytic aggregates. Acta Cytol 29: 554–558, 1985.
55. Oertel J, Oertel B, Kastner M, Lobeck H, Huhn D: The value of immunocytochemical staining of lymph node aspirates in diagnostic cytology. Br J Haematol 70: 307–316, 1988.
56. Orell S R, Skinner J M: The typing of non-Hodgkin's lymphoma using fine needle aspiration cytology. Pathology 14: 389–394, 1982.
57. Pitts W C, Weiss L M: Fine needle aspiration biopsy of lymph nodes. Pathol Annu 23 (pt 2): 329–360, 1988.
58. Pontifex A H, Klimo P: Application of fine needle aspiration cytology to lymphoma. Cancer 53: 553–556, 1984.
59. Qizilbash A H, Elavathil L J, Chen V, Young J E, Archibald S D: Aspiration biopsy cytology of lymph nodes in malignant lymphoma. Diagn Cytopathol 1: 18–22, 1985.
60. Radhika S, Gupta S K, Chakrabarti A, Rajwanshi A, Joshi K: Role of culture for mycobacteria in fine-needle aspiration diagnosis of tuberculous lymphadenitis. Diagn Cytopathol 5: 260–262, 1989.
61. Ramzy I, Rone R, Schultenover S J, Buhaug J: Lymph node aspiration biopsy. Diagnostic reliability and limitations — an analysis of 350 cases. Diagn Cytopathol 1: 39–45,1985.
62. Rilke F, Pilotti S, Carbone A, Lombardi L: Morphology of lymphatic cells and of their derived tumours. J Clin Pathol 31: 1009–1056, 1978.
63. Robey S S, Cafferty L L, Beschorner W E, Gupta P K: Value of lymphocyte marker studies in diagnostic cytopathology. Acta Cytol 31: 453–459, 1987.
64. Russell J, Orell S, Skinner J, Seshadri R: Fine needle aspiration cytology in the management of lymphoma. Aust NZ J Med 13: 365–368, 1983.
65. Shaha A, Webber C, Marti J: Fine needle aspiration in the diagnosis of cervical lymphadenopathy. Am J Surg 152: 420–423, 1986.
66. Silverman J F: Fine needle aspiration cytology of cat scratch disease. Acta Cytol 29: 542–547, 1985.

67. Sneige N, Dekmezian R H, Katz R L, Fanning T V, Lukeman J L, Ordonez N F, Cabanillas F F: Morphologic and immunocytochemical evaluation of 220 fine needle aspirates of malignant lymphoma and lymphoid hyperplasia. Acta Cytol 34: 311–322, 1990.
68. Söderström N: Fine-needle aspiration biopsy. Almqvist & Wiksell, Stockholm, 1966.
69. Spieler P, Schmid U: How exact are the diagnosis and classification of malignant lymphomas from aspiration biopsy smears? Path Res Pract 163: 232–250, 1978.
70. Spriggs A I, Vanhegan R I: Cytological diagnosis of lymphoma in serous effusions. J Clin Pathol 34: 1311–1325, 1981.
71. Stani J: Cytologic diagnosis of reactive lymphadenopathy in fine needle aspiration biopsy specimens. Acta Cytol 31: 8–13, 1987.
72. Strum S B, Park J K, Rappaport H: Observation of cells resembling Sternberg–Reed cells in conditions other than Hodgkin's disease. Cancer 26: 176–190, 1970.
73. Surbone A, Longo D L, DeVita V T Jr, Ihde D C, Duffey P L, Jaffe E S, Solomon D, Hubbard S M, Young R C: Residual abdominal masses in aggressive non-Hodgkin's lymphoma after combination chemotherapy: significance and management. J Clin Oncol 6: 1832–1837, 1988.
74. Tani E M, Christensson B, Porwit A, Skoog L: Immunocytochemical analysis and cytomorphologic diagnosis on fine needle aspirates of lymphoproliferative disease. Acta Cytol 32: 209–215, 1988.
75. Tani E, Löwhagen T, Nasiell K, Öst A, Skoog L: Fine needle aspiration cytology and immunocytochemistry of large cell lymphomas expressing the Ki-1 antigen. Acta Cytol 33: 359–362, 1989.
76. The non-Hodgkin's lymphoma pathologic classification project: National Cancer Institute sponsored study of classifications of non-Hodgkin's lymphomas. Summary and description of a working formulation for clinical usage. Cancer 49: 2112–2135, 1982.
77. Townsend R R, Laing F C, Jeffrey R B Jr, Bottles K: Abdominal lymphoma in AIDS: evaluation with US. Radiology 171: 719–724, 1989.
78. Turner R R, Martin J, Dorfman R F: Necrotizing lymphadenitis A study of 30 cases. Am J Surg Pathol 7: 115–123, 1983.
79. Wotherspoon A C, Norton A J, Lees Wr, Shaw P, Isaacson P G: Diagnostic fine needle core biopsy of deep lymph nodes for the diagnosis of lymphoma in patients unfit for surgery. J Pathol 158: 115–121, 1989.
80. Wright DH: The identification and classification of non-Hodgkin's lymphoma: a review. Diagn Histopathol 5: 73–111, 1982.
81. Zajdela A, Ennuyer A, Bataini P, Poncet P: Valeur du diagnostic cytologique des adenopathies par ponction aspiration. Confrontation cyto-histologique de 1756 cas. Bull Cancer (Paris) 63: 327–340, 1976.
82. Zajicek J: Aspiration biopsy cytology. Part I. Cytology of supradiaphragmatic organs. Karger, Basel, 1974.
83. Zornoza J, Cabanillas F F, Althoff T M, Ordonez N, Cohen M A: Percutaneous needle biopsy in abdominal lymphoma. AM J Roentgenol 136: 97–103, 1981.

6

THE THYROID GLAND

6 THE THYROID GLAND

CLINICAL ASPECTS

Fine needle aspiration (FNA) cytology of the thyroid gland is now firmly established as an important first-line diagnostic test for the evaluation of goitre and the single most effective test for the preoperative diagnosis of a solitary thyroid nodule. Abulcasim, a 10th century Arabian physician, was credited with using the technique by Anderson and Webb[3] but Scandinavian workers pioneered the modern use of FNA some four decades ago.[31,133] There is a large body of world literature attesting to its accuracy and advantages, although the need for caution in interpretation, meticulous attention to technique, and the limitations of diagnosis are also well documented.

Several advances have occurred in the last decade. A more critical analysis of the cost-effectiveness of FNA as a screening method for selecting cases for surgery has been undertaken.[4,5,78,115,130,136] Its use in conjunction with ultrasound imaging,[45,139] its particular value in areas of endemic goitre,[59,122,123] in the diagnosis of metastatic malignancy,[20,48,132,143,144] and in the goitre of pregnancy and childhood,[97,141] has been described, and a role suggested in the assessment of parathyroid disease.[24,28,41,46,75,104] Detailed analysis of the accuracy and complications compared with core needle biopsy has been performed.[13,17,108,129] There is a stronger realisation that a certain perhaps irreducible, false negative rate exists,[22,23,51,54] particularly in relation to cystic thyroid neoplasms,[22,105,117,121] requiring close cooperation between clinician and pathologist if delay in the diagnosis of neoplasia is to be avoided. It should be stressed, however, that FNA provides a more rapid, safe and accurate diagnosis of the solitary nodule than any other combination of clinical or laboratory tests and may well have reduced delays in diagnosis for many patients.[52] The use of the non-aspiration technique as an adjunct to aspiration has been outlined,[98,120] as well as the value of repeated sampling over a period of time to reinforce a benign diagnosis[3,52] or in 'indeterminate' cases.[10] Studies of the minimum amounts of material on which to make reliable diagnoses of benign lesions have led to a better appreciation of the 'satisfactory' smear.[43,55,57] Cell block techniques have been applied to the diagnosis of benign follicular lesions[77,86] and there has been wide discussion of the aims and limitations of cytological diagnosis in assessing follicular lesions.[5,83,94,103,138] In terms of descriptive morphology, the range of appearances and the diagnostic criteria of common neoplasms, and the common pitfalls in diagnosis,[51,54,63] are now well documented, along with some newer refinements. Grooved or folded nuclei have been recognized as a useful diagnostic feature in papillary carcinoma,[26,47,119,126] and the cytological findings in 'newer' histopathological entities such as hyalinising trabecular adenoma,[42] the tall cell variant[67] of papillary carcinoma and insular carcinoma[93] have been described. The value of immunoperoxidase techniques for identifying calcitonin[25,113] and thyroglobulin[37,150] in primary

and metastatic tumours has been emphasized, and, finally, the measurement of DNA ploidy levels,[6,7,14] particularly in papillary carcinomas, allows a more accurate prediction of biological behaviour which may be of value in determining therapy for individual patients.

The main indications for FNA remain:

1. The diagnosis of diffuse non-toxic goitre.
2. The diagnosis of the solitary or dominant thyroid nodule.
3. Confirmation of a clinically obvious thyroid malignancy.
4. To obtain material for ultrastructural study and clinical research.

Close cooperation is necessary between the pathologist and clinician so that the indications for the procedure, terminology used in reporting and the accuracy of the technique in one's own laboratory are clearly defined. Optimal results are achieved when an experienced cytopathologist performs the aspiration,[51] for he or she can best assess the adequacy of the particular biopsy and modify technique accordingly; however, good results are achieved by dedicated clinicians,[43,130] and where careful technique is combined with enthusiasm for FNA diagnosis, pathologists in the peripheral hospital setting achieve extremely good results.[110]

In our early experience we derived most benefit in diagnosing clinically obvious malignancy, in emptying simple thyroid cysts, and in the diagnosis of thyroiditis. The use of aspiration cytology to exclude malignancy is more difficult and an enlarging experience and full awareness of the pitfalls[51,54,63] are necessary to achieve low false negative rates.

The place of FNA in the investigative sequence

As with other superficial and easily accessible masses, thyroid aspiration is a simple office procedure which may be performed during the patient's first visit; it is an ideal first line diagnostic test.

In *diffuse non-toxic goitre* FNA offers the gold standard of an important and unequivocal distinction between colloid goitre and autoimmune thyroiditis, the latter requiring lifelong follow-up or treatment with thyroxin to shrink the gland and to avoid the subtle decline into hypothyroidism which is the natural history of the untreated disease. Antibody levels and TSH estimations will provide a diagnosis in 90–95% of cases at best.[50,149] Antibodies are positive in 60–80%[36,71] in some series, and in a smaller percentage in children or adolescents. Cases may be missed if antibody estimation is used as the sole screening indicator of disease; antibodies are also positive in up to 10–15% of patients without thyroiditis. FNA can provide a definitive diagnosis of Hashimoto's disease in aberrant clinical settings such as hyperthyroidism, or where there is dual disease, such as associated neoplasm.[8]

THE THYROID GLAND 6

The *solitary cold thyroid nodule* has become the main focus of attention for the use of FNA because of the potential to reduce the number of unnecessary operations for benign nodules. In 60% of patients with benign nodules, FNA can provide an unequivocal benign diagnosis and thus remove the need for operation, or allow more appropriate advice to be given to the patient and to the surgeon in planning operations.[43,92,145,146] Many authors report a fall in the proportion of patients operated on subsequent to the introduction of thyroid FNA to their hospitals;[43,61,101,115] in some series this fall is over 50%,[61,115] though others record a reduction of only 20%.[23] In the experience of some, the proportion of malignancies in surgically resected nodules from units with regular FNA services may be up to 40%[61] compared with 8–20% before the use of FNA, there being no obvious rise in the number of cases where treatment was delayed due to FNA.

A definitive FNA diagnosis of malignancy allows the patient to be informed that an operation for cancer is likely and preoperative staging procedures can be performed. The need for frozen section confirmation will depend on the experience of the pathologist; in the hands of the most experienced pathologists definitive typing of some neoplasms, for example papillary or medullary carcinoma, permits a one-stage surgical procedure without the need for histological verification of the diagnosis.

Confirmation of a *clinically obvious inoperable malignancy*, in particular spindle and giant cell carcinoma or malignant lymphoma, is valuable in sparing the patient additional invasive diagnostic procedures, thus allowing palliative therapy, to improve the symptoms of tracheal obstruction for example.

In general, aspiration cytology should be used in conjunction with other diagnostic methods such as antibody measurements, thyroid scanning and ultrasonography; it does not replace these tests. In the assessment of solitary nodules, FNA allows a far more specific diagnosis than scanning but many clinicians still prefer to have an overall assessment of glandular function by scanning in conjunction with FNA; demonstration of multinodularity or a 'hot' nodule by scanning may help in diagnosis where FNA findings are indeterminate. Some studies have shown increased accuracy in diagnosis by the combined use of cutting or core needle biopsy and FNA,[13,17,108] although large needle biopsy does not overcome the main deficiency of FNA, an inability to distinguish between follicular adenoma and carcinoma. For most clinicians and pathologists, the safety and ease of use of FNA and the possibility of repeated sampling without complications outweigh any increases in accuracy obtained by adding large needle biopsy.

Accuracy of diagnosis

FNA is highly accurate in the diagnosis of *thyroiditis*. In cases with histological follow up reported in the literature, virtually all cytological diagnoses of autoimmune thyroiditis were verified.[111] Lymphocytic infiltration of the gland in Graves' disease may result in an overlap in cytological appearances with Hashimoto's disease; because thyroiditis may be a patchy process or only affect one part of the thyroid gland, the affected area may not be adequately sampled even by a satisfactory technique. In up to 10% of cases of thyroiditis diagnostic material will not be obtained; repeat aspirations will reduce this false negative rate.[49,50,71,111,114,149]

Many studies of the accuracy of diagnosis of *solitary nodules* have been reported in the literature including comprehensive cytohistological correlation.[1,3,4,12,22,23,32,33,34,36,43,51,60,61,63,66,67,78,92,99,101,115,122,130]

In the reviews by Ashcroft and Van Herle[4] and by Frable[32] FNA is shown to achieve a diagnostic accuracy of over 90% in terms of predictive value, sensitivity, specificity and efficiency in the diagnosis of neoplasm and this has been confirmed in a number of recent studies.[3,32,43,63] In some series the sensitivity of diagnosis of malignancy can be close to 100%,[51,67,130] though this degree of accuracy is not recorded by most authors. False negative diagnoses arise from inadequate samples, geographic misses of the lesion, dual pathology and errors in interpretation.[51,54,63] False negative rates are reported in several ways. Where the total number of benign cases is used as the denominator, rates of less than 1–2% are reported. However, it must be realised that even in the hands of experienced cytopathologists approximately 5–10% of cancers, excluding occult types, will not be diagnosed by FNA.[32,92] A significant proportion of these are cases where a dominant nodule obscures a smaller or more diffusely growing carcinoma. Clinical findings and the results of thyroid scanning must therefore be taken into account in planning management.

Even in those series with extensive cytohistological correlation, large numbers of patients are not operated on, so precluding an exact assessment of a false negative rate. However, Boey et al,[12] countering this criticism, followed 365 patients with combined clinical and FNA diagnosis of benign nodules for 2.5 years; only two cases of carcinoma were subsequently diagnosed, both of which were cystic lesions. Nevertheless, cystic neoplasms provide a significant risk of diagnostic error; over 40% of cystic neoplasms in most series are not diagnosed by FNA and strict clinical–cytological criteria should be applied to avoid misdiagnosis (p. 104).[22,63,105,117,121]

Experience is an important factor in diagnosis, emphasised by the great improvement in accuracy reported over the course of some studies,[102] although some of these were involved in developing criteria for diagnosis which are now well documented, widely accepted and readily learned.[53] Individual centres must therefore establish their own false negative rates for the

6 THE THYROID GLAND

guidance of their clinicians and close cooperation between clinician and pathologist is necessary, particularly when the clinician or more than one clinician performs the aspirations. The pathologist must make it very clear to the clinician which aspirations are inadequate and which are adequate for assessment; there is a tendency for clinicians and pathologists alike to try to spare the patient further aspirations and the temptation to report on an inadequate specimen must be avoided. It has been suggested that 100–200 FNAs per year constitute reasonable continuing experience necessary to provide adequate samples for diagnosis.[43,136]

The reported false positive rate is usually low, being around 1–2% of the total number of malignancies. In some highly experienced centres the false positive rate approaches zero[1,92] and the cytological report can be used as a basis for definitive surgery. Some authors have compared FNA diagnosis with frozen section and advocate the former,[18,76] although frozen section or paraffin section confirmation would still be preferred by most pathologists, particularly as lesions such as follicular adenomas with marked nuclear atypia or unusual benign tumours such as hyalinising trabecular adenomas may be unavoidable sources of cytological error.[18] Frozen section has little to offer over FNA in the assessment of follicular neoplasms;[76] these require extensive sampling to exclude or prove capsular or vascular invasion. The value of smear imprints at the time of frozen section has however been noted,[123] particularly in the diagnosis of papillary carcinoma where recognition of a papillary growth or characteristic nuclear morphology may be difficult in frozen sections and much easier in smears.

Clinically obvious malignancies are usually easy to diagnose cytologically, most being anaplastic carcinomas or high grade lymphomas, where the risk of a false positive diagnosis is not high. Aspiration can be used safely in this area of diagnosis early in one's experience but there are difficulties in diagnosing widely invasive follicular carcinoma because of a lack of acceptable cytologic criteria of malignancy in this tumour, and in low or intermediate grade lymphoma, particularly in a background of Hashimoto's thyroiditis.

Contraindications

There are no contraindications to aspiration of a gland if the patient is co-operative. Aspiration may not be advisable in children or unco-operative adults if they are likely to move their head suddenly during the procedure.

Complications

Local haemorrhage into tissues may occur; we have seen haematomas within the thyroid gland and in adjacent subcutaneous tissue; these caused some discomfort to the patient but dissipated spontaneously over several days. Haemorrhage may make the meticulous surgery of parathyroidectomy more difficult and FNA should be performed with caution if parathyroidectomy is planned. Haemorrhage or necrosis due to FNA may occasionally obscure the histological pattern of thyroid lesions, particularly in adenomas;[69,74] this is rare, but endorses the need for careful technique. The use of multiangled or aggressive needling must be avoided; larger needles (21 gauge or larger) are probably more likely to cause this. Haemorrhage sufficient to cause tracheal compression has not been reported, but examples of transient laryngeal nerve paresis are reported.[130] Puncture of the trachea can cause a coughing spasm, and small amounts of blood may be coughed up; however, recovery occurs within a few minutes. Needling of the thyroid may be followed rarely by the formation of a hot nodule or conversion of a hot to a cold nodule on scan; if thought necessary, scans should probably be carried out before rather than after FNA. FNA can also cause elevated blood thyroglobulin levels.[88] Implantation or dissemination of tumour has not been reported with FNA of the thyroid gland.

Technical considerations

Taking the sample

The patient should be lying in the supine position. Placing a pillow under the neck tends to expose the gland more, bringing it away anteriorly from the sterno-mastoids and surrounding soft tissues — this is particularly useful when a small, diffuse goitre is being aspirated — it is also a useful manoeuvre during palpation of the gland.

During the procedure the patient is asked to lie still and to refrain from swallowing to prevent trauma to surrounding structures; this usually poses no problems because the needling should take only 5–10 seconds. Children may not tolerate the procedure; if, however, aspiration is absolutely essential, general anaesthesia may be required.

At least three aspirations are performed during a session. We use 25 gauge needles; 22 or 23 gauge needles do not cause significantly greater trauma, 25 gauge needles can provide perfectly adequate material. In diffuse goitres both sides are sampled and in nodules, material from several areas should be aspirated. It has been reported that six to eight passes with 25 gauge needles may reduce the number of indeterminate or false negative diagnoses[57] and may be of value in large lesions. Use of 22 or 21 gauge needles allows preparation of cell block samples which may be particularly valuable in the diagnosis of follicular lesions.[77,86]

It is rarely necessary to traverse the body of the sterno-mastoid; the depth of the underlying lesion becomes more difficult to judge if it lies beneath sterno-mastoid; depth is best judged in relation to the over-

THE THYROID GLAND 6

lying thyroid capsule; the skill of 'palpation with the needle tip' is also important and must be learnt over some time. In solitary masses the first needle pass should be designed to test whether the lesion is cystic. Cyst walls are sometimes fibrotic and difficult to enter and the depth required to reach the lesion may not be appreciated by beginners. If the lesion is not cystic the needle is moved to and fro for several millimetres in the same needle track; this manoeuvre must be performed rapidly because of the vascularity of the thyroid. Aspiration is stopped if any material appears in the hub of the needle or in the syringe. The presence of some material within the hub of the needle is, however, often impossible to prevent and this may be the source of an apparently inadequate aspiration. If possible, the material in the hub should be tapped onto a glass slide, aspirated with another needle, or removed with a small brush such as those used for endocervical sampling.

The non-aspiration technique of needle sampling is a useful recent innovation[120] and involves grasping the needle itself, without an attached syringe, and moving it rapidly within the lesion. The use of a syringe and aspiration first, particularly in nodules, allows testing for cystic change; however, if a lesion is not cystic, and particularly if aspirates are haemorrhagic, the non-aspiration technique may give better, cleaner and less haemorrhagic material. It also allows detection of more subtle differences in the texture of tissue and may allow smaller lesions to be sampled. It is especially valuable for clinicians who have not mastered the aspiration technique.

Repeat sampling some weeks or months after the initial aspiration is helpful in confirming the benign nature of nodules or in indeterminate cases and is preferable to immediate surgery.[10,52] Ultrasound imaging allows sampling of very small lesions, retrosternal or mediastinal lesions.[45,139] CT may be used for the same purpose, although the time taken to confirm correct placement of the needle often results in excessive haemorrhage and an unsatisfactory smear.

According to the clinical impression of the nature of a thyroid lesion the technique may need to be modified slightly. Some information may also be gained during the aspiration, for example, in Hashimoto's thryroiditis the gland is rather firm, is not very vascular, and tends to bleed less than other lesions so that more time may be spent obtaining material. Simple cysts may be aspirated completely. If any palpable lesion remains after cyst aspiration, re-aspiration of that site should be performed since neoplasms may be cystic; unfortunately, this sometimes leads to local haemorrhage and refilling of the cyst but this procedure should help to ensure that cystic neoplasms are not missed.

Colloid nodules may have a fibrous outer capsule but do not usually have a hard or firm centre; on aspiration they yield varying amounts of translucent or brown colloid of variable viscosity. Sometimes thick, inspissated colloid is removed which smears as a firm, jelly-like substance.

Follicular neoplasms usually have a firm capsule and the centre of the lesion may have a similar texture. These lesions are usually very vascular and it may be difficult to obtain material free of contaminating blood; therefore, when haemorrhage occurs easily in solitary lesions, the possibility of neoplasm should be considered. Very rapid aspiration may be needed in these cases, or the non-aspiration technique used. Primary hyperplasia also yields haemorrhagic aspirates. Carcinoma of medullary or giant cell type may be quite firm; papillary carcinomas are also usually firm but may be cystic.

Use of ancillary techniques

Cytochemistry[113]
Silver stains (Sevier-Munger or Grimelius) have been used to demonstrate argyrophilia in medullary carcinomas and in parathyroid neoplasms.[113] Askanazy cells may, however, be silver positive because of staining of granules. Mucin stains are of little help in diagnosing metastases or in distinguishing thyroid neoplasms of various types because papillary, follicular and medullary carcinomas of the thyroid may all secrete mucin.

Immunocytochemistry[25,27,37,38,113,140,150]
Antibodies to thyroglobulin[150] and calcitonin[25,113] are extremely useful in confirming the cell type in diagnostically difficult new growths and the technique will work successfully in destained smears.[38] Both are also particularly useful in examining tumour in metastatic sites. B- and T-cell antibodies or immunoglobulin light chain staining may help in establishing monoclonality in lymphoid infiltrations.[140] Typing of intermediate filaments is of limited value in thyroid diagnosis[25] except in displaying epithelial characteristics in anaplastic tumours.[27] Dual staining for keratin and vimentin is described in primary neoplasms of follicular and papillary type and in other benign processes.[25] Positive staining for lactoferrin, lactalbumin and secretory component would help rule out a thyroid neoplasm.[25]

Cell block preparations[77,86]
These are especially helpful for immunoperoxidase studies and histological examination alone may be of value in distinguishing follicular adenomas from colloid nodules.[86]

Nuclear morphometry[15,16]
The value of nuclear size measurements as a prognostic or diagnostic indicator in thyroid lesions is debated. Boon initially suggested that follicular adenomas and carcinomas could be separated by this method and has proposed that the variable results reported by different

6 THE THYROID GLAND

authors may be related to the selection and measurement of the material.[15,16,96]

DNA ploidy[2,6,7,14,62,73,137]

Backdahl and co-workers provided evidence that aneuploid papillary carcinomas have a higher rate of recurrence, morbidity and mortality compared with diploid lesions.[6,7] There were similar though less striking findings for other carcinomas.[14] These findings open the way for individualisation of patient management and in predicting the outcome of treatment, although ploidy studies are not helpful in distinguishing benign from malignant lesions;[137] some follicular adenomas are aneuploid[73] and many carcinomas are diploid.[6,7,14] DNA ploidy studies using archival paraffin embedded material and fresh smears or tissue show similar results,[62,85] although false aneuploid peaks have been described as a result of autolytic change in imperfectly preserved tissue.[2] Evaluation of S-phase component in paraffin-embedded material has also been undertaken[73] but may be more difficult technically.[62]

Intact follicles are st seen with an appearance like multinucleate giant cells. There are intact well defined follicles c̄ a sharply demarcated outline.

Colloid - varied appearances.
Thick or thin & wispy and v. difficult to make out - sp. if wispy in Paps.
- Pavementing; cracking artefacts; folds in a section sheet — are all terms to describe the varied appearance of colloid -

Unless otherwise stated the appearances described refer to MGG stained material.

The satisfactory smear

Hamburger et al[55,57] suggest that in the assessment of dominant nodules six clusters of benign cells in at least two slides prepared from separate aspirates constitute reasonable minimum material for satisfactorily diagnosing benign lesions. Using these criteria, they observed that of 100 satisfactory aspirates, 77% were achieved with two to four needle passes, whereas 23% required six to eight needle passes, and if lesser amounts of material were accepted as being satisfactory, higher rates of false negative diagnoses would have occurred. Other authors rely on similar criteria[43] (e.g. five to six groups of cells with more than 10 cells per group). In most series, approximately 80% of aspirates are satisfactory and this figure increases to 90% on repeat aspiration; those with the widest experience achieve over 97% of satisfactory samples.[51] We agree with these assessments but believe that a truly satisfactory smear contains many more than 12 benign cell clusters; abundant colloid is as important a requirement for the unequivocal diagnosis of a benign colloid nodule.

Normal structures (Fig. 6.1)

1. Small clusters and sheets of epithelial cells.
2. Small amounts of thin colloid.
3. C-cells.
4. Cartilage.
5. Tracheal epithelium.
6. Skeletal muscle.

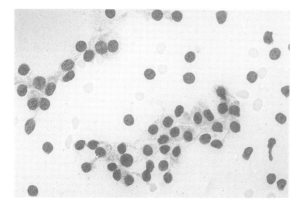

Fig. 6.1 Follicular epithelium
Uniform cells with fragile partially dispersed cytoplasm; bare lymphocyte-like nuclei in a background of thin colloid (MGG, HP)

In 'normal' thyroids, follicles are rarely removed intact. Sometimes fragments of follicles are large enough to form large two-dimensional flat sheets; they may also present as small, loose clusters. The cells are rather fragile and tend to disrupt easily so that bare nuclei are common; these are similar in size and appearance to normal lymphocytes. Nuclei are rounded or slightly oval with a regular nuclear outline. Small nucleoli may be evident. The cytoplasm stains pale blue with MGG and cell borders are indistinct or fuzzy. Sometimes coarse, blue intracytoplasmic granules are present (paravacuolar granules). Colloid in large amounts resembles varnish macroscopically; microscopically it stains blue to purple and forms a membrane-like coat often with folds and cracks. When diluted by blood it may be difficult to see and its appearance may mimic those of other protein-rich fluids including serum, which is also pale blue. Colloid, especially when it is thin, may be washed off the slide during processing. Sometimes a parched earth or 'crazy pavement' artefact may remain on the slide to signal the presence of colloid; red cells may be aligned with this 'crazy pavement' outline. Thicker colloid may present as clumps or inspissated globules. Colloid is more difficult to recognize in Pap or H & E stained smears, but presents as orangeophilic or eosinophilic homogeneous material, often with cracking artefact and clumping. Distinction of thin colloid from blood proteins is more difficult in Pap preparations.

Some authors report C-cells in aspirates of various thyroid conditions, identified by their resemblance to medullary carcinoma cells (p. 119). They are difficult to find in smears and only few may be present.

Puncture of the trachea may occur if the thyroid is only marginally enlarged. Sometimes a patient coughs when this happens and air will be aspirated into the syringe; more often there is no sign. Cytologically, small groups or single, ciliated columnar cells may be present with clumps of mucus. Cartilage appears as brilliant magenta flecks with fibrillar edges.

Distinction between hyalinized connective tissue, colloid, and other amorphous materials such as amyloid may be difficult at times (p. 120).

Simple colloid goitre

There is no clear cytological difference between the appearances of the normal thyroid gland and those of simple colloid goitre. There are few indications for aspirating normal-sized glands, so that the combination of a diffusely enlarged gland and 'normal cytological appearances' permits the diagnosis of simple colloid goitre. This entity is regarded by most authors as an early stage in the formation of nodular colloid goitre, colloid distension of follicles being the sole histological abnormality. The only cytological difference from normal may be the presence of colloid of varying thickness or excessively thick colloid.

6 *THE THYROID GLAND*

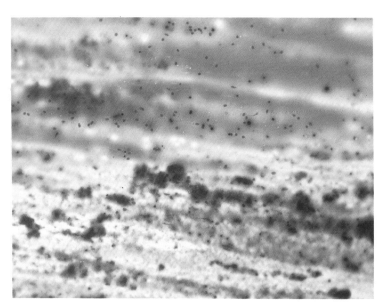

[handwritten note: long standing haemorrhage → macrophages containing coarse pigment later macrophages (haemosiderin)]

Fig. 6.2 Colloid, thick and thin
A varnish-like coat of variable density
with some thicker clumps (MGG LP)

Nodular colloid goitre (Figs 6.2–6.5)

Criteria for Diagnosis

1. Abundant colloid of both thick and thin types.
2. Follicular cells in sheets and clumps, with dissociation, and numerous bare nuclei.
3. Foamy cells.
4. Degenerating erythrocytes.
5. Hyalinised stroma.

[handwritten margin note: Cystic degeneration is common]

Abundant colloid is the most characteristic finding in nodular goitre and its presence is reassuring; abundant colloid with little epithelium is seldom a feature of malignancy (Figs 6.2, 6.3). One feature of the epithelial cells in nodular goitre is their fragility. Follicular cells show feathery cytoplasmic fragmentation and bare nuclei often dominate the smear. Epithelial cell nuclei may show more anisokaryosis than those of normal thyroid and some large nuclei may be present. Askanazy cell change may also occur (p. 106). Follicles may be removed intact by the needle; they can be seen either as small rings or as rounded syncytia at times resembling multinucleate giant cells (Fig. 6.15). Hyperplastic papillae containing follicles and intact dilated follicles in cell block preparations are supportive evidence of a colloid nodule. Small follicular or acinar formations in smears correspond to microfollicular structures in sections. Larger follicles are disrupted by aspiration and present as flat sheets of various size. The sheets are sometimes described as having a honeycomb structure,[10] though cell margins are not usually well defined and the cytoplasm often forms web-like extensions between cells. Foamy cells indicate degenerative change and are commonly seen in nodular goitre; they may contain blue-black stained debris including haemosiderin presumably

resulting from broken-down erythrocytes and other cells and they are, therefore, phagocytic (p. 103). Many others are probably derived from follicular epithelium, although it is impossible to distinguish them cytologically from cells of monocytic origin. Degenerative epithelial change manifests in several ways: the cytoplasm may be fragmented or show early foamy change; there may be small, dark-blue granules associated with cytoplasmic vacuoles (paravacuolar granules) representing lysosomal debris or lipofuscin. Epithelial cells may also become spindle-shaped, have more abundant cytoplasm and enlarged nuclei, giving the pathologist some cause for caution. Hyaline connective tissue presents as irregular, pale pink or mauve fragments of amorphous material, sometimes with adherent epithelial cells (Fig. 6.4). The predictive value of an unequivocal cytological diagnosis of colloid goitre can be up to 96%.[67]

Problems in diagnosis

1. Follicular neoplasms.
2. Askanazy cell change.
3. Papillary carcinoma (macrofollicular).
4. Atypical histiocytic or epithelial cells.
5. 'Hot' nodules.

The cytological appearances of nodules in colloid goitre form a continuum which merge with those of follicular adenoma, and in this grey area cytological criteria alone cannot reliably distinguish between the two. In a nodular goitre with hyperplastic areas composed of small follicles, for example, aspiration displays many small follicles or a repetitive pattern in smears, giving an impression of neoplasm.[29] If sampling throughout the lesion is performed, degenerative changes and the abundance of colloid elsewhere would

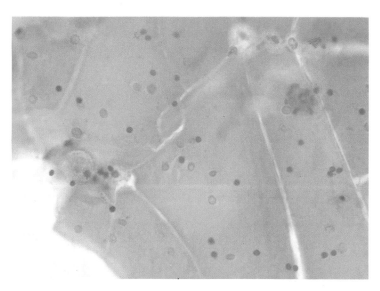

Fig. 6.3 Colloid
Cracking artefact (Pap, LP)

cystic deg. —common in
mng & colloid goitres.
There are —altered blood
↑ foamy macrophages
siderophages
crystals — seen at edges
of slide
sp. MGG
as empty spaces
c shape of dvd.
crystals.
Also can examine cyst fluid in
Polarized light.

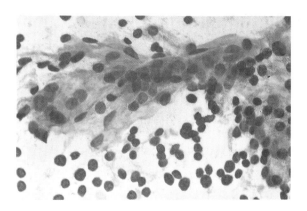

Fig. 6.4 Colloid goitre
Strands of pink stroma and adherent follicular cells (MGG, HP)

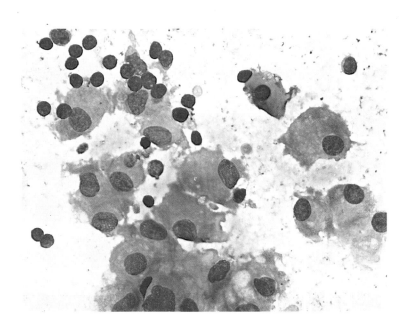

Fig. 6.5 Colloid goitre
Atypical histiocyte-like cells with abundant cytoplasm and enlarged, rather pleomorphic nuclei; bare nuclei of normal follicular cells (MGG, HP)

6 *THE THYROID GLAND*

indicate nodular goitre rather than neoplasm; however, where a nodule is composed exclusively of hyperplastic epithelium, cytological distinction from neoplasm (including carcinoma) is impossible. In cellular lesions where there is some colloid, a monolayered sheet arrangement of epithelial cells is said to be more characteristic of colloid nodule, and three-dimensional syncytial aggregates, of neoplasm.[5,59,83,109,138]

If Askanazy cell change is widespread these cells will dominate the smear; excision biopsy is necessary to exclude neoplasm (p. 111).

Occasionally, thyroid carcinoma may have macrofollicular areas and yield moderate amounts of colloid on FNA. We have seen this in several follicular variants of papillary carcinoma and in papillary carcinomas with degenerative change.

Small groups of large cells with pleomorphic nuclei are not infrequently found in nodular goitre and are probably related to degenerative change; their origin is uncertain; they may be histiocytic cells or possibly regenerating epithelial cells (Fig. 6.5). Some cell sheets resemble the appearance of epithelial 'repair'.

The value of cytological diagnosis in 'hot' or hyperfunctioning nodules is disputed by some authors; it is suggested that the cytologic atypia frequently displayed in these lesions may give rise to cytological misdiagnosis.[142] Others, however, conclude that FNA helps eliminate the rare possibility of malignancy in association with hot nodules[89,116] or can eliminate the need for scanning.

Cyst/haemorrhage into thyroid tissue[22,70,105,117,121]

Usual findings

1. Brown fluid.
2. Numerous foamy cells, many with ingested debris.
3. Sparse epithelium showing degenerative features.

Problems in diagnosis

1. Papillary carcinoma with cystic change.
2. Follicular neoplasm with cystic change.
3. Thyroglossal duct cyst.
4. Parathyroid cyst.

Cystic lesions of the thyroid pose diagnostic difficulties. Small foci of cystic change yielding a few drops of fluid on FNA commonly occur in nodular colloid goitre (up to 40% of cases);[22,63] and larger areas of cystic change, up to 3–4 ml or more, are also common. The pathogenesis of so-called simple cysts is uncertain but large cysts with or without associated haemorrhage may occur in a background of relatively normal thyroid. However, in one series, cystic change and/or haemorrhage in neoplasms was present in up to 25% of primary papillary carcinomas, in 20% of follicular neoplasms, and in 26% of follicular carcinomas.[63] In another series,

23% of malignant neoplasms were cystic.[22] Up to 50% of resected cystic lesions may be neoplastic[22,117] and according to some authors, the prevalence of malignancy in cystic lesions of thyroid is similar (10–15%) to that in solid nodules,[22,117,121] although such studies are of excised nodules which have been subjected to selection before surgery.

Nevertheless the mere identification of cystic change in thyroid tissue does not imply a benign lesion and further efforts must be made to establish the correct diagnosis. A definitive diagnosis of nodular goitre with cystic change requires adequate sampling of the wall of the lesion and adjacent tissue, and if only cyst fluid containing macrophages can be obtained after multiple aspirations it should be stressed that neoplasm with cystic change cannot be excluded. The gross appearance of cyst fluid is not an accurate guide to its nature; most cystic malignancies contained blood-stained fluid in one study,[22] in another there was little difference in the prevalence of neoplasm in association with blood-stained fluid, brown turbid fluid or straw-coloured fluid.[121]

Reasonable evidence of a benign lesion is established if a cystic lesion can be completely evacuated, no palpable nodule remains and the fluid shows no atypical epithelial elements.[70] The frequency of such completely evacuated cysts varies between series; according to some, as few as 4–12%[22] of cystic lesions may be permanently cured by FNA, while in others' experience, over 40%[121] of cystic lesions may disappear after aspiration, though some require repeat attendances. Such disparity presumably relates to case selection and how cysts are defined. Even in apparently simple cysts, a small percentage will harbour papillary carcinoma.[12] The potential for false negative diagnosis of cystic carcinoma appears in several series, in which at most 60% of such neoplasms were correctly identified by FNA,[22,105,117,121] emphasising the need for combined clinical/cytological strategies for selecting patients for surgery. Reaspiration of the cyst bed and multiple aspirations of any residual or recurrent swelling are advised. Recurrent cysts, incompletely decompressed lesions, lesions greater than 3–4 cm in diameter in which aspiration of several areas does not give good evidence of colloid nodule, and lesions in young males, have all been recommended as indications for surgical excision.[105,117,121]

The term 'colloid cyst' should probably be avoided in reporting because it may lead to confusion. A clear distinction between colloid nodule and a true focus of cystic change should be made and is most easily achieved by the aspirator although nodules containing thin colloid may cause difficulties.

Thyroglossal duct cysts may contain squamous or respiratory epithelium but one should be aware of the possibility of contamination from the skin or trachea before suggesting the diagnosis. These cysts usually yield clear or mucoid fluid in contrast with the discoloured brown fluid of thyroid cysts or the thick colloid of colloid nodules.

If crystal clear fluid emerges from a lateral cystic lesion, the possibility of a parathyroid cyst should be considered;[39] measurement of parathormone levels in the fluid may help confirm the diagnosis; evaluation of the C-terminal rather than the N-terminal end of the hormone is recommended to enhance the sensitivity of detection.[128]

Primary hyperplasia (Graves' disease)
(Figs 6.6 and 6.7)[72,107,111]

Usual findings

1. Blood-stained smear with little colloid.
2. Moderate amounts of epithelium and some follicular or ring structures.
3. Enlarged cells with more abundant cytoplasm; variation in nuclear size.
4. 'Fire flares'/'colloid suds'/'marginal vacuoles'.

The diagnosis of Graves' disease is best made by biochemical and serological tests; aspiration cytology has little value in establishing the diagnosis, although FNA in cases of diffuse goitre with thyrotoxicosis

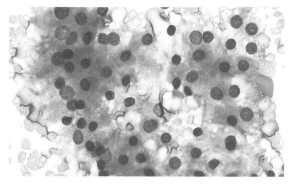

Fig. 6.6 1⁰ Hyperplasia
'Fireflares' at the periphery of loose sheets of epithelial cells with abundant pale cytoplasm (arrows) (MGG, HP)

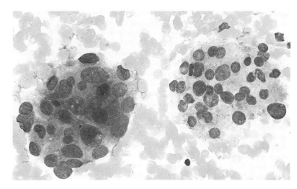

Fig. 6.7 1⁰ Hyperplasia
Striking nuclear atypia in a case of medically treated Graves' disease of long duration; subsequent surgical excision showed similar atypia but no evidence of malignancy (MGG, HP)

may occasionally reveal Hashimoto's thyroiditis, de Quervain's thyroiditis and, rarely, diffusely growing carcinomas. In Rieger's series of hyperthyroidism and concurrent malignancy,[16] FNA allowed preoperative diagnosis in most cases, though most neoplasms were in cold nodules within an enlarged gland and no carcinomas were found in association with true Graves' disease. If Graves' disease is unsuspected the cellularity of the smears may impart a false impression of neoplasm. 'Fire flares' or 'marginal vacuoles' are a common finding in hyperplastic cells.[72,107] They are pale violet or red vacuoles visible at the rim of the cytoplasm, measuring 1–7 μm in diameter and often possessing a pale centre (Fig. 6.6). Their relationship to the absorption vacuoles at the edges of follicles in histological sections is unknown; they may correspond to colloid droplets seen ultrastructurally or to dilated cisternae of endoplasmic reticulum. They are indicative of cellular hyperactivity and when they are seen in most cells in a smear, they are suggestive of hyperfunction; however, they may also be seen, for example, in Hashimoto's thyroiditis, diffuse nodular goitre and in neoplasms including carcinoma.[112] The variation in nuclear size which may occur in hyperplasia is well known; variation in nuclear size per se can *not* be used as a sign of neoplasia in the thyroid. Hyperplastic papillary structures may also appear in smears and give rise to a suspicion of papillary neoplasm. In some longstanding cases of medically treated Graves' disease, nuclear atypia may be very striking;[131] if there is a clinical suspicion of neoplasm excision will be necessary (Fig. 6.7). The same problem may be met in relation to *dyshormonogenetic goitre*.

Jayaram et al found epithelioid cells, scattered lymphocytes, and, occasionally, multinucleate giant cells in some cases of Graves' disease; Askanazy cell change occurred in some.[72] The relationship of these cases to Hashimoto's thyroiditis with hyperthyroidism is uncertain.

Acute suppurative thyroiditis

Criteria for diagnosis

1. Neutrophil granulocytes.
2. Evidence of tissue breakdown in the form of necrotic cells and cell debris.
3. Intracellular bacteria.

This lesion is uncommon; we have only seen a few cases. In two, including one which yielded a salmonella organism, the lesion was localised, perhaps arising in a degenerate nodule. Extreme tenderness, fever, debility and high ESR should enable a confident clinical diagnosis, however, the distinction from subacute thyroiditis or from a rapidly growing anaplastic carcinoma may sometimes be difficult clinically.

Neutrophils and debris dominate the smear and cytological diagnosis is usually not difficult. Intracellular

[handwritten margin note: These cytoplasmic vacuoles at cytoplasm rim are an imp. Dic feature. Vacuoles are bounded by red, granular appearance ↳ fire flares.]

6 THE THYROID GLAND

bacteria (usually Gram positive cocci) help confirm the diagnosis. Culture of the aspirate is probably the most useful part of the procedure.

Problems in diagnosis

1. Anaplastic carcinoma, giant-cell type.
2. Lymphadenitis with abscess formation.
3. Infected thyroid cyst.
4. Subcutaneous (phlegmonous) diffuse inflammation of the neck.

Giant cell anaplastic carcinoma may have an accompanying inflammatory infiltrate. The malignant cells may also have a histiocytic or fibroblastic appearance, enhancing the possibility of confusion with acute suppurative thyroiditis. The presence of bacteria in the MGG or Gram stain in thyroiditis, or bizarre giant cells and obvious features of malignancy in carcinomas will lead to the correct diagnosis. In the absence of identifiable thyroid tissue, infection outside the thyroid is difficult to exclude. For practical purposes the response to antibiotics should be dramatic in infective lesions.

Auto-immune thyroiditis (Hashimoto's thyroiditis; Lymphocytic thyroiditis) (Figs 6.8– 6.11)[35,49,50,71,80,111,114,149]

Criteria for diagnosis

Classical Hashimoto's thyroiditis

1. Askanazy cells.
2. Moderate numbers of mainly small lymphocytes and scattered plasma cells.
3. Small multinucleate giant cells; epithelioid histiocytes (variable).

Florid lymphocytic thyroiditis

1. Many lymphoid cells including small lymphocytes and centroblasts.
2. Little 'hypertrophic' or normal epithelium.

This disease is defined by the presence of antithyroid antibodies, particularly antimicrosomal antibodies, and intense lymphocytic infiltration of the gland associated with destruction and atrophy of thyroid epithelium; thyroid epithelial cells convert to a non-functioning form with plentiful eosinophilic cytoplasm — the Askanazy cell. The florid disease is common; based on follow-up studies and thyroid antibody distributions in 'normal populations', subclinical forms of the disease are also common. The earliest morphological stage of the disease is presumed to be lymphocytic infiltration gradually progressing to glandular destruction and atrophy; this progression results in a spectrum of morphological appearances: however, in cytological specimens two basic patterns can be recognised. We believe these correspond to different phases of the disease. 'Classical

Hashimoto's thyroiditis' generally occurs in older patients who are more often hypothyroid. The 'florid lymphocytic pattern' occurs in younger patients or those in whom the duration of the disease is shorter; they are usually euthyroid and more often have lower or negative antibody titres.[50,149]

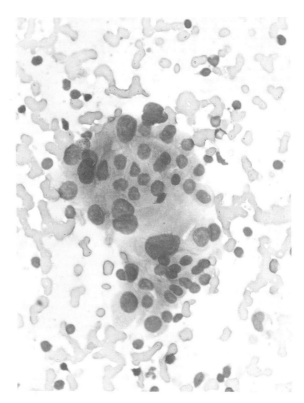

Fig. 6.8 Hashimoto's thyroiditis
Aggregate of Askanazy cells; background of blood and lymphocytes; note abundant cytoplasm and anisokaryosis (MGG, HP)

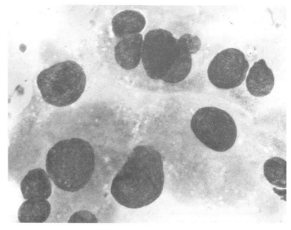

Fig. 6.9 Hashimoto's thyroiditis
Askanazy cells; abundant dense finely granular cytoplasm and anisokaryosis (MGG, HP Oil)

Askanazy cells in MGG–stained material present as enlarged cells with abundant grey blue cytoplasm and well defined borders. The cytoplasm is denser than in normal follicular epithelial cells and may show fine granularity either violet or magenta in colour. Nuclei are generally larger than normal and are more variable in size (Figs 6.8 and 6.9). Nuclei may show an increase of two, four or higher multiples of the normal follicular nuclear size. Nucleoli are often large. These cells may accompany follicular epithelium with a more normal appearance, some displaying evidence of hyperactivity. Small, mature lymphocytes have rounded nuclei and a short tail or sparse rim of eccentrically placed blue cytoplasm. When a moderate amount of blood is included in the smear, lymphocytes with prolonged tails are more common. Epithelioid cells are elongated and have oval or sandshoe-shaped nuclei and abundant pale cytoplasm. They are not uncommon and their significance is uncertain.

Centroblasts (large lymphoid cells), derived from germinal centres in lymphoid follicles in the gland, have paler staining nuclei and more abundant blue cytoplasm than small lymphocytes. Large immunoblasts may also be seen. The mixture of small and large cells is very characteristic of a reactive process (Fig. 6.10). Epithelial cells may be very sparse in the florid lymphocytic form; a thorough search may be necessary to be sure that the material has been taken from the thyroid.

Germinal centre histiocytes (dendritic reticulum cells) may also be found; these have plentiful pale violet cytoplasm and slightly oval or indented histiocytoid nuclei. They are often clustered and intimately associated with lymphocytes some of which lie within the cytoplasm of the histiocytes. Some histiocyte-lymphocyte rosettes may be seen. Such a close association is not seen between lymphocytes and epithelial cells despite the theoretical possibility of direct epithelial damage by lymphocytes.

Problems in diagnosis

1. Distinguishing bare thyroid nuclei from lymphocytes.
2. Lymphocytic infiltration in or around other lesions.
3. Lymphoma.
4. Problems with Askanazy cells.
5. Unilateral or focal auto-immune thyroiditis.
6. Giant cells in auto-immune thyroiditis.
7. 'Hyperthyroiditis'/'Hashitoxicosis'.
8. Proliferation of epithelial cells in florid lymphocytic thyroiditis.
9. Psammoma bodies.

It may be difficult to distinguish thyroid nuclei from lymphocytes especially when the material is poorly fixed or poorly air-dried. A thin rim of cytoplasm is characteristic of lymphocytes and this is not seen in single thyroid cells as they almost always have stripped nuclei.

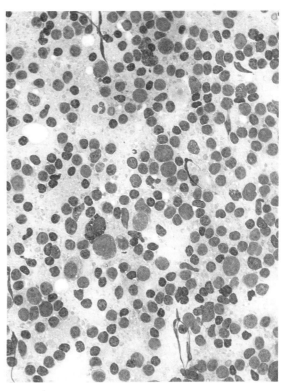

Fig. 6.10 Lymphocytic thyroiditis (florid)
Very cellular smear; pure population of lymphoid cells indistinguishable from reactive lymphadenitis (MGG, HP)

Thyroid nuclei are also slightly oval and more regular than lymphocytes having a more homogeneous chromatin pattern and a denser nuclear rim. Lymphocytes vary in size and larger, immature forms are usually present. Streaks of smeared lymphocytic nuclear material are often found; blue cytoplasmic fragments (lymphoid globules) are characteristic of lymphoid cell breakdown and do not derive from breakdown of thyroid cells (p. 68).

A lymphocytic infiltrate may co-exist with neoplasia,[49] particularly in the diffuse sclerosing form of papillary carcinoma. The pathologist must therefore rely on placing his needle accurately within the lesion and on the result of several punctures. There is a definite risk of missing small associated neoplasms.

Minor focal lymphocytic infiltration in an otherwise normal gland may be difficult to distinguish from patchy autoimmune thyroiditis in which sampling is inadequate and only few lymphocytes are removed. Follow up and re-aspiration may be necessary. Only a small percentage of cases with minor focal lymphocytic infiltration will show lymphocytes in their smears,[111] so that cytological over-diagnosis of Hashimoto's thyroiditis is most unlikely.

In some patients presenting with hyperthyroidism the aspiration may yield numerous lymphocytes.[71] The

6

THE THYROID GLAND

course of the disease in some of these patients may be a transition to destructive autoimmune lymphocytic infiltration ('Hashitoxicosis'), but in some the process may be self-limiting ('hyperthyroiditis'). Such cases have also been reported in postpartum patients. Clinical evidence of hyperthyroidism and serum thyroxin levels should alert the physician and cytologist to these uncommon entities which illustrate the close kinship of the various autoimmune thyroid diseases. The distinction between these cases and typical Graves' disease in which some lymphoid cells are aspirated may be difficult.

The cytological appearances of lymphocytic/autoimmune thyroiditis and lymphoma may overlap, and sometimes their cytological distinction is difficult. This applies in particular to follicular lymphomas with a mixed cell population. A monotonous, large lymphoid cell infiltration should lead to a suspicion of neoplasm. The 'florid lymphocytic pattern' with almost total absence of epithelial cells is common in younger age groups but is uncommon in elderly patients and should be diagnosed with caution in this age group. Approximately 75% of lymphomas arise in a background of autoimmune thyroiditis and may be initially focally distributed within the gland, making adequate sampling difficult. Immunocytochemistry or gene rearrangement studies of aspirated material may allow monoclonality to be detected.[140]

The degree of pleomorphism of Askanazy cells in thyroiditis may be extreme and may resemble a malignant process to the uninitiated. In so-called 'burnt out' Hashimoto's disease, and Hashimoto's disease with focal nodular hyperplasia of Askanazy cells, the aspirate may yield only Askanazy cells;[49,66,82] the cytological distinction from Askanazy cell neoplasia may be impossible so that surgical excision may be necessary. Again, multiple gland punctures offer the best chance of recognising the areas of lymphoid infiltration. Some authors have suggested that disorganised masses of Askanazy cells with prominent nucleoli are more indicative of neoplasm and that sheet-like structures with some infiltration by lymphocytes indicate hyperplasia,[114] however, we have found this distinction difficult on occasion. Nodular goitre may also yield numerous Askanazy cells in a smear. A mixture of colloid with normal follicular epithelium and Askanazy cells favours nodular goitre. Several other forms of large, non-lymphoid cells may be present in thyroid aspirates and may be confused with Askanazy cells. In the early stages of thyroiditis there may be many 'hypertrophic epithelial cells' with abundant cytoplasm. These are presumably TSH-stimulated cells. They do not have the dense cytoplasm and well-defined cytoplasmic borders of Askanazy cells and some may even have 'fire flares' (Fig. 6.6). Epithelioid-like cells may also be seen in some aspirates of Hashimoto's thyroiditis. These have an elongated, spindle-shaped cytoplasm and elongated or bean-shaped nuclei and may be very difficult to distinguish from Askanazy cells.

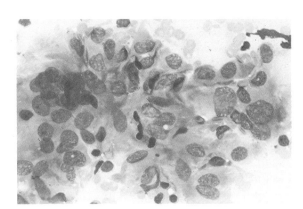

Fig. 6.11 Hashimoto's thyroiditis
Plump epithelioid-like cells forming a fairly tight cluster (MGG, HP)

Forms morphologically intermediate between these two types of cell may also be present (Fig. 6.11). Macrophage or dendritic reticulum cell clusters from germinal centres within the thyroid may also be confused with Askanazy cells.

Occasionally Hashimoto's disease presents as a nodule or solitary focus.[35] This clinical presentation should not prevent a cytological diagnosis, although the possibility of a neoplasm with surrounding thyroiditis should be considered, especially if a nodule yields abundant epithelium and lymphocytes.[80,82,114]

Giant cells are seen in 30% of Hashimoto's thyroiditis[111] and together with epithelioid cells[111] may cause confusion with De Quervain's thyroiditis. In our experience, an intense lymphocytic infiltration is not seen in subacute thyroiditis where a mixed inflammatory cell infiltrate with evidence of more severe tissue destruction is characteristic, although a few cases showing overlap in cytological features with Hashimoto's thyroiditis have been reported.[71]

Sometimes, and more often in younger patients with florid lymphocytic thyroiditis, abundant active-looking epithelium may be aspirated leading to a suspicion of neoplasm.

Psammoma bodies have been described in association with Hashimoto's thyroiditis[30] and can of course be seen in other benign processes; however, their presence in smears probably warrants surgical biopsy because they are much more likely to be associated with papillary carcinoma.

De Quervain's thyroiditis (Subacute thyroiditis; granulomatous thyroiditis) (Figs 6.12–6.14)[49,71,111]

Criteria for diagnosis

1. Multinucleate giant cells — large and numerous.
2. Inflammatory cells; macrophages and lymphocytes.
3. Degenerating follicular cells; cytoplasmic granules.
4. A dirty background with debris; abundant colloid.
5. Epithelioid cells.

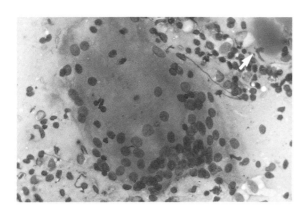

Fig. 6.12 De Quervain's thyroiditis
Huge multinucleated giant cell; some clumped colloid (arrow)
(MGG, MP)

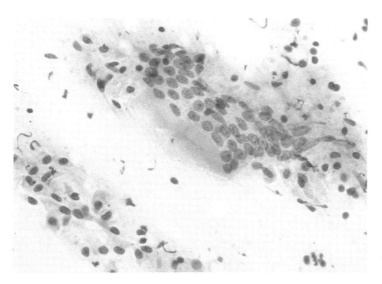

Fig. 6.13 De Quervain's thyroiditis
Multinucleate histiocyte, a loose aggregate
of thyroid epithelial cells, and scattered
nuclear fragments (Pap, HP)

Those follicular cells that are present often show degenerative features in the form of dark blue cytoplasmic granules representing lipofuscin or lysosomal debris and presenting in Pap-stained smears as fine golden pigment. These granules are not specific for De Quervain's disease and may be seen in nodular goitre and, occasionally, in association with papillary and follicular neoplasms.[127] Collections of stripped nuclei and crushed nuclei may also be seen. The histiocytic giant cells are usually very large and contain up to 200 nuclei. Some contain ingested, inspissated colloid. These cells are the hallmark of the disease (Figs 6.12 and 6.13), but the diagnosis may still be suggested should the other features of the disease be present (Fig. 6.14). In particular, a non-foamy macrophage and mononuclear cell reaction, and epithelial cell degeneration should alert one to the possibility of this diagnosis.

Problems in diagnosis

1. Multinucleate cells in other processes.
2. 'Pseudogiant cells'.

3. Nodular presentation.
4. Resolving phase of disease.

'Giant cells' may be found in other processes within the thyroid. Epithelioid histiocytes and giant cells, generally with small numbers of nuclei, may be a prominent finding in autoimmune thyroiditis and are seen occasionally in Graves' disease. 'Palpation thyroiditis', in which there is a macrophage reaction to ruptured follicles due to minor trauma, is probably only of theoretical interest although we have seen one case in which numerous giant cells were seen in a smear and at the margin of a neoplasm in the subsequent resection. Very rarely the thyroid may be affected by mycobacterial infection or other granulomatous processes.

If a follicle is withdrawn intact with its basement membrane, it may simulate a large, multinucleate giant cell; however, the rounded nature of the structure in contrast with the irregular, flat form of true histiocytic giant cells should prevent confusion (Fig. 6.15).

De Quervain's thyroiditis quite commonly presents as a firm focal lesion or a nodule and may simulate neo-

6 THE THYROID GLAND

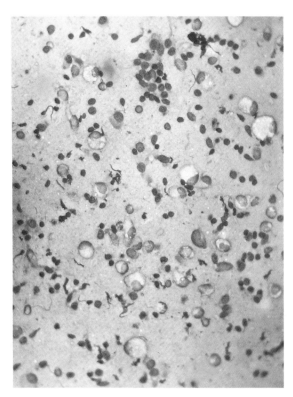

Fig. 6.14 De Quervain's thyroiditis
Mixed cell reaction; histiocytes, degenerating epithelial cells and some lymphocytes in a 'dirty' background with thin colloid (MGG, MP)

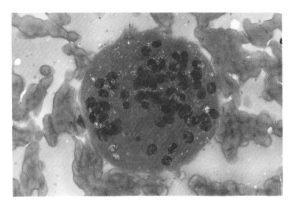

Fig. 6.15 'Pseudogiant cell'
Detached follicle with intact basement membrane but without visible cell borders; superficial resemblance to a multinucleated giant cell (MGG, HP)

plasm clinically. We have also seen examples in which the nodule was mistaken clinically for a lymph node near the thyroid. The disease may also be painless and clinically resemble so-called silent thyrotoxic thyroiditis ('Hyperthyroiditis'). Carcinomatous involvement of the gland can mimic subacute thyroiditis clinically.[118,144]

In later resolving phases of the disease process, the characteristic cytological features may not be present.

Follicular neoplasm (Figs 6.16–6.25)[5,59,82,83,94,103,138]

Criteria for diagnosis

1. Cellular smear.
2. Many equal-sized cell clusters scattered throughout the smear.
3. Disorganized syncytial cell aggregates.
4. Scanty colloid.
5. Askanazy cell change/clear cell change (variable).

Microacinar or rosette-like clusters are derived from follicles (Figs 6.16, 6.17 and 6.18). This finding applies

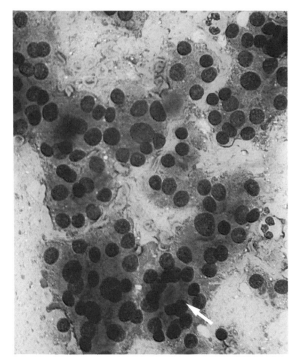

Fig. 6.16 Follicular adenoma
Equisised cell clusters representing microfollicles; small amounts of inspissated colloid (arrow) (MGG, HP)

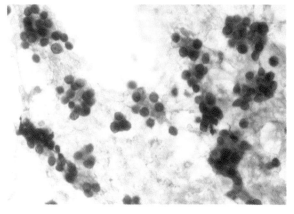

Fig. 6.17 Follicular adenoma
Microfollicular aggregates (Pap, HP)

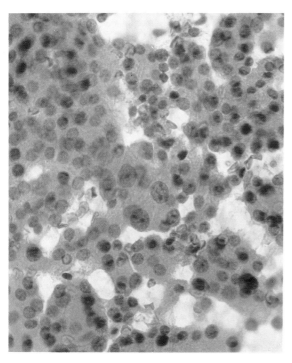

Fig. 6.18 Follicular adenoma
Cellular smear; some tendency to microfollicular formation; moderate anisokaryosis (H & E, HP)

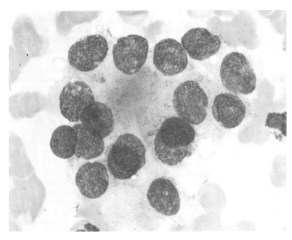

Fig. 6.19 Follicular adenoma
Microfollicular cell cluster (MGG, HP Oil)

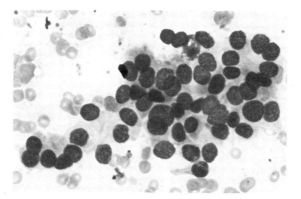

Fig. 6.20 Follicular carcinoma
Aspirate of distant lymph nodal metastasis of follicular carcinoma from a patient with skeletal dissemination; note small uniform nuclei (MGG, HP)

particularly to microfollicular neoplasms (Fig. 6.l9). Neoplasms with trabecular or solid growth pattern do not yield these structures although a repetitive pattern may still be evident in smears. Cell clusters in more solid neoplasms are usually more variable in size and are densely cellular, often having a disorganised or syncytial appearance. Sometimes small blood vessels of capillary or venular size may be included with adherent epithelial cells (Fig. 6.21).

The cytological appearances of follicular adenoma and follicular carcinoma are very similar. In general, carcinoma will be more cellular and will be composed of crowded disorganised clusters of cells with larger nuclei, more prominent nucleoli and a more irregular chromatin pattern than follicular adenoma;[109,138] however, these differences may be subtle and very difficult to appreciate subjectively. Attempts to separate the two cytologically have met with varying success; some authors diagnose over 75% of follicular carcinomas[103] and it may well be that critical attention to cytological criteria allows selection of a group at particular risk of carcinoma.[103,109,138] However, most authors are content to use cytology to select microfollicular, trabecular or solid lesions for surgical excision, and leave exact classification to histological assessment of capsular and vascular invasion. The ultimate biological behaviour of microfollicular, solid or trabecular adenomas is uncertain, and these should probably be excised, adding further reasons for a conservative approach to FNA diagnosis. Morphometric analysis may enable a distinction to be made and there are promising studies along these lines; yet, other studies found little of value in the method,[14,96,137] although it has been suggested that differences in technical methodologies may explain these variable results.[15] We have found morphological nuclear criteria to be unhelpful in separating adenoma from carcinoma; indeed, in one of our cases the nuclei of cells aspirated from a distant lymph node metastasis of a follicular carcinoma were of equal size to those of normal follicular cells (Fig. 6.20).

Follicular neoplasms with Askanazy cell (Hurthle cell) change (Figs 6.21–6.23) usually yield abundant material. The Askanazy cell change is usually diffuse, so that a mixture of these and 'normal' epithelial cells is more a feature of nodular goitre.[66] There may be nuc-

6 *THE THYROID GLAND*

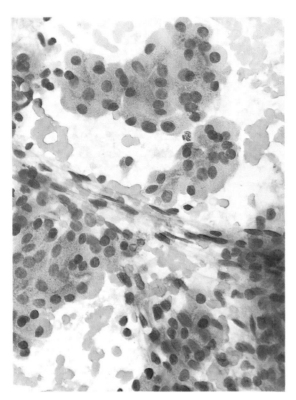

Fig. 6.21 Follicular oxyphil adenoma
Sheets of Askanazy cells adherent to capillary blood vessels
(MGG, HP)

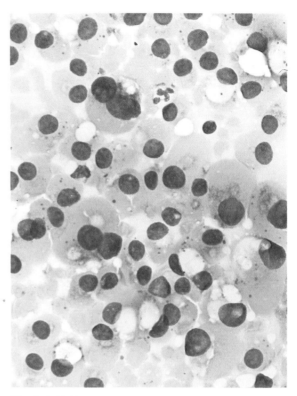

Fig. 6.22 Follicular oxyphil carcinoma
Dispersed cells of Askanazy type; nuclear enlargement and
anisokaryosis (MGG, HP)

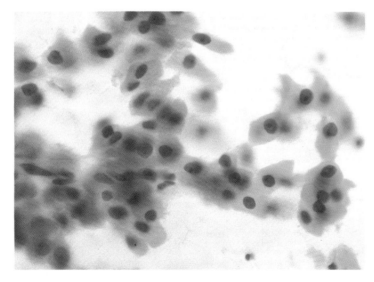

Fig. 6.23 Follicular oxyphil carcinoma
Loosely adherent Askanazy cells
(Pap, HP)

lear pleomorphism; however, nuclei are often more uniform in size in neoplasms than in Hashimoto's thyroiditis with prominent Askanazy cell change.[29,82] Flat sheets are said to be more characteristic of thyroiditis than the syncytial poorly orientated aggregates of neoplasms.[114] The distinction between benign and malignant lesions of Hurthle cell type is particularly difficult (Figs 6.21, 6.22 and 6.23).[14]

Neoplasms with clear-cell change in histological sections appear in MGG–stained smears with abundant cytoplasm of variable density.[68] Clearing is often not evident in smears, however, if this change can be identified, excision of the lesion should be advised; clear-cell carcinoma cannot be distinguished from adenoma and metastatic clear-cell carcinoma will also need to be considered.[48]

HISTOLOGICAL DIAGNOSIS	COLLOID NODULE	MACROFOLLICULAR ADENOMA	MICROFOLLICULAR ADENOMA	TRABECULAR ADENOMA	FOLLICULAR CARCINOMA
CYTOLOGICAL CATEGORY	COLLOID NODULE		FOLLICULAR NEOPLASM		
MORPHOLOGICAL FEATURES	⟶ INCREASING CELLULARITY ⟶ ⟶ MICROFOLLICULAR STRUCTURES ⟶ ⟶ DECREASING AMOUNTS OF COLLOID ⟶ ⟶ INCREASING NUCLEAR SIZE ⟶				

Fig. 6.24 Follicular neoplasms
Rationale for cytological diagnosis

From 70 to 90% of follicular neoplasms are detected by cytology and the proportion of carcinoma in lesions designated as follicular neoplasms ranges from 14 to 44% in large series.[29,59,92,103]

Problems in diagnosis

1. Nodular goitre.
2. Vascularity.
3. Papillary carcinoma.
4. Atypical adenomas.
5. Parathyroid adenoma.
6. Askanazy cell change (p. 104).
7. Inspissated colloid mimicking psammoma bodies.
8. Chemodectoma (paraganglioma).
9. Widely invasive follicular carcinoma.
10. Cystic change.

Distinguishing between follicular neoplasm and nodular goitre represents the most common differential diagnostic problem when a solitary nodule is found. Because the cytological appearances of these lesions overlap, it will be impossible to differentiate between them in some cases;[5] it must be acknowledged that in solitary adenomas composed of large follicles containing abundant colloid an incorrect cytological diagnosis of 'colloid goitre' will be given. The false negative rate of FNA in the diagnosis of follicular neoplasm may therefore be 30% or more[23] because of the inability to recognise macrofollicular neoplasms. However, the main aim of the procedure is to detect carcinoma; most follicular carcinomas will be either micro-follicular, trabecular or solid and contain little colloid, and there is much less danger of these lesions being missed by cytology. The argument is depicted in Figure 6.24. Although the false negative rate in the diagnosis of follicular carcinoma is up to 20% in several series,[23] (including cystic lesions and geographical sampling errors), some authors achieve an extremely high sensitivity of diagnosis with false negative rates as low as 0–2%[3,67,123,130] and believe that the threshold criteria for selecting cases for surgery can be set so as to minimise false negative errors.[123]

Follicular neoplasms are often vascular. Aspiration may produce excessive contamination of the smear by blood and make diagnosis difficult. One should beware of ascribing an excessively blood-stained smear to poor technique and bear in mind the possibility of vascular neoplasm. The non-aspiration technique is of value in this situation.

In lesions having mixed follicular and papillary growth pattern, the component cells will usually still display cytological features of papillary carcinoma even though areas with papillary structures might not be sampled. According to some, 60–90% of the pure follicular variant of papillary carcinoma may be diagnosed

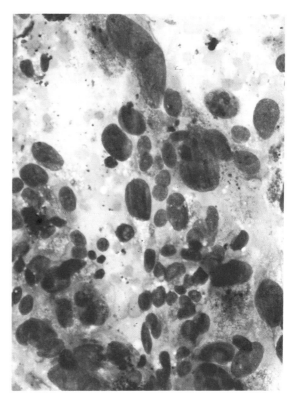

Fig. 6.25 Atypical adenoma
Severe nuclear pleomorphism; histology showed similar epithelial atypia but no capsular or vascular invasion (MGG, HP)

6 THE THYROID GLAND

by FNA,[81,102] through recognition of intranuclear inclusions and pale nuclei with nuclear grooves; however, we have found this diagnosis difficult cytologically. In a few of these lesions, we and others[64] have seen abundant colloid in smears derived from macrofollicular areas of tumour.

In some papillary carcinomas the density of the cytoplasm may mimic Askanazy cell change and the tumour may be wrongly diagnosed as follicular.

Some adenomas may be composed of pleomorphic cells and give a cytological impression of malignancy (Fig. 6.25) although in fact pleomorphism is not a particular feature of most follicular carcinomas. These tumours are not designated as carcinoma histologically unless there is capsular or vascular invasion; caution in making a cytological diagnosis of malignancy, particularly in follicular lesions, is warranted.

There are no reliable cytological criteria which distinguish parathyroid adenoma from follicular thyroid neoplasm;[104] the problem is rarely faced as most parathyroid adenomas do not present as palpable nodules. Nevertheless, we have misdiagnosed several of these.

Colloid in small follicles is often very dense and may be laminated, but the regular edge is unlike that of a psammoma body. The latter also stains poorly with MGG and appears refractile and glass-like rather than dense blue like colloid.

One limitation of FNA lies in the diagnosis of widely invasive follicular carcinoma. These neoplasms may be obviously malignant to the clinician but may lack reliable cytological criteria on which to base a diagnosis.

Papillary carcinoma
(Figs 6.26–6.35)[44,63,81,100,102,105,124]

Criteria for diagnosis

1. Cellular smears.
2. Papillary clusters of cells.
3. Monolayered sheets of cells with dense cytoplasm and distinct intercellular borders.
4. Pale nuclei, indistinct nucleoli; intranuclear cytoplasmic invaginations; nuclear grooves; irregular nuclear outlines.
5. Variation in cell size and Askanazy cell-like change, especially in monolayered sheets.
6. Viscous colloid (chewing gum-like or stringy).
7. Psammoma bodies.
8. Macrophages and debris (evidence of cystic degeneration).
9. Multinucleate giant cells.

Papillary clusters are among the most characteristic features of papillary neoplasms; however, there are sometimes problems in recognizing them in smears. Most papillae are not removed intact by the needle and they usually form monolayered sheets with irregular 'papillaroid' outlines (Fig. 6.26). If they have not been

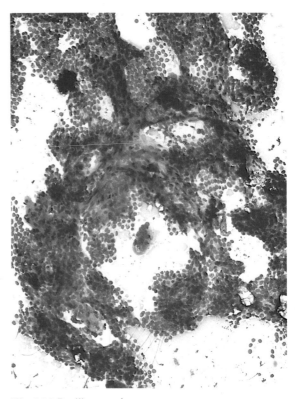

Fig. 6.26 Papillary carcinoma
Highly cellular smear; sheets and papillae with vascular cores (MGG, LP)

disrupted they may present as finger-like aggregates of cells (Fig. 6.27) with a well-defined 'anatomical' edge to the cluster, corresponding presumably to the tip of the papilla (Fig. 6.28). The accompanying fibro-vascular core of the papilla is rarely seen in cytological material, but it may be present; however, a vascular core covered by cells does not necessarily mean that the lesion is papillary, because follicular neoplasms may yield similar structures when the epithelial cells adhere to small, central vessels. The density of the cytoplasm in the monolayered sheets may be quite striking and may resemble squamous metaplasia or Askanazy cell change (Figs 6.30a and 6.34).

Intranuclear cytoplasmic inclusions (Figs 6.29 and 6.31) have been regarded as pathognomonic of papillary carcinoma and are seen in up to 90% of these carcinomas and in up to 5% of the cells.[21,134] However, they are occasionally seen in anaplastic carcinoma, medullary carcinoma, and follicular neoplasms,[40,87] and have been described in non-neoplastic conditions,[29,150] in lesions seen near the thyroid such as paraganglioma,[65] and in metastatic renal cell carcinoma within the thyroid.[48]

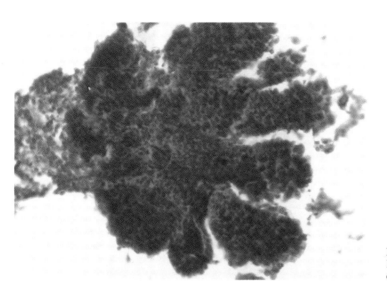

Fig. 6.27 Papillary carcinoma (Blunted papillae)
Finger-like papillae with 'anatomical edges' (H & E, IP)
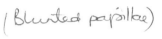

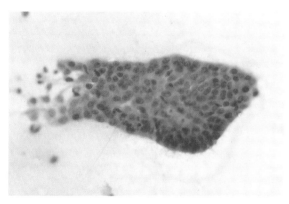

Fig. 6.28 Papillary carcinoma
Finger-like papilla; note peripheral palisading (H & E, MP)

Intranuclear inclusions manifest as areas of nuclear clearing with sharp well-defined margins (Figs 6.29 and 6.31). Inclusions are similar in colour and texture to cytoplasm although they are sometimes paler. Interestingly, they may not contain thyroglobulin in immunoperoxidase studies,[37] although the cytoplasm of the same cell may be positive. They can be mimicked by artefacts in both Pap and MGG-stained material,[21,51] however, artefactual vacuoles appear empty and have less distinct outlines. Irregularity of nuclear outline is a feature of the cells of papillary carcinoma. It is likely that the invaginations or inclusions represent cytoplasm entrapped within deep nuclear folds, although inclusions and nuclear creases seldom co-exist.[26] Ground glass nuclei are distinct from intranuclear vacuoles. They may be seen in some cases in alcohol-fixed Pap or H & E stained material but are generally not well demonstrated in cytological preparations and are prominent only in formalin fixed, paraffin embedded material.[58,87]

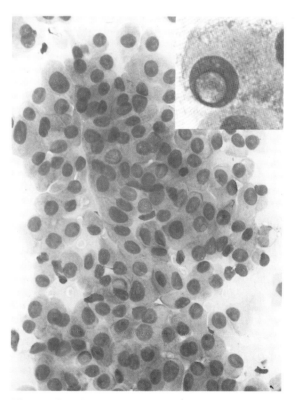

Fig. 6.29 Papillary carcinoma
Flat monolayered sheet; dense cytoplasm with well defined cell borders; large pale nuclei (MGG, HP). Inset: intranuclear vacuole (MGG, HP Oil)

Attention has been drawn to the longitudinal nuclear groove or nuclear crease (Fig. 6.32) as a helpful feature in the diagnosis of papillary carcinoma in smears and sections.[26,47,119,126] The grooves are seen easily only in

6

THE THYROID GLAND

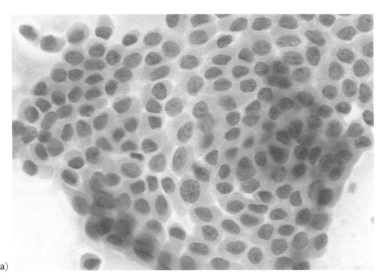

(a)

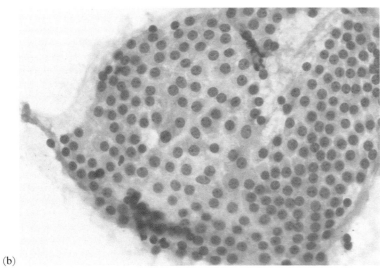

(b)

Fig. 6.30 (a) **Papillary carcinoma**
Flat monolayered sheet; dense cytoplasm
with well-defined cell borders; irregular
nuclear outlines (H & E, HP)
(b) **Colloid nodule**
Disrupted macrofollicle forming a flat
monolayered sheet with a honeycomb
structure and rounded nuclei.
(H & E, HP)

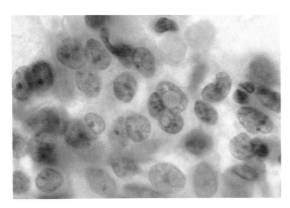

Fig. 6.31 Papillary carcinoma
Pale nuclei with rather irregular outlines; a few intranuclear
vacuoles (H & E, HP Oil)

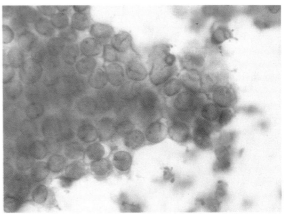

Fig. 6.32 Papillary carcinoma
Pale overlapping nuclei with prominent longitudinal grooves
(Pap, HP)

alcohol-fixed material and are difficult to discern in MGG preparations. They may be confused with overlying structures and strict criteria for recognition have been suggested: continuous grooves or creases, clearly defined and running the length of the nucleus.[47] When present in most cells of a sheet or group of cells or in most fields examined[119] they constitute strong supportive evidence of papillary carcinoma, although small numbers of longitudinal grooves are found in 70–80% of non-papillary neoplasms and 50–60% of non-neoplastic thyroid lesions.[47]

The 'chewing gum' colloid presents as thin or thick strands or chunks of dense, darkly staining colloid, being rather unlike the colloid found in other thyroid diseases. Macrophages and cell debris may be very prominent especially when there is associated cystic change; multinucleate giant cells, probably of histiocytic origin rather than epithelial origin, may also be seen.

Psammoma bodies are present in only a small percentage of aspirates. In MGG-stained material they are difficult to discern and have a glassy, refractile appearance. They may rarely be seen in benign processes[30] (Fig. 6.36).

Squamous metaplasia (Fig. 6.34), even including keratinisation, may occasionally be observed cytologically; neoplasms with this change apparently show no different biological behaviour.

Logistic regression analysis of the various criteria for the diagnosis of papillary carcinoma suggested that a combination of intranuclear cytoplasmic inclusions, papillary structures without adherent blood vessels, and dense 'metaplastic' cytoplasm, were the three most important variables.[100] A combination of any of these two gave 100% predictive value. The sensitivity and predictive value of cytological diagnosis in several other large series ranged from 60% to over 90%.[63,81,100,102,124]

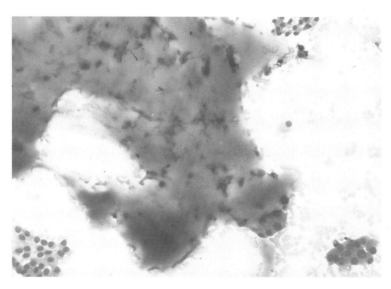

Fig. 6.33 Papillary carcinoma
Thick colloid from an area of tumour with macrofollicular growth; loose aggregates of epithelial cells (MGG, LP)

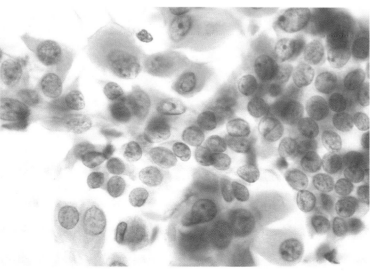

Fig. 6.34 Papillary carcinoma
Sheets and loose aggregates of cells including some with dense 'metaplastic' cytoplasm (Pap, HP)

6 THE THYROID GLAND

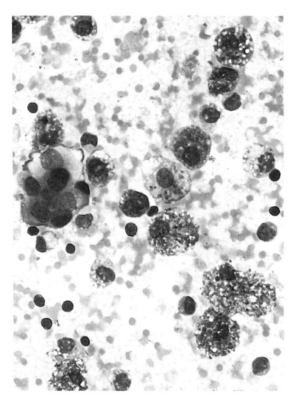

Fig. 6.35 Cystic papillary carcinoma
Cystic change in a lymph nodal metastasis; mainly
haemosiderin containing foamy cells; one small cluster of
atypical epithelial cells (MGG, HP)

Problems in diagnosis

1. Cystic change.
2. Lymphocytic infiltration.
3. Mixed patterns of growth (p. 113).
4. Askanazy cell-like change (p. 114).
5. Papillary adenoma.
6. Hyalinising trabecular adenoma.
7. Oxalate crystals; calcific debris; inspissated colloid.

The fluid aspirate from cystic papillary tumours is
usually brown, darkly stained or haemorrhagic[22] and is
identical to material from many simple or degenerative
cysts. Cytologically, there is a risk of overlooking papillary carcinoma if macrophages and debris predominate
(Fig. 6.35).[22,44,63,70,105,117,121] Large atypical cells with
enlarged nuclei and foamy cytoplasm may sometimes be
the only indicator of neoplasm; however, similar cells
may also be seen in some benign cysts. If there is
abundant epithelium within the material, caution should
be exercised in reporting. The sensitivity of FNA
diagnosis in cystic neoplasms may be as low as
40%[22,105,117,121] and all cystic lesions should be managed
carefully in accordance with clinical and cytological
criteria to exclude cancer (p. 104). Using such criteria
some authors identify most cystic neoplasms.[70]

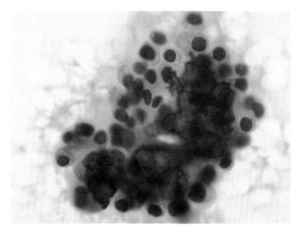

Fig. 6.36 Colloid nodule with cystic change
Several calcific (psammoma) bodies surrounded by epithelial
cells (Pap, HP)

There may be a diffuse lymphocytic infiltrate in papillary carcinoma, particularly in the diffuse sclerosing
variant. If there is prolific epithelium in an aspirate
containing lymphoid cells, the possibility of papillary
carcinoma should be entertained. A histiocytic and giant
cell reaction to neoplasm together with lymphocytes
may also mimic thyroiditis. The abundance of the
epithelium and the other features of papillary tumours
should prevent misdiagnosis.

The follicular variant of papillary carcinoma may
display intranuclear inclusions, nuclear grooves, and
psammoma bodies; however, some may present with
cytological features more akin to follicular neoplasms.[64]
Some show macrofollicular areas and yield abundant
colloid. In several series 70–100% were diagnosed by
FNA.[100,102,103]

Askanazy cell-like change in papillary tumours may
make distinction from follicular neoplasm difficult; true
Askanazy cell change may also be found.

The existence of papillary adenoma is disputed by
some pathologists, although it is acknowledged as an
entity by international authorities. Because of this possibility and the occurrence of papillae in degenerating
colloid nodules,[128] and in primary hyperplasia or
pregnancy,[9] the presence of even indisputable papillary
elements is therefore not pathognomonic of malignancy.
The identification of follicles within papillary structures
in cell block preparations may help in distinguishing
hyperplastic from neoplastic papillae.[86]

Goellner and Carney[42] drew attention to an unusual,
apparently benign neoplasm, the hyalinising trabecular
adenoma which may closely mimic carcinoma cytologically. Intranuclear inclusions and nuclear grooves were
present in aspirates in one of their cases, while another
with poorly cohesive spindle cells was more suggestive
of medullary carcinoma. One of our cases had the
cytological features of follicular neoplasm. 'Tall cell'

carcinoma[67] and tumours of 'insular' type are also described cytologically.[93]

Oxalate crystals are often present in benign thyroid lesions and may mimic psammoma bodies in smears; birefringence excludes the latter possibility. Calcific debris and inspissated colloid may also be difficult to distinguish from psammoma bodies.

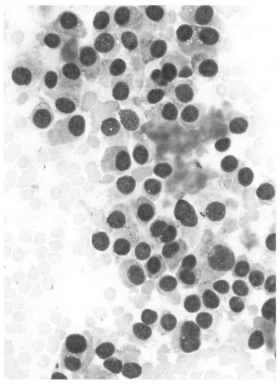

Fig. 6.37 Medullary carcinoma
Dispersed epithelial cells with abundant well defined cytoplasm and eccentric moderately pleomorphic nuclei; note the fragment of amyloid (MGG, HP)

Medullary carcinoma (Figs 6.37–6.43)[11,38,84,91,135]

Criteria for diagnosis

1. Dispersed cell pattern.
2. Cuboidal or rounded cells with oval, eccentric, pleomorphic nuclei uniform hyperchromasia and stippled chromatin; abundant grey-blue cytoplasm. Bi- and multinucleate forms.
3. Spindle-cell forms with elongated cytoplasm.
4. Red cytoplasmic granularity (MGG).
5. Fragments of amorphous pink/violet background material (amyloid).

In the past few years many histological growth patterns of this type of carcinoma have been described and spindle-cell, small cell, follicular, tubular and giant cell variants are accepted. Amyloid is not necessarily present in the stroma of the tumour. Some other poorly differentiated thyroid carcinomas may show features of medullary carcinoma when examined ultrastructurally.[106] In these poorly differentiated or unusual forms, the findings in the aspirate alone may not be sufficient for diagnosis. However, in the classical and spindle-cell varieties they may be diagnostic. The neoplastic cells have low cohesiveness and, although tissue clumps may be present, there is a tendency to cell dispersal. Cell cytoplasm is not particularly fragile so that most dispersed cells are intact. Nuclei are usually eccentrically placed within the more epithelioid cell types. In these tumours the cytoplasm is moderately dense and has fairly well-defined cytoplasmic borders; the cell is sometimes described as being triangular[135] (Fig. 6.37). In the spindle-cell form, which may be the most common in some authors' experience,[38] the nucleus is more central and the cytoplasm less distinct. Some spindle cell tumours have a distinctly mesenchymal appearance (Figs 6.41–6.43).[11] Cytoplasmic granularity is usually fine and may not be present in all cells. In most cases one can find scattered cells with prominent

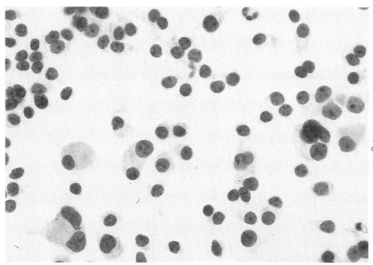

[handwritten note:] Amyloid mb difficult to make out. In wet fixed smears - has a pale blue appearance (Paps) and also shows birefringence in Paps cout staining for Congo red.

Fig. 6.38 Medullary carcinoma
Dispersed cells with a 'plasmacytoid' appearance and several binucleate forms (Pap, HP)

6 THE THYROID GLAND

granularity — multinucleate cells more often show this feature (Fig. 6.39). The granules are invisible in alcohol-fixed Pap stained smears. This granularity is a helpful diagnostic feature, but has been observed in some apparently follicular tumours[91,94] and in some anaplastic carcinomas. Immunological studies show calcitonin mainly in the granular cells so these are probably associated with neurosecretion. At the ultrastructural level, neurosecretory granules are very variable in size, some cells having abundant large granules (Fig. 6.41).

Boey et al[12] observed that amyloid may sometimes be recognisable grossly as chalky white material. It appears in smears as amorphous clumps which stains variable shades of pink or violet with MGG (Fig. 6.37) and is orangeophilic with Pap staining[63,95] (Fig. 6.40). Cracking artefact may be seen. Congo red staining and dichroism confirm the nature of the material which otherwise might be confused with connective tissue or colloid.

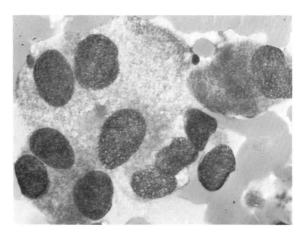

Fig. 6.39 Medullary carcinoma
Tumour cells containing many relatively coarse, red granules (MGG, HP Oil)

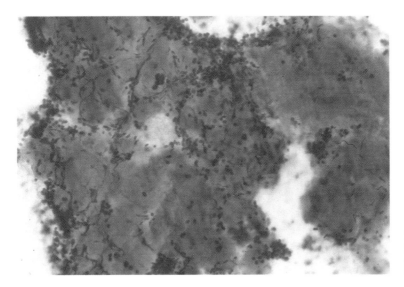

Fig. 6.40 Medullary carcinoma; amyloid
Irregular fragment with adherent epithelial cells and cells within clefts (Pap, LP)

In a series of 16 cases of medullary carcinoma, 10 were recognised by FNA and the remainder were thought cytologically to be either anaplastic carcinomas or follicular or papillary tumours. Of 19 cases in which the diagnosis was suggested, 50% were correct and the remainder Hurthle cell or papillary tumours.[84]

Problems in diagnosis

1. Variants of medullary carcinoma.
2. Askanazy cell neoplasms.
3. Follicular neoplasms.

It is unlikely that the small-cell, giant-cell, poorly differentiated spindle cell forms or other rare variants[79] of medullary carcinoma will be recognised solely on cytological criteria; other primary or secondary spindle-cell masses such as fibroblastic tumours and melanoma

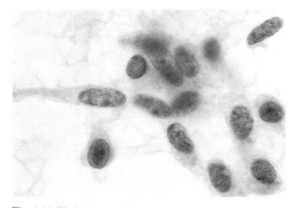

Fig. 6.41 Medullary carcinoma; spindle-cell form
Dispersed cells with elongated nuclei and speckled nuclear chromatin (Pap, HP Oil) (case of Dr E. Waters and Dr J. Armstrong)

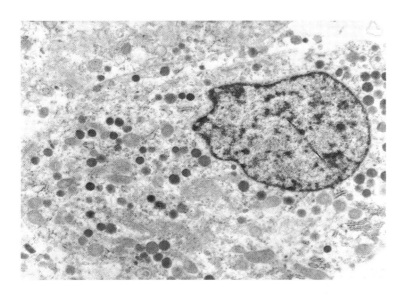

Fig. 6.42 Medullary carcinoma; spindle-cell form
Pleomorphic neurosecretory granules in aspirated tumour cell; same case as Figure 6.41 (EM × 9500)

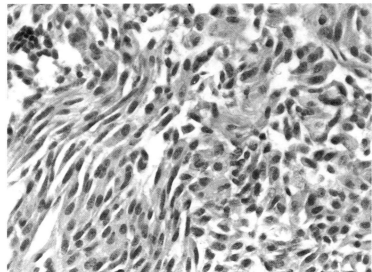

Fig. 6.43 Medullary carcinoma; spindle-cell form
Tissue section; same case as Figures 6.41 and 6.42 (H & E, MP)

may have a similar appearance. Definitive diagnosis can be provided by immunoperoxidase staining for calcitonin,[25] which can be carried out on destained smears, or ultrastructural analysis of a fine needle aspirate (Fig. 6.41).

Sometimes the tumour cells may resemble Askanazy cells. The cytoplasm in medullary carcinoma is, however, less dense; the granules which are often present in Askanazy cells are violet in contrast to the red granules of medullary carcinoma. Nunez suggests that macronucleoli are more characteristic of Askanazy cells and are less often seen in medullary carcinoma.[109]

Tumour cells may be arranged in small follicular clusters resembling follicular neoplasm. Conversely, in some follicular neoplasms, cell dissociation may occur, mimicking medullary carcinoma. We have seen two cases of mixed medullary/follicular carcinoma. Both

were diagnosed by FNA as medullary carcinoma with some unusual features. Simultaneous staining for calcitonin and thyroglobulin might have suggested a mixed pattern, although it would be difficult cytologically to exclude the possibility of residual thyroglobulin secreting epithelial cells being trapped within the neoplasm.

Giant-cell anaplastic carcinoma (spindle and giant-cell carcinoma) (Figs 6.44–6.46).[29,94,123]

Criteria for diagnosis

1. Bizarre, large malignant cells with a macrophage-like appearance; multinucleate malignant cells.
2. Malignant spindle-cells with a mesenchymal appearance.
3. Necrotic cell fragments, debris and dirty background.

6 *THE THYROID GLAND*

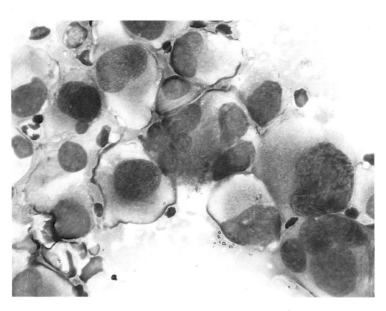

Fig. 6.44 Anaplastic giant-cell carcinoma
Giant mononuclear and multinucleated tumour cells (MGG, HP)

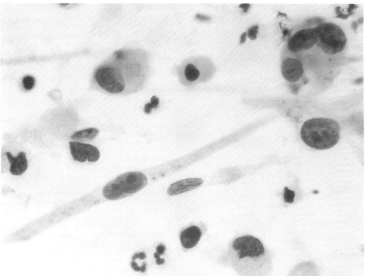

Fig. 6.45 Spindle- and giant-cell carcinoma
Histiocyte-like giant cells; fibroblastoid spindle cells (Pap, HP)

The bizarre nature of the tumour cells together with the clinical history of a rapidly enlarging mass generally make this diagnosis easy and permit palliative treatment without operative intervention (Figs 6.44–6.46). Residual areas of differentiated papillary or follicular cancer may also be sampled.

Problems in diagnosis

1. Sampling problems.
2. Fibroblastic and histiocytic cells in other lesions.
3. Variants of giant-cell anaplastic carcinoma.
4. Mesenchymal neoplasms.
5. Follicular adenoma with severe nuclear atypia.
6. Metastatic tumours.

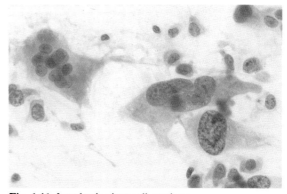

Fig. 6.46 Anaplastic giant cell carcinoma
Malignant giant cells together with an osteoclastic cell (Pap, HP)

Obtaining diagnostic material may be difficult because of fibrosis or extensive necrosis and accompaning inflammation.

Resolving suppurative thyroiditis and De Quervain's thyroiditis may contain fibroblastic cells some with atypia; conversely, in the more spindle and fibrous forms of anaplastic carcinoma many of the tumour cells may not appear overtly malignant; a search for diagnostic cells may be necessary.

On one occasion we have seen an entirely encapsulated follicular neoplasm with areas of bizarre giant cells whose nuclear features suggested malignancy; this would be a rare cause of a 'false positive' diagnosis.

There is wide variation in the morphology of anaplastic spindle and giant-cell carcinoma. Some may contain remnants of pre-existing follicular or papillary neoplasms; others may be cytologically indistinguishable from pleomorphic mesenchymal neoplasms such as malignant fibrous histiocytoma (Fig. 6.45); however, sarcomas are extremely rare within the thyroid. Sometimes benign looking osteoclast-like giant cells may be found (Fig. 6.46), and one well-recognised variant of giant-cell anaplastic carcinoma contains many such cells[147] in contrast to the bizarre malignant cells usually composing this tumour. The prognosis in these cases is similar to the usual form.

Metastatic anaplastic malignancy, e.g. of renal or lung origin, may be impossible to distinguish from primary neoplasm without ancillary testing.

Lymphoma[90,140]

Although primary lymphomas of the thyroid are uncommon, the gland is prey to the development of most of the morphological varieties of non-Hodgkin's lymphoma including low-grade and high-grade forms. Lymphomas usually occur in glands affected by Hashimoto's thyroiditis and can be difficult to distinguish clinically and cytologically from this disease. The low-grade lymphomas, for example follicular lymphomas (centrocytic/centroblastic), are especially difficult to diagnose because their mixed cell population may closely resemble florid reactive processes. The higher grade lesions, e.g. centroblastic or immunoblastic neoplasms, are the most common and will generally present with a rapidly enlarging gland suggesting malignancy; the monotonous and atypical cytological picture in these cases enables an easier diagnosis of malignancy and the definitive diagnosis of lymphoma. Hodgkin's lymphoma can also present in the thyroid occasionally. Diagnostic criteria are similar to those of lymphoma in other sites (see Ch. 5).

Problems in diagnosis

1. Thyroiditis.
2. Small cell anaplastic carcinoma.

Distinguishing non-Hodgkin's lymphoma from a reactive process is covered in the section on lymph nodes (p. 68). As a rule, predominance of a small lymphocytic population with some large lymphoid cell indicates a reactive process no matter how 'atypical' or activated single lymphoid cells may be. In coexistent thyroiditis and lymphoma, there is a distinct possibility of inadequate sampling. Multiple aspirations will help to overcome this problem; however, cytological diagnosis will remain difficult. Immunoperoxidase studies to prove monoclonality[140] or DNA studies to detect immunoglobulin or T-receptor gene rearrangements may be useful.

In ultrastructural and immunological studies, most small-cell malignancies of the thyroid are shown to be lymphoid in origin; apart from the rare small-cell medullary carcinoma, true anaplastic small-cell carcinoma is extremely rare. It is interesting that most such 'carcinomas' had been described as having cytological features which suggested a lymphoid origin.[31] Abundance of round fragments of pale blue cytoplasm in the background (lymphoid globules) is the most reliable sign of a lymphoid origin. Cell clustering, nuclear moulding and engulfment and tear-drop cells are more typical of small cell anaplastic carcinoma.

Metastatic malignancies[20,48,118,132,143,144]

The thyroid is a relatively common site for metastasis in disseminated malignancy and occasionally a metastasis will present as an apparent primary mass[132] or even as 'thyroiditis'.[118] Breast, kidney, melanoma, lung and lymphoid tumours are among the most frequently met[20,132] and in patients with a prior malignancy of these types, metastatic tumour may be as likely as a new thyroid primary tumour. Renal cell carcinoma may be particularly difficult to diagnose because of its resemblance to follicular neoplasms;[48] thyroglobulin staining helps to confirm a primary lesion[37] and electron microscopy may also be helpful. Poorly differentiated metastatic tumours may be extremely difficult to distinguish from anaplastic thyroid tumours.

Squamous cell carcinoma may rarely occur as a primary lesion. We have also seen thyroid metastases from squamous cell carcinoma of the lung and from the direct spread of laryngeal tumours infiltrating through the cartilage and presenting clinically as apparent thyroid primary lesions.

Parathyroid diseases[24,28,41,46,75,104]

Several authors now suggest a role for FNA in the evaluation of parathyroid disease. FNA appears to be of limited value in the preoperative assessment of patients with hyperparathyroidism, but in patients in whom surgery failed to locate a parathyroid adenoma[46] FNA in conjunction with ultrasound examination of the neck[45,46,75] or CT of the mediastinum[28] may be useful. High cellularity, fragments of cohesive cells having small nuclei 6–8 μm in diameter with coarse granular chromatin, some larger nuclei 10–30 μm, scattered

6 *THE THYROID GLAND*

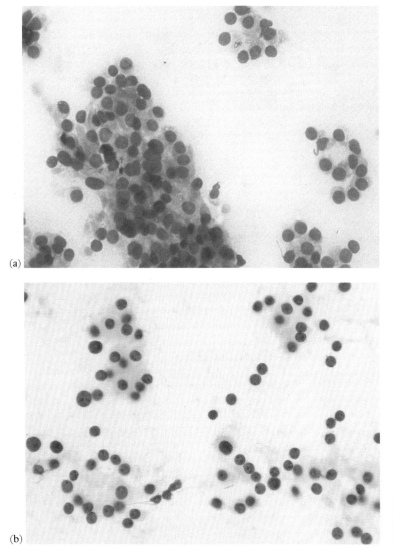

(a)

(b)

Fig. 6.47 Parathyroid adenoma
Microfollicular structures with small
nuclei and pale cytoplasm. (a) MGG, HP.
(b) Pap, HP.

oxyphil cells and absence of colloid or macrophages, are described as cytological criteria for identifying parathyroid cells;[24,41] others found numerous bare nuclei in smears of adenomas.[104] Monolayered sheets and microfollicular structures are said to be more characteristic of thyroid disease;[24] however, most authors have found it difficult on cytological grounds to distinguish parathyr-

oid from thyroid tissue. We have seen parathyroid adenomas with a microfollicular structure (Figs 6.47) and papillary structures have also been described in some.[24] Positive staining with silver (argyrophilia), immunoperoxidase positivity for parathormone and biochemical estimations of aspirated material have all been used in diagnosis.[28]

THE THYROID GLAND 6

REFERENCES

1. Akerman M, Tennvall J, Biorklund A, Martensson H, Moller T: Sensitivity and specificity of fine needle aspiration cytology in the diagnosis of tumours of the thyroid gland. Acta Cytol 29: 850–855, 1985.
2. Alanen K A, Joensuu H, Khlemi P J: Autolysis is a potential source of false aneuploid peaks in flow cytometric DNA histograms. Cytometry 10: 17–25, 1989.
3. Anderson J B, Webb A J: Fine needle aspiration biopsy and the diagnosis of thyroid cancer. Br J Surg 74: 292–296, 1987.
4. Ashcroft M W and Van Herle A J: Management of thyroid nodules II. Head Neck Surg 3: 297–322, 1981.
5. Atkinson B, Ernest C S, Li Volsi V: Cytologic diagnosis of follicular tumours of the thyroid. Diagn Cytopathol 2: 1–5, 1986.
6. Backdahl M, Carstensen J, Auer G, Tallroth E. Statistical evaluation of the prognostic value of nuclear DNA content in papillary, follicular and medullary thyroid tumours. World J Surg 10: 974–980, 1986.
7. Backdahl M, Wallin G, Lowhagen T, Auer G, Granberg P O. Fine needle biopsy cytology and DNA analysis. Their place in the evaluation and treatment of patients with thyroid neoplasms. Surg Clin North Am 67: 197–211, 1987.
8. Beecham J E: Coexistent disease as a complicating factor in the fine needle aspiration diagnosis of papillary carcinoma of the thyroid. Acta Cytol 30: 435–438, 1986.
9. Betsill W: Thyroid fine needle aspiration in pregnant women. Diagn Cytopathol 1: 53–54, 1985.
10. Block M A, Dailey G E, Robb J A. Thyroid nodules indeterminate by needle biopsy. Am J Surg 146: 72–76, 1983.
11. Blonk D I, Talerman A, Visser-van Dijk M N: The cytology of medullary carcinoma of the thyroid with spindle cell pattern. Arch Geschwulstforsch 48: 313–317, 1978.
12. Boey J, Hsu C, Collins R J: False-negative errors in fine needle aspiration biopsy of dominant thyroid nodules: A prospective follow up study. World J Surg 10: 623–630, 1986.
13. Boey J, Hsu C, Collins R J, Wong J. A prospective controlled study of fine needle aspiration and Tru-cut needle biopsy of dominant thyroid nodules. World J Surg 8: 458–465, 1984.
14. Bondeson L, Azavedo E, Bondeson A G, Caspersson T, Ljungberg O: Nuclear DNA content and behavior of oxyphil thyroid tumours. Cancer 58: 672–675, 1986.
15. Boon M E, Kok L P. An explanation for the reported variability of nuclear areas in air dried Romanowsky-Giemsa stained smears of follicular tumours of the thyroid. Acta Cytol 31: 527–530, 1987.
16. Boon M E, Lowhagen T, Cardozo P L, Blonk D I, Kurver P J, Baak J P. Computation of preoperative diagnosis probability for follicular adenoma and carcinoma of the thyroid on aspiration smears. Anal Quant Cytol 4: 1–5, 1982.
17. Broughan T A, Esselstyn C B Jr. Large needle thyroid biopsy: still necessary. Surgery 100: 1138–1141, 1986.
18. Bugis S P, Young J E, Archibald S D, Chen V S. Diagnostic accuracy of fine needle aspiration biopsy versus frozen section in solitary thyroid nodules. Am J Surg 152: 411–416, 1986.
19. Carney J A, Brendan Moore S, Northcutt R C, Woolner L B, Stillwell G K. Palpation thyroiditis (multifocal granulomatous folliculitis). Am J Clin Pathol 64: 639–647, 1975.
20. Chacho M S, Greenebaum E, Moussouris H F, Schreiber K, Koss L G: Value of aspiration cytology of the thyroid in metastatic disease. Acta Cytol 31: 705–712, 1987.
21. Christ M L, Haja J H: Intranuclear cytoplasmic inclusions (invaginations) in thyroid aspirations; frequency and specificity. Acta Cytol 23: 327–331, 1979.
22. Cusick E L, McIntosh C A, Krukowski Z H, Matheson N A: Cystic change and neoplasia in isolated thyroid swellings. Br J Surg 75: 982–983, 1988.
23. Cusick E L, MacIntosh C A, Krukowski Z H, Williams V M M, Ewen S W B, Matheson N A. Management of isolated thyroid swellings: a prospective six year study of fine needle aspiration cytology in diagnosis. Br Med J 301: 318–321, 1990.
24. Davey D D, Glant M D, Berger E K: Parathyroid cytopathology. Diagn Cytopathol 2: 76–80, 1986.
25. Davila R M, Bedrossian C W, Silverberg A B: Immunocytochemistry of the thyroid in surgical and cytological specimens. Arch Pathol Lab Med 112: 51–56, 1988.
26. Deligeorgi-Politi H: Nuclear crease as a cytodiagnostic feature of papillary thyroid carcinoma in fine needle aspiration biopsies. Diagn Cytopathol 3: 307–310, 1987.
27. Domagala W, Lasota J, Wolska H, Lubinski J, Weber K, Osborn M. Diagnosis of metastatic renal cell and thyroid carcinomas by intermediate filament typing and cytology of tumour cells in fine needle aspirates. Acta Cytol 32: 415–421, 1988.
28. Doppman J L, Krudy Ag, Marx S J, Saxe A, Schneider P, Norton J A, Spiegel A M, Downs R W, Schaaf M, Brennan M E, Schnedier A B, Aurbach G D. Aspiration of enlarged parathyroid glands for parathyroid hormone assay. Radiology 148: 31–35, 1983.
29. Droese M: Cytological aspiration biopsy of the thyroid gland. F K Schattauer, Stuttgart, 1980.
30. Dugan J M, Atkinson B F, Avitabile A, Schimmel M, LiVolsi V A: Psammoma bodies in fine needle aspirate of the thyroid in lymphocytic thyroiditis. Acta Cytol 31: 330–334, 1987.
31. Einhorn J, Franzen S. Thin-needle biopsy in the diagnosis of thyroid disease. Acta Radiol 58: 321–336, 1962.
32. Frable W J. The treatment of thyroid cancer. The role of fine needle aspiration cytology. Arch Otolaryngol Head Neck Surg 112: 1200–1203, 1986.
33. Frable W J, Frable M A: Fine needle aspiration biopsy of the thyroid. Histopathologic and clinical correlations. Progress in Surgical Pathology Vol. 1, Masson, New York, 1980.
34. Freidman M, Shimoaka K, Getaz P. Needle aspiration of 310 thyroid lesions. Acta Cytol 23: 194–203, 1979.
35. Friedman M, Shimoaka K, Rao V. Diagnosis of chronic lymphocytic thyroiditis (nodular presentation) by needle aspiration. Acta Cytol 25: 513–522, 1981.
36. Gagneten C B, Roccatagliata G, Lowenstein A, Soto F, Soto R. The role of fine needle aspiration biopsy cytology in the evaluation of the clinically solitary thyroid nodule. Acta Cytol 31: 595–598, 1987.
37. Gal R, Aronof A, Gertzmann H, Kessler E: The potential value of the demonstration of thyroglobulin by immunoperoxidase techniques in fine needle aspiration cytology. Acta Cytol 31: 713–716, 1987.
38. Geddie W R, Bedard Y C, Strawbridge H T G: Medullary carcinoma of the thyroid in fine needle aspiration biopsies. Am J Clin Pathol 82: 552–558, 1984.
39. Ginsberg J, Young J E, Walfish P G. Parathyroid cysts; medical diagnosis and management. JAMA 240: 1506–1507, 1978.

6 *THE THYROID GLAND*

40. Glant M D, Berger E K, Davey D D: Intranuclear cytoplasmic inclusions in aspirates of follicular neoplasms of the thyroid. Acta Cytol 28: 576–579, 1989.

41. Glenthoj A, Karstrup S. Parathyroid identification by ultrasonically guided aspiration cytology. Is correct cytological identification possible? APMIS 97: 497–502, 1989.

42. Goellner J R, Carney J A: Cytologic features of fine needle aspirates of hyalinizing trabecular adenoma of the thyroid. Am J Clin Pathol 91: 115–119, 1989.

43. Goellner J R, Gharib H, Grant C S, Johnson D A: Fine needle aspiration cytology of the thyroid, 1980 to 1986. Acta Cytol 31: 587–590, 1987.

44. Goellner J R, Johnson D A: Cytology of cystic papillary carcinoma of the thyroid. Acta Cytol 26: 797–808, 1982.

45. Goldfinger M, Rothberg R, Stoll S. Sonographic guidance of thyroid needle biopsy. J Can Assoc Radiol 37: 186–188, 1986.

46. Gooding G A, Clark O H, Stark D D, Moss A A, Montgomery C K. Parathyroid aspiration biopsy under ultrasound guidance in the postoperative hyperparathyroid patient. Radiology 155: 193–196, 1985.

47. Gould E, Watzak L, Chamizo W, Albores-Saavedra J: Nuclear grooves in cytologic preparations. A study of the utility of this feature in the diagnosis of papillary carcinoma. Acta Cytol 33: 16–20, 1989.

48. Gritsman A Y, Popok S M, Ro J Y, Dekmezian R H, Weber R S: Renal cell carcinoma with intranuclear inclusions metastatic to thyroid: a diagnostic problem in aspiration cytology. Diagn Cytopathol 4: 125–129, 1988.

49. Guarda L A, Baskin H J: Inflammatory and lymphoid lesions of the thyroid gland. Cytopathology by fine needle aspiration. Am J Clin Pathol 87: 14–22, 1987.

50. Gutteridge D H, Orell S R: Non-toxic goitre: diagnostic role of aspiration cytology, antibodies and serum thyrotrophin. Clin Endocrinol 9: 505–514, 1978.

51. Hall T L, Layfield L J, Philippe A, Rosenthal D L: Sources of diagnostic error in fine needle aspiration of the thyroid. Cancer 63: 718–725, 1989.

52. Hamburger J I: Consistency of sequential needle biopsy findings for thyroid nodules. Management implications. Arch Intern Med 147: 97–99, 1987.

53. Hamburger J I: Is expertise in cytology diagnosis on thyroid nodules transferable? Diagn Cytopathol 4: 88–89, 1988.

54. Hamburger J I, Hamburger S W: Fine needle biopsy of thyroid nodules: avoiding the pitfalls. NY State J Med 86: 241–249, 1986.

55. Hamburger J I, Husain M: Semiquantitative criteria for fine needle biopsy diagnosis: reduced false negative diagnoses. Diagn Cytopathol 4: 14–17, 1988.

56. Hamburger J I, Miller J M, Kini S R: Clinico-pathological evaluation of thyroid nodules: Handbook & Atlas. Southfield, MI, 1979.

57. Hamburger J I, Husain M, Nishiyama R, Nunez C, Solomon D. Increasing the accuracy of fine needle biopsy for thyroid nodules. Arch Pathol Lab Med 113: 1035–1041, 1989.

58. Hapke M R, Dehner L P. The optically clear nucleus. A reliable sign of papillary carcinoma of the thyroid? Am J Surg Pathol 3: 31–38, 1979.

59. Harach H R. Usefulness of fine needle aspiration of the thyroid in an endemic goiter region. Acta Cytol 33: 31–35, 1989.

60. Harsoulis P, Leontsini M, Economou A, Gerasimidis T, Smbarounis C: Fine needle aspiration biopsy cytology in the diagnosis of thyroid cancer: comparative study of 213 operated patients. Br J Surg 73: 461–464, 1986.

61. Hawkins F, Bellido D, Bernal C, Rigopoulou D, Ruiz Valdepenas M P, Lazaro E, Perez-Barrios A, De Agustin P: Fine needle aspiration biopsy in the diagnosis of thyroid cancer and thyroid disease. Cancer 59: 1206–1209, 1987.

62. Hostetter A L, Hrafnkelsson J, Wingren S O W, Ernestrom S, Nordenskjold B. A comparative study of DNA cytometry methods for benign and malignant thyroid tissue. Am J Clin Pathol 89: 760–763, 1988.

63. Hsu C, Boey J: Diagnostic pitfalls in the fine needle aspiration of thyroid nodules. A study of 555 cases in Chinese patients. Acta Cytol 31: 699–704, 1987.

64. Hugh J C, Duggan M A, Chang-Poon V: The fine needle aspiration appearance of the follicular variant of thyroid papillary carcinoma: a report of three cases. Diagn Cytopathol 4: 196–201, 1988.

65. Jacobs D M, Waisman J. Cervical paragangalioma with intranuclear vacuoles in a fine needle aspirate. Acta Cytol 31: 29–32, 1987.

66. Jayaram G: Problems in the interpretation of Hurthle cell populations in fine needle aspirates from the thyroid. Acta Cytol 27: 84–85, 1983.

67. Jayaram G: Fine needle aspiration cytologic study of the solitary thyroid nodule. Profile of 308 cases with histologic correlation. Acta Cytol 29: 967–973, 1985.

68. Jayaram G: Cytology of clear cell carcinoma of the thyroid. Acta Cytol 33: 135–136, 1989.

69. Jayaram G, Aggarwal S: Infarction of thyroid nodule; a rare complication following fine needle aspiration. Acta Cytol 33: 940–941, 1989.

70. Jayaram G, Kaur A: Cystic thyroid nodules harbouring malignancy. A problem in fine needle aspiration cytodiagnosis. Acta Cytol 33: 941–942, 1989.

71. Jayaram G, Marwaha R K, Gupta R K, Sharma S K: Cytomorphologic spects of thyroiditis. A study of 51 cases with functional, immunologic and ultrasonographic data. Acta Cytol 31: 687–693, 1987.

72. Jayaram G, Singh B, Marwaha R K: Graves' disease. Appearance in cytologic smears from fine needle aspirates of the thyroid gland. Acta Cytol 33: 36–40, 1989.

73. Joensuu H, Klemi P J, Eeorola E. Diagnostic value of flow cytometric DNA determination combined with fine needle aspiration biopsy in thyroid tumors. Anal Quant Cytol Histol 9: 328–334, 1987.

74. Jones J D, Pittman D L, Sanders L R: Necrosis of thyroid nodules after fine needle aspiration. Acta Cytol 29: 29–32, 1985.

75. Karstrup S, Glenthoj A, Torp-Pedersen S, Hegedus L, Holm H H. Ultrasonically guided fine needle aspiration on suggested enlarged parathyroid glands. Acta Radiol 29: 213–216, 1988.

76. Keller M P, Crabbe M M, Norwood S H. Accuracy and significance of fine needle aspiration and frozen section in determining the extent of thyroid resection. Surgery 101: 632–655, 1987.

77. Kern W H, Haber H. Fine needle aspiration minibiopsies. Acta Cytol 30: 403–408, 1986.

78. Khafagi F, Wright G, Castles H, Perry-Keene D, Mortimer R: Screening for thyroid malignancy: the role of fine needle biopsy. Med J Aust 149: 302–307, 1988.

79. Kimura N, Ishioka K, Miura Y, Sasano N, Takaya K, Mouri T, Kimura T, Nakazato Y, Yamada R. Melanin-producing medullary thyroid carcinoma with glandular differentiation. Acta Cytol 33: 61–66, 1988.

80. Kini S R, Miller J M, Hamburger J I: Problems in the cytologic diagnosis of the 'cold' thyroid nodule in patients with lymphocytic thyroiditis. Acta Cytol 25: 506–512, 1980.

81. Kini S R, Miller J M, Hamburger J I, Jane Smith M: Cytopathology of papillary carcinoma of the thyroid by fine needle aspiration. Acta Cytol 24: 511–521, 1980.

82. Kini S R, Miller J M, Hamburger J I: Cytopathology of

Hurthle cell lesions of the thyroid gland by fine needle aspiration. Acta Cytol 25: 647–652, 1981.

83. Kini S R, Miller J M, Hamburger J I, Smith-Purslowe M J: Cytopathology of follicular lesions of the thyroid gland. Diagn Cytopathol 1: 123–132, 1985.

84. Kini S R. Miller J M, Hamburger J I, Smith-Purslowe J: Cytopathologic features of medullary carcinoma of the thyroid. Arch Pathol Lab Med 108: 156–159, 1984.

85. Klemi P J, Joensuu H. Comparison of DNA ploidy in routine fine needle aspiration biopsy samples and paraffin-embedded tissue samples. Anal Quant Cytol Histo 10: 195–199, 1988.

86. Kung I T, Yuen R W: Fine needle aspiration of the thyroid. Distinction between colloid nodules and follicular neoplasms using cell blocks and 21-gauge needles. Acta Cytol 33: 53–60, 1989.

87. Lew W, Orell S R, Henderson D W: Intranuclear vacuoles in non-papillary carcinoma of thyroid: a report of 3 cases. Acta Cytol 28: 581–586, 1984.

88. Lever E G, Refetoff S, Scherberg N H, Carr K: The influence of percutaneous fine needle aspiration on serum thyroglobulin. J Clin Endocrinol Metab 56: 26–29, 1983.

89. Liel Y, Zirkin H J, Sobel R J: Fine needle aspiration of the hot thyroid nodule. Acta Cytol 32: 866–867, 1988.

90. Limonova Z, Nenwintova R, Smejkal V: Malignant lymphoma of the thyroid. Exp Clin Endocrinol 90: 113–119, 1987.

91. Ljungberg O: Cytologic diagnosis of medullary carcinoma of the thyroid gland. Acta Cytol 16: 253–255, 1972.

92. Lowhagen T, Granberg P-O, Lundell G, Skinnari P, Sundblad R, Willems J-S: Aspiration biopsy cytology (ABC) in nodules of the thyroid gland suspected to be malignant. Surg Clin North Am 59: 3–18, 1979.

93. Lowhagen T, Linsk J. Aspiration biopsy cytology of the thyroid gland. In: Clinical Aspiration Cytology, 2nd edn. Linsk J A, Franzen S. (eds) Lippincott, New York, 1989.

94. Lowhagen T, Sprenger E: Cytologic presentation of thyroid tumours in aspiration biopsy smears. Acta Cytol 18:'192–197, 1974.

95. Lucas A, Sanmarti A, Salinas I, Llatjos M, Foz M: Amyloid goitre. Diagnosis by fine needle aspiration biopsy of the thyroid. J Endocrinol Invest 12: 43–46, 1989.

96. Luck J B, Mumaw V R, Frable W J. Fine needle aspiration of the thyroid. Differential diagnosis by videoplan image analysis. Acta Cytol 26: 793–796, 1982.

97. Mahoney C P. Differential diagnosis of goiter. Pediatr Clin North Am 34: 891–905, 1987.

98. Mair S, Dunbar F, Becker P J, Du Plessis W: Fine needle cytology — Is aspiration suction necessary. A study of 100 masses in various sites. Acta Cytol 33: 809–813, 1989.

99. Mazzaferri E L, de los Santos E T, Rofagha-Keyhani S. Solitary thyroid nodule: diagnosis and management. Med Clin North Am 72: 1177–1211, 1988.

100. Miller T R, Bottles K, Holly E A, Friend N F, Abelle J S: A step-wise logistic regression analysis of papillary carcinoma of the thyroid. Acta Cytol 30: 285–293, 1986.

101. Miller J M, Hamburger J I, Kini S R. Thyroid needle biopsy. Arch Intern Med 145: 764–765, 1985.

102. Miller J M, Hamburger J I, Kini S R: The needle biopsy diagnosis of papillary thyroid carcinoma. Cancer 48: 989–993, 1981.

103. Miller J M, Kini S R, Hamburger J I: The diagnosis of malignant follicular neoplasms of the thyroid by needle biopsy. Cancer 55: 2812–2817, 1985.

104. Mincione G P, Borelli D, Cicchi P, Ipponi P L, Fiorini A: Fine needle aspiration cytology of parathyroid adenoma: A review of seven cases. Acta Cytol 30: 65–70, 1986.

105. Muller N, Cooperberg P L, Suen K C H, Thorson S C: Needle aspiration biopsy in cystic papillary carcinoma of the thyroid. Am J Roentgenol 144: 251–253, 1985.

106. Niewenhuijzan Kruseman A C, Bosman F T, Van Bergen Henegouw J C, Cramer-Knijnenburg G, de la Riviere G B. Medullary differentiation of anaplastic thyroid carcinoma. Am J Clin Pathol 77: 541–547, 1982.

107. Nilsson G: Marginal vacuoles in fine needle aspiration biopsy smears of toxic goiters. Acta Pathol Microbiol Scand A 80: 289–293, 1972.

108. Nishiyama R H, Bigos S T, Goldfarb W B, Flynn S D, Taxiarchis L N. The efficacy of simultaneous fine needle aspiration and large needle biopsy of the thyroid gland. Surgery 100: 1133–1137, 1986.

109. Nunez C, Mendelsohn G: Fine needle aspiration and needle biopsy of the thyroid gland. Pathol Annu 24 Pt 1, 24: 161–198, 1989.

110. Pepper G M, Zwickler D, Rosen Y. Fine needle aspiration biopsy of the thyroid nodule. Results of a start-up project in a general teaching hospital setting. Arch Intern Med 149: 594–596, 1989.

111. Persson P S: Cytodiagnosis of thyroiditis. A comparative study of cytological histological immunological and clinical findings in thyroiditis. Acta Med Scand (Suppl) 483: 7–100, 1968.

112. Pitts W C, Berry G J: Marginal vacuoles in metastatic thyroid carcinoma: a case report. Diagn Cytopathol 5: 200–202, 1989.

113. Rastad J, Wilander E, Lindgren P G, Ljunghall S, Stenkvist B G, Akerstrom G: Cytologic diagnosis of a medullary carcinoma of the thyroid by Sevier-Munger silver staining and calcitonin immunocytochemistry. Acta Cytol 31: 45–47, 1987.

114. Ravinsky E, Safneck J R: Differentiation of Hashimoto's thyroiditis from thyroid neoplasms in fine needle aspirates. Acta Cytol 32: 854–861, 1988.

115. Reeve T S, Delbridge L, Sloan D, Crummer P: The impact of fine needle aspiration biopsy on surgery for single thyroid nodules. Med J Aust 145: 308–311, 1986.

116. Rieger R, Pimpl W, Oney S, Rettenbacher L, Galvan G. Hyperthyroidism and concurrent thyroid malignancies. Surgery 106: 6–10, 1989.

117. Rosen I B, Provias J P, Walfish P G: Pathologic nature of cystic thyroid nodules selected for surgery by needle aspiration biopsy. Surgery 100: 606–616, 1986.

118. Rosen I B, Strawbridge H G, Walfish P G, Bain J. Malignant pseudothyroiditis: a new clinical entity. Am J Surg 136: 445–449, 1978.

119. Rupp M, Ehya H: Nuclear grooves in the aspiration cytology of papillary carcinoma of the thyroid. Acta Cytol 33: 21–26, 1989.

120. Santos J E, Leiman G: Nonaspiration fine needle cytology. Application of a new technique to nodular thyroid disease. Acta Cytol 32: 353–356, 1988.

121. Sarda A K, Bal S, Dutta Gupta S, Kapur M M: Diagnosis and treatment of cystic disease of the thyroid by aspiration. Surgery 103: 593–596, 1988.

122. Schmid K W, Hofstadter F, Propst A Jr, Ladurner D, Zechmann W. A fourteen year practice with the fine needle aspiration biopsy of the thyroid in an endemic area. Pathol Res Pract 181: 308–310, 1986.

123. Schmid K W, Ladurner D, Zechmann W, Feichtinger H. Clinicopathologic management of tumours of the thyroid gland in an endemic goiter area. Combined use of preoperative fine needle aspiration biopsy and intraoperative frozen section. Acta Cytol 33: 27–30, 1989.

124. Schmid K W, Lucciarini P, Ladurner D, Zechmann W, Hofstadter F: Papillary carcinoma of the thyroid gland. Analysis of 94 cases with preoperative fine needle aspiration cytologic examination. Acta Cytol 31: 591–594,

6 THE THYROID GLAND

1987.

125. Schneider V, Frable W J: Spindle and giant cell carcinoma of the thyroid. Cytologic diagnosis by fine needle aspiration. Acta Cytol 24: 184–189, 1980.

126. Shurbaji M S, Gupta P K, Frost J K: Nuclear grooves: a useful criterion in the cytopathologic diagnosis of papillary thyroid carcinoma. Diagn Cytopathol 4: 91–94, 1988.

127. Sidaway M K, Costa M. The significance of paravacuolar granules of the thyroid. A histologic, cytologic and ultrastructural study. Acta Cytol. 33: 929–934, 1989.

128. Silverman J F, Prabhaker K G, Morris M T. Parathyroid hormone (PTH) assay of parathyroid cysts examined by fine needle aspiration biopsy. Am J Clin Pathol 86: 776–780, 1986.

129. Silverman J F, West R L, Finley J L, Larkin E W, Park H K, Swanson M S, Fore W W: Fine needle aspiration versus large needle biopsy or cutting biopsy in evaluation of thyroid nodules. Diagn Cytopathol 2: 25–30, 1986.

130. Silverman J F, West R L, Larkin E W, Park H K, Finley J L, Swanson M S, Fore W W. The role of fine needle aspiration biopsy in the rapid diagnosis and management of thyroid neoplasm. Cancer 57: 1164–1170, 1986.

131. Smejkal V, Smejkalova E, Rosa M, Zeman V, Smetana K: Cytologic changes simulating malignancy in thyrotoxic goitres treated with carbimazole. Acta Cytol 29: 173–179, 1985.

132. Smith S A, Gharib H, Goellner J R: Fine needle aspiration. Usefulness for diagnosis and management of metastatic carcinoma to the thyroid. Arch Intern Med 147: 311–312, 1987.

133. Soderstrom N. Puncture of goiters for aspiration biopsy. A preliminary report. Acta Med Scand 144: 235–244, 1952.

134. Soderstrom N, Bjorklund A. Intranuclear cytoplasmic inclusions in some types of thyroid cancer. Acta Cytol 17: 191–197, 1973.

135. Soderstrom N, Telenius B M, Akerman M: Diagnosis of medullary carcinoma of the thyroid by fine needle aspiration biopsy. Acta Med Scand 197: 71–76, 1975.

136. Solomon D H: Cost effective analysis of the evaluation of the thyroid nodule. Ann Int Med 96: 221–232, 1982.

137. Sprenger E, Lowhagen T, Vogt-Schaden M. Differential diagnosis between follicular adenoma and follicular carcinoma of the thyroid by nuclear DNA determination. Acta Cytol 21: 528–530, 1977.

138. Suen K C: How does one separate cellular follicular lesions of the thyroid by fine needle aspiration biopsy? Diagn Cytopathol 4: 78–81, 1988.

139. Sutton R T, Reading C C, Charboneau J W, James E M, Grant C S, Hay I D. US-guided biopsy of neck masses in postoperative management of patients with thyroid cancer. Radiology 168: 769–772, 1988.

140. Tani E, Skoog L: Fine needle aspiration cytology and immunocytochemistry in the diagnosis of lymphoid lesions of the thyroid gland. Acta Cytol 33: 48–52, 1989.

141. Van Vliet G, Glinoer D, Verelst J, Spehl M, Gompel C, Delange F. Cold thyroid nodules in childhood: is surgery always necessary? Eur J Pediatr 146: 378–382, 1987.

142. Walfish P G, Strawbridge H T G, Rosen I B. Management implications from routine needle biopsy of hyperfunctioning thyroid nodules. Surgery 1179–1186, 1985.

143. Watts N B: Carcinoma metastatic to the thyroid: prevalence and diagnosis by fine needle aspiration cytology. Am J Med Sci 293: 13–17, 1987.

144. Watts N S, Sewell C W. Carcinomatous involvement of the thyroid presenting as subacute thyroiditis. Am J Med Sci 296: 126–128, 1988.

145. Willems J S, Lowhagen T: Fine needle aspiration cytology in thyroid diseases. Clin Endocrinol Metab 10: 247–266, 1981.

146. Willems J S, Lowhagen T: The role of fine needle aspiration in the management of thyroid disease. Clin Endocrinol Metab 10: 267–273, 1981.

147. Willems J S, Lowhagen T, Palombini L: The cytology of a giant cell osteoclastoma-like malignant thyroid neoplasm. Acta Cytol 23: 214–216, 1979.

148. Wilson R A, Gartner W S Jr: Teflon granuloma mimicking a thyroid tumor. Diagn Cytopathol 3: 156–158, 1987.

149. Yuen R W M, Whitaker D, Sterrett, G: Aspiration cytology in the diagnosis of autoimmune thyroiditis. Med J Aust 2: 561–564, 1976.

150. Zirkin H J, Hertzanu Y, Gal R. Fine needle aspiration cytology and immunocytochemistry in a case of intrathoracic thyroid goiter. Acta Cytol 31: 694–698, 1987.

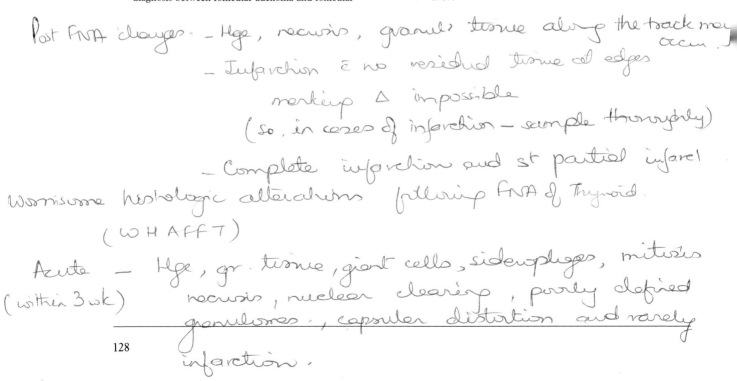

Post FNA changes. - Hge, necrosis, granul. tissue along the track may occur.

- Infarction c no residual tissue at edges making Δ impossible

(So, in cases of infarction - sample thoroughly)

- Complete infarction and st partial infarct

Worrisome histologic alterations following FNA of Thyroid.

(WHAFFT)

Acute — Hge, gr. tissue, giant cells, siderophages, mitosis
(within 3 wk) necrosis, nuclear clearing, poorly defined granulomes, capsular distortion and rarely infarction.

BREAST

With Karin Lindholm

contd.

Chronic

Linear fibrosis near siderophages,
Oncocytic metaplasia, spindle cell & sq. type also.
Infarction
Pseudo invasion of the capsule.
Significant random nuclear atypia.
Cyst formation
Papillary apparent
Calcification.

However, all above events do occur spont in goitres

H. cell neoplasms were found to be more prone
to infarction

7 BREAST

CLINICAL ASPECTS

A palpable breast lump is a common diagnostic problem both to the general practitioner and to the surgeon. Excisional biopsy of all breast lumps has long been the generally accepted practice, particularly in the older age groups where the incidence of malignancy is high. Although this should continue to apply with clearly definable breast lumps unless the FNA diagnosis is of a specific benign lesion such as a cyst or a fibroadenoma, there will be many less discrete mass lesions where, with the additional help of mammography and cytology, a safe policy of more selective surgical excision can be followed, particularly in younger women. In the past, where a cancer was suspected clinically, definitive treatment was often undertaken as a one-step procedure, ablative surgery following directly upon frozen section confirmation. Staging investigations then had to be carried out before a histological diagnosis had been established, which meant that they were often performed unneccessarily. The alternative of a two-step protocol of open biopsy for histology followed by ablative surgery as a second procedure after completion of the staging investigations, involved two separate operations with the additional delay caused by the staging investigations. This, to many surgeons, was the preferred option. A pre-operative diagnosis by means of a less invasive method therefore offers several advantages:

1. Immediate diagnosis relieves patient anxiety and saves time.
2. The definitive treatment can be planned in advance with the informed consent of the patient.
3. If cancer is confirmed, staging investigations (bone scan, liver scan, etc.) can be arranged without delay.
4. Some benign conditions can be confidently diagnosed and surgery avoided.
5. Hospital facilities can be more economically used if the degree of urgency and the extent of surgery are known beforehand.
6. The need for frozen section diagnosis is reduced.

Since the works of Martin and Ellis in the early 1930s, a vast experience of the diagnosis of breast lumps by needle biopsy has been accumulated in many parts of the world. Some prefer tissue fragments obtained with larger needles (e.g. Tru-cut or drill biopsy[25]) but FNA for cytologic preparations is now by far the most frequently adopted method.[41,75] Although FNA has important limitations, particularly related to the representativity of samples and to the exact typing of various hyperplastic and neoplastic processes, many centres have recorded a very high level of diagnostic accuracy with this technique. Once accepted by local surgeons, breast aspirates constitute the majority of FNA smears in most cytology laboratories.

As a result of recent advances in mammographic techniques and of the rapidly increasing experience in mammographic diagnosis, the use of FNA and mammography in parallel as complements to clinical examination (triple diagnosis) has become the standard approach to the investigation of palpable breast lumps. This has to some extent overcome the limitations of FNA cytology mentioned above and has lead to further improvement in preoperative diagnosis. The modern trend towards more conservative surgery and individualised treatment has increased the significance of tumour typing and grading and the importance of close correlation of mammographic, cytological and histological findings. The cytology of nodules in irradiated breast tissue is a relatively new problem created by the conservative treatment of cancer in the form of lumpectomy followed by irradiation.

Another recent development is the use of aspirated cell material for hormone receptor analysis based on immunohistochemical methods, and for various quantitative investigations such as morphometry, DNA measurement and cell kinetics, in an attempt to obtain more objective and reproducible indicators of prognosis. Finally, FNA has an important role to play in the investigation of small, impalpable lesions detected by mammographic screening of asymptomatic women. This has opened up a new field to cytological diagnosis; the very small cancers, an increasing proportion of in situ carcinoma in relation to invasive cancer, and a variety of proliferative processes suspected of having a premalignant potential.[64]

The place of FNA in the investigative sequence

The advantage of FNA over other biopsy methods is the simplicity of the technique. The biopsy is readily accepted by patients, the equipment is simple and inexpensive, and the whole procedure including fixation and staining is so quick that a report can be issued in a few minutes. To make the most of these advantages, a FNA biopsy should be performed in every patient presenting with a palpable breast lump. In doubtful cases, this should if possible follow mammographic examination, as the radiological findings may influence the choice of the area to be biopsied. Moreover, the fine needle biopsy may, on occasions, lead to changes which, although minor, may affect the interpretation of the films. If there is easy access to the cytology laboratory, the smears should be stained and read immediately while the patient is waiting. Further steps can then be discussed with her on the basis of the preliminary cytology report and this will relieve anxiety and avoid unnecessary delay.[23,27]

The main indication for FNA biopsy of breast lumps is to confirm cancer pre-operatively. A second consideration is to avoid unnecessary surgery in some benign conditions.[89,91] The indications can be specified as follows and applied so as to suit local experience and requirements:

1. The diagnosis of simple cysts.

2. The investigation of suspected recurrence or metastasis in cases of previously diagnosed cancer.
3. The confirmation of inoperable, locally advanced cancer.
4. The pre-operative confirmation of clinically suspected cancer.
5. The investigation of any palpable lump, clinically benign or malignant.
6. As a complement to mammography in the screening situation.
7. To obtain tumour cells for special analysis and research, e.g. hormone-receptor studies,[77] DNA analysis, immunohistochemistry and cell kinetics.

The place of FNA in non-palpable breast lesions

The main goal of cytological investigation is to reduce time, surgery and anxiety on the way to correct diagnosis — without causing delay in treatment. In healthy women, mammography will detect palpable and non-palpable lesions. The radiologist can select the patients for further investigation in different ways and with different accuracy depending on experience. The proportion of benign lesions should be as small as possible among those finally selected for surgery. As stated above, triple diagnosis for palpable lesions is well established and in the last decade several centres have reported good results with the combination of guided FNA and mammography also for non-palpable lesions.[21,28,33,51]

There are four main types of mammographic abnormalities:

1. Well circumscribed lesions.
2. Spiculated lesions.
3. Microcalcifications.
4. Asymmetrical parenchymal lesions.

The first group includes cysts and fibroadenomas as well as single small cancers. The benefit of combined cytology and mammography in this group is to reduce unnecessary surgery. The spiculated lesions on the other hand, are highly suspicious of malignancy from a mammographic point of view, surgery is nearly always recommended and the benefit of a FNA biopsy is the clear-cut diagnosis of cancer as a basis for definitive, therapeutic surgery. Clustered microcalcifications are suspicious of intraductal carcinoma — DCIS. Intraductal cancers can be of different types and of different grades. The large cell pleomorphic cancer of comedo type is easily recognised as cancer cytologically, while cribriform and papillary cancers present differential diagnostic difficulties in relation to benign atypical intraductal epithelial proliferations. Borderline cases can be a problem both for cytology and for histology. The question whether invasion is present or not is obviously a problem specific to cytology. In the fourth group,

asymmetrical parenchymal lesions, guiding the biopsy is difficult and the results of FNA are still uncertain.

In summary, the role of FNA cytology in the management of mammographically detected non-palpable lesions is still being evaluated. Multidisciplinary case conferences are the best approach to individual case management.

FNA as a sampling method for prognostication

Many institutions have reported their experience with the use of cell samples obtained by FNA for prognostication in breast cancer. Subjective cytological grading of routine smears shows some correlation with prognosis[58] but objective measuring of a number of variables in a sufficiently large cell sample is likely to provide more consistent, reproducible and reliable indicators of prognosis.[87] A number of quantitative methods have been applied to FNA samples, such as microspectrophotometry,[2] flow cytometry,[47] video image analysis[13] and cell kinetics. Many authors have shown a good correlation of ploidy and different DNA distribution patterns in breast cancer aspirates with hormone receptor content and with survival. Immunohistochemical demonstration and quantitation of hormone receptors at the cellular level using the ERICA technique[35] is one of the most important new developments in breast pathology. The demonstration of heterogeneity of receptor content in a tumour cell population made possible by this technique has opened a new and interesting approach to the understanding of response to hormone therapy.

However, a word of caution may be appropriate. To date, pre-operative prognostication by FNA has not yet proved to be of practical value. The diagnosis of cancer based on routine morphology always comes first and sampling for prognostic studies must never interfere with this principle.

FNA in the follow up of breast cancer

The diagnosis by FNA of recurrence or metastasis in cases of confirmed breast cancer following mastectomy with or without post-operative radiotherapy used to be straightforward, simply a distinction between cancer and suture granuloma, fat necrosis and scarring. The occurrence of atypical fibroblasts post radiation is well recognised. The introduction of conservative surgery followed by postoperative radiation with its effects on the remaining benign glandular epithelium has created new difficulties and a risk of overdiagnosis of radiation-induced epithelial atypia.[11,67] However, with experience and with the application of triple diagnosis in this situation, a high level of diagnostic accuracy has been achieved.[97]

7 BREAST

[handwritten margin notes: sensitivity 95% / obviate F/S]

Accuracy of diagnosis

The sensitivity of FNA biopsy in the diagnosis of breast cancer reported in the literature varies from just over 50% to approximately 95% (90–95% in most series). The aim should be a sensitivity of no less than 95%, and this can be achieved with increasing experience. The predictive value of a positive diagnosis is close to 100% in most reports.[6,16,19,34,41,48,65,74,76,80,98] There are many factors which may influence diagnostic accuracy. Skill and experience are, of course, important both in performing the biopsy and in the preparation and reading of the smear. Results will not be satisfactory if aspirates and smears are not consistently of a high quality.[43] Although the technique is simple, it requires a lot of training and practice to acquire and to maintain skill. It has been shown that results can vary considerably depending on the person who performed the biopsy, all other factors being equal.[6] Several centres recorded a significant improvement of diagnostic accuracy as a result of increasing experience.[19,36,99] Because microscopy gives an immediate feedback information of the quality of the smears, any pathologist who practises FNAC soon learns to improve his technique. Consequently, the best results are achieved if the pathologist who reads the smears also performs the biopsies. Patient selection is another factor; diagnostic accuracy is naturally influenced by the size of the tumour.[41,43]

A positive cytological diagnosis with a similar confidence level to a frozen section diagnosis is possible in 75–80% of cancer cases. In these cases decisions on definitive treatment can be based on the cytological diagnosis without the need of confirmation by frozen section, provided that the cytological diagnosis is in harmony with clinical and with mammographic assessment. As a rule, histological confirmation prior to definitive treatment should be obtained whenever there is disagreement between cytology and mammography. It must be acknowledged that additional information regarding tumour type is sometimes provided by frozen section and that this may influence surgical management.[7] In situ carcinoma constitutes a special problem since it is not possible to decide if invasion is present or not by cytological examination;[16,49] an unqualified cancer diagnosis by FNAC in a case of in situ carcinoma could lead to inappropriate treatment. Large cell intraduct carcinoma (classical comedocarcinoma) is easily recognised as malignant in FNA smears. Certain cytologic features (large, pleomorphic malignant cells, prominent necrosis and many foamy macrophages, see p. 150) are suggestive of large cell in situ carcinoma and, seen in combination with the absence of a discrete mass on palpation and with the characteristic calcifications in the mammogram, they provide fairly good evidence that this is the most likely diagnosis. The surgeon may decide to postpone definitive treatment and to do a limited excision waiting for the histological examination to show

if there is a component of invasive cancer, and if so in what proportion. Small cell intraduct carcinomas of papillary or cribriform type may not show an obviously malignant cytological pattern but smears are cellular and atypical enough to be reported as suspicious or atypical with a recommendation for open biopsy. The presence of necrotic debris, granular calcification and a characteristic microarchitectural pattern are suggestive of DCIS (see p. 151).[68]

Indecisive reports such as 'suspicious of malignancy' or 'cytological atypia not diagnostic of malignancy' are recorded differently by different authors. This to some extent explains the wide variation in false negative and false positive rates reported in the literature. In a practical sense such reports are neither false negative nor false positive diagnoses and should be understood as expressing the need for a formal surgical biopsy. A positive report should never be issued if smears are quantitatively or qualitatively unsatisfactory or if there is the slightest doubt. Such a policy inevitably results in a number of indecisive reports inversely proportional to experience. There should be no false positive diagnoses, although it must be acknowledged that human error can never be entirely eliminated. Detractors of FNA cytology should be reminded that even histopathological examination of a surgically excised breast lump is not infallible; occasional false positive diagnoses are sometimes revealed when histological slides are re-examined.[94]

[handwritten margin note: False + Pitfall]

In our experience, the greatest risk of making a false positive diagnosis is in the uncommon case of fibroadenoma with prominent epithelial atypia particularly in the higher age group. This problem will be further discussed on page 141. A summary of diagnostic pitfalls is presented at the end of this chapter on page 165.

The false negative rate is usually between 5 and 10%, although lower figures have been reported. Can a cytology report of a benign breast lesion therefore ever be regarded as diagnostic? Under certain conditions which will be discussed later, well-circumscribed lesions such as simple cysts, lipomas, most fibroadenomas, intramammary lymph nodes and fat necrosis can be diagnosed with confidence. Poorly circumscribed lesions — the common hormonal mastopathy–fibrocystic disease–fibroadenosis–mammary dysplasia — cannot be confidently diagnosed by FNA to the exclusion of malignancy. This is even more true in the complex lesions with epithelial hyperplasia and adenosis. However, if multiple aspirates with a satisfactory yield of cells are obtained from different parts of the lesion, and if the result is consistent with the clinical and mammographic evaluation, conservative management based on clinical follow up is justified.[10,89,91]

Triple diagnosis is the combination of clinical examination, mammography and FNA biopsy. The advances in mammographic technique are impressive and this facility has become available in most major hospitals and in clinics specialising in breast disease. The use of all three modalities in parallel has lead to further improvement of preoperative diagnosis. If all three investigations are in agreement that a lesion is either benign or malignant, diagnostic accuracy is over 99%.[10,90] The diagnostic accuracy of stereotactically guided FNA biopsy of impalpable lesions detected by mammography has been reported from several centres with a long experience (see above). These reports show that with the triple diagnostic approach, the rate of negative surgical biopsies can be reduced by 90%.

The unsatisfactory sample

When should a FNA sample of a breast lesion be regarded as unsatisfactory? What is the definition of a satisfactory sample? These are frequently asked questions to which there is no simple answer. Obviously, one cannot expect to obtain many cells from a fibrous mastopathy, from a sclerosed fibroadenoma, from a carcinoma with a highly desmoplastic stroma, or from hypertrophic adipose tissue. An acellular smear from such a lesion is therefore not unsatisfactory but it must of course be evaluated in conjunction with the clinical findings and, very importantly, with the feel of the consistency of the tissue through the biopsy needle. This is not a problem if the same person takes the biopsy and reads the smear but it becomes difficult when smears are sent to a laboratory for diagnosis. Poorly prepared smears with crush or drying artefacts or ,with cells trapped in clotted blood must of course be rejected as unsatisfactory.

Complications

Significant complications are extremely rare. Minor haematomas may occasionally follow biopsy but major haematomas are exceptional. Septic complications are rare. Pneumothorax caused by perforating the pleura with the biopsy needle is a rare but important complication which can occur in very thin patients and in the biopsy of lesions in the axilla. Tumour implantation in the needle-track has not been recorded in the breast. Long-term follow up of large series of cases has not shown any adverse influence of FNA on tumour spread and prognosis.[9]

Contra-indications

There are no contraindications to FNA of breast lumps.

Technical considerations

Aspirates suitable for cytological preparation are best obtained with needles of 21–23 gauge. Fine needle biopsy without aspiration (see Ch. 2) is preferable for benign and malignant breast lesions with a high cell

content. The difference in tissue consistency between for example a ductal carcinoma of the usual type, a scirrhous cancer, a medullary carcinoma, a fibroadenoma, adipose tissue and a cyst wall, which can be felt when the needle is held directly with the fingertips, is a very valuable piece of information. With experience, one comes to regard the special sensitivity offered by this technique as indispensable. This sensitivity, which also helps to secure a representative specimen, is lost to a significant degree if the needle is attached to a syringe. It is therefore recommended that needle biopsy without aspiration is tried first (except in cysts), and that aspiration is used only if the sample by the needle alone is insufficient. Lesions which are predominantly fibrous and are poor in cells require the additional force of the negative aspiration pressure for a sufficient number of cells to be sampled. Large needle core biopsy requires local anesthesia and stricter sterility control and carries a higher incidence of local complications. Also, it may be technically impossible to obtain a core biopsy from small lumps and multiple biopsies from different parts of larger lesions may not be acceptable. On the other hand, in scirrhous carcinoma and other fibrous lesions it may be impossible to obtain a sufficient number of cells with a fine needle, and a core needle biopsy may be the only alternative to a formal surgical biopsy.

Cyst fluid is processed in a similar manner to effusions (cytocentrifuge). An aspirate from a carcinoma not infrequently consists mainly of blood. Satisfactory direct smears can still be made with the two-step smearing technique (see Fig. 2.6) but it is usually best to repeat the biopsy from another angle. The practice recommended by some authors of routinely rinsing the needle and syringe with fixative which is then filtered through a Millipore or a Nucleopore filter has been discussed in Chapter 2.[17,75] We feel this is an unnecessary complication and an inferior alternative to direct smearing of a correctly performed biopsy.

The choice of fixation and staining depends on personal experience and preference. As breast carcinoma may show little cytologic atypia in the usual sense, the exaggeration of differences in nuclear size by air-drying is helpful. Also, stromal components are better seen in air-dried Giemsa-stained smears. On the other hand, the nuclear chromatin pattern is seen more distinctly in alcohol-fixed preparations. If possible, both alcohol-fixed and air-dried smears should be studied.

Non-palpable lesions detected by mammography can be sampled by FNA using special localising techniques as described by Nordenström.[61] Less elaborate instruments for guiding, such as a coordinate grid or simple stereotactic instruments adaptable to the ordinary mammography equipment have been used successfully.[51] In many centres the guided FNA is performed by the radiologist assisted by a cytopathologist, a cytotechnologist or a radiographer specially trained to take care of the aspirated sample. Some centres have organised

7 BREAST

special clinics to make it possible to perform selected mammography, guided FNA, cytological diagnosis and clinical examination including information to the patient, all in one day. This is of course a matter of resources and staffing. However, the value of an extremely fast investigation of any abnormality detected by screening to immediately direct the woman into the clinical patient situation seems to have been overemphasised. Precise information at each step and time to grasp the situation is probably of greater importance.

The common benign pattern (Figs 7.1–7.3)

Components of normal breast gland tissue

1. Overall low cell yield.
2. Sheets of ductal and aggregates of ductular epithelial cells with small uniform nuclei.
3. Myoepithelial nuclei visible among epithelial cells in aggregates.
4. Single, bare, oval nuclei separate from epithelial aggregates.

This pattern is common to normal, resting glandular breast tissue and to various forms of hormonal mastopathy. Quantitative variations occur with the menstrual cycle and with the age of the patient, depending upon the variable proportions between cells and fibrous stroma. The yield of the needle biopsy is usually poor and multiple biopsies should always be made to increase the likelihood of obtaining representative material.

The bimodal pattern of aggregates of epithelial cells and scattered single, bare nuclei is characteristic.[50,99] Ductular epithelial cells — this term is used here to designate cells from the intralobular epithelial structures of the resting breast which differ distinctly from the acinar epithelial cells seen in pregnancy and lactation as described below — occur in small cohesive aggregates. These aggregates represent casts of terminal ductules and are therefore often multilayered and are sometimes branching. The nuclei are irregularly distributed within the aggregates and may appear crowded, they are small, ovoid or round, dark with a finely granular chromatin. Nucleoli are not visible or are very small. There may be minor variation in nuclear size and shape. Cytoplasm is scanty, clearly visible but without distinct cell borders, it is pale and may show a fine blue granulation in

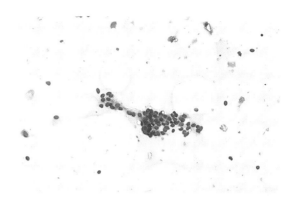

Fig. 7.1 The common benign pattern
Rather sparsely cellular smear with a ductal cell cluster and scattered bare oval nuclei
(MGG, LP)

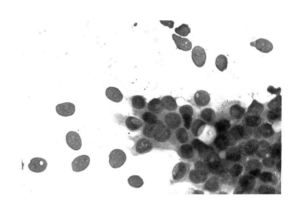

Fig. 7.2 The common benign pattern
Regular cohesive ductal cells with a rather high N/C ratio; bare oval nuclei (MGG, HP)

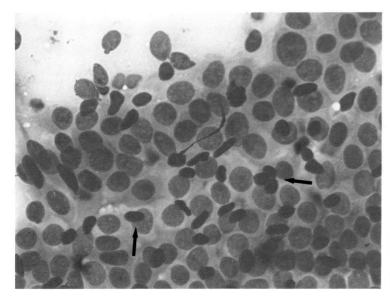

Fig. 7.3 The common benign pattern
Sheet of cohesive ductular epithelial cells. Note smaller and darker nuclei of myoepithelial cells scattered between the ductular cells (arrows) (MGG, HP)

7 BREAST

Giemsa-stained smears. Epithelial fragments from larger ducts are sometimes seen. They appear as monolayered sheets of regularly arranged, slightly larger cells with uniform nuclei. The single, bare nuclei scattered in the background are of the same size or a little smaller than those of the epithelial cells. They have a bipolar shape and a smooth, very distinct nuclear outline. The chromatin is dense and homogenous and nucleoli are not seen (Fig. 7.2). These cells sometimes wash off in heavily blood-stained and in wet-fixed smears. Nuclei of similar appearance can also be seen scattered between the cells of the epithelial aggregates, distinguishable from these by their smaller size and darker staining (Fig. 7.3). These nuclei no doubt represent the myoepithelial cells, whereas the single nuclei in the smear background may be either of myoepithelial or of fibroblastic origin derived from the specialised, intralobular connective tissue. The number of single nuclei seems to parallel the cellularity of the intralobular connective tissue and staining for alkaline phosphatase is negative.[53,92] Small fragments of collagen may be seen in the smears, particularly if larger calibre needles have been used, but are usually inconspicuous, whereas fragments of adipose tissue are more common.

The most common malignant pattern — infiltrating duct carcinoma NOS (Figs 7.4–7.8)

Criteria for diagnosis

1. A high cell yield.
2. A single population of atypical epithelial cells.
3. Irregular, angulated clusters of atypical cells.
4. Reduced cohesiveness of epithelial cells.
5. Nuclear enlargment and irregularity of variable degree.

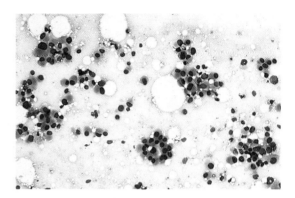

Fig. 7.4 The common malignant pattern
Moderately cellular smear; cell dispersal with some loose aggregates (MGG, LP)

6. Single cells with intact cytoplasm.
7. Absence of single bare nuclei of benign type.
8. Necrosis — important if present.

Usually, needle biopsy of a carcinoma yields a much larger number of cells than normal glandular tissue (compare Figs 7.1 and 7.4). A scirrhous cancer may, however, yield very few cells or no cells at all. The consistency of these desmoplastic tumours felt through the needle is usually so characteristic that this is a suspicious finding on its own, which leads to a recommendation of open biopsy even if no cells are obtained.

Architectural features are important to observe at low power. Aggregates of atypical cells are irregular and often have an angular contour, small clusters and groups and single files of cells are often seen as well as single cells. Many duct carcinomas show obvious cytological criteria of malignancy such as nuclear enlargment and

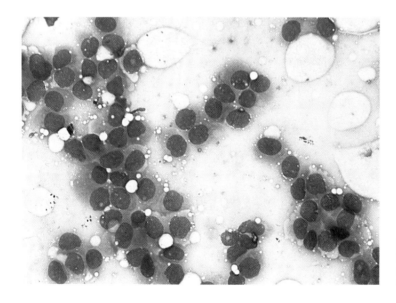

Fig. 7.5 The common malignant pattern
Poorly cohesive cells with abundant cytoplasm and enlarged eccentric nuclei; absence of bare oval nuclei (MGG, HP)

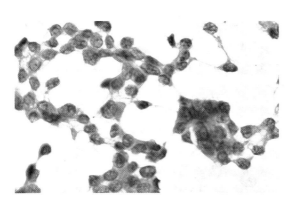

Fig. 7.6 The common malignant pattern
Poorly cohesive cells with enlarged nuclei, irregular nuclear
outlines and abnormal granular chromatin pattern
(H & E, HP)

pleomorphism, irregular distribution of nuclear chromatin, prominent nucleoli, nuclear crowding within aggregates of cells and diminished cell cohesion.[24] Nuclei of irregular shape and with irregular contours (buds, indentations, sharp angles, folds, etc.) are important indicators of malignancy. However, the cell population can be quite monomorphous in breast cancer, and nuclear abnormalities may be subtle.[38,41,43,66] The two most important criteria of malignancy are nuclear enlarge-

ment, which is exaggerated and therefore easier to appreciate in air-dried smears, and the breaking up of epithelial aggregates into single cells and small groups of cells in combination with the absence of the single, bare nuclei characteristic of benign breast tissue (Figs 7.5–7.7). In poorly differentiated carcinomas, dissociation of cells may be total and the smear pattern may resemble that of large cell lymphoma (Fig. 7.8). More often the malignant cells are seen both in aggregates and lying single. Nuclei are irregularly distributed and overlapping within aggregates of tumour cells and a tendency to microacinar groupings is not uncommon. Single carcinoma cells usually and characteristically have well-defined cytoplasm, but there are exceptions to this rule, particularly infiltrating lobular carcinoma (see below). Collagen fragments and adipocytes may be intimately associated with the cancer cells but stromal components are on the whole inconspicuous. Nuclei of lymphocytes and of fibroblasts or fibrocytes derived from the tumour stroma may be present and these must not be mistaken for the bipolar, naked nuclei characteristic of benign lesions.

The presence of necrosis is strong evidence in favour of malignancy. It is particularly characteristic of and more commonly found in in situ duct carcinoma than in invasive carcinoma. The importance of distinguishing tumour necrosis from condensed secretion in duct ectasia is discussed on page 147.

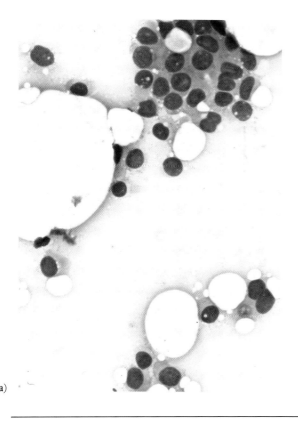

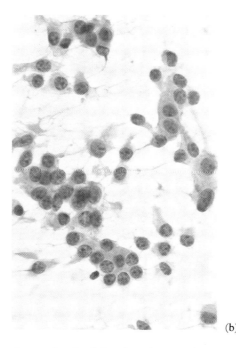

(a)

(b)

Fig. 7.7 Small cell ductal carcinoma
Small regular cells with only minor nuclear atypia; note the
single cells with intact cytoplasm and the absence of bare oval
nuclei (a. MGG, HP; b. H & E, HP)

7 BREAST

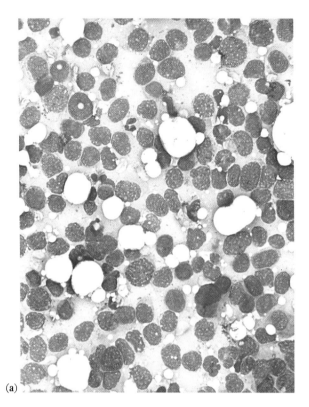

(a)

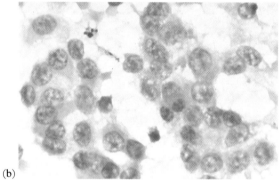

(b)

Fig. 7.8 Poorly differentiated carcinoma
Dispersed population of pleomorphic cells with irregular nuclear chromatin and fragile largely disrupted cytoplasm. Nucleoli are prominent in b (a. MGG, HP; b. H & E, HP)

Problems in diagnosis

1. Representativity of the sample.
2. Smearing artefacts.
3. Small cell carcinoma.
4. Desmoplastic cancers.
5. In situ and low grade carcinoma.

Obviously, malignancy cannot be ruled out solely on the basis of finding only the common benign pattern in smears from a suspicious lump, since the aspirate may represent the normal breast tissue next to a carcinoma.

Small carcinomas, or tumours obscured by surrounding fibrous tissue, or by an adjacent, dominant benign lesion such as a cyst or a lipoma, can of course be missed by the needle. Mammography is an important means of overcoming this problem. The combination of clinical examination, mammography and FNA biopsy is the only way to achieve a close to 100% diagnostic accuracy.

Artefacts (crush artefacts in air-dried smears, drying artefacts in alcohol-fixed smears) may cause nuclei of benign epithelial cells to look larger and irregular so that they could be mistaken for malignant cells. In addition, too much pressure exerted in smearing may cause artefactual dissociation of cell aggregates. One should therefore disregard those parts of a smear in which fixation and cell preservation is poor. When benign epithelial cells are mixed with an abundance of fat, the nuclei may become deformed and distorted by the fat droplets, an artefactual pleomorphism which can be quite confusing. The negative pressure should therefore be released while the needle is still in the target lesion so that aspiration of the surrounding fat is avoided.

Smears from small cell carcinomas with a desmoplastic stroma (mainly infiltrating lobular but also some duct carcinomas) may, seen with low magnification, simulate the benign pattern. However, under high power it becomes obvious that the single cells are not the single, bare nuclei of benign breast tissue but are dissociated malignant cells similar to those forming clusters, and that the cells have nuclei of irregular shape and usually some visible cytoplasm (Figs 7.7 and 7.51).

Very fibrous acellular lesions such as scirrhous (desmoplastic) carcinomas and sclerotic fibroadenomas may not yield sufficient cells to allow a diagnosis by FNA. The best chance of obtaining cells from a desmoplastic cancer is from its periphery. This is true also of cancers with extensive central necrosis. It is sometimes difficult to distinguish tumour necrosis from thick inspissated secretion derived from ectatic ducts. A thorough search for preserved malignant or benign ductal epithelial cells is necessary (see p. 147 and Figs 7.30 and 7.31).

In situ duct carcinoma causes special problems in cytological diagnosis. The cells of large cell in situ duct carcinoma of comedo type are readily recognised as malignant in FNA smears. Certain cytological features listed on page 152 are suggestive of an invasive component but focal invasion can obviously never be ruled out. Small cell in situ intraduct carcinoma of papillary or cribriform type are more often reported cytologically as epithelial hyperplasia with atypia, or as suspicious but not diagnostic of malignancy (see p. 152). It is doubtful if lobular carcinoma in situ can be diagnosed by FNA. Most cases are probably interpreted cytologically as atypical epithelial hyperplasia.[49,68] However, Salhany and Page[72] recently studied a series of such cases and listed features indicative of this diagnosis. Low grade, tubular invasive carcinoma can also be difficult to distinguish from epithelial hyperplasia particularly since naked nuclei of benign type, presumably derived from remnants of specialised lobular stroma, are often found in the smears (see p. 153).[12]

When a FNA smear from a breast lesion is examined microscopically, the overall pattern observed under low power (cellularity, presence or absence of a bimodal cell population, cell cohesiveness, size and shape of cell aggregates and stromal components) is as important as cellular and nuclear detail observed under high power. The general pattern cannot be evaluated if the sample is too scanty and if smears are poor in cells. This is why a confident cytological diagnosis depends to a high degree on the adequacy of the sample. A repeat FNA or an open biopsy and histological examination is mandatory if cytological atypia is noted in scanty smears. Nuclear enlargement, chromatin clumping, poor cell cohesion,

and above all an irregular nuclear outline, constitute significant atypia which can be recognised even in smears with a poor cell content. A less common feature which is a strong indicator of malignancy in individual cells is intracytoplasmic neolumina (Fig. 7.52a)

The diagnostic pitfalls in FNAC of palpable breast lumps are summarised at the end of this chapter.

Other benign patterns

Fibroadenoma (Figs 7.9–7.16)

Criteria for diagnosis

1. A high cell yield.
2. Large, branching, monolayered sheets of uniform epithelial cells.

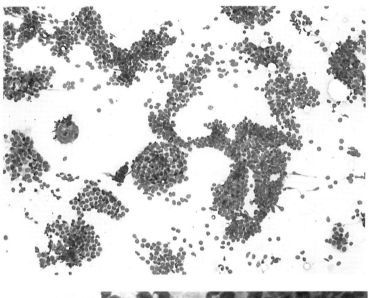

Fig. 7.9 Fibroadenoma
Highly cellular smear; numerous monolayered sheets or finger-like structures and many dispersed bare oval nuclei (MGG, LP)

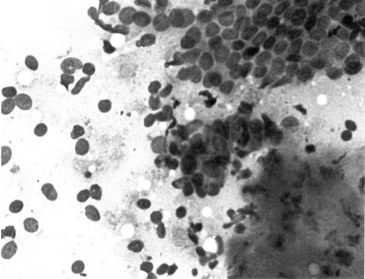

Fig. 7.10 Fibroadenoma
Cohesive ductal cells, bare oval nuclei and a fragment of myxoid stromal tissue (MGG, HP)

7 BREAST

3. Numerous single, bare nuclei of benign type.
4. Fragments of fibromyxoid stroma.

Fibroadenomas are usually well-circumscribed lesions and have a characteristic consistency which differs from normal breast tissue and from fibroadenosis. It is therefore possible to be confident that the aspirate is representative and to exclude malignancy in most cases.

Smears show a similar bimodal pattern as normal breast tissue but are much more cellular (Fig. 7.9).[50] The monolayered sheets of regularly arranged epithelial cells are usually large and branching, reflecting the appearance in histological sections. The nuclei of the epithelial cells are slightly larger than those of normal ductular epithelial cells. They are uniform, have a uniform finely granular chromatin pattern and often one or two small nucleoli. Single, bare nuclei are typically numerous, scattered in the background. Sometimes, epithelial cells of apocrine differentiation, also forming sheets, may be prominent, and large numbers of foamy macrophages may suggest a cystic component. Fibromyxoid stromal fragments are frequently seen. They are pink to bright red in MGG-stained smears, have a fibrillary structure and contain spindle fibroblastic nuclei (Fig. 7.10). There may be a thin film of myxoid ground substance in the background. Smears from fibroadenomas with abundant collagenous stroma and scanty epithelium are less characteristic and the pattern approaches that of hormonal mastopathy.[14,96]

Benign phyllodes tumour (giant fibroadenoma)[99] has a similar cytological appearance to the common fibroadenoma but the stromal elements tend to predominate over the epithelial elements in FNA smears. Single bare nuclei are generally more numerous than in the common fibroadenoma — there is an overlap, fibroadenomas can also be very cellular — and a proportion of them are spindle shaped nuclei of fibroblastic type (Figs 7.11 and 7.12). Occasionally, only the epithelial component of a phyllodes tumour is represented in the smears. The cytological pattern is thus not specific or diagnostic and the clinical presentation and the size of the tumour must be taken into account. In some cases, cohesive fragments of highly cellular stroma of spindle cells may be found and if there is nuclear pleomorphism malignancy may be suspected (Fig. 7.65, see page 163). Conversely, focal malignant transformation can be missed by FNA in large tumours.

Problems in diagnosis
Since a confident diagnosis of fibroadenoma usually means no excision and no further follow up, diagnostic criteria must be strictly observed. These include the clinical or mammographic presentation of a well defined mass. The cytological pattern of epithelial hyperplasia seen in FNA smears can resemble that of fibroadenoma, although fragments of myxoid stroma are not present and single bare nuclei are less numerous. Epithelial

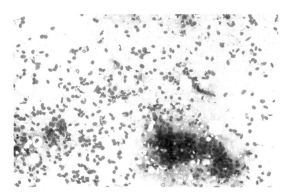

Fig. 7.11 'Giant' fibroadenoma
Cellular smear with a large component of dispersed bare oval nuclei; relative paucity of ductal cells (MGG, LP)

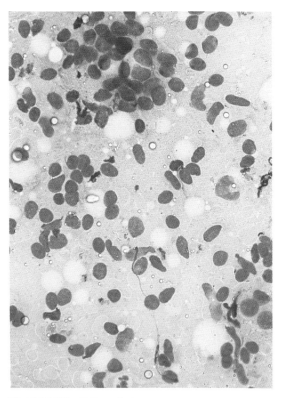

Fig. 7.12 'Giant' fibroadenoma
Slightly irregular bare spindle-shaped and oval nuclei (MGG, HP)

hyperplasia, especially if atypical, often accompanies malignancy, and if seen in a FNA biopsy requires mammographic examination and follow up.

Some fibroadenomas, probably those in a growing phase, may show nuclear enlargment and anisokaryosis which may be further exaggerated by crush or drying artefacts. Such findings could be mistaken for malignancy. In addition, epithelial sheets can be broken up by

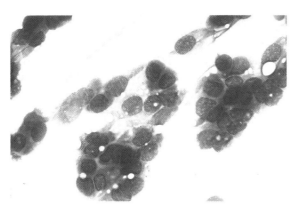

Fig. 7.13 Fibroadenoma
Dissociation of ductal cells brought about by too vigorous smearing; note the strands of smeared nuclear material in the background (MGG, HP)

too firm smearing pressure to simulate malignant dissociation (Fig. 7.13). We have seen a few fibroadenomas in women over 40 years of age, in which cellular atypia was severe and worrying both in smears and in histological sections but in which the histology was typical of fibroadenoma in every other respect with no evidence of malignancy (Figs 7.14–7.16). Some of these fibroadenomas in fact showed an aneuploid pattern (video image analysis, unpublished results). A false positive cytological diagnosis in these uncommon cases can only be avoided if one pays attention to the overall pattern, in particular to the presence of single bare nuclei of benign type and of fragments of the characteristic myxoid stroma. An unqualified diagnosis of cancer should never be made in the presence of a bimodal pattern, even if epithelial atypia is severe. Since carcinoma can arise in a fibroadenoma, albeit rarely[56], and since fine needle aspirates from tubular

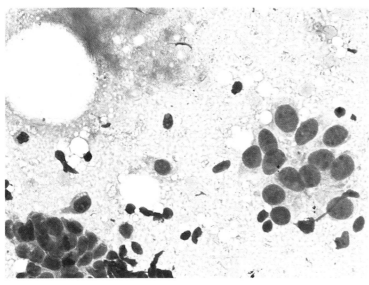

Fig. 7.14 Fibroadenoma
Cluster of atypical enlarged cells together with some cohesive ductal cells of usual type; some bare nuclei and myxoid ground substance (MGG, HP)

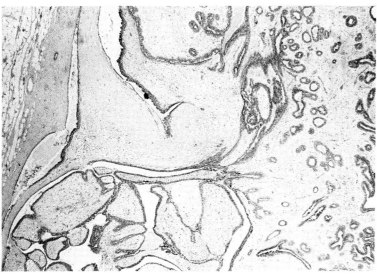

Fig. 7.15 Fibroadenoma
Tissue section — same case as Figure 7.13; typical pattern (H & E, LP)

7 BREAST

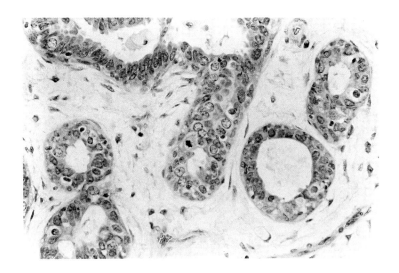

Fig. 7.16 Fibroadenoma
Tissue section — same case as Figure 7.13; atypical epithelial proliferation with mitoses within small ducts (H & E, HP)

carcinoma can occasionally mimic fibroadenoma, a recommendation of excision biopsy is justified in the presence of obvious atypia.

The problem of ruling out malignancy (sarcoma) in very large giant fibroadenomas has been mentioned above.

Gynaecomastia[71]

The cytological pattern of gynaecomastia is not specific and the clinical presentation must be known to allow a diagnosis. The pattern is intermediate between that of fibroadenosis and of fibroadenoma. Smears are moderately cellular, epithelial sheets are often large and there are many single bare nuclei. Moderate nuclear variation and atypia can be allowed in the presence of a benign bimodal pattern. Fragments of fibromyxoid stroma may be seen.

Fibrocystic change

This is a variant of the common benign pattern in which 'cyst macrophages' and sheets of ductal epithelial cells of oxyphil or apocrine type are found in addition to the usual bimodal cell population of ductular epithelium and single bare nuclei. The former components may be numerous and may dominate the smears. Fluid from dilated ducts tend to increase the volume of the aspirate. The 'macrophages' have an abundant, finely vacuolated cytoplasm which may contain pigment, and small round central nuclei. It is likely that these cells are in fact degenerating epithelial cells exfoliating from the lining of dilated ducts, rather than true macrophages. The ductal epithelial cells of oxyphil or apocrine type have abundant, dense, finely granular eosinophilic cytoplasm which stains grey-blue with MGG. The nuclei are round, nuclear size may vary considerably, and nucleoli are often prominent. However, the nuclear outline is smooth and even and the chromatin pattern is uniformly finely granular. These cells should therefore not give

rise to a suspicion of malignancy. Cells from a duct carcinoma with apocrine differentiation have large, pleomorphic, obviously malignant nuclei.

Fibrocystic change is not a cytological diagnosis. These changes are usually poorly circumscribed and the adjacent tissue may harbour hyperplasia, atypia or even malignancy. Malignancy can only be ruled out in the tiny area biopsied and the cytological report should be seen in the context of clinical and mammographic findings.

Simple cyst (Figs 7.17–7.20)

Criteria for diagnosis

1. Complete disappearance of the lump following aspiration of the fluid.
2. Absence of blood in the aspirated fluid.
3. Debris, 'cyst macrophages' and oxyphil/apocrine epithelial cells.

This is the most common situation in which malignancy can be excluded by FNA and a surgical excision avoided. To many general practitioners this is still the only indication for FNA of breast lumps.

The aspirated fluid may be thin, clear or turbid, straw-coloured, brown or green. Smears may be practically cell free or may contain large numbers of 'cyst macrophages' (Fig. 7.17) and epithelial cells, usually of oxyphil type and often degenerating (Fig. 7.18). Numerous polymorphs are sometimes found in the cyst fluid in cases with no clinical signs of inflammation.

Problems in diagnosis

1. A carcinoma may be present adjacent to a cyst and obscured by this. If any residual lump can still be felt after the cyst has been emptied, a repeat needle biopsy must be made from the solid area.

2. It has been said that malignancy can safely be

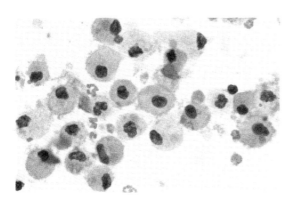

Fig. 7.17 Simple cyst
Cyst 'macrophages' (Pap, HP)

excluded if no abnormality is felt after the cyst has been emptied, provided the fluid is not bloody, and that examination of the fluid is therefore not necessary.[18] We have seen two cases of non-palpable, microscopical invasive carcinoma in the cyst wall with malignant cells present in the fluid (Fig. 7.19). This is, however, an extremely rare finding which hardly justifies routine cytological examination of all clear, non-haemorraghic cyst fluids. Blood stained fluids should always be carefully examined.[15,57,89]

3. Atypia shown by degenerating or regenerating oxyphil cells is commonly seen. The atypia may be bizarre and worrying (Fig. 7.20). It can sometimes mimic squamous differentiation. However, if all other findings are typical of a simple cyst, and in the absence

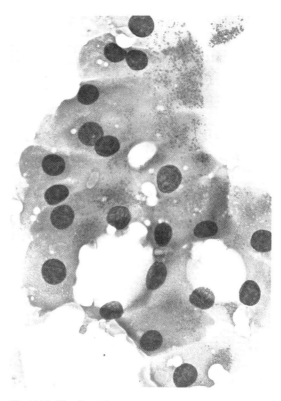

Fig. 7.18 Simple cyst
Epithelial cells of apocrine type; abundant dense cytoplasm and coarse cytoplasmic granularity; large nuclei with a solitary, usually central nucleolus (MGG, HP)

Background may contain altered blood as granules, necrotic material and orange RBC. St — spindle cells are seen in cysts — these are from granular tissue at edges.

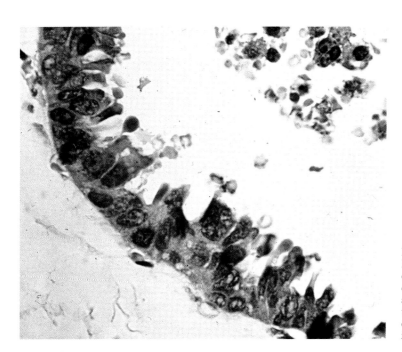

Fig. 7.19 Malignant cells lining a cyst
In this case, the cyst was completely emptied by aspiration; highly atypical cells were observed in smears of the fluid and excision was advised; histologically the lesion was judged to be an intracystic carcinoma, with a microscopic focus of invasion (H & E, HP)

7 *BREAST*

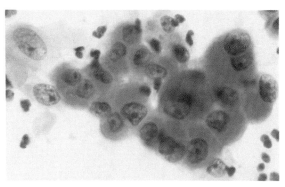

Fig. 7.20 Simple cyst
Although the nuclear atypia of these ductal epithelial cells of oxyphil type is prominent and worrying, the cells derive from a simple benign cyst (Pap, HP)

of altered blood or necrotic debris, or of a residual mass after the fluid has been drained, there is no indication for further investigation.

Benign epithelial hyperplasia, adenosis, etc.
(Figs 7.21–7.26)

Common findings

1. A high yield of epithelial cells.
2. A bimodal population of sheets and clusters of epithelial cells and single bare nuclei.
3. 'Cyst macrophages' and/or epithelial cells of oxyphil or apocrine type.
4. Mild epithelial atypia (variable).
5. Stromal fragments often present (intraduct papillary projections).

Again, it must be clearly understood that this is *not* a cytological diagnosis. In this section, we simply describe

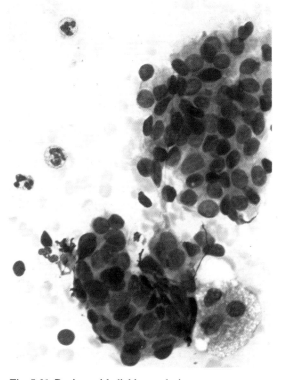

Fig. 7.21 Benign epithelial hyperplasia
Large slightly disorganised clusters of ductal cells; a foamy cell and several bare oval nuclei lie in the background (MGG, HP)

the cytological patterns which correspond to benign epithelial proliferations of different types seen in histological sections.[42,64]

There is a spectrum of changes in complex lesions of glandular tissue in which there is epithelial hyperplasia

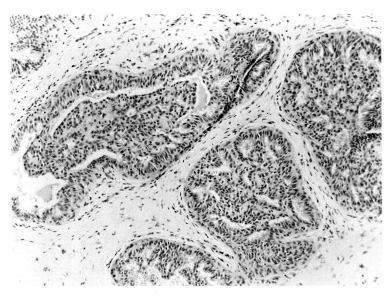

Fig. 7.22 Benign epithelial hyperplasia
Tissue section; same case as Figure 7.19; Epitheliosis; papillomatosis (H & E, IP)

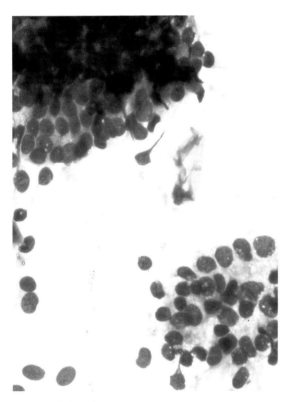

Fig. 7.23 Adenosis
Microacinar pattern within epithelial cell aggregates; bare oval nuclei (MGG, HP)

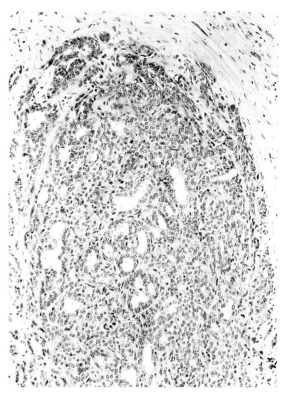

Fig. 7.24 Adenosis
Tissue section; same case as Figure 7.23; sclerosing adenosis (H & E, IP)

of ductal, lobular or mixed types of variable degree and extent. Many terms have been used to describe these changes, such as mammary dysplasia, epitheliosis and papillomatosis. The hyperplastic epithelium may or may not show cytological atypia (Figs 7.21, 7.22 and 7.25). Epithelial hyperplasia and atypia is often seen in relation to malignancy, particularly in situ carcinoma, and close correlation with clinical and mammographic findings is essential — malignancy can never be ruled out by FNA alone.

Although histologically separated from epithelial hyperplasia, *sclerosing adenosis* (Figs 7.23 and 7.24) and other forms of adenosis are included under this heading, since they cannot be clearly distinguished cytologically. A tendency to a microacinar pattern in epithelial aggregates may be seen, but in general, type specific diagnoses are not possible within this group of conditions. Open biopsy should be recommended whenever there is a significant degree of cytological atypia.

In *subareolar duct papillomatosis* (Fig. 7.26) cytological material can either be obtained by scraping the nipple or by FNA depending on the depth of the lesion. In scrape smears, squamous epithelium and some inflammatory cells are mixed with aggregates of mildly atypical epithe-

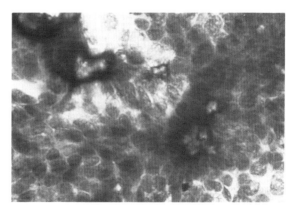

Fig. 7.25 Atypical hyperplasia
Large cluster of mildly atypical epithelial cells; some loss of cohesion; note presence of calcification (MGG, HP)

lial cells of ductal type showing little tendency to dissociation. These are quite different from the single large malignant cells seen in Paget's disease. Single, bare nuclei of benign type may be inconspicuous (Fig. 7.26).[88]

7 BREAST

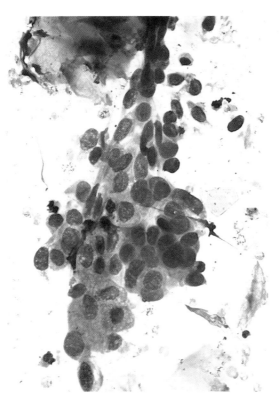

Fig. 7.26 Benign epithelial hyperplasia
Subareolar duct papillomatosis in nipple scraping; cohesive, but somewhat atypical epithelial cells with enlarged nuclei and abundant cytoplasm; background of keratin flakes and some inflammatory cells (MGG, HP)

Problems in diagnosis
Mild nuclear atypia is frequently present in the form of some nuclear enlargment, variation in nuclear size and an irregular arrangement of nuclei, but there is no dissociation of epithelial aggregates, the shape of the nuclei is regular, the nuclear contour is smooth, and nucleoli are not prominent, except in cells of oxyphil type. If epithelial atypia is more obvious, an open biopsy should be recommended since it may be difficult or impossible to distinguish cytologically betwen atypical hyperplasia (Fig. 7.25), lobular carcinoma in situ, small cell ductal carcinoma in situ and some low grade invasive carcinomas, for example tubular carcinoma. On the other hand, over-diagnosis of cancer is avoided by paying attention to the benign single bare nuclei present in the background. In the presence of this bimodal pattern, a definitive diagnosis of malignancy should never be made, regardless of the presence of epithelial atypia.

Post-radiation effects (Figs 7.27 and 7.28)

Common findings

1. Anisocytosis but preserved N/C ratio.
2. Hyperchromasia but structureless chromatin.

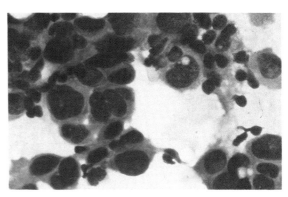

Fig. 7.27 Radiation induced atypia
The epithelial cells in this irregular cluster show considerable nuclear enlargment, pleomorphism and hyperchromasia, but also some degenerative changes (MGG, HP)

3. Cytoplasm abundant, vacuolated, indistinct, or basophilic-amphophilic hyaline.
4. Preserved spatial arrangement of cells.
5. Little dissociation of epithelial cells.
6. Presence of myoepithelial cells.
7. Clean background.

These features apply to irradiated glandular breast tissue left by conservative surgery. The appearance of atypical fibroblasts in irradiated connective tissue is well known and need not be described here. Some of the findings listed above are controversial, and the reader is also referred to the papers by Zajdela & Maublanc,[97] by Bondeson,[11] and by Peterse et al.[67]

The key to a correct distinction cytologically between post-radiation atypia and recurrent malignancy is above all the awareness of this pitfall and the experience of benign reactive cellular changes from other fields of cytology.

Breast tissue in pregnancy and lactation
(Fig. 7.29)[26,30]
Retention cysts (galactocele) and abscesses present no difficulties. The cytological pattern of solid lumps of fibroadenosis/adenoma type is quite different from the usual when they occur in a pregnant or lactating breast. Smears show large numbers of cells most of which are acinar epithelial cells. These have an abundant, fragile cytoplasm showing prominent vacuolation and a fine granularity. Nuclei are round, central and have distinct small nucleoli. Cell cohesion is poor and many single cells occur (Fig. 7.29). These features may induce a suspicion of malignancy, particularly as there is also a variation in nuclear size and as the single, bare nuclei of the benign pattern are inconspicuous. However, the nuclear chromatin is finely granular and evenly distributed, and the nuclei are uniformly round, with a smooth outline. The background of abundant lipid secretion in the form of numerous vacuoles is characteristic and immediately gives away the fact that the smear

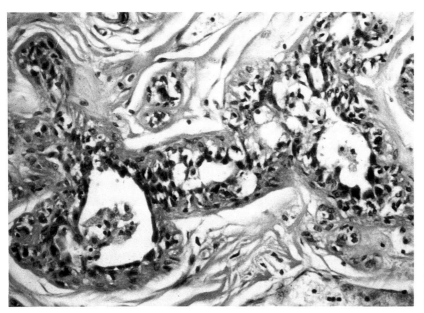

Fig. 7.28 Radiation induced atypia
Tissue section, same case as Figure 7.27. Similar nuclear atypia seen in ductules of normal breast tissue (H & E, IP).

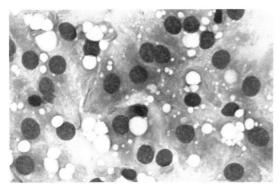

Fig. 7.29 Lactating breast
Dispersed acinar cells with abundant cytoplasm, rounded nuclei and central nucleoli; background of lipid secretions (MGG, HP)

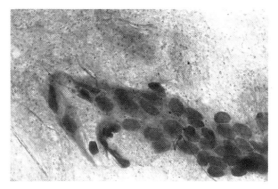

Fig. 7.30 Duct ectasia
Cohesive sheet of uniform ductal cells in a background of amorphous material (MGG, HP)

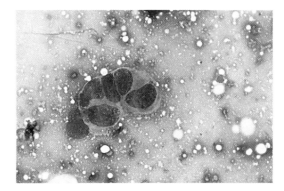

Fig. 7.31 Necrotic carcinoma
Small group of malignant cells in background of necrotic debris (MGG, HP)

derives from an actively secreting breast gland in case this information has not been supplied by the clinician. Surgical biopsy may occasionally be necessary to exclude malignancy in the rare cases with marked cytological atypia.

Duct ectasia (Fig. 7.30)

Criteria for diagnosis

1. A thick, creamy or cheesy aspirate.
2. Amorphous material and debris.
3. Chronic inflammatory cells.
4. Occasional monolayered sheets of uniform duct epithelium which may be of oxyphil type.

Problems in diagnosis

It can be difficult to distinguish duct ectasia from massive central necrosis in a carcinoma (Figs 7.30 and 7.31). The total absence of nuclear debris in the condensed secretion of duct ectasia is a clue. Smears of thick, amorphous material with debris but with few

BREAST

preserved cells should be screened carefully for atypical cells which could indicate necrotic carcinoma. If no well preserved cells are found, aspiration should be repeated aimed at the periphery of the lesion. It is important to correlate the cytological findings with the clinical presentation. Duct ectasia is usually located close to the nipple and is an unlikely diagnosis in lesions located peripherally in the breast.

Mastitis (Fig. 7.32)[52,93]

Common findings

1. A benign bimodal pattern.
2. Inflammatory cells, chronic and/or acute.
3. Regenerative epithelial atypia.
4. Epithelioid histiocytes, multinucleated giant cells and many plasma cells (granulomatous mastitis).

The diagnosis of acute mastitis and abscess presents no problems. Chronic localised inflammation in the breast gland is uncommon. It may be the result of persistence of an acute mastitis, a reaction to retained secretion in fibrocystic disease or duct ectasia, or secondary to previous surgery. Its importance to the cytologist is the occurrence of regenerative epithelial atypia which sometimes can cause diagnostic difficulties.

The cytological findings in non-specific *granulomatous mastitis* and in *tuberculous mastitis* have been described.[52,93]

Problems in diagnosis

Regenerative atypia of epithelium lining larger ducts can look worrying and suspicious (Fig. 7.32). In addition, the nuclei of reactive histiocytes may appear large and atypical, particularly in air-dried smears. However, large numbers of acute and chronic inflammatory cells are rarely seen in carcinoma. In medullary carcinoma with lymphocytic infiltration and in comedocarcinoma, in which lymphocytes and histiocytes are mixed with the carcinoma cells, the latter dominate and show obvious malignant features. The presence of necrotic cell debris should evoke a suspicion of malignancy.

Recurring subareolar abscess (lactiferous duct fistula)[62,81]

The finding of mature or anucleate squamous cells in greater numbers than could be explained by contamination from the skin, and pus, in an aspirate from an abscess deep to the areola enables this diagnosis to be made. A specific cytologic diagnosis is of clinical significance, since these lesions require surgical treatment. Infected or ruptured epidermal cysts may produce a similar cytological picture, but are likely to occur more laterally.

Fat necrosis (Figs 7.33–7.35)

Criteria for diagnosis

1. A background of granular debris, fat and fragments of adipose tissue.
2. Foamy macrophages, multinucleated giant cells and adipocytes with bubbly cytoplasm.
3. Chronic inflammatory cells.
4. Absence of epithelial cells.

The site of the lesion can give a clue to the diagnosis since many of these lesions are caused by seat belt injury. The aspirate is usually scanty and consists mainly of fat with some foamy macrophages or altered, vacuolated adipocytes (Fig. 7.33) and multinucleated histiocytic giant cells. The untidy background of granular debris represents the actual necrosis and is therefore an important finding (Fig. 7.35).

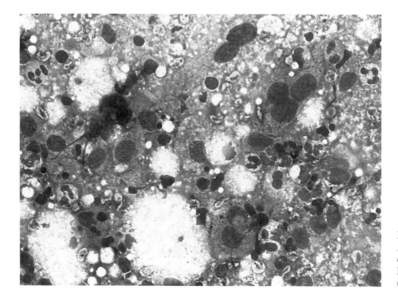

Fig. 7.32 Acute mastitis
Atypical, presumably regenerative epithelial cells in a background of histiocytes, inflammatory cells and debris (MGG, HP)

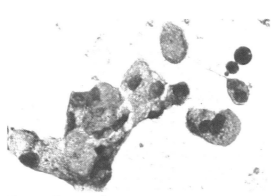

Fig. 7.33 Fat necrosis
Foamy cells, either macrophages or altered adipocytes
(MGG, HP)

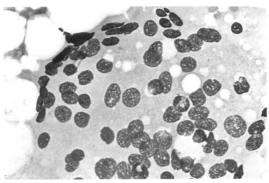

Fig. 7.34 Fat necrosis
Multinucleate macrophage (MGG, HP)

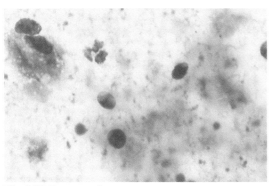

Fig. 7.35 Fat necrosis
'Dirty' background of necrotic debris; macrophages with
vacuolated cytoplasm (MGG, HP)

Nodules or lumps are sometimes felt adjacent to silicone implants. One must carefully avoid puncturing the prosthesis when such nodules are biopsied. Histiocytes and foreign body giant cells containing vacuoles where the lipid-like material has been dissolved in processing are seen if the nodule is a reaction to escaped silicone (see Fig. 5.13). Biopsy is important; we have diagnosed a few unexpected carcinomas in this situation.

'Lipoma'

Criteria for diagnosis

1. A well-defined, rounded, soft mass.
2. 'Empty' sensation on needling.
3. Fat only in multiple aspirates — fat vacuoles and/or fragments of adipose tissue.

Lesions of this type in the breast are not true lipomas but focal hypertrophy of fat tissue. Contained within a fibrous compartment of the breast, focal fat hypertrophy presents as a discrete, rounded, relatively soft mass which is often tender. When the needle is introduced, the resistance of the thin fibrous capsule may be felt, but the mass itself has a soft, 'empty' feeling to the needle. This condition is commonly seen also in postmenopausal women. Correlation with mammography is important to ascertain that the biopsy is representative.

Intramammary lymph nodes
Lymph nodes are not uncommonly found within the breast, usually in the axillary tail, but occasionally more centrally, and may clinically simulate a fibroadenoma or a cyst. It should be kept in mind that a mass in the breast can, albeit rarely, be the first presentation of malignant lymphoma. The principles applied in the differential diagnosis between a reactive lymph node and lymphoma are described in detail in Chapter 5.

Variants of primary carcinoma

A correlation between cytological patterns in FNA smears and prognosis in breast carcinomas has been reported from some centres. Whilst mastectomy remained the standard treatment for breast carcinoma, cytological subtyping had little influence on the further management of the case. Furthermore, accurate typing requires histological examination of multiple blocks of tissue in view of the variation from one part to another seen in many tumours. Histological assessment is also necessary to distinguish between invasive and non-invasive ductal carcinoma (p. 132). However, with increasing patient demand for the full discussion of all treatment options prior to surgery, subtyping may provide firmer ground on which to base such discussions. Cytological subtyping can also provide valuable help in correlating the radiological findings with the expected histopathology. This applies particularly to those types of carcinoma in which the anatomical extent correlates poorly with the clinical and mammographic findings, e.g. invasive lobular carcinoma and the micropapillary/cribriform small cell variants of ductal carcinoma in situ. In these circumstances, breast conservative surgery may not be feasible or appropriate. However, in the majority of cases, parameters other than tumour type, such as tumour size and grade, clinical stage, hormone

7 BREAST

receptor content and other biological factors, will determine the extent of surgery and the need for adjuvant therapy.[3,87] Nevertheless, familiarity with all the various cancer patterns found in the breast is a prerequisite to achieve a high level of accuracy in the cytological diagnosis of breast cancer.[44] The basic diagnostic criteria previously given for infiltrating duct carcinoma (the most common malignant pattern) are to some extent applicable to all subtypes.

Ductal carcinoma in situ (DCIS)[49,83,95]

Large cell type (comedocarcinoma) (Fig. 7.36)

Usual findings

1. Variable cell yield.
2. Neoplastic cells in irregular aggregates and single.
3. Large, pleomorphic cells showing obvious malignant features.
4. Necrotic debris, lymphocytes and vacuolated macrophages.

The cells of DCIS of large cell (comedo) type are large, pleomorphic and show all the usual cytological criteria of malignancy. The cytoplasm may be abundant and eosinophilic as in oxyphil cells. The diagnosis of carcinoma is easy even when only a few cells are present in the smears. The abundant necrotic debris and the vacuolated macrophages often containing hemosiderin pigment represent the 'comedo' plugs seen in tissue sections and are characteristic of comedocarcinoma. Calcification may be seen also in smears. Invasive growth may be suggested by certain cytological features listed below, but can obviously never be excluded by FNA biopsy. The absence of a well defined palpable mass on clinical examination, and the presence of characteristic calcifications in the mammogram together with the cytologic features described, strongly suggest that the carcinoma is at least predominantly in situ. The definitive assessment whether invasive growth is present or not can only be made by histological examination of an open biopsy.

Papillary type (Fig. 7.37)[59]

Usual findings

1. Highly cellular smears.
2. Papillary aggregates, sometimes with a central fibrovascular core.
3. Columnar cells in rows, palisades and single.

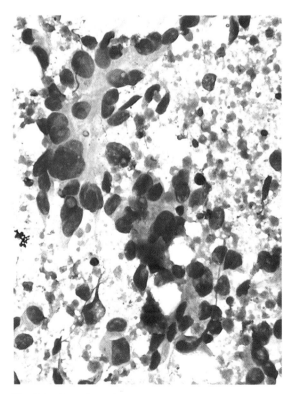

Fig. 7.36 Comedocarcinoma
Pleomorphic malignant cells with a background of necrotic debris (MGG, HP)

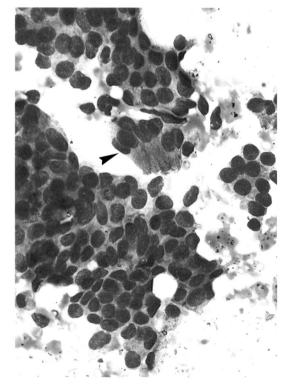

Fig. 7.37 Papillary carcinoma
Cellular smear; large cells with evidence of palisading (arrow) and a tendency to dissociation (MGG, HP)

4. Variable nuclear enlargment, pleomorphism and atypia.
5. Bare nuclei of benign type absent.
6. Macrophages and epithelial cells with cytoplasmic vacuoles.
7. Necrotic debris.

It is difficult to distinguish well-differentiated papillary carcinoma, in situ or invasive, from intraduct papilloma. The presence of myoepithelial nuclei strongly suggests benign papilloma, while nuclear enlargment, nuclear pleomorphism, poor cell cohesion and the presence of necrosis favour a malignant diagnosis. Also, it is not possible to predict if a well-differentiated papillary carcinoma is invasive or non-invasive on the basis of cytological criteria. For these reasons, the cytological diagnosis of a papillary tumour is only preliminary and the definitive diagnosis must await histological examination.

Cribriform type (Figs 7.38–7.40)

Usual findings

1. Epithelial cells relatively cohesive forming large monolayered sheets, balls or papillary fragments.
2. Variable, relatively mild epithelial atypia.
3. Necrotic debris often calcified.
4. Macrophages, often with haemosiderin pigment.

The microarchitectural pattern seen in smears is a result of epithelial proliferation taking place in a preformed lumen. It is not in itself an indicator of malig-

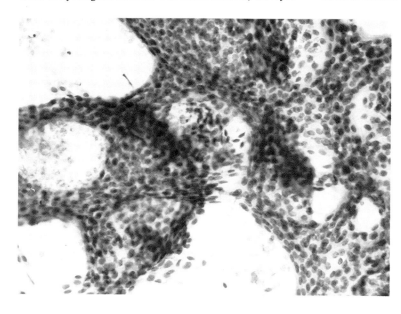

Fig. 7.38 DCIS, cribriform type
Large, monolayered sheet of uniform epithelial cells with rounded spaces like those seen in sections; some granular debris (Pap, IP)

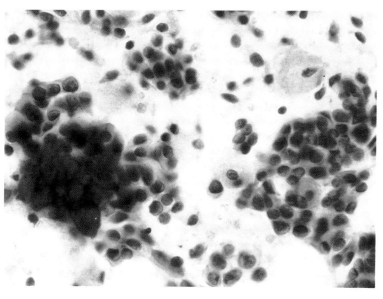

Fig. 7.39 DCIS, cribriform type
Aggregates of mildly atypical cells; some loss of cohesion; foamy macrophages, debris, microcalcification (Pap, HP)

7 BREAST

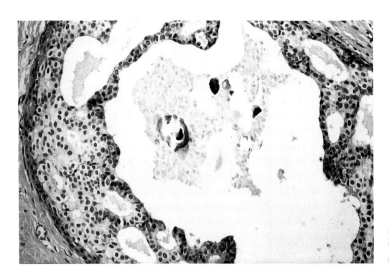

Fig. 7.40 DCIS, cribriform type
Tissue section, same case as Figure 7.38
(H & E, IP)

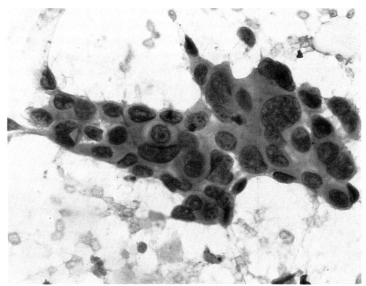

Fig. 7.41 Comedocarcinoma with invasion
This cluster of malignant cells with an angular contour in a smear from a DCIS of large cell type is suggestive of an invasive component (Pap, HP)

nancy. Malignancy is suggested by cytological atypia and, above all, by the presence of necrosis. Myoepithelial cells are absent within the sheets of atypical epithelial cells. Large epithelial sheets can sometimes show round holes suggestive of a cribriform pattern (Fig. 7.38), but a similar appearance can be caused by artefacts in other forms of hyperplasia and it is therefore not a reliable diagnostic criterium. Calcifications may be present. Distinction from epithelial hyperplasia, particularly from atypical epithelial hyperplasia, is difficult or impossible; correlation with the mammogram is essential, and definitive diagnosis must usually be deferred to histology.

The following features are indicators of invasive growth in any of the variants of DCIS.

1. Angulated, irregular aggregates of epithelial cells (Fig. 7.41).

2. Irregular stromal fragments, particularly if closely related to irregular epithelial fragments.
3. Fibroblasts/cytes dispersed in the background — to distinguish from the single bare nuclei of the benign pattern.
4. Single malignant cells or groups of cells in a fatty, vacuolated (non-necrotic) background.

Lobular carcinoma in situ (LCIS)

We have not been able to define cytological criteria for this diagnosis in FNA smears. The reader is referred to the interesting paper by Salhany and Page.[72] These authors point to intracytoplasmic neolumina as the most useful clue to the cytologic recognition of both invasive and noninvasive lobular lesions.

Variants of invasive carcinoma

Tubular carcinoma (Figs 7.42–7.45)[12]

Usual findings

1. Moderately cellular smears.
2. Cells predominantly in cohesive clusters — dissociation not prominent.
3. Epithelial clusters with an angular shape and a tubular pattern.
4. Mainly, uniform, mildly atypical epithelial cells.
5. Single bare nuclei of benign type often present.

Problems in diagnosis

Only pure tubular carcinomas have a favourable prognosis which allows a more conservative treatment.

However, tubular carcinoma not infrequently constitutes a variable proportion of an infiltrating duct carcinoma which is otherwise of the common type. Both components may not be represented in a FNA biopsy, a type-specific diagnosis by cytology can therefore only be tentative, and correlation with the mammographic findings is important. The FNA diagnosis is more reliable in very small tumours.

Nuclear morphology is usually bland. Nuclear grooves and intracytoplasmic vacuoles have been found to be suggestive but not diagnostic features.[12] Many tubular carcinomas have a loose, cellular stroma similar to normal intralobular connective tissue and smears may contain single, bare nuclei of benign type, probably derived from this stroma. In the presence of such a bimodal cell population, a definitive diagnosis of carci-

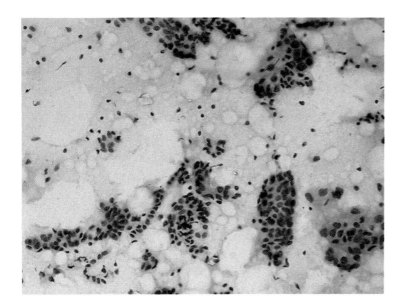

Fig. 7.42 Tubular carcinoma
Angular clusters of mildly atypical epithelial cells; single files; note single bare nuclei in background (Pap, IP)

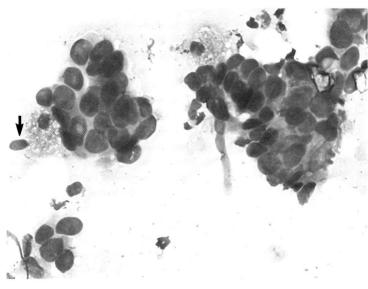

Fig. 7.43 Tubular carcinoma
Angular clusters; mild atypia; occasional single bare nuclei (arrow) (MGG, HP)

7 *BREAST*

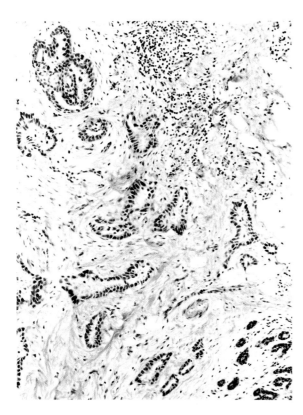

Fig. 7.44 Tubular carcinoma
Tissue section; same case as Figure 7.43; infiltrating tubules of regular cells; adjacent benign ductular structures (H & E, IP)

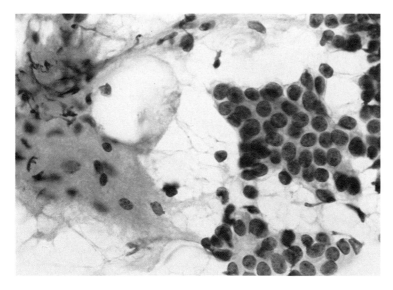

Fig. 7.45 Tubular carcinoma
Angular clusters of mildly atypical epithelial cells; some single bare nuclei; fragment of fibrous stroma (Pap, HP)

noma should, generally speaking, not be made cytologically, but await open biopsy and histology. However, a cytological diagnosis is possible in many cases of tubular carcinoma, in which case surgery can be planned as a therapeutic rather than as a diagnostic procedure.

To the radiologist, the main differential diagnosis is the radial scar. This can be a difficult problem since both tubular carcinoma and radial scars often occur in a complex glandular tissue with intraductal epithelial hyperplasia and variable cytological atypia. If the benign epithelial proliferation is the dominant component of the smear, the cancer can easily be missed.

Occasionally, tubular carcinoma may have large, cohesive, monolayered sheets of epithelial cells which can be mistaken for fibroadenoma, particularly since nuclear enlargement and atypia may occur in both con-

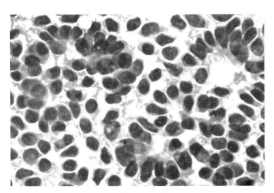

Fig. 7.46 Invasive cribriform carcinoma
Rather dispersed population of small monomorphic cells, often columnar in shape and forming a micro-acinar pattern (MGG, HP)

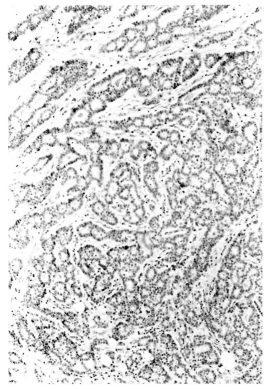

Fig. 7.47 Invasive cribriform carcinoma
Tissue section; same case as Figure 7.46 (H & E, IP)

ditions (see p. 141). However, single, bare nuclei are absent or sparse, as are fragments of myxoid stroma.

Infiltrating cribriform carcinoma is another variant of low grade breast cancer related to tubular carcinoma. In keeping with its histological growth pattern, smears from a cribriform carcinoma are usually highly cellular but the neoplastic cells are bland as in tubular carcinoma, cuboidal or columnar, and show an obvious tendency to an acinar or microglandular arrangement (Figs 7.46 and 7.47).

Mucinous (colloid) carcinoma (Fig. 7.48)[22,86]

Usual findings

1. Abundant background mucin (usually seen macroscopically).
2. Atypical cells in small solid aggregates, single files and single.
3. Cellular monomorphism.

Mucinous carcinomas may be round, well circumscribed lesions and may clinically be mistaken for fibroadenoma or cyst. Nuclear enlargment and pleomorphism is usually only mild to moderate. The tumour cells have abundant cytoplasm. The mucin stains violet to blue with MGG but is less conscpicuous in smears stained with H & E or Pap. Some mucinous carcinomas have intracytoplasmic mucin and the cells may have a signet-ring appearance. Distinction from metastatic carcinoma of, for example, gastrointestinal origin can occasionally be a problem. Cell aggregates of metastatic adenocarcinoma usually show microglandular patterns, while cells of mucinous carcinoma tend to form solid cords and files.

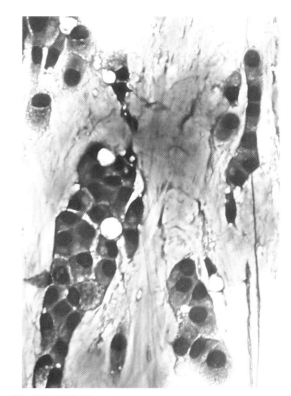

Fig. 7.48 Colloid carcinoma
Rather regular ductal cells with abundant cytoplasm suspended in mucus; note single files (MGG, HP)

7 *BREAST*

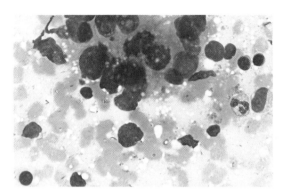

Fig. 7.49 Medullary carcinoma
Cluster of large malignant cells and scattered lymphoid cells
(MGG, HP)

Medullary carcinoma (Fig. 7.49)

Usual findings

1. Highly cellular smears.
2. Irregular cell aggregates and single cells.
3. Large, pleomorphic, obviously malignant nuclei.
4. Many lymphocytes (medullary carcinoma with lymphocytic infiltration).

Like mucinous carcinoma, medullary carcinoma also tends to be rounded and well circumscribed and to have a soft 'empty' feel to the needle. It often bleeds easily. The cytology is quite similar to that of comedocarcinoma. The cells of both these tumours have abundant cytoplasm and large, pleomorphic, obviously malignant nuclei. Necrotic debris and foamy macrophages are more typical of comedocarcinoma but may be found also in medullary carcinoma. Loss of cell cohesion is greater in medullary carcinoma. The presence of numerous lymphocytes in the smears may only reflect focal lymphocytic infiltration and is not reliable evidence of true medullary carcinoma. The current criteria for a diagnosis of medullary carcinoma, which take both circumscription, tumour cell cytology and lymphocytic infiltration into account, thus require histological examination of the whole tumour.

Paget's disease of the nipple (Fig. 7.50)

Criteria for diagnosis

1. Background of keratin, squamous cells and inflammatory cells (scrape smears from nipple).
2. Large malignant cells, single and in small groups.
3. Abundant pale cytoplasm with distinct borders.
4. Obvious nuclear features of malignancy.

The preparation of scrape smears from the nipple is an excellent method to diagnose Paget's disease. First, any crust or exudate must be removed carefully. The clean surface is then scraped with a scalpel blade held at

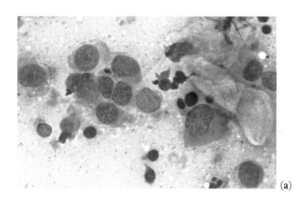

(a)

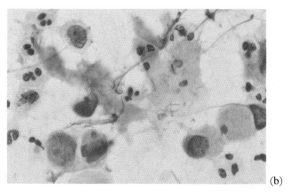

(b)

Fig. 7.50 Paget's disease of the nipple
Nipple scraping; large pale malignant cells and some anucleate squamous cells and inflammatory cells (a) MGG, HP.
(b) Pap, HP.

a blunt angle. Both alcohol-fixed and air-dried smears should be made. If there is any palpable mass in the breast, this should also be biopsied.

Problems in diagnosis

The main differential diagnosis is subareolar duct papillomatosis (Fig. 7.26). In this condition, the epithelial cells form cohesive aggregates, they are smaller and more uniform in size and they do not show malignant nuclear characteristics.

Another differential diagnosis is a subareolar in situ or invasive carcinoma arising from a major duct just below the nipple and secondarily erupting onto the nipple, but not infiltrating the epidermis in a true Pagetoid fashion. In such a case, scrape smears from the nipple contain numerous malignant cells which have a much greater tendency to form cohesive clusters than the cells of true Paget's disease. Also, there is not the intimate mixture of carcinoma cells and squamous epithelial cells typical of Paget's disease.

Infiltrating lobular carcinoma (Figs 7.51–7.53)

Usual findings

1. A varible, often very poor cell yield.
2. Cells single and in small clusters, short single files common.

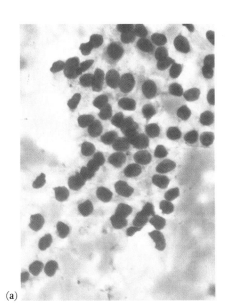

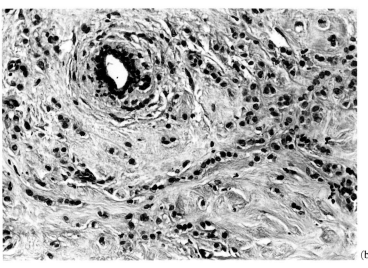

(a)

(b)

Fig. 7.51 Infiltrating lobular carcinoma
(a) Poorly cohesive cluster; single files; uniformly small nuclei with some irregularity of shape; indistinct cytoplasm (MGG, HP).
(b) Tissue section, same case as (a) (H & E, IP).

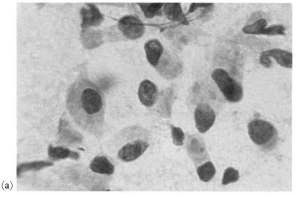

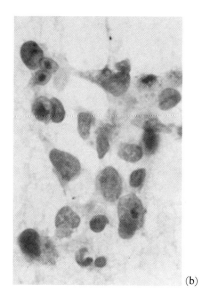

(a)

(b)

Fig. 7.52 Infiltrating lobular carcinoma
(a) The malignant cells have intracytoplasmic neolumina
(H & E, HP). (b) Small malignant cells with intracytoplasmic
mucin vacuoles (alcohol-fixed PAS, Oil).

3. Cytoplasm scanty, indistinct, often missing.
4. Small dark nuclei of relatively uniform size.
5. Irregularity of nuclear shape.

The majority of infiltrating lobular carcinomas have an abundant desmoplastic stroma. The neoplastic cells are seen as small groups and single files, strangled, as it were, by the coarse collagenous stroma. Smears are therefore usually very poor in cells which are both single and forming small clusters and single files (Fig. 7.51). The small cancer cells have often lost their cytoplasm and often show nuclear moulding, particularly within single files of cells. The nuclei are only slightly larger than those of benign cells and do not vary much in size. Although variation in nuclear size may be slight, nuclear outline is characteristically irregular, angular rather than rounded, with folds, buds and indentations. Fragments of collagen may be seen associated with the tumour cells.

The cells of some lobular carcinomas have abundant cytoplasm and intracytoplasmic mucin droplets and have the appearance of signet ring cells (Fig. 7.52b).

7 BREAST

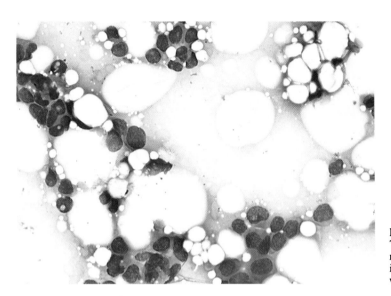

Fig. 7.53 Infiltrating lobular carcinoma
This pattern of clusters of relatively small, moderately pleomorphic malignant cells is indistinguishable from duct carcinoma with small cells (MGG, HP)

Problems in diagnosis

A smear from a lobular carcinoma, poor in cells, showing small clusters of cells as well as single naked nuclei, can easily be mistaken for benign mammary dysplasia. Lobular carcinomas constitute the majority of false negative diagnoses in breast cytology if non-representative biopsies are not included.[38,41,44] However, on close examination with high power, it becomes evident that all the cells are tumour cells with abnormal although small nuclei, and that the single nuclei are identical to those of cells forming clusters. Naked, bipolar nuclei of benign type are absent.

The distinction between lobular and ductal carcinoma is not always possible and may be difficult also in histological sections. Some ductal carcinomas have equally small, relatively uniform neoplastic cells and, conversely, lobular carcinoma may have larger cells similar to those of ductal carcinoma NOS (compare Figs 7.7 and 7.53).

Some uncommon variants of carcinoma

Breast carcinoma in the male[71]

Most breast cancers in male patients are infiltrating ductal carcinoma NOS, identical to the common ductal carcinoma in women. One should remember that metastatic cancer is perhaps as common as primary carcinoma in the male. The distinction from gynecomastia presents no difficulties.

Adenoid cystic carcinoma (Fig. 7.54)[45]

This uncommon subtype is important to recognise in FNA smears as the prognosis is significantly better than for other invasive carcinomas. The cytological pattern is identical to that of adenoid cystic carcinoma in other sites, such as salivary glands, lung, etc. (see Figs 4.41

and 4.42). Hyaline globules resembling those of adenoid cystic carcinoma can occasionally be seen in benign epithelial hyperplasia, so called *collagenous spherulosis* (Figs 7.55 and 7.56). Nuclear atypia — moderate enlargement and hyperchromasia — is therefore also required to make a diagnosis of adenoid cystic carcinoma.

'Inflammatory' carcinoma

The clinical presentation of 'inflammatory' carcinoma is a diffuse increase in the consistency of the breast without a distinct mass, and thickening and erythema of the skin due to extensive intralymphatic spread of tumour causing lymph stasis and oedema. Random sampling from central parts of the breast usually produces enough malignant cells to allow a confident diagnosis. Intracutaneous sampling with a 25 gauge needle introduced tangentially, has also been recommended. The cytological pattern is similar to that of the common infiltrating duct carcinoma. Inflammatory cells are not seen.

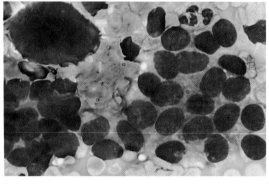

Fig. 7.54 Adenoid cystic carcinoma
Dense cluster of small uniform cells; one hyaline globule (MGG, HP)

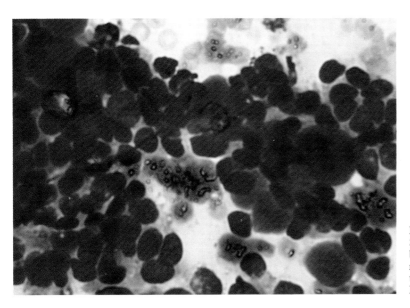

Fig. 7.55 Collagenous spherulosis
Sheet of epithelial cells with uniform bland nuclei. Several globules of hyaline material staining bright red, similar to those of adenoid cystic carcinoma (MGG, HP)

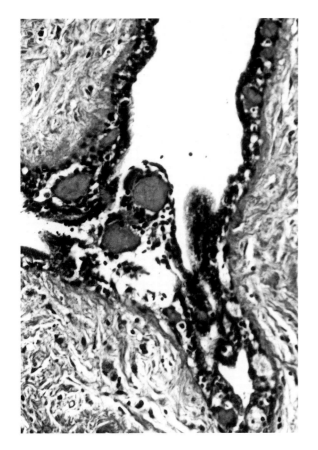

Fig. 7.56 Collagenous spherulosis
Tissue section; same case as Figure 7.55. Rounded clumps of hyaline matieral among the epithelial cells lining a duct (H & E, IP)

Carcinoma with apocrine (oxyphil) differentiation
(Figs 7.57 and 7.58)[37]

Pure carcinomas of this cell type are rare; however, focal apocrine differentiation or oxyphil change in duct carcinoma is not uncommon. Cancer cells of oxyphil type have large, pleomorphic nuclei, a coarse and irregular nuclear chromatin and large nucleoli. In comparison to the common duct carcinoma cells, the nuclear/cytoplasmic (N/C) ratio is relatively low and the cytoplasm is dense eosinophilic and granular. Benign ductal epithelial cells of apocrine (oxyphil) type as seen in cyst fluids, fibrocystic disease, in many lesions with epithelial hyperplasia and in some fibroadenomas may show marked anisokaryosis and may have prominent nucleoli. Irregular nuclear shape, irregular chromatin distribution, some cells with a high N/C ratio, loss of cell cohesion, necrosis and the absence of bland ductular epithelial cells and of single nuclei of the benign type, are all features in favour of carcinoma.

Clear cell (glycogen-rich) carcinoma
(Figs 7.59 and 7.60)

Smears show a dispersed cell population. The cells have abundant, fragile, pale cytoplasm which tends to disperse into a 'tigroid' background. Nuclear structures are similar to those of most duct carcinomas. In paraffin sections carcinomas of this type show a clear cell pattern due to the high glycogen content.

Other uncommon variants

We have no personal experience of *secretory carcinoma* in FNA smears and the reader is referred to several case reports in the literature.[1,60] We have seen one example

7 *BREAST*

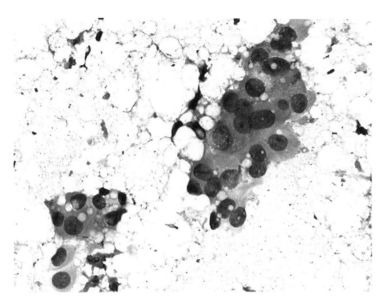

Fig. 7.57 Carcinoma with apocrine differentiation
Groups of malignant cells with abundant finely granular dense cytoplasm and irregular pleomorphic nuclie; some background nuclear debris indicating necrosis (MGG, HP)

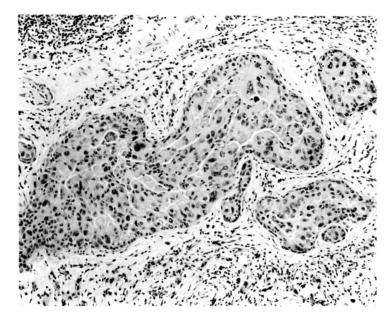

Fig. 7.58 Carcinoma with apocrine differentiation
Tissue section; some case as Figure 7.57; focus of apocrine differentiation in infiltrating duct carcinoma (H & E, IP)

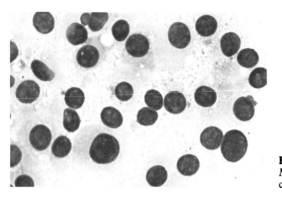

Fig. 7.59 Glycogen-rich carcinoma
Mainly dispersed malignant cells with abundant pale fragile cytoplasm (MGG, HP)

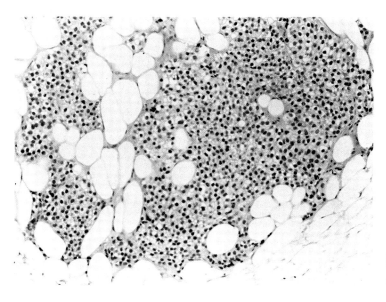

Fig. 7.60 Glycogen-rich carcinoma
Tissue section; same case as Figure 7.59
(H & E, IP)

of a *small cell carcinoma* of neuroendocrine type in the breast, in which the cells were shown to contain dense core granules by electron microscopy. The smear pattern was similar to that of small cell carcinoma of bronchogenic origin. Squamous differentiation is sometimes seen in poorly differentiated duct carcinoma. Pure *squamous carcinoma* has been described[46] but is very rare. Duct *carcinoma with osteoclast-like, multinucleated giant cells* without osteoid or chondroid material tends to be well circumscribed and can mimic fibroadenoma mammographically. The giant cells have been shown to be of histiocytic type by electron microscopy and appear to be of stromal origin (Figs 7.61 and 7.62). There are

several variants of *'metaplastic' carcinoma*.[85] Spindle cell carcinoma can be difficult to distinguish from sarcoma. Figures 7.63 and 7.64 illustrate an example of a metaplastic carcinoma showing both mucinous and chondrosarcomatous differentiation.

Other malignant tumours

Metastatic malignancy[73,78,84]
Malignant tumours of extramammary origin occasionally metastasise to the breast and may present clinically as a solitary lump which suggests primary breast carcinoma. If the cytological pattern does not fit any of the

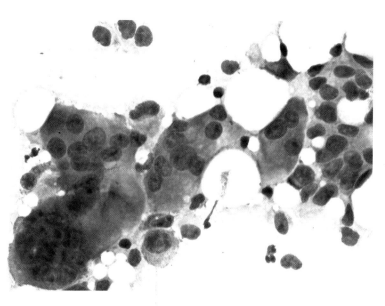

Fig. 7.61 'Metaplastic' carcinoma
Poorly differentiated ductal carcinoma
with osteoclast-like giant cells (MGG, HP)

7 BREAST

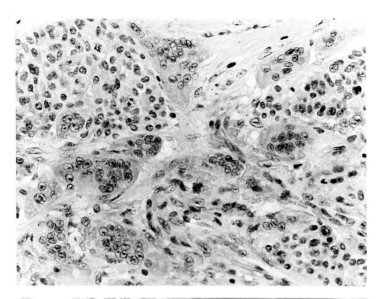

Fig. 7.62 'Metaplastic' carcinoma
Tissue section; same case as Figure 7.61
(H & E, IP)

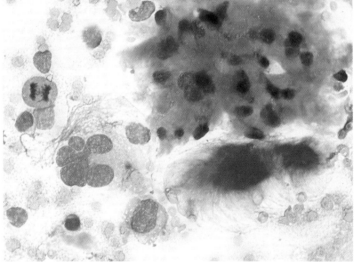

Fig. 7.63 'Metaplastic' carcinoma
Carcinoma with chondrosarcomatous
areas; note the dense clump of chondroid
ground substance, together with myxoid
stromal tissue and epithelial cells
(MGG, HP)

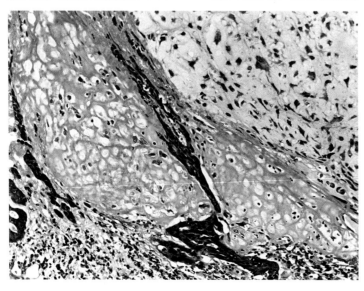

Fig. 7.64 'Metaplastic' carcinoma
Tissue section; same case as Figure 7.63
(H & E, IP)

subtypes of primary breast cancer, the possibility of metastatic malignancy should be considered. Malignant melanoma is probably the most common metastatic malignancy seen in the breast (see p. 305). We have also seen metastatic tumours in the breast from squamous carcinoma of the uterine cervix, small cell anaplastic carcinoma of lung, mucin-secreting adenocarcinoma of stomach, ovarian adenocarcinoma and alveolar rhab-domyosarcoma.

Lymphoma

Malignant lymphoma may rarely present as a primary breast tumour. The differential diagnosis of malignant lymphoma and reactive lymphoid tissue is described in Chapter 5. Large cell lymphoma (centroblastic and im-munoblastic) may closely resemble poorly differentiated breast carcinoma with a completely dispersed cell population. In large cell lymphoma, nuclear size, shape and chromatin pattern is usually more variable, many cells have a basophilic cytoplasm, eccentric nucleus and a perinuclear halo, and nucleoli characteristic of either centroblasts or immunoblasts are present. The presence in the background of round basophilic cytoplasmic fragments (lymphoid globules) is a useful indicator of the lymphoid nature of the cells.

Sarcoma (Figs 7.65–7.69)[70,79,82]

The biological behaviour of a *phyllodes tumour* is difficult to predict on the basis of histologic appearances. Architectural features such as size, tumour margins and relative lack of an epithelial component, as well as mito-tic counts, have shown some correlation with recurrence

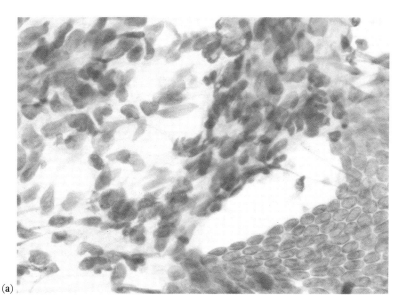

(a)

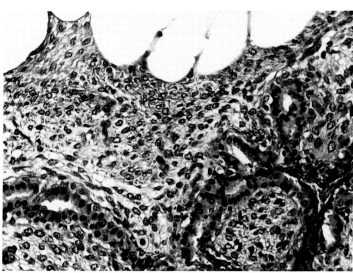

(b)

Fig. 7.65 Malignant phyllodes tumour
(a) Monolayered sheet of bland epithelial cells; fragment of cellular spindle cell stroma showing nuclear enlargment and pleomorphism (Pap, HP). (b) Tissue section, same case as (a) (H & E, IP).

7 BREAST

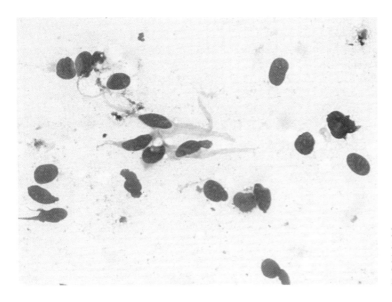

Fig. 7.66 Malignant phyllodes tumour
Moderately cellular smear with a
predominance of fibroblastoid spindle
cells. This tumour recurred repeatedly
requiring total mastectomy (MGG, HP)

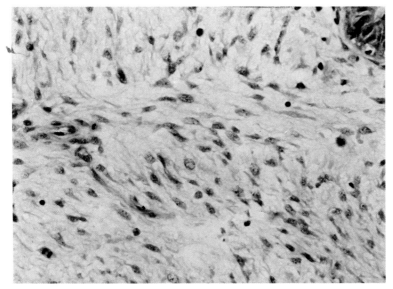

Fig. 7.67 Malignant phyllodes tumour
Tissue section; same case as Figure 7.66
(H & E, IP)

rate. These parameters can obviously not be assessed in
FNA smears. Smears from a tumour at the malignant
end of the spectrum contain fragments of highly cellular
stromal tissue of spindle cells which may show nuclear
atypia and pleomorphism similar to a spindle cell sarcoma (Fig. 7.66). In addition, there is a variable number
of sheets of epithelial cells (Fig. 7.65). The latter may
appear atypical but do not show malignant criteria. In
such a case, the cytology report should suggest a phyllodes tumour with stromal atypia suspicious of malignancy but a definitive diagnosis of sarcoma should not
be made, no matter how atypical the spindle cell component may appear. The definitive diagnosis must await
histological examination. Smears from a tumour at the

benign end of the spectrum may suggest fibroadenoma,
but contain larger numbers of spindle-shaped stromal
nuclei while epithelial cells are relatively sparse. If mitotic figures and stromal nuclear atypia are found, a suspicion of borderline or malignant phyllodes tumour
should be expressed. Prominent squamous metaplasia of
the epithelial component is sometimes seen in phyllodes
tumours. It should be remembered that the histological
pattern may be variable within the same tumour, and
the FNA biopsy may therefore not necessarily be representative, particularly if the tumour is large.

In *angiosarcoma* of the breast, aspiration yields plenty
of blood and tumour cells may be few in numbers and
difficult to find. This is particularly the case with low-

grade tumours which consist mainly of wide, anastomosing vascular channels and in which the malignant endothelial cells show little tendency to form solid proliferations.[20] High grade, mainly solid tumours are more easily recognised as sarcomas cytologically. The tumour cells are spindle-shaped, they have an attenuated basophilic cytoplasm without distinct borders and dark pleomorphic, elongated or plump spindle nuclei. Most cells form syncytial clusters but some are single (Figs 7.68 and 7.69).[54] Fat tissue fragments may be a conspicuous component of the aspirate due to the tendency of the neoplastic vascular channels to invade the fat tissue widely.

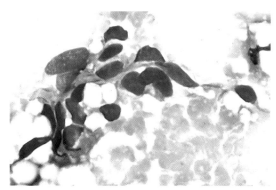

Fig. 7.68 Angiosarcoma
Heavily blood-stained smear; few groups of pleomorphic spindle cells of malignant appearance (MGG, HP)

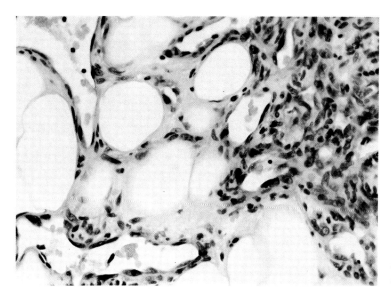

Fig. 7.69 Angiosarcoma
Tissue section; same case as Figure 7.68
(H & E, IP)

Diagnostic pitfalls in breast FNAC

Conditions in which there is a risk of making a false positive diagnosis

1. Papillary lesions
The difficult distinction between intraduct papilloma, in situ papillary carcinoma and invasive papillary carcinoma has been discussed on page 151.

2. Atypical epithelial hyperplasia
The large number of epithelial cells, a proportion of which have enlarged, atypical nuclei, may raise a suspicion of malignancy, but the presence of single bare nuclei of benign type prevents a cancer diagnosis. Open biopsy and histological examination should follow (see p. 145).

3. Fibroadenoma
Epithelial atypia can be extremely worrysome in some fibroadenomas. Again, the presence of single benign nuclei should prevent a false positive diagnosis. The myxoid stroma characteristic of fibroadenoma is also a very helpful sign (p. 141).

4. Regenerative epithelial atypia
In the presence of inflammatory cells, particularly of polymorphs, epithelial atypia should be interpreted with caution (p. 148).

5 Pregnancy and lactation
The smear pattern of dispersed cells resembles cancer at low power but the uniformly round nuclei, the bland

7 BREAST

nuclear chromatin and, above all, the lipid secretion in the background prevent misdiagnosis (p. 146).

6. *Atypia of ductal epithelium in cysts*
Ductal epithelial cells of oxyphil type seen in cyst fluid can look very atypical. If the fluid is not haemorrhagic, and if there is no residual lump following evacuation of the fluid, there is practically no probability at all of malignancy (p. 143).

7. *Skin adnexal tumours*
The smear pattern of a syringocystadenoma papilliferum imitates that of breast cancer closely. The following case illustrates this rare problem.

The patient, a 60-year-old woman, presented with a subcutaneous lump in the right axilla. She had a history of right mastectomy for cancer 4 years ago. A FNA smear from the lump contained numerous epithelial cells, both single and in clusters. The cells had a moderate amount of cytoplasm of a vaguely oxyphil appearance and moderately atypical nuclei. The pattern was considered to be in keeping with metastatic breast cancer, but histological examination of the excised lesion showed this to be a syringocystadenoma papilliferum.

Conditions in which there is a risk of making a false negative diagnosis

1. *Tumours with central necrosis or sclerosis*
Smears are practically acellular and the distinction between scirrhous cancer and sclerosed fibroadenoma, and between necrotic cancer and duct ectasia may require an open biopsy (p. 147).

2. *A small carcinoma obscured by a dominant benign lesion*
The benign lesion could be a 'lipoma', a cyst, or a lumpy fibroadenosis. This problem can only be overcome by the consistent use of mammography.

3. *Complex proliferative lesions*
Representative sampling can never be assured in poorly defined complex lesions with epithelial hyperplasia with and without atypia, which may include foci of in situ or even invasive carcinoma. Close correlation with clinical and mammographic findings is crucial.

4. *Low grade carcinoma*
Tubular carcinoma in particular can be a problem, since single, bare, stromal nuclei of benign type are often present in smears from such tumours and epithelial atypia may be minimal. In most cases the overall architectural pattern is sufficiently atypical to suggest an open biopsy (p. 153).

5. *Small cell carcinoma*
Cells of infiltrating lobular carcinoma often have uniformly small nuclei and the cell yield is poor due to the extremely desmoplastic stroma. The irregular shape of the nuclei, the tendency to form single files or clusters with nuclear moulding and the absence of single, bare nuclei of benign type are diagnostic features (p. 157). Some ductal cancers also have uniformly small neoplastic cells.

REFERENCES AND SUGGESTED FURTHER READING

1. d'Amore E S, Maisto L, Gatteschi M B, Toma S, Canavese G: Secretory carcinoma of the breast. Report of a case with fine needle aspiration biopsy. Acta Cytol 30: 309–312, 1986.
2. Auer G, Caspersson T, Wallgren A: DNA content and survival in mammary carcinoma. Anal Quant Cytol 2: 161–165, 1980.
3. Auer G, Tribukait B: Comparative single cell and flow DNA analysis in aspiration biopsies of breast carcinomas. Acta Path Microbiol Scand A 88: 355–358, 1980.
4. Azavedo E, Fallenius A, Svane G, Auer G: Nuclear DNA content, histological grade, and clinical course in patients with nonpalpable mammographically detected breast adenocarcinomas. Am J Clin Oncol 13: 23–27, 1990.
5. Azavedo E, Svane G, Auer G: Stereotactic fine-needle biopsy in 2594 mammographically detected non-palpable lesions. Lancet 1: 1033–1036, 1989.
6. Barrows G H, Anderson T J, Lamb J L, Dixon J M: Fine-needle aspiration of breast cancer. Relationship of clinical factors to cytology results in 689 primary malignancies. Cancer 58: 1493–1498, 1986.
7. Bauermeister D E : The role and limitations of frozen section and needle aspiration biopsy in breast cancer diagnosis. Cancer 46: 947–949, 1980.
8. Bell D A, Hajdu S I, Urban J A, Gaston J P: Role of aspiration cytology in the diagnosis and management of mammary lesions in office practice. Cancer 51: 1182–1189, 1983.
9. Berg J W, Robbins G F: A late look at the safety of aspiration biopsy. Cancer 15: 826–827, 1962.
10. Bicker T, Schondorf H, Naujoks H: Long-term follow-up in patients with mammary gland changes found unsuspicious by aspiration cytology. Cancer Detect Prev 11: 319–322, 1988.
11. Bondeson L: Aspiration cytology of radiation-induced changes of normal breast epithelium. Acta Cytol 31: 309–310, 1987.
12. Bondeson L, Lindholm K: Aspiration cytology of tubular breast carcinoma. Acta Cytol 34: 15–20, 1990.
13. Boon M E, Trott P A, van Kaam H, Kurver P J, Leach A, Baak J P: Morphometry and cytodiagnosis of breast lesions. Virchows Arch (Pathol Anat) 396: 9–18, 1982.
14. Bottles K, Chan J S, Holly E A, Chiu S H, Miller T R: Cytologic criteria for fibroadenoma. A step-wise logistic regression analysis. Am J Clin Pathol 89: 707–713, 1988.
15. Ciatto S, Cariaggi P, Bulgaresi P: The value of routine cytologic examination of breast cyst fluids. Acta Cytol 31: 301–304, 1987.
16. Ciatto S, Cecchini S, Grazzini G, Iossa A, Bartoli D, Cariaggi M P, Bulgaresi P: Positive predictive value of fine needle aspiration cytology of breast lesions. Acta Cytol 33: 894–898, 1989.
17. Coleman D, Desai S, Dudey H, Hollowell S, Hulbert M: Needle aspiration of palpable lesions: a new application of the membrane filter technique and its results. Clin Oncol 1: 27–32, 1975.
18. Cowen P N, Benson E A: Cytologic study of fluid from breast cysts. Br J Surg 66: 209–211, 1979.
19. Dixon J M, Anderson T J, Lamb J, Nixon S J, Forrest A P: Fine needle aspiration cytology, in relationships to clinical examination and mammography in the diagnosis of a solid breast mass. Br J Surg 71: 593–596, 1984.
20. Donnell R M, Kay S, Rosen P P, Braun D W Jr, Lieberman P H, Kinne D W, Kaufman R J: Angiosarcoma and other vascular tumours of the breast. Am J Surg Pathol 5: 629–642, 1981.
21. Dowlatshahi K, Gent H J, Schmidt R, Jokich P M, Bibbo M, Sprenger E: Nonpalpable breast tumours: diagnosis with stereotaxic localization and fine-needle aspiration. Radiology 170: 427–433, 1989.
22. Duane G B, Kanter M H, Branigan T, Chang C: A morphologic and morphometric study of cells from colloid carcinoma of the breast obtained by fine-needle aspiration. Distinction from other breast lesions. Acta Cytol 31: 742–750, 1987.
23. Duguid H L D, Wood R A B, Irving A D, Preece P E, Cuschieri A: Needle aspiration of the breast with immediate reporting of material. Br Med J 2: 185–187, 1979.
24. Dziura B R, Bonfiglio T A: Needle cytology of the breast. A quantitative and qualitative study of the cells of benign and malignant ductal neoplasia. Acta Cytol 23: 320–340, 1979.
25. Elston C W, Cotton R E, Davies C J, Blamey R W: A comparison of the use of the Tru-Cut needle and fine needle aspiration cytology in the preoperative diagnosis of carcinoma of the breast. Histopathology 2: 239–254, 1978.
26. Finley J L, Silverman J F, Lannin D R: Fine-needle aspiration cytology of breast masses in pregnant and lactating women. Diagn Cytopathol 5: 255–259, 1989.
27. Frable W J: Needle aspiration of the breast. Cancer 53: 671–676, 1984.
28. Frisell J, Eklund G, Nilsson R, Hellström L, Somell A: Additional value of fine-needle aspiration biopsy in a mammographic screening trial. Br J Surg 76: 840–843, 1989.
29. Gal R, Gukovsky-Oren S, Lehman J M, Schwartz P, Kessler E: Cytodiagnosis of a spindle-cell tumor of the breast using antisera to epithelial membrane antigen. Acta Cytol 31: 317–321, 1987.
30. Grenko R T, Lee K P, Lec K R: Fine needle aspiration cytology of lactating adenoma of the breast. A comparative light microscopic and morphometric study. Acta Cytol 34: 21–26, 1990.
31. Grubb C: Colour atlas of breast cytopathology. Heyden, London, 1981.
32. Gupta R K, Naran S, Buchanan A, Fauck R, Simpson J: Fine-needle aspiration cytology of breast: its impact on surgical practice with an emphasis on the diagnosis of breast abnormalities in young women. Diagn Cytopathol 4: 206–209, 1988.
33. Helvie M A, Baker D E, Adler D D, Andersson I, Naylor B, Buckwalter K A: Radiographically guided fine-needle aspiration of nonpalpable breast lesions. Radiology 174: 657–661, 1990.
34. Hiller G, Harney M, Legg S, Hart S A: Fine needle aspiration cytology in breast disease management — a 4 year experience. Aust NZ J Surg 57: 239–242, 1987.
35. Horsfall D J, Jarvis L R, Grimbaldeston M A, Tilley W D, Orell S R: Immunocytochemical assay for oestrogen receptor in fine needle aspirates of breast cancer by video image analysis. Br J Cancer 59: 129–134, 1989.
36. Ingram D W, Sterrett G F, Sheiner H J, Shilkin K B: Fine needle aspiration cytology in the management of breast masses. Med J Aust 2: 170–173, 1983.
37. Johnson T L, Kini S R: The significance of atypical apocrine cells in fine-needle aspirates of the breast. Diagn Cytopathol 5: 248–254, 1989.
38. Kern W H: The diagnosis of breast cancer by fine-needle aspiration smears. J A M A 241: 1125–1127, 1979.
39. King E B, Chew K L, Duarte L, Hom J D, Mayall B H, Miller T R, Petrakis N L: Image cytometric classification

7 BREAST

of premalignant breast disease in fine needle aspirates. Cancer 162: 114–124, 1988.

40. Kline T S: Masquerades of malignancy. A review of 4,242 aspirates from the breast. Acta Cytol 25: 263–266, 1981.

41. Kline T S, Kline I K: Guides to clinical aspiration biopsy. Breast. Igaku-Shoin, New York, 1989.

42. Kreuzer G: Aspiration biopsy cytology in proliferating benign mammary dysplasia. Acta Cytol 22: 128–131, 1978.

43. Kreuzer G, Zajicek J: Cytologic diagnosis of tumours from aspiration biopsy smears. III. Studies of 200 carcinomas with false negative or doubtful cytologic reports. Acta Cytol 16: 249–252, 1972.

44. Lamb J, Anderson T J: Influence of cancer histology on the success of fine needle aspiration of the breast. J. Clin Pathol 42: 733–735, 1989.

45. Lamovec J, Us-Krasovec M, Zidar A, Kljun A: Adenoid cystic carcinoma of the breast; a histologic, cytologic, and immunohistochemical study. Semin Diagn Pathol 6: 153–164, 1989.

46. Leiman G: Squamous carcinoma of the breast. Diagnosis by aspiration cytology. Acta Cytol 26: 201–209, 1982.

47. Levack P A, Mullen P, Anderson T J, Miller W R, Forrest A P: DNA analysis of breast tumour fine needle aspirates using flow cytometry. Br J Cancer 56: 643–646, 1987.

48. Lew W Y, Lee W H: Fine needle aspiration cytology: its role in the management of breast tumours. Aust NZ J Surg 58: 941–946, 1988.

49. Lindholm K: Cytology versus histology in carcinoma in situ of the breast and the role of fine-needle aspiration cytology in the treatment of carcinoma in situ. In: Goerttler K, Feichter GE, Witte S (eds) New frontiers in cytology. Modern aspects of research and practice. Springer, Berlin, 1988.

50. Linsk J, Kreuzer G, Zajicek J: Cytologic diagnosis of mammary tumours from aspiration biopsy smears. II. Studies on 210 fibroadenomas and 210 cases of benign dysplasia. Acta Cytol 16: 130–138, 1972.

51. Löfgren M, Andersson I, Bondeson L, Lindholm K: X-ray guided fine-needle aspiration for the cytologic diagnosis of nonpalpable breast lesions. Cancer 61: 1032–1037, 1988.

52. Macansh S, Greenberg M, Barraclough B, Pacey F: Fine needle aspiration cytology of granulomatous mastitis. Report of a case and review of the literature. Acta Cytol 34: 38–42, 1990.

53. Marasa L, Tomasino R M: Aspiration cytology of the breast. II. Significance of bipolar naked nuclei. Pathologica 74: 193–200, 1982.

54. Masin M, Masin F: Cytology of angiosarcoma of the breast. A case report. Acta Cytol 22: 162–164, 1978.

55. McDivitt R W, Boyce W, Gersell D: Tubular carcinoma of the breast. Clinical and pathological observations concerning 135 cases. Am J Surg Pathol 6: 401–411, 1982.

56. McDivitt R W, Stewart F W, Farrow J H: Breast carcinoma arising in solitary fibroadenomas. Surg Gynecol Obstet 125: 572–576, 1967.

57. McSwain G R, Valicenti J F, O'Brien P H: Cytologic evaluation of breast cysts. Surg Gynecol Obstet 146: 921–925, 1978.

58. Mouriquand J, Bolla M, Gabelle P, Geindre M, Sage J C, Mouriquand C: Le grade cytologique facteur de pronostic dans le cancer du sein. J Gynecol Obstet Biol Reprod (Paris) 11: 471–476, 1982.

59. Naran S, Simpson J, Gupta R K: Cytologic diagnosis of papillary carcinoma of the breast in needle aspirates. Diagn Cytopathol 4: 33–37, 1988.

60. Nguyen G K, Neifer R: Aspiration biopsy cytology of secretory carcinoma of the breast. Diagn Cytopathol 3: 234–237, 1987.

61. Nordenström B, Ryden H, Svane G: Stereotaxic breast biopsy. In: Percutaneous needle biopsy. Zornoza J (ed.) Williams & Wilkins, Baltimore, 1980.

62. Oertel Y C, Galbum L I: Fine needle aspiration of the breast: diagnostic criteria. Pathol Annual 18: 375–407, 1983.

63. Oertel Y C: Fine needle aspiration of the breast. Butterworth, Boston, 1987.

64. Page D, Anderson T: Diagnostic histopathology of the breast. Churchill Livingstone, Edinburgh, 1987.

65. Patel J J, Gartell P C, Smallwood J A, Herbert A, Royle G, Buchanan R, Taylor I: Fine needle aspiration cytology of breast masses: an evaluation of its accuracy and reasons for diagnostic failure. Ann R Coll Surg Engl 69: 156–159, 1987.

66. Peterse J L, Koolman-Schellekens M A, van de Peppel-van de Ham T, van Heerde P: Atypia in fine-needle aspiration cytology of the breast: a histologic follow-up study of 301 cases. Semin Diagn Pathol 6: 126–134, 1989.

67. Peterse J L, Thunnissen F B, van Heerde P: Fine needle aspiration cytology of radiation-induced changes in nonneoplastic breast lesions. Possible pitfalls in cytodiagnosis. Acta Cytol 33: 176–180, 1989.

68. Pilotti S, Rilke F, Delpiano C, Di Pietro S, Guzzon A: Problems in fine needle aspiration biopsy cytology of clinically or mammographically uncertain breast tumours. Tumori 68: 407–412, 1982.

69. Remvikos Y, Magdellenat H, Zajdela A: DNA flow cytometry applied to fine needle sampling of human breast cancer. Cancer 15: 1629–1634, 1988.

70. Rupp M, Hafiz M A, Khalluf E, Sutula M: Fine needle aspiration in stromal sarcoma of the breast. Light and electron microscopic findings with histologic correlation. Acta Cytol 32: 72–74, 1988.

71. Russin V L, Lachowicz C, Kline T S: Male breast lesions: gynecomastia and its distinction from carcinoma by aspiration biopsy cytology. Diagn Cytopathol 5: 243–247, 1989.

72. Salhany K E, Page D L: Fine-needle aspiration of mammary lobular carcinoma in situ and atypical lobular hyperplasia. Am J Clin Pathol 92: 22–26, 1989.

73. Schmitt F C, Tani E, Skoog L: Cytology and immunocytochemistry of bilateral breast metastases from prostatic cancer. Report of a case. Acta Cytol 33: 899–902, 1989.

74. Schondorf H: Aspiration cytology of the breast. Saunders, Philadelphia, 1978.

75. Shabot M M, Goldberg I M, Schick P, Nieberg R, Pilch Y H: Aspiration cytology is superior to Tru-Cut needle biopsy in establishing the diagnosis of clinically suspicious breast masses. Ann Surg 196: 122–126, 1982.

76. Sheikh F A, Tinkoff G H, Kline T S, Neal H S: Final diagnosis by fine-needle aspiration biopsy for definitive operation in breast cancer. Am J Surg 154: 470–474, 1987.

77. Silfversward C, Gustafsson J A, Gustafsson SA, Nordenskjöld B, Wallgren A, Wrange O: Estrogen receptor analysis on fine needle aspirates and on histologic biopsies from human breast cancer. Eur J Cancer 16: 1351–1357, 1980.

78. Silverman J F, Feldman P S, Covell J L, Frable W J: Fine needle aspiration cytology of neoplasms metastatic to the breast. Acta Cytol 31: 291–300, 1987.

79. Silverman J F, Geisinger K R, Frable W J: Fine-needle aspiration cytology of mesenchymal tumors of the breast. Diagn Cytopathol 4: 50–58, 1988.

80. Silverman J F, Lannin D R, O'Brien K, Norris H T: The triage role of fine needle aspiration biopsy of palpable breast masses. Diagnostic accuracy and cost-effectiveness. Acta Cytol 31: 731–736, 1987.

81. Silverman J F, Lannin D R, Unverferth M, Norris H T:

Fine needle aspiration cytology of subareolar abscess of the breast. Spectrum of cytomorphologic findings and potential diagnostic pitfalls. Acta Cytol 30: 413–419, 1986.

82. Simi U, Moretti D, Iacconi P, Arganini M, Roncella M, Miccoli P, Giacomini G: Fine needle aspiration cytopathology of phyllodes tumor. Differential diagnosis with fibroadenoma. Acta Cytol 32: 63–66, 1988.

83. Sneige N, White V A, Katz R L, Troncoso P, Libshitz H I, Hortobagyi G N: Ductal carcinoma-in-situ of the breast: fine-needle aspiration cytology of 12 cases. Diagn Cytopathol 5: 371–377, 1989.

84. Sneige N, Zacharia H, Fanning T V, Dekmezian R H, Ordornez N G: Fine-needle aspiration cytology of metastatic neoplasms in the breast. Am J Clin Pathol 92: 27–35, 1989.

85. Stanley M W, Tani E M, Skoog L: Metaplastic carcinoma of the breast: fine-needle aspiration cytology of seven cases. Diagn Cytopathol 5: 22–28, 1989.

86. Stanley M W, Tani E M, Skoog L: Mucinous breast carcinoma and mixed mucinous-infiltrating ductal carcinoma: a comparative cytologic study. Diagn Cytopathol 5: 134–138, 1989.

87. Stenquist B, Bengtsson E, Eriksson O, Jarkrans T, Nordin B: Image cytometry in malignancy grading of breast cancer. Results in a prospective study with seven years of follow up. Analyt Quant Cytol 8: 293–300, 1986.

88. Stormby N, Bondeson L: Adenoma of the nipple. An unusual diagnosis in aspiration cytology. Acta Cytol 28: 729–732, 1984.

89. Strawbridge H T G, Bassett A A, Foldes I: Role of cytology in management of lesions of the breast. Surg Gynecol Obstet 152: 1–7, 1981.

90. Thomas J M, Fitzharris B M, Redding W H, Williams J E, Trott P A, Powles T J, Ford H T, Gazet J C: Clinical examination, xeromammography and fine-needle aspiration

cytology in diagnosis of breast tumours. Br Med J 2: 1139–1141, 1978.

91. Trott P A, McKinna J A, Gazet J C: Breast aspiration cytology. Lancet 1: 40, 1981.

92. Tsuchiya S, Maruyama Y, Koike Y, Yamada K, Kobayashi Y, Kagaya A: Cytologic characteristics and origin of naked nuclei in breast aspirate smears. Acta Cytol 31: 285–290, 1987.

93. Vassilakos P: Tuberculosis of the breast: Cytologic findings with fine-needle aspiration. Acta Cytol 17: 160–165, 1973.

94. Wallgren A, Silfverswärd C, Hultborn A: Carcinoma of the breast in women under 30 years of age. A clinical and histopathological study of all cases reported as carcinoma to the Swedish cancer registry, 1958–1968. Cancer 40: 916–923, 1977.

95. Wang H H, Ducatman B S, Eick D: Comparative features of ductal carcinoma in situ and infiltrating ductal carcinoma of the breast on fine-needle aspiration biopsy. Am J Clin Pathol 92: 736–740, 1989.

96. Wilkinson S, Anderson T J, Rifkind E, Chetty U, Forrest A P: Fibroadenoma of the breast: a follow-up of conservative management. Br J Surg 76: 390–391, 1989.

97. Zajdela A, de Maublanc M A: Valeur et intéret de la ponction cytologique dans la surveillance des cancers mammaires irradiés. Bull Cancer (Paris) 66: 107–112, 1979.

98. Zajdela A, De Maublanc M A, Pilleron J P: La fiabilité de l'examen des tumeurs mammaires par cytoponction. Experience de l'Institut Curie. Chirugie 107: 193–198, 1981.

99. Zajicek J: Aspiration biopsy cytology. Part I. Cytology of supradiaphragmatic organs. Monographs in Clinical Cytology, Vol. 4. S Karger, Basel, 1974.

8

LUNG, MEDIASTINUM, CHEST WALL AND PLEURA

8 LUNG, MEDIASTINUM, CHEST WALL AND PLEURA

CLINICAL ASPECTS

LUNG

Although sporadic reports of the diagnosis of lung carcinoma by fine needle aspiration (FNA) appeared as early as 1886,[76] the impetus for widespread use of the technique only arose with the development of image intensifiers and television viewing which allowed localisation of small parenchymal lesions.[32] Recognition of the accuracy of cytological diagnosis based on material obtained from the fine needle technique,[32] and simpler methods of treating pneumothorax brought the method within the reach of most hospital radiologists and pathologists. Infection and other benign processes may be proven by FNA, but the main indication is for the diagnosis of localised intrathoracic lesions suspected of being malignant, particularly when less invasive investigations prove negative.[72,106]

Several changes have occurred in the last few decades. The emphasis has shifted from the diagnosis of malignancy in inoperable patients and confirmation of metastatic tumour to its use as a definitive diagnostic procedure on which crucial management decisions are based.[106] All intrathoracic sites, including mediastinum and deep hilar lung lesions, are now routinely and safely sampled using fine (less than 20 G) needles and with increased flexibility and accuracy when used with CT[114,174] with or without stereotaxic guidance,[24] and in selected cases, ultrasound guidance.[179,180] Lung function studies and radiology are used to predict accurately the risk of pneumothorax[41,78] allowing safer selection of patients for outpatient FNA.[98] Small chest tubes are a safe and easy method of treating pneumothorax.[91] Transbronchial FNA[55,108,112,144,145] permits sampling of submucosal tumours and mediastinal lesions, enhances the role of FNA in the staging of lung cancers,[111] and may be used for the diagnosis of pulmonary infection[73] and cysts.[113] The use of the non-aspiration technique,[2] coaxial needle sampling,[23,48] fine cutting needles,[48] and screw needles,[10,127] allows the selection of sampling devices for particular purposes. The presence of the pathologist at the procedure leads to a reduction in the number of needle passes and may decrease the pneumothorax rate[58] and increase sensitivity.[23,79] Intraoperative FNA and rapid diagnosis may be of value to the surgeon for lesions which are difficult or hazardous to biopsy by standard methods,[21,35] or provide educational benefits for cytology and radiology staff.[79] There is more accurate knowledge of the cost-effectiveness of FNA[47,69,106] and, along with greater expectations by clinicians about tumour typing, extremely high rates of cytohistological correlation for common tumours have occurred.[59,80,96] Precise criteria for the verification of diagnosis in follow up studies have been constructed.[18]

The value and accuracy of FNA in diagnosis in areas such as the spectrum of neuroendocrine tumours,[45,61,129] and mediastinal[155,156,163,170,175] and pleural[177,178,181,182] tumours is accepted particularly when allied with cell block preparations,[96] plastic embedded semi-thin sections[37] immunoperoxidase studies[67,130] and electron microscopy.[34,52,102,152] Ancillary tests are now widely used and are indispensable to diagnosis in selected cases. The cytological findings in less common tumours such as sarcomas,[28,66] lymphoid lesions,[12,42] and a wide range of metastatic tumours[93] are now documented as well as the important role of FNA in the diagnosis of second primary tumours.[44,93]

The place of FNA in the investigative sequence

There is wide agreement that FNA complements other diagnostic methods.[60,72] Among invasive techniques, we believe FNA to be the one of first choice in lesions which are in the pulmonary apex, medial upper lobe[106] or periphery, particularly small lesions 1 cm or so in diameter, and in the mediastinum. Fibreoptic bronchoscopy (FOB) with brushings and biopsy are most effective in diagnosing more centrally placed pulmonary lesions; FNA also has especial value in cases in which FOB is not diagnostic.[72]

Some authors advocate diagnostic thoracotomy for lesions undiagnosed by non-invasive methods; others have found that a choice between strategies of immediate FNA, open thoracotomy, or a wait-and-see approach may not be so different in terms of overall patient survival,[29] but that there is value in preoperative diagnosis for individual patients.[106] For example, thoracotomy is generally contraindicated for small cell anaplastic carcinoma, metastatic tumours, or infection. A confident diagnosis of benign lesions like tuberculosis or chondroid hamartoma makes surgical intervention unnecessary;[36] a definitive diagnosis of malignancy in patients who are operative risks allows surgeons to operate without the fear that it might be unnecessary or harmful.[69,106] FNA has been shown to be a cost-effective method of diagnosis,[47] leading to shorter hospitalisation, lower costs and a reduction in diagnostic thoracotomies and in studies using decision analysis[69] and methods of estimating how FNA influences post-test probability of disease,[140] a critical evaluation of the place of FNA in diagnosis has taken place.

The technique may be the only way of providing a diagnosis in inoperable patients and perhaps the greatest value to the clinician is still in these cases.[151] An unequivocal diagnosis of carcinoma and distinction between well-differentiated squamous cell carcinoma, small cell anaplastic carcinoma, and large cell carcinoma of other types, gives the clinician sufficient information to select appropriate therapy.

FNA can also be useful intraoperatively to replace frozen section when incisional or large needle biopsy is contraindicated.[21,35,79] During bronchoscopy, transbronchial aspiration allows sampling of submucosal tumours not accessible to brushing or biopsy, or of subcarinal, paratracheal or hilar nodes and mediastinal structures.[144,145]

Accuracy of diagnosis

The sensitivity of FNA, including transbronchial FNA[55] in the diagnosis of malignant pulmonary neoplasms is over 80% in most series;[59,60,96,109,123,128,140] this varies according to the size and site of the mass and the experience of the radiologist[95] and the pathologist. In selected series it reaches over 90%.[23,48,126] A nonspecific negative result on FNA does not exclude malignancy[15,72,151] and in this event a repeat aspiration, careful clinical follow-up, or additional diagnostic procedures are necessary. The rate of false positives is usually less than 0.5%; however, a few false diagnoses of malignancy are still reported,[62] associated with chondroid hamartomas,[30,96] reactive bronchiolar epithelial proliferation, squamous metaplasia[62] and reactive mesothelial cell proliferation,[59] associated with lesions such as tuberculosis or pulmonary infarcts. 'False positive' diagnosis due to contamination of transbronchial aspirates by intrabronchial tumours has been described.[27,111] Although there are pitfalls and limitations to FNA diagnosis,[132] Tao[133] stresses the need for caution in assuming that a lack of cytological, clinical or histological correlation is a result of false positive cytological diagnosis; he introduced the term 'false false positives' for cases where longer clinical follow up or closer histological examination confirms the cytological diagnosis; very well differentiated adenocarcinomas or very small tumours within larger areas of radiological opacity are particularly prone to this error.[132] Caya[18] advocates the following criteria in diagnosing cases as 'benign' or 'malignant' to improve the statistical reliability of follow up studies of accuracy: for benign lesions — either open lung biopsy or autopsy proof, or a minimum of 6 months follow up with clinical data compatible with infection or infarction or the like, or resolution of any radiographic abnormality; and for malignancy — biopsy or autopsy proof of primary or metastatic disease or chest X-ray, scans, or CT evidence of lung involvement by malignant newgrowth, or strong clinical evidence such as SVC obstruction, or recurrent laryngeal nerve palsy.

Experienced cytopathologists identify the histological type of 75–90%[59,80,96,126] of primary lung tumours and approximately 80% of their predictions of type are correct[32,59,80,96,126] (figures similar to those achieved with bronchial biopsy[89,96]). Some authors attribute high levels of cyto-histological correlation to the combined use of smears and cell-blocks which can be prepared from needles as fine as 23 G, and allow better assessment of tissue architecture,[96] or by using larger cutting needles,[64] though others show no particular advantage

from fine cutting needles.[149,153] Rapid scrutiny of material in the radiology theatre may enhance accuracy of typing by allowing selection of particular ancillary techniques which aid in diagnosis. Most cases of small cell anaplastic carcinoma,[80,122,129,148] well-differentiated adenocarcinoma, including bronchiolo-alveolar carcinoma[57,74,115,116,134] and squamous cell carcinoma are easily identified, but poorly differentiated tumours of glandular or squamous origin, and large cell anaplastic carcinoma are more difficult to separate. Most chondroid hamartomas[30,31,36,38,50,100,124] are accurately diagnosed; however, other benign neoplasms are difficult to type because their cohesiveness prevents aspiration of adequate material.[15] This problem may be overcome by using larger needles,[48] the Rotex screw needle[10,127] or cell block preparations[96] making histological assessment of tissue fragments possible.[77,109] Some authors assert that 70–90% of benign lesions overall may be diagnosed by these methods.[3,64] Cytological evidence of infection including tuberculosis may be gained in up to 80% of cases.[6,33,103] Very fine needles have been used with a high degree of accuracy to diagnose bacterial, fungal, or pneumocystis infection in immunosuppressed patients;[8,142] indeed, larger needles are contraindicated in these patients because of the danger of severe bleeding.

Complications

Fatalities are rare but have occurred when 20 gauge or larger needles are used; most patients were either terminally ill or had severe underlying pulmonary disease or infection.[128] The most common cause of death was haemorrhage, although some died from air embolism and tension pneumothorax;[123] recently further cases of air embolism have been reported[1,8,22] including one fatality[1] using a 22 G needle. It was suggested that biopsy of cavities, or during coughing or deep inspiration should be avoided and that hyperbaric oxygen facilities should be available for treatment of such cases.[8,22] A mortality rate of 0.2% is quoted in one combined series of 1562 patients,[53] but no deaths have occurred in our experience of over 3000 cases, and we know of only two other examples of death associated with the use of 22 G or finer needles.

The rate of pneumothoraces reported in the literature varies from 6 to 57% and those requiring intercostal catheterization from 1.5 to 20%.[9,128] In many cases, thin catheters may be used to remove pleural air safely,[91] and these can be inserted either in the radiology theatre or the ward. Emphysema, deep lesions, multiple punctures, older patients, and inexperienced operators,[46] all contribute to a higher rate.[41,78,95,99,121] There is a linear relationship between the degree of severity of chronic obstructive airways disease (emphysema) as judged by lung function tests and radiological assessment and the

LUNG, MEDIASTINUM, CHEST WALL AND PLEURA

prevalence of pneumothorax.[41,78] Young fit patients without emphysema have a low risk and FNA is sometimes performed as an outpatient procedure in this group.[41] Several small studies claim that the use of very fine needles or coaxial techniques may reduce the incidence, but this is disputed by other workers. Examination of material in the radiology theatre allows the number of needle passes to be reduced, and so reduces the rate of pneumothorax.[58] Several other methods of reducing the rate have been suggested, including the use of autologous blood injected into the pleura after FNA to provide a 'blood patch', and pure O_2 breathing. In controlled trials neither has been proven to be of value,[13,99] although O_2 breathing may reduce the size of a pneumothorax, increase the resorption rate, and diminish the need for intercostal drainage.[99] Other complications like pneumomediastinum, air embolism, and haemothorax are extremely rare after fine needle aspiration of lung. Less than 5% of patients complain of minor haemoptysis. A small haemorrhage into the surrounding lung occurs in up to 10% of cases without being detrimental to the patient. Only a few cases of neoplastic implantation along a thoracic needle track have been reported,[81,83,125] and one case of skin implantation with fungal organisms.[17] Bacteraemia may occasionally be induced.[147]

Contraindications

Patients who do not have a cough reflex, who are unconscious, or who cough intractably, should not be aspirated. Vascular lesions like arteriovenous malformation or aneurysm are usually excluded before attempting a puncture and hilar lesions are avoided by some workers because of the supposed risk of damaging large vessels; however, the risk of bleeding, even from large vessels, is minimal when fine needles are used. Nevertheless, there is an increased risk of bleeding in patients with pulmonary hypertension, bleeding disorders, or undergoing anticoagulant therapy, and these should be assessed for needle aspiration only in exceptional circumstances, for example, in immunosuppressed patients where a positive diagnosis of an infection may lead to curative therapy.[8] Most authors do not recommend aspiration of suspected hydatid cysts for fear of anaphylactic reaction to leaking cyst fluid or implantation of germinal epithelium. Bilateral aspirations are also not recommended.

Technical considerations

Obtaining material

Most workers use simple, thin-walled, long bevelled needles of less than 20 gauge, with a central stylet, such as the 'Chiba needle', although we feel that the bevel angle in commercially available needles is not acute enough. Shorter needles used for injection seem to have

the optimal bevel angle, an impression reinforced by some scientific studies which suggest that thin core needles or short bevel needles yield less material than those with a longer bevel although larger core short bevel needles may be more successful.[5,48] Modifications like the Hayata brush[62] and the Rotex needle[10,127] may increase the amount of material obtained and are useful in special situations such as hard or cohesive tumours,[127] but they are not any more successful than FNA if employed routinely,[10] and we use them only as second line needles. The use of 22–23 G needles provides satisfactory material for most malignant tumours, and they are perfectly adequate for making cell block preparations. We have generally used finer needles to lessen tissue damage, although their flexibility may reduce the chance of successful puncture in very deep lesions. Larger needles may be used more safely in pleural based or chest-wall lesions.

The puncture site is marked on the skin and local anaesthetic introduced down to the pleura. A short guide needle is inserted which makes aiming of the aspiration needles easier, reduces the risk of bending of flexible needles, and precludes contamination of the aspirate with chest wall tissues.[23,82] By carefully positioning this needle immediately above the lesion, the aspiration needle can be directed down to the lesion usually without needing biplane imaging. It is debatable whether introducing the guide needle through the pleura increases or decreases the rate of pneumothorax. Coaxial techniques have been advocated where an outer needle is passed down to the lesion allowing multiple sampling by a fine central needle without multiple transgressions of the pleura.[23,48] They do, however, involve the use of outer needles larger than 20 G, and some risk of pleural tearing if wide respiratory excursions or coughing occurs. Non-aspiration techniques can yield quite adequate material[2] and may be particularly useful in haemorrhagic lesions (e.g. metastatic tumours such as renal cell carcinomas).

TV-fluorography is the simplest and most convenient method of imaging, and is much less time-consuming than CT guidance; however, CT is useful in small peripheral lesions, in some cases where the lesion is difficult to visualise by image intensifier, or in a juxtavascular location in the mediastinum,[139,174] and is extremely useful in the preaspiration assessment of the depth and location of deep lesions and lesions which move excessively with respiration. Stereotactic CT[24] is used by some for localising deep lesions and ultrasound may be suitable for apical or chest wall tumours.[179,180]

The contribution of operator expertise to increasing the sensitivity of the diagnosis of malignancy and in reducing pneumothorax rate has been studied by Philips et al[95] and Sinner.[121] In several other series in which large numbers of operators are involved in an aspiration service, the sensitivity has been around 75–80%,[90] although in one of these there was no significant differ-

LUNG, MEDIASTINUM, CHEST WALL AND PLEURA

ence between trainees and qualified radiologists.[82] In the teaching hospital setting, some compromise of sensitivity may be unavoidable.

Carcinomas may be soft, or have a 'gritty' feel when the needle enters; however, metastases, carcinoid tumour, and non-Hodgkin's lymphoma are said to lack this sensation. Chondroid hamartomas may sometimes be recognised by the operator by their rubbery resistance[31] and old scars, Hodgkin's lymphoma, and 'rounded atelectasis', may be very hard.[64] Aspiration of neural tumours may cause intense pain during aspiration in contrast to carcinoma and most benign lesions.[157]

Adequacy of material is assessed in the Radiology Theatre by a member of the Pathology Department after rapid H & E or MGG staining and microscopic scrutiny. The needling may be repeated up to three or four times until adequate material for diagnosis is obtained; often one puncture suffices. If the material is heavily blood-stained, collection on to a watch glass may be helpful. Small clumps of tumour may be recognised as bright translucent fragments against the red background. To reduce blood contamination these may be selected and smeared on a slide. By lysing red blood cells Carnoys' fixative is also helpful. Material is taken for ultrastructural study or culture if appropriate, and for special stains or cell blocks in *all* cases if it can be obtained safely. Plastic embedding may permit a combination of thin histological and electron microscopical examination to be performed on adjacent sections, enhancing diagnostic accuracy.[37] For those centres without on-site pathology services, pre-fixation of aspirated material in 50% alcohol can be used for preserving material for transport.

Some authors report the development of significant numbers of pneumothoraces up to 24 hours after the procedure; they therefore recommend serial radiographs until this time.[9] Others have found that an X-ray 1 hour after the procedure shows most pneumothoraces.[91] If symptoms of pain or shortness of breath develop after this time, further X-rays are performed. Occasionally, we perform aspirations on outpatients, but generally observe them for at least several hours after the procedure.[91,98] There are thus a wide range of imaging techniques, needle types, needle sizes and options for particular contingencies; close co-operation between the radiologist and pathologist is essential to ensure the most efficient use of this flexibility.

Use of ancillary techniques

Cell-block preparations

The microanatomical details evident in cell blocks[96] or plastic embedded sections[37] aid in typing large cell carcinomas, and also provides the basis for controlled studies by cytochemistry and immunocytochemistry in an appraisal of diagnostically difficult lesions.[177]

Cytochemistry

We routinely apply mucin stains to smears and cell-block preparations to aid in subtyping large cell carcinomas and in distinguishing between some primary and metastatic tumours; for example, in excluding renal cell or adrenal carcinoma. Detection of hyaluronic acid in the epithelial cells in mesothelioma has proven useful in a few cases (see Fig. 8.74).[182] Demonstration of argyrophilia is said to help distinguish between atypical carcinoid and small cell carcinoma,[129] or carcinoid and non-neuroendocrine tumours, but we have not found these stains easy to apply in smears.

Immunocytochemistry[7,67,130]

In the diagnosis of thoracic lesions we have found the range of uses for immunocytochemistry in FNA cell block preparations similar to those in histological specimens. Monoclonal antibodies to keratins of various molecular weights, epithelial membrane antigen, (EMA), CEA (see Fig. 8.73), S-100, leucocyte common antigen, and, more recently LeuM-1 and 44-3A6,[7] can separate most poorly differentiated carcinomas, melanomas, and lymphomas, and aid in the diagnosis of mesothelioma. We have applied neuroendocrine markers such as synaptophysin, bombesin, chromogranin, and NSE in studying neuroendocrine tumours, but found limited value in using them to separate small-cell from non-small cell tumours. The use of panels of monoclonal antibodies against ultrastructurally characterised small cell carcinomas has suggested a significant association between keratin-staining and extent of disease, raising the possibility of using these markers as prognostic indicators.[130] Specific markers, e.g. for prostate specific antigen, breast cyst fluid protein and thyroglobulin, are extremely useful in selected cases; oestrogen receptor staining may also be of limited value in identifying metastases of breast carcinoma. Chess and Hajdu reported a high proportion of unexpected positive and negative findings in their studies of smears (see Ch. 3) and we have avoided smear preparations for IPOX studies for this reason although other authors have found that even smears stained previously with Papanicolaou are suitable. Gustafsson (see Ch. 2) advocated washing of cells and paying critical attention to the type and time of fixation to avoid excessive background staining and to increase sensitivity and specificity of staining. Nordgren's filter block preparations may aid in preserving all material for study (see Ch. 2). Enhanced sensitivity may derive from adding another antibody layer to the avidin–biotin system (see Ch. 2). The use of various monoclonal antibodies such as B72.3, 44-3A6,[7] CE407,[62] and BL99-57,[67] may aid in subtyping of large cell carcinoma, and in excluding other poorly differentiated tumours.

Electron microscopy[34,52,102,152]

This modality is increasingly used in association with

LUNG, MEDIASTINUM, CHEST WALL AND PLEURA

FNA of all sites, but, in particular, deep aspirations. In Silverman's experience (see Ch. 2) FNA samples are the most frequent non-renal samples sent for EM in his department, and we agree that this technique has a uniquely valuable role in diagnostically difficult tumours. Along with other authors, we select cases for those studies by an initial evaluation of the material in the radiology theatre. Many methods of preparing and processing tissue are suggested, mainly with the aim of separating tumour from contaminating red cells (see Ch. 2). We use Lazaro's method of cell concentration and in some 150 cases from various sites, 100 contained adequate well-preserved material for assessment. In 60% of these cases EM only confirmed the LM diagnosis, but in 40%, the findings were diagnostic per se. In our experience most value is obtained in recognising neuroendocrine tumours (see Fig. 8.29) and in the specific diagnosis of melanoma, mesothelioma (see Fig. 8.76) and some carcinomas, including metastases where immunocytochemistry often cannot provide such positive diagnostic features. Accurate subtyping of small-cell carcinomas by EM or immunohistochemistry may carry prognostic implications, and an accurate distinction between carcinoid, atypical carcinoid, and small cell tumours is facilitated by EM. As detailed by Taccagni, EM is particularly useful in mediastinal lesions such as thymomas.[172]

Cytometry

DNA cytometry has been applied to lung lesions,[20] though without clear evidence of diagnostic or prognostic value at present.

MEDIASTINUM

The differential diagnosis of mediastinal lesions is extensive; a proper appraisal of the radiological appearance of the lesion is necessary to narrow the list of possible diagnoses, before any assessment can be made on cytological material. Clinical and laboratory findings are often helpful; for example, the presence of high levels of circulating human chorionic gonadotrophin and alpha-fetoprotein in germ cell tumours, or the presence of myasthenia gravis or the detection of circulating anti-striated muscle antibody in thymoma may virtually establish the diagnosis before morphological study. Specific diagnoses of lesions such as thymic carcinoma are impossible without clinico-radiological exclusion of

tumours of other primary sites. Fine needle aspiration findings are now accepted as a basis for definitive therapy, for example, in the confirmation of metastatic small cell carcinoma or other types of lung carcinoma; but the main role of aspiration in primary mediastinal lesions is often to give the clinician a guide to the nature of the lesion before surgical intervention. Most malignant lesions will be diagnosed and accurate tumour typing is often possible.[155,156,163,170,175,176] Thymomas, particularly biphasic tumours, are easily diagnosed cytologically, and by a combination of immunoperoxidase and ultrastructural study, most variants can be recognised by FNA.[158,167,168,170,173] Complications of aspiration of this site are probably no more frequent than in lung;[155,175] and even when superior vena caval obstruction is present aspiration appears to be very safe.[155] CT has great value in this site, as it can localise the needle tip within the lesion far better than fluoroscopy[155] (see Ch. 3); such rare complications as cardiac tamponade could be avoided using this method.[68] Transbronchial or transcarinal FNA are useful in diagnosing and staging metastatic disease. Mediastinal cystography can generally give a strong guide to the nature of cysts.[162,166]

CHEST WALL AND PLEURA

Chest wall is included here to emphasise that the exact site of origin of lesions in this region may be difficult to ascertain; those arising in rib, chest wall soft tissues, pleura or even breast may extend to underlying lung tissues and may be confused with primary lung lesions. Contaminating bone marrow from rib may give rise to concern. We have seen several cases of myeloma in the chest wall in which the cells were pleomorphic and which could have been mistaken for an undifferentiated lung carcinoma. Anaplastic tumours, particularly spindle cell neoplasms, provide considerable difficulty in distinguishing between mesothelioma, anaplastic carcinoma, melanoma, and sarcomas of the chest wall. A chondrosarcoma arising in rib caused difficulty in diagnosis because the site of origin was not appreciated. On the other hand, a malignant mesothelioma growing along a chest drain site was considered clinically to be a primary breast lesion until aspiration biopsy was performed. Larger needles may be more safely used because the risk of pneumothorax and bleeding is much less than in deeper lesions. Ultrasonic guidance may occasionally be a worthwhile adjunct in this site.[179,180] Most lesions of this region are described in Chapter 11.

LUNG, MEDIASTINUM, CHEST WALL AND PLEURA 8

CYTOLOGICAL FINDINGS

LUNG

The satisfactory smear

A specific benign diagnosis by FNA is generally restricted to the identification of infection, chondroid hamartomas, cysts, and a few other disease processes. Non-specific negative findings do not exclude malignancy[15,72,151] and can only be used for management in conjunction with clinical findings, and when a precise statistical assessment of accuracy rates for a radiology department and a laboratory are known. In a sense, the only satisfactory sample is one which contains material permitting a specific diagnosis. Nevertheless, many workers would use a negative result on three passes where the needle was shown to be in an accurate position by radiology, as sufficient evidence for conservative management unless there were other clinical indications for subsequent investigation.[106]

Normal structures (Figs 8.1–8.3)

1. Bronchial epithelium.
2. Bronchiolar epithelium.
3. Mesothelium.
4. Macrophages.
5. Fat tissue (chest wall).
6. Cartilage/bone marrow (rib).

Bronchial epithelium is occasionally seen and may be present abundantly if the needle traverses a medium-sized bronchus or tracks along a bronchial lumen. Bronchial epithelium appears as small palisaded clusters with a ciliated border. In large aggregates the cells may present as flat sheets with a pavement-like aspect, but ciliated cells can usually be observed at the edges of these sheets.

Bronchiolar epithelium or non-ciliated epithelium is seen commonly as sheets of various size (Fig. 8.1). They usually have irregular edges and the component cells display variable cell separation. The nuclei are generally small and there is a low nuclear–cytoplasmic ratio. Sometimes the nuclear outlines are slightly irregular and small intranuclear cytoplasmic invaginations are observed. Occasionally, atypia of bronchiolar epithelium may be quite pronounced, for example in reactive or inflammatory processes; however, the number of atypical cells is usually small. A diagnosis of malignancy should not be based on small numbers of cells, unless nuclear features of malignancy are unequivocal.

Mesothelium is easily distinguished from bronchiolar epithelium. It is seen as various-sized, flat, monolayered sheets; there is usually more cell separation than in bronchiolar epithelium which sometimes gives a sponge-like appearance. The cells may appear to be joined by intercellular bridges similar to those of squamous epithelium (Fig. 8.2).

Macrophages are almost invariably present in smears, except when pure newgrowth is aspirated (Fig. 8.3). An aspirate from normal lung yields a population of macrophages widely dispersed over the slide; these contain small particles of brown or black particulate matter some of which is inhaled dust, especially in smokers. Many haemosiderin-laden macrophages usually imply

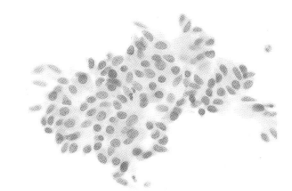

Fig. 8.1 Bronchiolar epithelium
Small sheet of regular glandular cells (H & E, HP)

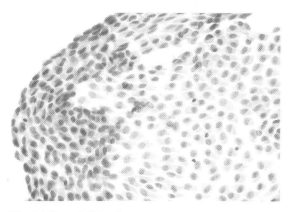

Fig. 8.2 Mesothelial cells
Monolayered sheet of cells showing 'spongiotic' separation of individual cells within the sheet (H & E, HP)

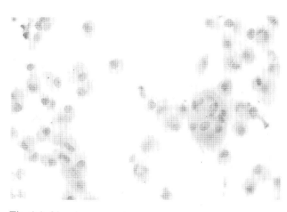

Fig. 8.3 Alveolar macrophages
Dispersed cells, including some with intracytoplasmic pigment and multinucleate forms (H & E, HP)

8 *LUNG, MEDIASTINUM, CHEST WALL AND PLEURA*

tissue or blood breakdown near the lesion and may add to a suspicion of pulmonary infarction should the clinical background be appropriate.

If stylets are not used, contamination of smears by chest wall tissues such as fat, cartilage, and bone marrow may occur. Occasionally, intrapulmonary lymph nodes may be aspirated and recognised by cytoradiological correlation. Aspirations near the diaphragm can contain liver or splenic tissue, and cause concern unless the possibility of inadvertent puncture of abdominal organs is appreciated.

Inflammatory/non-neoplastic processes

Acute inflammatory material

Common findings

1. Several drops of viscous purulent material.
2. Many polymorphs.
3. Granular and amorphous debris.
4. Macrophages, lymphocytes, and plasma cells in varying numbers.
5. Bacteria.

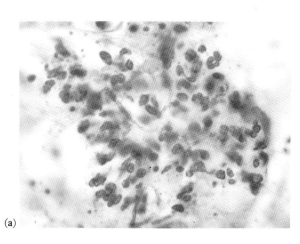

(a)

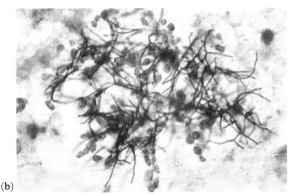

(b)

Fig. 8.4 Neutrophil rosette
(a) Clump of neutrophils (H & E, HP Oil). (b) Fine branching filaments of Nocardia (Methemamine silver, HP Oil).

These findings are not specific unless bacteria are evident, but they can suggest an acute infection. It is worth repeating the aspiration, sending all the material obtained for aerobic and anaerobic culture. Associated vegetable material may suggest aspiration as a cause.

Problems in diagnosis

1. Squamous cell carcinoma with necrosis.
2. Caseous necrosis.
3. Fungal infection.

When the centre of a necrotic carcinoma is aspirated, particularly those of squamous type, acute inflammatory material may result. Macroscopically this may resemble pus and microscopically few squamous cells may be present. Small squamous cells with pyknotic nuclei may be difficult to distinguish from degenerate macrophages.

Polymorphonuclear leukocytes are not uncommonly seen in tuberculosis and the background debris may also be rather 'watery' similar to that in some acute inflammatory processes. We stain all inflammatory smears with the Ziehl-Neelsen (ZN) stain.

A high polymorph content is usually present in the inflammatory reaction to fungi. A search for a granulomatous component and fungal organisms is mandatory if acute inflammatory material is obtained. In several of the cases of fungal infection we have seen, fungi (and bacteria) have been identifed in the centre of distinctive, cohesive neutrophil clusters or rosettes after silver impregnation; this clustering, therefore, may be a clue to such infection (Fig. 8.4).

Granulomatous inflammation (Figs 8.5–8.7)[6,101,103,118]

Criteria for diagnosis

1. Epithelioid histiocytes.
2. Few non-pigmented multinucleate histiocytes.
3. Granular, calcific, mucoid or acute inflammatory debris (corresponding to caseous necrosis in TB).
4. Lymphocytes.

Many conditions are associated with a granulomatous reaction in lung tissue.[88] Cytological findings may be helpful and one can make a confident diagnosis of a 'granulomatous process' on aspirated material; however, a more important aspect of the aspiration in these cases is to obtain an adequate sample for staining for acid fast bacilli and for culture, particularly to distinguish between 'typical' and 'atypical' mycobacteria.[118] It is best to have a large sample for this purpose and we have not found much value in washings of the needle after a cytology smear has been made; the whole aspirate needs to be sent for culture. Culture is more successful in cases with necrotic and inflammatory debris.

Epithelioid histiocytes are fairly cohesive and tend to form collections with a granuloma-like appearance (Fig. 8.5). Epithelioid cells have an elongated or bean-shaped

LUNG, MEDIASTINUM, CHEST WALL AND PLEURA 8

but sometimes outlines of necrotic cells may be prominent (Fig. 8.7b) and often the appearances are merely of non-descript debris, histocytes and neutrophils. Dahlgren cites granular calcific material as a common accompaniment.[33] Lymphocytes may be plentiful in granulomatous inflammation.

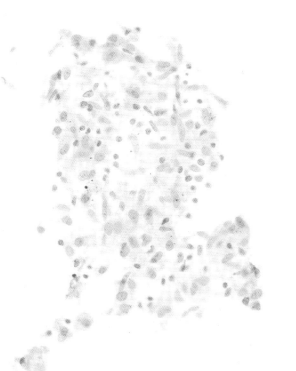

Fig. 8.5 Granuloma
Clustered epithelioid histiocytes and lymphocytes (H & E, HP)

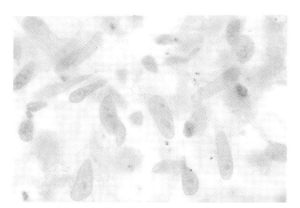

Fig. 8.6 Epithelioid histiocytes
Elongated foot print shaped nuclei; pale cytoplasm with indistinct borders (H & E, HP Oil)

(a)

(b)

Fig. 8.7 Caseation necrosis
(a) Amorphous and granular debris (H & E, MP). (b) Single cell pattern of necrosis (H & E, HP).

nucleus and abundant cytoplasm which is rather pale and indistinct both in Pap and H & E stained specimens (Fig. 8.6). The cytoplasmic density is higher in MGG-stained material. Multinucleated histiocytes are seen but are usually sparse. They are mainly free of intracyto-plasmic pigment or birefringent material, unlike the multinucleated histiocytes seen in non-specific reactions in pulmonary tissue. Caseous necrosis has a very variable appearance; there may be an amorphous and granular background with little cell outline visible (Fig. 8.7a),

LUNG, MEDIASTINUM, CHEST WALL AND PLEURA

Bailey diagnosed 28 of 34 cases of TB by either auramine rhodamine fluorescence or positive culture; AFBs were seen in only 38% of cases.[6]

Problems in diagnosis

1. Identification of epithelioid histiocytes.
2. Giant cells in non-specific inflammation.
3. Giant cell reaction to neoplasm.
4. Tumour necrosis mimicking caseation and vice versa.
5. Neutrophil reaction in tuberculosis.

Epithelioid histiocytes may resemble fibroblasts, smooth muscle cells, or endothelial cells; they are most characteristically found in clusters and can rarely be identified if they lie singly.

Giant cells which contain pigment are more in keeping with a non-specific reaction than a true granulomatous process.

A granulomatous reaction may develop at the edge of a carcinoma or other neoplasm, particularly squamous cell carcinoma forming keratin; this reaction may be a foreign body giant cell reaction and yield many multinucleated cells. Histiocytic giant cell reactions also occur in fungal infections, e.g. cryptococcosis[117,143] or histoplasmosis,[118] so the cytoplasm of any giant cells present should be closely examined. Tuberculosis may, of course, co-exist with carcinoma.

Necrotic tumour may be homogeneous or granular and resemble caseous material. Conversely, in one of our cases of tuberculosis, the necrosis consisted of necrotic single cells distributed across the smear and closely resembled necrotic tumour necrosis (Fig. 8.7b).

As has been pointed out by several authors, acid-fast bacilli were more often seen in cytological material characterised by a mixture of neutrophils, histiocytes, mucoid, or necrotic material than in those lesions with a prominent epithelioid cell component,[6,101] though culture is positive in a similar percentage of cases with and without epithelioid cells.[6] In our cases, necrotic debris has macroscopically sometimes resembled pus, or mucoid material, or thin watery fluid. Whenever necrotic debris is seen, we restain smears with ZN stains.

Other specific infections

In Aspergillus and Phycomycete infections in the lung, fungal hyphae are easily visible in H & E stained material. In one of our cases of Cryptococcosis, organisms were only seen within multinucleated cells.[150] In some fungal infections, particularly histoplasmosis, and in Actinomycosis and Nocardiosis, organisms may only be seen in methenamine silver preparations although the Pap stain is a superb technique for identifying most organisms including the filamentous higher bacteria. Destained H & E or Pap stained smears are as suitable as unstained material for special stains. Culture is neces-

sary for the exact classification of the organism in most of these cases.

Multiple and unusual infections may be met with in AIDS[49] and percutaneous FNA has a place in well patients without significant respiratory compromise;[142] Pneumocystis organisms and CMV effect are easily recognised cytologically. Coccidioidomycosis[43] and Dirofilariasis[51] have been described in needle biopsy samples, though the latter was diagnosed with a cutting needle.

Oxalate crystals are produced by several species of Aspergillus and if identified in cytological material should lead to a search for organisms.[39,70]

Pneumoconioses

Identification of birefringent silica and collagenous tissue, or asbestos bodies may help confirm silicosis or exposure to asbestos,[104] however, as pointed out by Leiman et al,[71] concomitant malignancy, tuberculosis, or other infections, may be the cause of the localized lung lesion sampled in these patients.

Pulmonary infarct

Silverman describes sheets of metaplastic squamous cells showing regeneration, and histiocytes containing clumped refractile haemosiderin in a clinically unsuspected infarct, in which FNA findings led to the diagnosis being suggested.[120]

Common primary carcinomas

Squamous cell carcinoma (Figs 8.8–8.12)

Criteria for diagnosis

Keratinising

1. Single cell presentation.
2. Keratinised malignant cells; cytoplasm refractile and eosinophilic (Pap, H & E); dense, pure blue (MGG).
3. Perinuclear halo.
4. Bizarre cell shapes, spindle and caudate cells.
5. Irregular angular, densely hyperchromatic nuclei.
6. Necrosis.

Non-keratinising

1. Irregular solid cohesive fragments; absence of flat sheets.
2. Elongated or spindle shaped nuclei.
3. Variable chromatin density in adjacent cells.

Well differentiated squamous cell carcinomas with keratinising cells and bizarre cell shapes are not difficult to recognise. The malignant cells are usually dispersed especially when they are very well differentiated (Fig. 8.8); necrosis is a common accompaniment. Single keratinising cells are the most reliable indicators of squamous differentiation; when keratinisation is not ob-

LUNG, MEDIASTINUM, CHEST WALL AND PLEURA   8

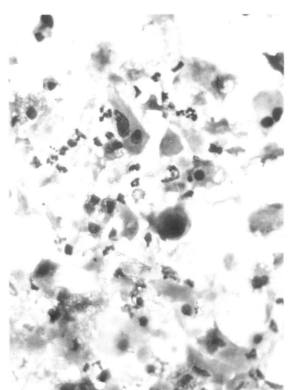

Fig. 8.8 Squamous cell carcinoma
Dispersed keratinising malignant cells and necrotic debris
(MGG, HP)

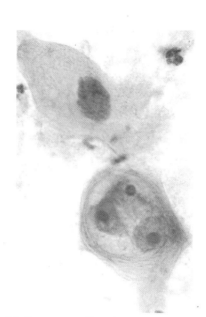

Fig. 8.9 Squamous cell carcinoma
Keratinised squamous cell, and a cell with a prominent
perinuclear halo (H & E, HP Oil).

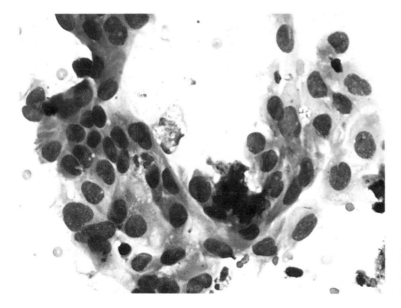

Fig. 8.10 Squamous cell carcinoma
Irregular clump of relatively cohesive
non-keratinising cells; variation in
chromatin density (MGG, HP).

vious, a perinuclear halo within the cytoplasm and con-
densation of peripheral cytoplasm are helpful guides to
squamous differentiation (Fig. 8.9). This halo corre-
sponds to a clearer cell appearance in sections and often
represents intracytoplasmic glycogen. Non-keratinising

tumours are usually more cohesive and present as multilayered fragments. Their nuclei are usually spindle
shaped or elongated with dense, irregularly distributed
chromatin. There is often conspicuous variation in the
degree of chromasia of nearby nuclei. Nucleoli vary in

8 *LUNG, MEDIASTINUM, CHEST WALL AND PLEURA*

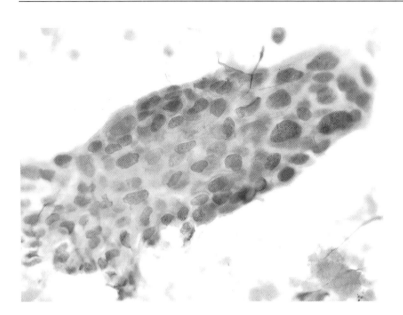

Fig. 8.11 Squamous cell carcinoma
Cohesive fragment of pleomorphic
non-keratinising cells; necrotic debris
(H & E, HP)

size and number (Figs 8.10 and 8.11). Dense cytoplasm and well-defined cell borders are indicators of squamous differentiation but some adenocarcinomas may have strikingly well-defined borders and very dense cytoplasm.

Problems in diagnosis

1. Necrosis in other carcinomas simulating keratinisation.
2. Other poorly differentiated large cell carcinomas.
3. Inflammation and necrosis, especially in cavitating lesions.
4. Giant-cell reaction to tumour.
5. Very well differentiated squamous cell carcinoma.
6. Teratoma.
7. Mucoepidermoid tumours.

Misinterpreting the cytoplasmic eosinophilia of necrosis for keratinisation is a common source of error.[80] Necrosis can also impart an angular hyperchromatic appearance to nuclei, similar to squamous carcinomas. These are less of a problem when Pap staining is used because orangiophilia distinguishes between necrosis and keratin better than H & E; where possible, we try to keep some material for Pap staining.

There is an overlap between the appearances of poorly differentiated squamous cell carcinoma, large cell anaplastic carcinoma, and poorly differentiated or solid adenocarcinoma in aspirated material. They all present as large, multilayered fragments corresponding to the solid growth of these carcinomas. Squamous cell carcinoma is over-diagnosed in some series because adenocarcinoma in aspirates may present as pavement-like sheets, mimicking the appearance that squamous cell carcinoma has in sections. The pavement-like appearance of squamous cell carcinoma results only from thin

sectioning and does not occur in aspirated material. Palisading of cells which may occur at the margins of lobules of non-keratinising squamous tumours may give rise to a false impression of the margin of a gland in smears. There is also a tendency to over-estimate the grade of tumour in aspirated material, perhaps because viable rather than maturing or exfoliating newgrowth is removed. Diagnostic malignant squamous cells may be difficult to find when there is associated acute inflammation and abundant necrosis, especially in cavitating tumours (Fig. 8.8).

Keratinising squamous cell carcinoma more than other carcinomas tends to produce a giant-cell response in nearby tissues and a false impression of a granulomatous process may be gained (Fig. 8.12). A variegated population of many and different types of inflammatory cells, foamy macrophages, mast cells, and alveolar cells

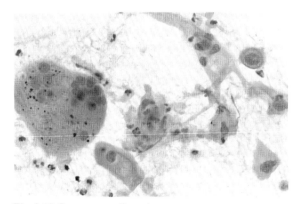

Fig. 8.12 Squamous cell carcinoma
Granulomatous reaction to tumour; multinucleate macrophages and a few atypical squamous cells (H & E, HP)

LUNG, MEDIASTINUM, CHEST WALL AND PLEURA 8

may also be present, resulting from bronchial obstruction associated with the carcinoma. Other types of carcinoma, especially adenocarcinomas, do not usually show this extensive inflammatory reaction.

Occasionally only keratinous debris or very well differentiated cells may be removed from a squamous cell carcinoma and cells with diagnostic malignant nuclei may be absent. The location of the lesion within pulmonary parenchyma and other clinical features may then aid in diagnosis.

Teratoma enters the differential diagnosis, particularly when a lesion has a mediastinal component. In the aspirate from the only mature teratoma we have seen, the squamous epithelium was very cohesive in contradistinction to the dispersed cells of well differentiated squamous cell carcinoma.

Low grade mucoepidermoid tumours have been described in FNA samples.[86]

Adenocarcinoma 'bronchogenic' (Figs 8.13–8.18)

Criteria for diagnosis

1. Medium sized to large cells with abundant delicate cytoplasm.
2. Flat sheets.
3. Rosettes, acinar structures, or cell clusters/balls.
4. Columnar cells.
5. Round to oval eccentric nuclei with large solitary nucleoli.

The cellular morphology of bronchogenic adenocarcinoma is similar to that described in brush material. Rosettes, acinar formations (Fig. 8.13), or cohesive cell clusters represent anatomical structures removed from the tumour by the needle and these can be correlated with their histological counterparts.

The larger the gland formations the less likely they are to be removed intact and when only partly removed deposit on the slide as flat sheets in a monolayer (Fig. 8.15): this feature is also a very useful indicator of

glandular differentiation. Artefactual spaces are often seen in large tissue fragments and may be misinterpreted as acinar structures; however, where the spaces have an 'anatomical' rigidity, they may indicate glandular differentation. Mucin secretion is difficult to identify without special stains (Fig. 8.16) and vacuolation of the

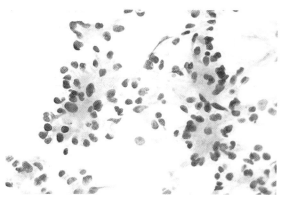

Fig. 8.13 Adenocarcinoma 'bronchogenic'
Rosette or acinus-like structures (H & E, HP)

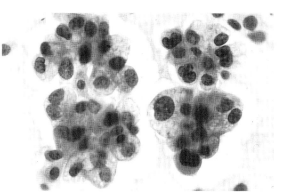

Fig. 8.14 Adenocarcinoma 'bronchogenic'
Cell clusters/cell balls (H & E, HP)

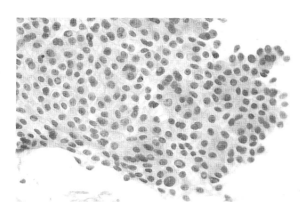

Fig. 8.15 Adenocarcinoma 'bronchogenic'
Flat monolayered sheet of moderately pleomorphic glandular cells (H & E, MP)

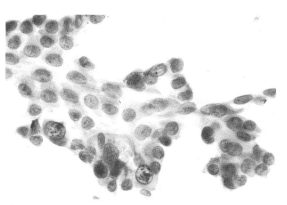

Fig. 8.16 Adenocarcinoma 'bronchogenic'
Intracytoplasmic mucin (PAS/diastase, HP)

8 *LUNG, MEDIASTINUM, CHEST WALL AND PLEURA*

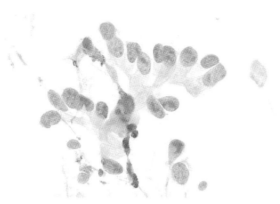

Fig. 8.17 Adenocarcinoma 'bronchogenic'
Group of palisaded columnar cells (H & E, HP)

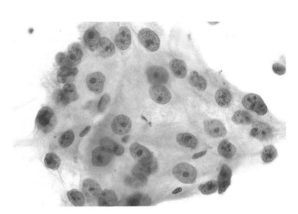

Fig. 8.18 Adenocarcinoma 'bronchogenic'
Delicate cytoplasm, rounded nuclei with single prominent central nucleoli (H & E, HP)

cytoplasm may occur as a result of degeneration or the presence of glycogen. In H & E or Pap stained material vacuoles with a central, inspissated, eosinophilic or orangiophilic centre are very suggestive of mucin secretion and correspond to the intracellular lumina described ultrastructurally in adenocarcinomas. With MGG staining mucin may be visible as magenta or purple material within the cytoplasm either homogeneously or as red granules within a pale vacuole (Figs 4.46 and 4.49). Well-formed columnar cells or groups of palisaded cells may also be a guide to glandular differentiation and terminal plates/bars may also be present (Fig. 8.17).

Problems in diagnosis

1. Other poorly differentiated large cell carcinomas.
2. Bronchiolo-alveolar carcinoma.
3. Metastatic adenocarcinoma.
4. Neuroendocrine tumour (p. 193).

In those adenocarcinomas with meagre mucin secretion and little or no glandular formation the possibility of accurate diagnosis by aspiration cytology is low. The cytoplasmic and nuclear features of large cell anaplastic and of some poorly differentiated squamous cell carcinomas may also closely resemble adenocarcinoma, although if the tumour cells are fairly regular and the nuclei are rounded with large central nucleoli they are more likely to be glandular; this is not, however, a completely reliable criterion (Fig. 8.18).

The cytological appearances of bronchogenic adenocarcinoma overlaps with that of bronchiolo-alveolar carcinoma, particularly when the tumour is composed of large glands or has a papillary structure.

There are no absolute criteria for separating primary from secondary adenocarcinomas, although there may be features indicative of a particular organ of origin (see Ch. 5, p. 77).

Bronchiolo-alveolar carcinoma (BAC)
(Figs 8.19–8.25)[57,74,115,116,134]

Criteria for diagnosis

1. Profuse amounts of material.
2. Large, cohesive, monolayered sheets.
3. Papillary processes, cell balls and clusters.
4. Variability in amount of pleomorphism and nuclear atypia.
5. Intranuclear cytoplasmic inclusions.
6. Psammoma bodies.

This subgroup of adenocarcinoma of the lung is usually well differentiated and situated peripherally. It tends to spread through the lung using the existing alveolar walls as a support, often with a superimposed papillary pattern. Ultrastructurally, neoplasms with this pattern of growth are extremely heterogeneous and may be composed of mucin-secreting cells, Clara cells, type II alveolar lining cells, bronchial columnar cells,[52] or other cell types, and, rarely, may show neuroendocrine features. This pattern of growth is quite commonly seen as a component of lung adenocarcinomas, but is uncommon in pure form.

Some BACs are highly differentiated and in these the malignant characteristics of nuclear atypia, stromal invasion, and metastasis may be absent; in others, the cytological and histological attributes of malignancy are more obvious. These variations are also reflected in cytological material, and some BAC has been subdivided into 'secretory', 'non-secretory' and 'pleomorphic' types using cytological criteria.[134] The more pleomorphic or poorly differentiated forms of BAC are said to have a worse prognosis than those with more uniform cells.[134]

Despite these variations the cytological characteristics of BAC can be distinctive in material obtained by FNA and the correct tumour typing may often be predicted.

LUNG, MEDIASTINUM, CHEST WALL AND PLEURA 8

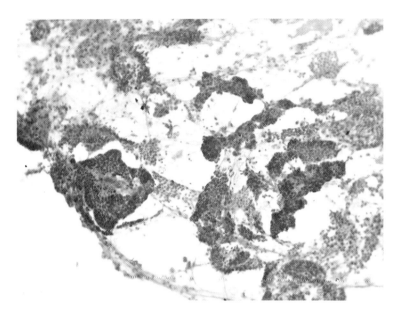

Fig. 8.19 Bronchiolo-alveolar carcinoma
Sheets and 'papillaroid' structures; highly cellular smears (II & E, LP)

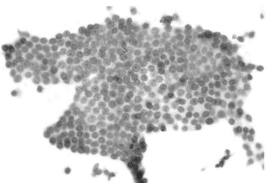

Fig. 8.20 Bronchiolo-alveolar carcinoma
Flat monolayered sheet regular benign looking cells (H & E, MP)

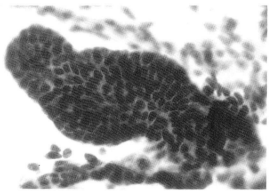

Fig. 8.21 Bronchiolo-alveolar carcinoma
Fingerlike papilla (H & E, HP)

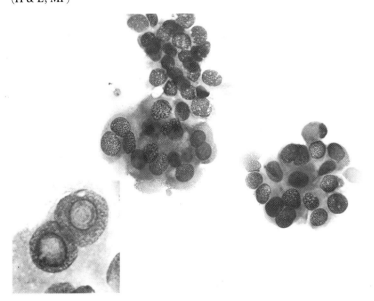

Fig. 8.22 Bronchiolo-alveolar carcinoma
Clusters of regular small cells (MGG, HP).
Inset: intranuclear vacuoles (MGG, HP Oil).

8 LUNG, MEDIASTINUM, CHEST WALL AND PLEURA

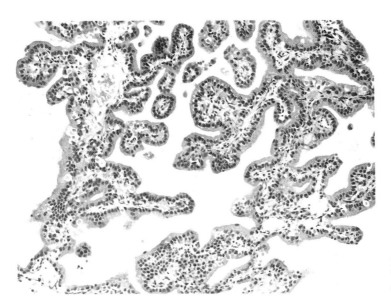

Fig. 8.23 Bronchiolo-alveolar carcinoma
Tissue section; well-differentiated 'non-secretory' form; (H & E, MP)

Aspirates usually provide abundant cellular material which is readily seen on low-power microscopic examination (Fig. 8.19). In our experience the material consists mainly of aggregates and a few single cells. The aggregates frequently form flat sheets containing upward of 200 cells which reflect the growth of neoplastic cells in a monolayer along alveolar walls (Fig. 8.20). Although flat sheets are characteristic, many of the aggregates are three-dimensional and form papillary processes or cell balls. The finger-like projections no doubt represent a papillary growth pattern within air spaces, the cell balls and clusters corresponding to the tips of papillae or detached groups of cells within alveolar lumina (Figs 8.21 and 8.22). In the so-called secretory variant the component cells have abundant cytoplasm and are arranged in honeycomb-like sheets

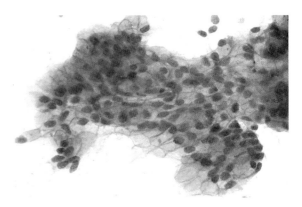

Fig. 8.24 Bronchiolo-alveolar carcinoma
Tumour of 'secretory' type; honeycomb-like sheet; columnar cells (H & E, HP)

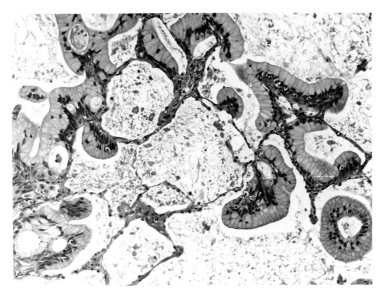

Fig. 8.25 Bronchiolo-alveolar carcinoma
Tissue section; well-differentiated secretory form (H & E, MP)

(Fig. 8.24), although a mixture of secretory, non-secretory and pleomorphic cells is common.[74]

In Silverman's detailed study,[115] BAC had a varied cytological presentation: the most common included three-dimensional cell clusters similar to those seen in sputum, and many dispersed cells resembling atypical macrophages; fewer cases showed prominent two-dimensional sheets; an arrangement of malignant cells along alveolar septal structures was observed in smears in some cases.

We have been struck by the tendency of the neoplasm to yield material in which the degree of atypia varies in different parts of the smear and to a lesser extent within single aggregates; larger and more pleomorphic cells, including multinucleated cells, are commonly seen. Throughout the smear one can often trace a progression from cells with small nuclei and small amounts of cytoplasm closely resembling bronchial epithelium to cells with more abundant densely staining cytoplasm with large nuclei in which there are malignant nuclear features.

Intranuclear cytoplasmic inclusions occur in many neoplasms (melanoma, papillary carcinoma of thyroid, and anaplastic carcinomas for example). They may also be seen in pleomorphic, large cell carcinomas of the lung, in bronchogenic adenocarcinoma,[137] especially papillary types, and in benign bronchiolar epithelium, including that associated with hamartomas. We have found them more frequently in BAC than in other pulmonary neoplasms and view them as a helpful diagnostic indicator (Fig. 8.22, inset). They may be associated with optically clear nuclei in BAC.[116] Psammoma bodies are occasionally found.[116] Ultrastructural identification of 'surfactant' bodies in unequivocally neoplastic cells allows identification of a tumour as being of primary lung origin, although few cases will possess this characteristic. Most tumours are positive for CEA, keratin and vimentin, although this observation is of limited value in differential diagnosis.[74]

Almost all BACs are diagnosed by FNA in the largest series.[74,134]

Problems in diagnosis

1. Reactive bronchiolar epithelium.
2. Other primary lung neoplasms.
3. Metastatic well differentiated adenocarcinoma.
4. Mesothelioma.

A common difficulty we have met is in diagnosing well differentiated BAC when the degree of nuclear atypia is insufficient to allow an unequivocal diagnosis of malignancy. The material may mimic the appearance of benign bronchiolar epithelium, especially when occurring in sheets. Abundant material should raise the index of suspicion, as should papillae or cell balls. A thorough search of the material is mandatory. Sometimes there may be only small numbers of diagnostic

cells so that an overall impression of variation in atypia can be important in reaching a conclusion. Aspirates from non-malignant lesions of the lung frequently contain bronchiolar epithelium sometimes showing nuclear atypia.[115] Reactive sheets, however, are usually small and few;[57] they often have more irregular borders than malignant sheets. Jarrett and Betsill considered that high cellularity, architectural three-dimensionality, intranuclear cytoplasmic inclusions and large nucleolar size were the most helpful features in distinguishing BAC from reactive bronchiolar proliferations.[57] Silverman found a lack of hyperchromasia, prominence of cell borders, presence of terminal plates, goblet cells, and nuclear moulding, to be more characteristic of benign reactive epithelium.[115]

Confusion with other primary pulmonary neoplasms may occur. Lesions such as well-differentiated bronchogenic adenocarcinoma, carcinoid tumours and rare tumours such as sclerosing hemangioma[146] yield a uniform cell population similar to that of BAC. Carcinoid tumours, however, usually consist of regular cells which are smaller than those of BAC, are more dispersed, and their round nuclei have a characteristic stippled 'neuroendocrine', chromatin pattern (see Figs 8.38, 8.39).

The metastatic well-differentiated neoplasms we have studied include an endometrial carcinoma whose cytological features resembled BAC quite closely and in which cytological atypia was slight. A lack of flat sheets and the presence of markedly elongated nuclei, sometimes in palisades, were findings unlike those of BAC (p. 198).

The distinction between a peripheral, well-differentiated adenocarcinoma and the epithelial form of malignant mesothelioma is difficult. This diagnosis should always be considered when an aspirate from a lesion close to the pleura reveals a papillary or acinus-forming tumour. Immunoperoxidase and ultrastructural studies can exclude this possibility conclusively.

Small cell anaplastic carcinoma
(Figs 8.26–8.35)[80,122,129,148]

Criteria for diagnosis

1. Small or medium sized cells with little or no cytoplasm (larger than in sputum).
2. Dispersed cell presentation; some clusters, including some small tight groups.
3. Nuclear moulding and engulfment; irregular nuclei (Fig. 8.20).
4. Tear drop cells, smeared cells, and streaks of nuclear material.
5. Coarsely granular nuclear chromatin; small nucleoli.

This group of lung carcinomas is the most aggressive of the common types, having a mean survival of less than 6 months without treatment. From the clinical point of view, it is most important to categorise this newgrowth accurately because it is to date the only one

8 LUNG, MEDIASTINUM, CHEST WALL AND PLEURA

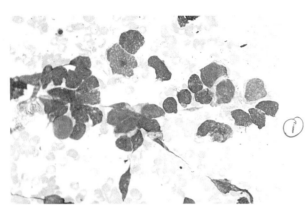

Fig. 8.26 Small cell anaplastic carcinoma
Pleomorphic poorly cohesive cells with little or no cytoplasm; nuclear moulding (MGG, HP)

in which chemotherapy produces an improvement in survival time. The group is fairly homogenous in terms of its biology, but is more heterogenous morphologically. Attempts at subclassification into oat cell, polygonal cell, and fusiform cell types have been made and there were initial suggestions of a correlation between histological subtypes and prognosis; however, even the larger 'intermediate' and smaller 'oat cell' subtypes are not reliably separable by expert pathologists, and have not been shown to have significantly different behaviour or response to therapy.

Cytology is very successful in diagnosing small cell carcinoma in sputum and pleural fluid; in fact, sputum cytology may be more accurate than FNA in typing this lesion, and the appearances more characteristic than in bronchial or pleural biopsies which are often subject to crush-artefact. The criteria for the diagnosis of small

cell carcinoma in aspirated material are similar to those in other sites, but there are some important differences.

Material is usually aspirated from the neoplasm easily and if smeared correctly without too much pressure the appearances are characteristic. Cell pleomorphism is so distinctive that a diagnosis of malignancy is seldom in doubt. The most immediate impression is the absence or sparseness of cytoplasm rather than the small size of the neoplastic cell (Fig. 8.26); in fact, the cell nuclei may appear larger than similar cells in sputum and this may mislead one into making a diagnosis of anaplastic carcinoma of non-small cell type. This difference in size between sputum and aspirated material is recorded by other authors and is presumably due to degenerative changes and shrinkage in sputum specimens. It is sparseness of cytoplasm rather than size which is the most helpful initial clue in differentiating the lesion from other pulmonary carcinomas.

The combination of dispersal with clustering is also important, especially when other small cell newgrowths enter the differential diagnosis (Fig. 8.27). Lymphomas generally do not display such cell cohesion, although large fragments may be dislodged and in some cases there may be clustering or packeting within the aspirated material (Fig. 8.34).

Fragility of nuclei is emphasised by tear drop cells or streaks of smeared nuclear material, and the close nuclear apposition and moulding so commonly seen in sputum is also evident (Fig. 8.28). Coarsely granular nuclear chromatin is also a well recognised feature of this cancer in other sites, but one point of difference from sputum is the frequency of small nucleoli in aspirated material; they are less commonly seen in sputum; this may also be related to the better preservation of cells removed directly from tumour; small nucleoli are also often seen in bronchial brush material.

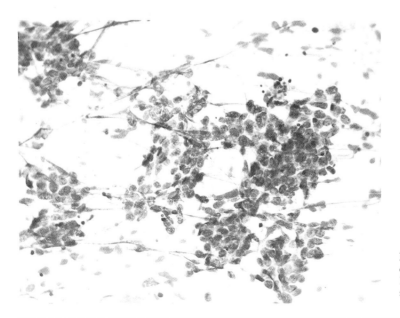

Fig. 8.27 Small cell anaplastic carcinoma
Loose clusters with some dispersal and smearing artefact (Pap, HP)

LUNG, MEDIASTINUM, CHEST WALL AND PLEURA   8

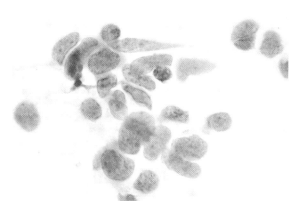

Fig. 8.28 Small cell anaplastic carcinoma
Small loose cluster showing absence of cytoplasm, nuclear moulding, teardrop cells and inconspicuous nucleoli (H & E, HP oil)

In the largest series the predictive value of a diagnosis by FNA is over 90%,[80,122,148] and the sensitivity 80%;[122,148] however, there are few series with complete histological follow up and recently some small series where accuracy was low.[90] Reasonable experience with cytological diagnosis in general and FNA diagnosis in particular is necessary before the diagnosis can be assumed to be as reliable as by biopsy or sputum cytology.

Problems in diagnosis

1. 'Intermediate' small cell carcinoma.
2. Other poorly differentiated primary carcinomas.
3. 'Combined' small cell carcinoma.
4. Complement of large cells; mixed small and large cell carcinoma.

5. Low grade carcinomas, e.g. carcinoid tumour (including spindle-cell carcinoid, and atypical carcinoid), adenoid cystic carcinoma.
6. Other carcinomas with excessive artefactual smearing.
7. Lymphoma.
8. Mixtures with inflammatory material.
9. Metastatic tumours (e.g. melanoma).

Although 'intermediate' small cell carcinoma is no longer recognised as a separate category in international classifications, we find it a useful concept to preserve, to highlight the occasional difficulty in distinguishing between small cell and poorly differentiated non-small cell carcinomas (Figs 8.29–8.31). There is overlap in nuclear size between some small and some large cell carcinomas, and a tendency to incude tumours with larger than expected nuclei, in the non-small cell category. Critical attention to nuclear morphology is of value. In general, if the nuclear features of a problematical tumour are those of small cell carcinoma — that is

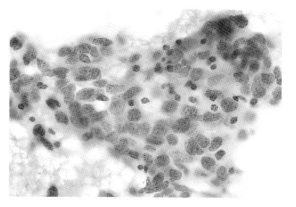

Fig. 8.29 Small cell anaplastic carcinoma
(a) 'Intermediate' variant showing more cohesion and larger cells than usual; note the granular 'neuroendocrine' chromatin pattern; tumours of this appearance are difficult to distinguish from atypical carcinoid/well-differentiated neuroendocrine carcinoma (H & E, HP). (b) Neurosecretory granules in cytoplasm of aspirated cells (EM).

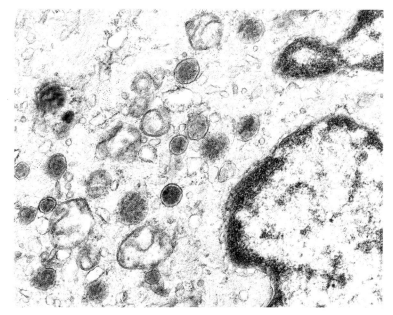

8 LUNG, MEDIASTINUM, CHEST WALL AND PLEURA

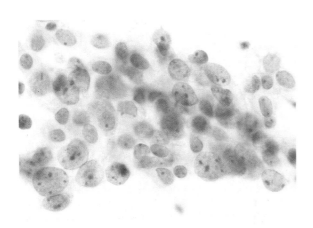

Fig. 8.30 'Borderline' tumour
Minimal cytoplasm; pale nuclei of intermediate size, with inconspicuous nucleoli; difficult to exclude small cell carcinoma cytologically; classified as large cell anaplastic carcinoma when resected (Pap, HP).

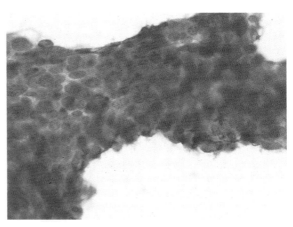

Fig. 8.31 Basaloid squamous cell carcinoma
Metastatic tumour from a pharyngeal primary; a cohesive aggregate with a sharply defined border (H & E, HP)

coarsely granular chromatin without prominent nucleoli — the neoplasm will fall into the small cell carcinoma group histologically; vesicular nuclei with prominent nucleoli would generally be evidence of non-small cell tumour (Fig. 8.30), though we have seen exceptions. Cell cohesion is not a feature of small cell cancer and, when present, some caution should be adopted; differentiation from other poorly differentiated carcinomas, in particular squamous cell carcinoma with minimal cytoplasm, may be especially difficult (Fig. 8.31). 'Borderline' newgrowths are also found, where there may be difficulty deciding even histologically between a diagnosis of so-called intermediate small cell and large cell carcinoma.

Combined tumours may occasionally be diagnosed by cytology[107] but discrepancies between cytological and histological classification can also occur because of combined or collision tumours or separate synchronous primaries where cytological sampling may not reveal all tumour elements. Roggli and others have shown frequent heterogeneity in lung cancers; 10% of predominantly non-small cell tumours may have a small cell component histologically when the whole mass is available for study.[105]

A few very large cells are occasionally seen in typical oat cell tumours. These usually lie singly and scattered across the smear; however, when clusters of larger cells are present or when these cells are numerous, caution should be exercised (Fig. 8.33). Combined tumours of mixed small and large cell type are said to have a worse prognosis and to be less sensitive to therapy. Further biopsy or ultrastructural assessment may be advisable to confirm them if suspected cytologically.

Our approach to problem cases has generally been to request more biopsy or cytological material and to submit some for electron microscopy, cell block and im-

munoperoxidase studies. Reinforcement of a diagnosis of small cell carcinoma may be possible by demonstrating evidence of neuroendocrine differentiation or other forms of differentiation using the electron microscope (Figs 8.29 and 8.32). On the other hand, detection of squamous or glandular differentiation by EM does not necessarily exclude small cell carcinoma, and some large

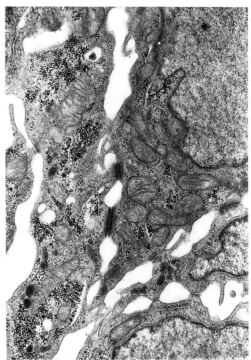

Fig. 8.32 Basaloid squamous cell carcinoma
Prominent desmosomes and intracytoplasmic glycogen; absence of neurosecretory granules (EM)

LUNG, MEDIASTINUM, CHEST WALL AND PLEURA 8

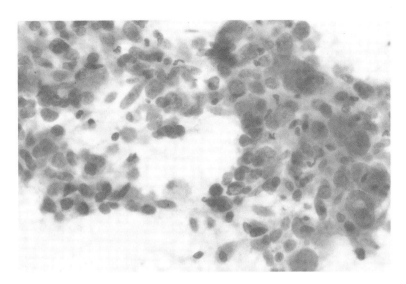

Fig. 8.33 Mixed small and large cell carcinoma
Disorganised aggregates of pleomorphic large cells and a population of smaller cells; the small cell component was prominent in cell block preparations (H & E, HP)

cell tumours ultrastructurally have neuroendocrine features. EM diagnosis, therefore, also requires considerable judgement and experience in difficult cases. Immunoperoxidase studies are also helpful, although neuroendocrine antigens show variable preservation in routinely fixed material. Specific markers for small cell cancer are not readily available. Poorly differentiated carcinomas which do not quite conform to the diagnosis of small cell anaplastic carcinoma may have a similar biological behaviour, but in 'operable' stage I tumours or peripheral tumours large biopsy or lobectomy is advisable when diagnostic difficulty is not resolved by repeated FNA or FOB because some of these tumours will be well-differentiated neuroendocrine carcinomas, best treated by surgery (see Fig. 8.43).[45]

Low grade carcinomas, e.g. those of carcinoid or adenoid cystic type, are also composed of small cells. The cohesiveness, regularity, and intact cytoplasm of the former should prevent misdiagnosis. In our cases of metastatic adenoid cystic carcinoma to the lung, the appearances are essentially similar to those seen in salivary gland, and this has been the experience of other authors;[4,86] however, we have seen one poorly differentiated primary salivary gland adenoid cystic carcinoma in which the cytological appearances were similar to small cell anaplastic carcinoma. Other lesions such as spindle-cell carcinoid, atypical carcinoid, and hemangiopericytoma should be considered when the morphology, or location of the tumour, or clinical features are unusual, for example, in small peripheral lesions, massive lung tumours, polypoid intrabronchial lesions, or in non-smokers.[25]

Although atypical carcinoid/well-differentiated neuroendocrine carcinomas are identifiable cytologically,[45,61,129] some may closely resemble small cell carcinoma (see

Fig. 8.43). The distinction from atypical carcinoid is based on the presence of prominent nuclear moulding and pleomorphism, abundant mitotic activity, and necrosis, including single cell necrosis, in small cell carcinoma;[129] however, it is safe to heed Frierson et al's,[45] and Gould's advice, that small, peripheral or stage I tumours thought to be small cell carcinoma on cytological or small biopsy histological examination, should be further evaluated, because at least some of these would be classified as atypical carcinoids/well-differentiated neuroendocrine carcinoma or 'peripheral small cell carcinoma of lung resembling carcinoid tumour' if resected, and might be cured by this method of management.[45]
by this method of management.[45]

When only small amounts of material are aspirated, artefactual smearing is more common; in these cases the loss of cytoplasm and the disruption of nuclei occurring in other poorly differentiated carcinomas may mimic small cell carcinoma.

It may sometimes be very difficult to distinguish small cell carcinoma from lymphomas particularly those of follicular centre cell origin with pronounced cell pleomorphism and nuclear irregularity (Fig. 8.34). Cell dispersal together with a rim or a tail of intact cytoplasm in individual cells and a background of round, cytoplasmic fragments staining blue with MGG (lymphoid globules) are helpful features in making a diagnosis of lymphoma. Dispersed cells of small cell carcinoma are usually bare nuclei.

An inflammatory reaction associated with neoplastic cells may obscure the latter, although this tumour does not characteristically produce a marked local reaction.

We have seen one case of metastatic melanoma in which FNA material was virtually indistinguishable from small cell carcinoma (Fig. 8.35).

8 *LUNG, MEDIASTINUM, CHEST WALL AND PLEURA*

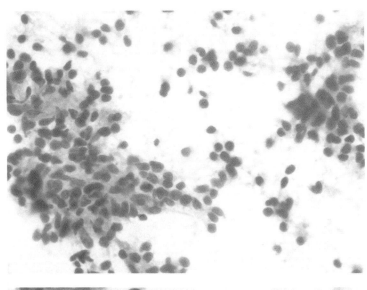

Fig. 8.34 Non-Hodgkin's lymphoma, mixed small and large cell (centroblastic/centrocytic)
Several aggregates of lymphoid cells (H & E, HP)

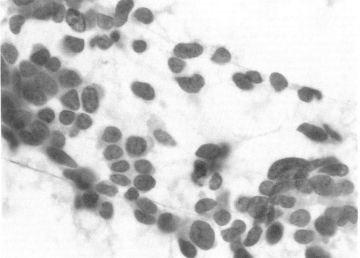

Fig. 8.35 Metastatic melanoma
Small tumour cells closely resembling small cell carcinoma (H & E, HP)

Poorly differentiated large cell carcinomas
(Figs 8.36 and 8.37)

Usual findings

1. Large highly pleomorphic cells with abundant cytoplasm.
2. Large multilayered fragments of malignant tissue.
3. Tumour giant cells.
4. Polymorph ingestion.
5. Fragile cytoplasm.

Large cell anaplastic carcinoma is a diagnosis of exclusion in that features of squamous or glandular differentiation are absent in a non-small cell tumour. It may be necessary to examine large areas histologically to ensure that differentiation is lacking. Because FNA samples only small amounts of newgrowth, this diagno-

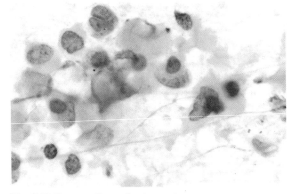

Fig. 8.36 Large cell anaplastic carcinoma
Necrosis; eosinophilia and nuclear pyknosis simulating squamous differentiation (H & E, HP)

LUNG, MEDIASTINUM, CHEST WALL AND PLEURA

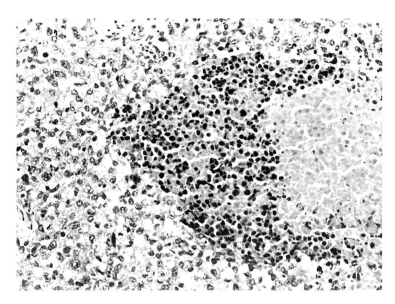

Fig. 8.37 Large cell anaplastic carcinoma
Tissue section; same case as Fig. 8.31; necrosis imparting a squamous appearance to the cells (H & E, MP)

sis can never be established by aspiration alone. Instead, we use the category of 'poorly differentiated large cell carcinoma' to designate large cell tumours in which further subtyping is not possible. Many of these prove to be squamous cell carcinoma or adenocarcinoma after histological examination, and the category is virtually eliminated if typing by electron microscopy is used. In addition, because of the problem of sampling and the difficulty of subtyping, *adenosquamous carcinoma* is uncommonly diagnosed cytologically. *Carcinosarcoma*[40] or *blastoma* are other considerations in poorly differentiated tumours with a spindle component.

The findings in poorly differentiated large cell carcinoma are very variable; the foregoing are common features but have little specific diagnostic value and other cytological patterns may occur. For example, cell dispersal may be striking in some cases and an appearance resembling melanoma may be observed (see Fig. 8.49). Polymorph ingestion appears to be linked to an abundance of cytoplasm and cell pleomorphism rather than any particular form of differentiation. Any tumour may demonstrate the phenomenon and we have also seen it in bronchiolo-alveolar carcinoma.

Pure giant cell carcinomas may occur and have been diagnosed or suggested cytologically.[26] They are usually peripheral highly aggressive neoplasms.

Problems in diagnosis

1. Poorly differentiated squamous cell carcinoma and adenocarcinoma.
2. Metastatic neoplasms and other poorly differentiated malignancies.
3. Small cell carcinoma (p. 190)

The cytological findings in poorly differentiated squamous cell carcinomas and adenocarcinomas overlap with those of large cell anaplastic carcinoma. In particular, highly eosinophilic cytoplasm simulating squamous differentiation may occur because of necrosis (Fig. 8.37) and is a common source of error in classification.

Metastatic neoplasms, especially other anaplastic carcinomas, melanoma, sarcoma and carcinosarcoma[40,110] may have similar cytological findings; large cell pulmonary neoplasms may have strikingly similar cytological features to melanoma (see Ch. 11, p. 306).

Megakaryocytes, seen in FNA samples of lung either due to contamination from bone marrow or from pulmonary capillaries[19] or extramedullary haematopoesis[141] may give rise to suspicion of neoplasia.

Carcinoid tumours (Figs 8.38–8.46)[25,45,46,54,65,129]

Typical carcinoid[129]

Usual findings

1. Dispersed cell population with some trabecules or palisades, and small cell clusters.
2. A uniform population of small neoplastic cells with small amounts of intact cytoplasm.
3. Rounded or oval nuclei with stippled nuclear chromatin and small but prominent nucleoli.
4. Background of small blood vessels; adherence of cells to vascular cores.

In the cases of typical carcinoid tumour we have aspirated, material was easily obtained and the cytological findings distinctive enough to permit the diagnosis in virtually all, although we have often confirmed the

8 *LUNG, MEDIASTINUM, CHEST WALL AND PLEURA*

diagnosis by ultrastructural assessment before open surgery.

The round or oval nuclei with stippled nuclear chromatin are distinctive in smears; the chromatin pattern may be rather similar to the 'clock face' chromatin of plasma cells (Figs 8.38 and 8.39); this combination of nuclear morphological findings is a clue to neuroendocrine tumours in general. Although the cells are not particularly cohesive, small groups and clusters are quite common, the cells retaining their rim of cytoplasm. Leashes of small venules or vascular cores with adherent tumour cells are a feature of bronchial carcinoids (Fig. 8.39) and are very seldom seen in small cell carcinomas. The amount of cytoplasm varies from case to case and we have seen examples with abundant glassy or pale cytoplasm. In a few cases we have observed intracytoplasmic densities corresponding to intermediate

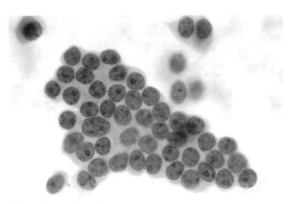

Fig. 8.38 Carcinoid tumour
Small sheet of cells with stippled nuclear chromatin and small distinct nucleoli (H & E, HP Oil)

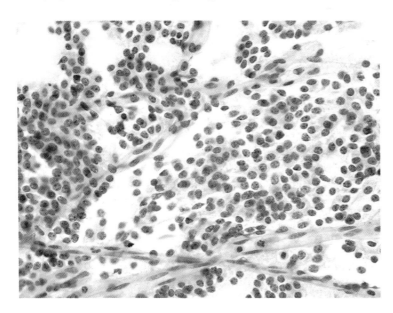

Fig. 8.39 Carcinoid tumour
Loose aggregates of regular tumour cells in company with small capillary blood vessels (H & E, HP)

filament 'buttons' ultrastructurally and similar to those seen in pituitary adenomas and Merkel cell tumours. Intracytoplasmic mucin is present in some.

Problems in diagnosis

1. Small-cell anaplastic carcinoma.
2. Bronchiolo-alveolar carcinoma.
3. Hamartoma.
4. Other small-cell tumours.

Small cell anaplastic carcinoma is usually distinguishable by the pleomorphism, absence of cytoplasm, mitotic rate, and other features of this tumour, unless material is minimal or poorly preserved. As advised by Frierson et al,[45] in small peripheral tumours or apparent stage I small cell tumours, a diagnosis of small cell

carcinoma should be given cautiously as several of these tumours are better classified as atypical carcinoids and treated surgically.

Bronchiolo-alveolar carcinoma may be composed of very uniform cells; however, the cells are usually much larger having more abundant cytoplasm and more cohesion than those of carcinoids. Some carcinoids of ordinary type can simulate adenocarcinoma (Fig. 8.45) and show acinar formations or sheets or three-dimensional structures without characteristic neuroendocrine nuclear features.

The epithelial cells of hamartomas may bear some resemblance to carcinoid cells; other small cell lesions such as adenoid cystic carcinoma should be taken into account in the differential diagnosis of small cell tumours;[4] bronchiolar cells and plasma cells may also resemble neuroendocrine cells.[129]

LUNG, MEDIASTINUM, CHEST WALL AND PLEURA

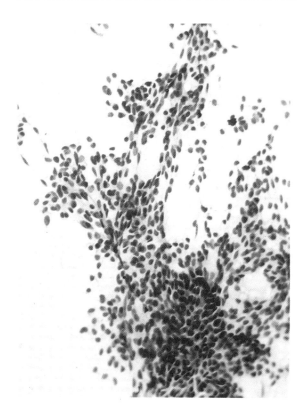

Fig. 8.40 Carcinoid tumour; spindle cell form
Aggregate of well-preserved slightly irregular spindle cells in a clean background; note tumour cell adherence to capillaries (H & E, MP)

Spindle cell carcinoid[25,129]

Peripheral location of a spindle or small cell tumour should lead one to suspect this possibility. We have seen cytological material from several spindle cell carcinoid tumours in which uniformity of nuclear size was a feature which, together with absence of nuclear smearing and background debris, excluded small cell anaplastic carcinoma. Cell clumps were present to a varying degree (Fig. 8.40) and in some smears, cell dispersal was more evident. Adherence to proliferative vascular cores led to an appearance much like a vascular tumour in one case. Ultrastructural examination of aspirated material was particularly helpful in confirming the neuroendocrine nature of one of the lesions before excision, and it would help exclude other spindle-cell lesions, for example haemangiopericytoma.[25]

Atypical carcinoid (Well-differentiated neuroendocrine carcinoma)[45,61,129]

These tumours occupy a position between carcinoid tumours and small cell carcinoma in the spectrum of

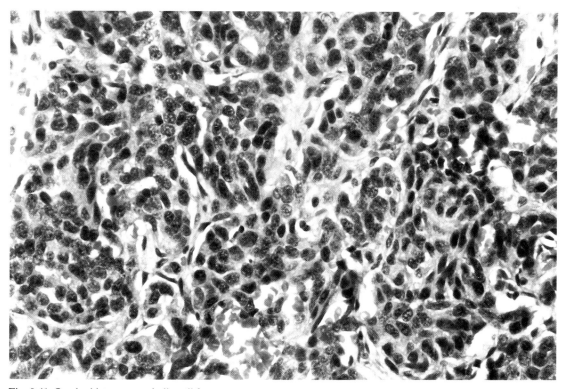

Fig. 8.41 Carcinoid tumour; spindle cell form
Tissue section; same case as Fig. 8.45, (H & E, HP)

8 *LUNG, MEDIASTINUM, CHEST WALL AND PLEURA*

neuroendocrine carcinomas of lung both in terms of morphology and biological behaviour.[16] There are examples which are difficult to categorise even when all of the tumour is available for study,[45] and individual cases may contain mixtures of typical and atypical carcinoid or even foci indistinguishable from small cell carcinoma. Nevertheless, in recent years, several papers detailing their cytological appearances have appeared,[45,61] and we have recognised some examples by FNA. They usually possess neuroendocrine cytological characteristics including rounded or oval nuclei with coarse chromatin stippling, and dispersed cells with intact cytoplasm. Increased pleomorphism, a few mitoses, and focal necrosis, distinguish the better differentiated forms from typical carcinoids (Fig. 8.42), and the absence of widespread moulding, smeared fragile nuclei, abundant single cell necrosis, or abundant mitoses, and the pre-

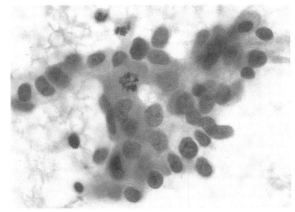

Fig. 8.42 Atypical carcinoid tumour
Aggregate of small cells with a small amount of cytoplasm, resembling typical carcinoid and with little pleomorphism but mitotically active (H & E, HP)

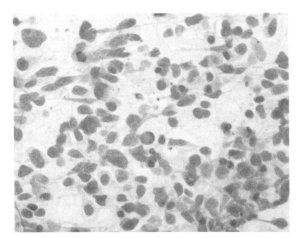

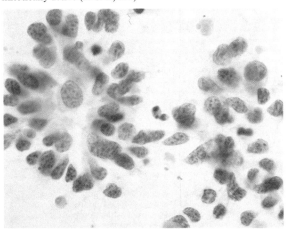

Fig. 8.43 Atypical carcinoid/well differentiated neuroendocrine carcinoma
(a) Foci closely resembling small cell carcinoma including single cell necrosis, and pleomorphic fragile cells with minimal cytoplasm (H & E, HP). (b) Same case; foci of cohesive acinar and rosette-like structure (Pap, HP).

sence of cohesive acinar rosette-like or sheet-like groupings with palisading (Fig. 8.43)[45,61] help exclude small cell carcinoma. However, sampling from partly necrotic, mitotically active foci or more poorly differentiated forms may yield smears closely resembling those of small cell carcinoma.[45] Metastatic tumours such as breast carcinoma or prostatic carcinoma may cause differential diagnostic problems.[129]

Adenocarcinoid[87,97]
Tumours with prominent glandular differentiation but showing ultrastructural neuroendocrine features are well described[87,97,129] and may not be recognisable as being neuroendocrine cytologically (Figs 8.45 and 8.46); similar difficulties may be encountered in large cell carcinomas with neuroendocrine differentiation.

Argyrophilia in Grimelius or Sevier-Munger stains is a feature of typical carcinoids, carcinoid variants and some atypical carcinoids, and is not seen in small cell carcinomas;[129] however, we have not found this technique easy to apply. Neuroendocrine markers such as bombesin, synaptophysin, and chromogranin are all relatively insensitive in detecting neuroendocrine differentiation in our experience without special attention to fixation, and neuron-specific enolase, although useful in some author's hands, has not been specific enough for routine use in ours. Ultrastructural study has however been of great benefit as it allows the reliable detection of neuroendocrine differentiation and an evaluation of numbers, size, and location of neurosecretory granules, cell processes and junctions, and nuclear morphology, which may be crucial in subtyping these lesions.[130]

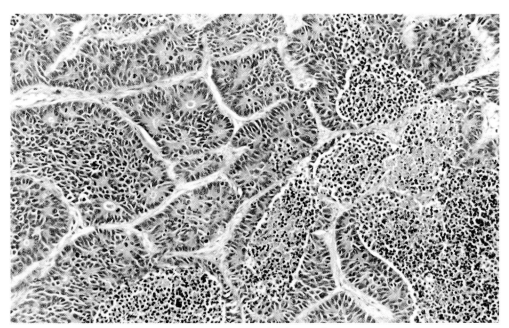

Fig. 8.44 Atypical carcinoid/well differentiated neuroendocrine carcinoma
Tissue section; same tumour as Fig. 8.43; necrosis and prominent acinar and rosette-like structures (H & E, × 160)

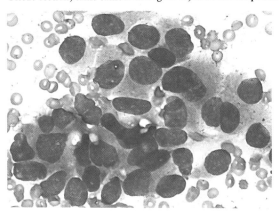

Fig. 8.45 Carcinoid tumour
A cohesive cell cluster; nuclear pleomorphism, and more abundant cytoplasm than usual; histologically this was a carcinoid with some well formed gland structures and some intracellular mucin (MGG, HP)

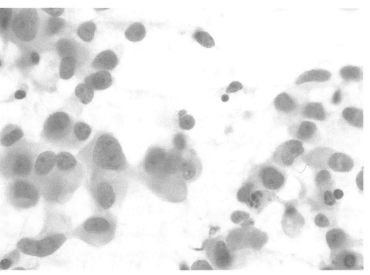

Fig. 8.46 Adenocarcinoid
Poorly cohesive malignant cells including columnar forms with abundant cytoplasm; ultrastructurally neuroendocrine and histologically a poorly differentiated carcinoma with glandular features (H & E, HP)

8 LUNG, MEDIASTINUM, CHEST WALL AND PLEURA

Metastatic malignancy[93]

As pointed out by Johnson[59] the approach to the diagnosis of metastatic newgrowth by FNA is similar to that of the surgical pathologist. Detailed knowledge of the clinical history must be available together with earlier cytological and histological preparations, for review and comparison with current material. Using these principles, the diagnosis is usually achieved with a high degree of reliability, although some caution is necessary because of the ability of lung carcinoma to mimic other tumours including sarcomas. Even if the aspirated material resembles a previous malignancy at another site cytologically, a new primary tumour may still be difficult to exclude completely and more so in the case of adenocarcinoma. Pilotti et al,[96] Perry,[93] and Freidman et al[44] drew attention to the relatively common occurrence of new primary tumours when metastases were suspected clinically.

Metastatic well-differentiated adenocarcinoma (e.g. colon) (Figs 8.47 and 8.48)

Helpful findings

1. Necrosis.
2. Palisading of nuclei; elongated nuclei.
3. Large, elongated columnar cells.

Metastatic well-differentiated adenocarcinoma from colon, endometrium, endocervix, and ovary may show the above features, but in particular the colon.

We have seen significant necrosis in only one case of very well-differentiated, apparently primary carcinoma of the lung. The histological appearances in this case were strikingly similar to those of colonic carcinoma. In all other cases of well-differentiated adenocarcinoma of bronchogenic or bronchiolo-alveolar type, there has been no necrosis seen in smears. Palisading of elongated nuclei of columnar cells has also been a feature in some of the metastatic carcinomas, in particular colonic carcinoma, but not in bronchogenic adenocarcinoma or bronchiolo-alveolar carcinoma, except perhaps for uncommon secretory forms. In cases of metastatic colonic carcinoma, glandular structures, very similar to those seen when normal colonic mucosa is smeared, may also be evident (Figs 8.47 and 8.48) and the demonstration of a clear apical space and a brush border in the tumour cells is another characteristic of colonic carcinoma (Fig. 8.48).[77] EM demonstration of junctional complexes and cell surface features of hind-gut type in colonic cancer is also helpful;[35] other ultrastructural features may aid in deciding a primary site for, e.g., cervix or lung. Breast carcinoma has relatively distinctive attributes as does renal cell carcinoma,[84] although we have seen adrenal metastases essentially similar in appearance and staining properties to renal cell tumours, and benign clear cell

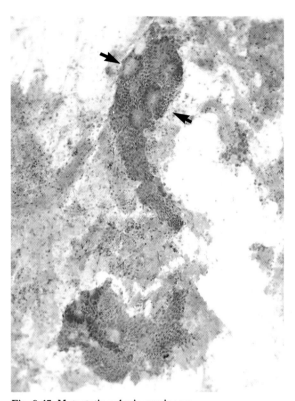

Fig. 8.47 Metastatic colonic carcinoma
Well-differentiated tumour with gland formations (arrow) and a background of necrotic tumour (H & E, LP)

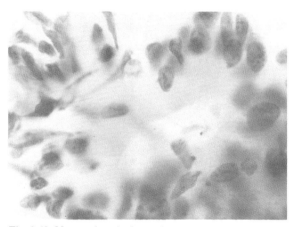

Fig. 8.48 Metastatic colonic carcinoma
A gland structure demonstrating palisading of elongated nuclei and abundant apical cytoplasm with a well-defined lumenal border (Pap, HP)

('sugar') tumours might provide difficulties.[85] Ancillary studies may again be valuable.

Melanoma (Fig 8.50 and Ch. 11, Figs 11.6–11.10)[92]

Despite the rather distinctive cytological features of melanoma, an unequivocal diagnosis of metastatic mela-

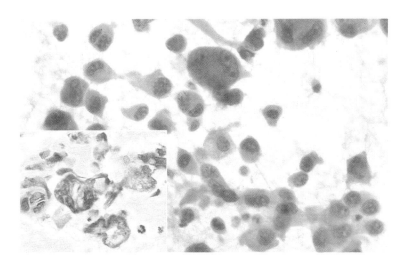

Fig. 8.49 Large cell anaplastic carcinoma
Dispersed cell population including multinucleate cells, resembling melanoma (H & E, HP). Inset: cell block preparation; positive staining of tumour cells with AE1/AE3 monoclonal antibodies to keratin (IPOX HP).

noma by FNA alone is difficult without identifiable pigment in tumour cells; in Perry's series of 120 cases of melanomas 60% were amelanotic in FNA samples.[92] If the cells can be compared with those of the original tumour, a more confident opinion may be given, but large cell anaplastic carcinomas of lung may exhibit very similar cytological features to melanoma (Fig. 8.49) as may other metastatic carcinomas and sarcomas.

Identification of melanin itself may be difficult. Melanoma cells commonly shed their pigment which is taken up by surrounding macrophages, leaving few or no malignant cells containing pigment. Melanin within macrophages cannot be reliably distinguished from lipofuscin or hematoidin. We have found that using the Masson-Fontana stain on smears, especially when alcohol-fixed, is less effective than in sections; the stained pigment is often rather pale brown and may be indistinguishable from lipofuscin or haematoidin. MGG does not distinguish the various pigments as almost all brown pigments stain blue-black. Formalin-induced fluorescence (Ch. 2, App. 1) and S-100 staining of tumour cell nuclei adds conviction to a diagnosis of melanoma. Ultrastructural diagnosis is extremely useful and we have been repeatedly surprised by melanoma when submitting tumours with unusual cytological appearances for EM.

Spindle-cell melanoma should be considered when *any* spindle-cell malignancy is encountered, and especially when there is little or no accompanying connective tissue stroma and when the cells are monotonous or easily dispersed. Some melanomas may closely mimic sarcomas (Fig. 8.50) and possess very fragile, elongated cytoplasmic tails. *Other variants* are also described, including cohesive tumours, and small cell tumours which may resemble lymphoma[92] or small cell carcinoma (Fig. 8.35).

Sarcomas in the lung

Several series of FNA of primary or metastatic sarcomas of lung or pleura, have been documented,[28,66] and there are reports of small numbers of such lesions as malignant schwannoma,[119] malignant fibrous histiocytoma,[63] and dermatofibrosarcoma protruberans.[94] An awareness of the full spectrum of cytological appearances of sarcomas is necessary. Spindle shaped cells with fragile cytoplasm, which are poorly cohesive and form rather flat cellular aggregates and display many single cells; nuclei with finely granular chromatin and small nucleoli; and bizarre multinucleated cells are all suggested as general indicators of mesenchymal malignancy[28,66] in contrast to three dimensional cell aggregates and coarsely granular nuclear chromatin of carcinoma.

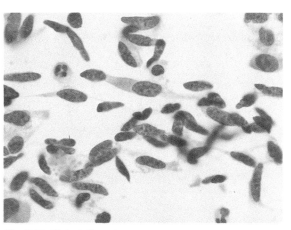

Fig. 8.50 Metastatic melanoma
Spindle cell tumour including cells with fragile cytoplasmic tails resembling a mesenchymal neoplasm (H & E, HP)

8 LUNG, MEDIASTINUM, CHEST WALL AND PLEURA

In individual cases, definitive diagnosis may be extremely difficult. In distinguishing between, e.g. malignant fibrous histiocytoma, melanoma, spindle cell or sarcomatoid carcinoma,[110] and mesothelioma, ultrastructural study is by far the most helpful single ancillary test overall, although immunoperoxidase tests may often give answers to specific diagnostic questions.

Benign neural tumours in particular may show alarming nuclear atypia and are a possible source of false positive diagnoses of malignancy (see also Ch. 11).

Other primary lesions of lung

Chondroid hamartoma
(Figs 8.51–8.55)[30,31,36,38,50,100,124]

Criteria for diagnosis

1. Mature cartilage.
2. Myxoid connective tissue/'immature cartilage'.
3. Sheets of bronchiolar epithelium.
4. Fat.

Chondroid hamartomas represent approximately 8% of coin lesions.[36] The peripheral location of this lesion and its rounded, well-demarcated border and so-called 'popcorn' calcification or CT densitometric appearances may lead to a strong suspicion of the diagnosis solely by X-ray[36] and, if the aspiration needle is deflected by the lesion or bends when inserted into it, this impression is reinforced. Despite its firmness, presumably related to the cartilage, a good sample of material is often obtained. Aspirated chondroid material, however, is difficult to express onto the slide. It has an opaque 'glassy' colour, is firm to gelatinous in consistency, and gives a gritty sensation on being smeared. The cytological features are distinctive, corresponding to the components of the lesion found in histological sections.

Mature cartilage has a homogeneous waxy, purple-grey appearance in H & E stained material (Fig. 8.51). It is sparsely cellular; chondrocytes may be seen in lacunae, but are difficult to recognise. In contrast, the immature cartilage or myxoid connective tissue has a fibrillar texture (Fig. 8.52). It is pale staining in H & E, bright red in MGG (Fig. 8.53), and poorly cellular, resembling mucus at first glance. There is, however, a component of spindle cells, and the material is usually more cellular than mature cartilage. This material is the most useful diagnostic indicator of hamartoma.[31,38] The bronchiolar epithelial sheets are usually small and may show some differences from normal bronchiolar epithelium. There is more abundant pale cytoplasm with less obvious borders; multinucleation may be present. Nuclei are usually rounded, but may be quite large and variable in size. Large intranuclear cytoplasmic inclusions may be evident. Mature fat may or may not be present.

Fig. 8.51 Chondroid hamartoma
Fragment of hyaline cartilage (H & E, HP)

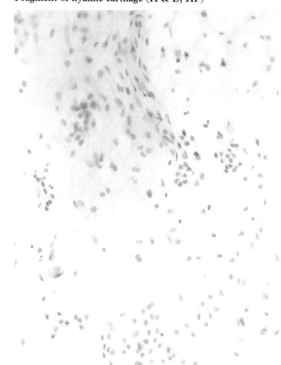

Fig. 8.52 Chondroid hamartoma
Myxoid connective tissue and some bronchiolar epithelial sheets (H & E, MP)

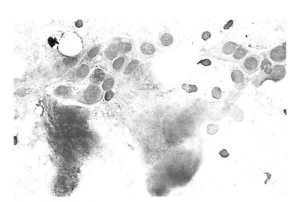

Fig. 8.53 Chondroid hamartoma
Purple myxoid connective tissue and bronchiolar epithelium
(MGG, HP)

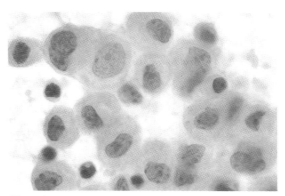

Fig. 8.54 Chondroid hamartoma
Atypical bronchiolar/alveolar epithelium (H & E, HP Oil)

In the largest series, over 90% of chondroid hamarto-mas are recognised by FNA,[31,36,38] or core needle biopsy[50] and diagnosis by these methods is now widely used to justify conservative management,[36,50] or, in lesions which continue to grow, enucleation rather than lobectomy.

An associated lymphocytic and macrophagic component may be present.

Problems in diagnosis

1. Tissue from chest wall or bronchus.
2. Atypia in the cartilaginous or epithelial component.
3. Difficulty in recognizing myxoid material.

It is possible to aspirate material from the costochon-dral junctions, especially if a stilette or guide needle is not used; and if found in an aspirate with fat, a diagnosis of hamartoma may be incorrectly assumed.[38] We have seldom found cartilage from normal bronchi in our aspirations, although if larger needles or the Rotex device are used this is encountered.

In one of our cases, the variation in nuclear size and large intranuclear inclusions were sufficient to lead to a false positive diagnosis of carcinoma; this should not occur if the other components of the lesion are recognised (Figs 8.54 and 8.55),[32] but this is a *common* source of error in the literature.[30]

It may be difficult to discern the myxoid material or cartilage in smears unless one is familiar with its appearances. The material resembles the myxoid stroma of other entities, for example fibroadenoma of the breast. It is conceivable that other lesions, such as mixed salivary tumours of the bronchial wall and myxoid fibrous neoplasms or amyloidosis[56] might produce similar cytological pictures but both are extremely rare; the combination of appearances listed above is diagnostic for practical purposes.

Inflammatory pseudotumour (plasma cell granuloma)
(Figs 8.56–8.58)[75,135]
We have seen three examples of this entity in FNA smears. In two cases, the lesions offered firm resistance to the needle and aspirates were scanty. The Rotex screw needle, which was not available for two of the

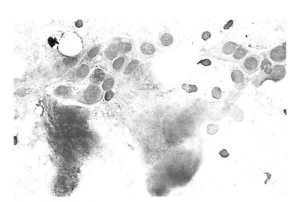

Fig. 8.55 Chondroid hamartoma
Tissue section; same case as Fig. 8.54; atypical bronchiolar/alveolar epithelial proliferation near the advancing edge of an actively growing lesion with prominent myxoid stromal tissue (H & E, HP)

8 *LUNG, MEDIASTINUM, CHEST WALL AND PLEURA*

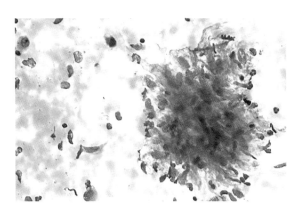

Fig. 8.56 Inflammatory pseudotumour
Fragment of fibroblastic tissue with abundant intercellular collagen (MGG, MP)

cases, would seem to be particularly suitable for firm lesions of this type. In one case the aspirate was very poorly cellular and contained only histiocytes, lymphocytes, and plasma cells. In another, smears showed minimal tissue fragments and single cells of histiocytes and fibroblasts with prominent intercellular collagen, lymphocytes, and plasma cells (Figs 8.56 and 8.57). A few large, ganglion-like cells were seen which had large, pale nuclei and prominent nucleoli. The diagnosis was based on the clinical findings of a solitary, peripheral, coin lesion in a young patient together with the cytological findings and was later confirmed histologically.

In a third case, a recurrence, the aspirate consisted of plump fibroblastic cells with large nuclei and prominent nucleoli in a background of lymphocytes and plasma cells, closely resembling the original lesion (Fig. 8.58). The FNA diagnosis was confirmed histologically. Our

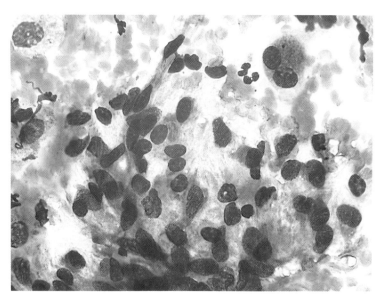

Fig. 8.57 Inflammatory pseudotumour
Cohesive fibroblastic and histiocytic cells, lymphocytes and pink intercellular collagen (MGG, HP)

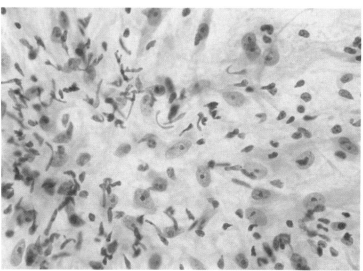

Fig. 8.58 Inflammatory pseudotumour
Loosely aggregated fibroblastic cells and lymphocytes (Pap, HP)

LUNG, MEDIASTINUM, CHEST WALL AND PLEURA 8

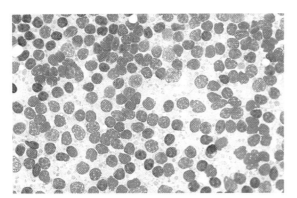

Fig. 8.59 Low grade lymphocytic lymphoma
Monotonous population of small lymphoid cells; this patient
had a pleural effusion, multiple intrapulmonary lesions and a
circulating IgM paraprotein (MGG, HP)

findings are similar to those reported by others;[75,135] in
general, however, the above findings are not specific;
histological examination of the whole lesion will be
necessary to exclude a reaction to other benign or malignant processes.

Lymphoid lesions in lung and pleura (Fig. 8.59)[12,42]
Differential diagnosis revolves first around whether the
lesion lies in the mediastinum, within the lung, or is
associated with the pleura; radiological methods can
usually separate these broad areas. Even when accurate
localisation is made, caution in diagnosis is usually
necessary because of the wide range of possible causes
ranging from chronic inflammatory or infective lesions
such as tuberculosis, through lymphoid hyperplasia and
lymphoid interstitial pneumonia to lymphoproliferative
disorders like lymphomatoid granulomatosis (angiocen-
tric T-cell lymphoma).[12] Abundant lymphocytes usually
mean that a significant lymphoid lesion is present; we
have not seen them in large numbers in non-specific
reactive processes or adjacent to neoplasms in either
lung or pleura.

Where the desired objective is to confirm spread of
lymphoma which has been previously diagnosed, cytological diagnosis may be relatively simple. As in other
sites, large cell lymphomas are usually diagnosed, small
cell or mixed cell tumours present more problems. In
Bonfiglio's series,[12] eight of 10 cases were diagnosed,
and in two the findings were used as a basis for definitive therapy. In Flint's series of 13 cases of previously
diagnosed Hodgkin's disease affecting lung
secondarily[42] all were diagnosed by FNA. We have only
diagnosed a few cases of primary lung non-Hodgkin's
lymphoma, all of which were confirmed histologically
before definitive therapy.

Problems in diagnosis

1. Mixture of inflammatory cells and carcinoma cells.
2. Low grade lymphoproliferative disorders.

In small cell anaplastic carcinoma the neoplastic cells
may be the size of lymphocytes and become obscured by
debris and inflammatory cells. Apart from this uncommon problem we have not found a significant lymphocytic reaction to other tumours.

The distinction between lymphoid interstitial
pneumonia, pseudolymphoma, and low grade non-
Hodgkin's lymphoma (Fig. 8.59) is extremely difficult
even in histological sections. Cytological findings are
unlikely to be diagnostic because these lesions are all
composed of small 'mature' cells. Sending material for
immunological assessment or for detecting clonal rearrangements of immunoglobulin, or T-receptor genes
will be required.

MEDIASTINUM

Thymoma (Figs 8.60–8.66)[158,167,168,170,171,173]

Criteria for diagnosis

1. Cohesive tissue fragments with bland, oval or spindle
   'epithelial' cells (rarely, Hassall's corpuscles).
2. Lymphoid cells (lymphoepithelial thymoma).

There is wide variation in the morphological appearance of thymomas. Tao lists small cell, intermediate,
large, spindle-cell, and pleomorphic types,[171] with
various proportions of accompanying lymphocytic
infiltration.

In the benign thymomas we have seen the epithelial
cells are extremely cohesive (Figs 8.60 and 8.66). With
the usual smearing methods virtually no free epithelial
cells are identified separate from cell fragments. Epithelial cells are not immediately evident in the lymphoepithelial lesions at low power but are discernible
without difficulty using the high power objective. The

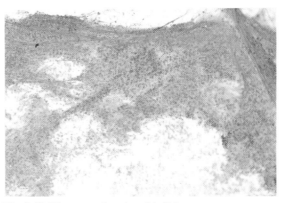

Fig. 8.60 Thymoma; lymphoepithelial
Dense cohesive fragments of tumour tissue in a background of
lymphoid cells (H & E, LP)

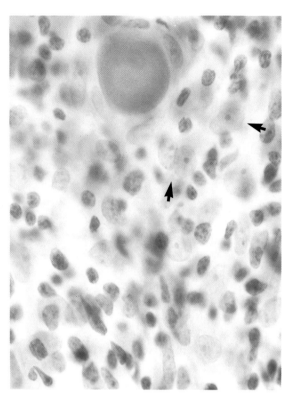

Fig. 8.61 Thymoma; lymphoepithelial; metastatic within lung
A bi-phasic cell population of lymphocytes and epithelial cells with pale nuclei, small nucleoli and indistinct cytoplasm; note the Hassall's corpuscle (Pap, HP Oil)

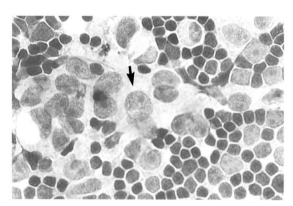

Fig. 8.62 Thymoma; lymphoepithelial
Lymphoid cells surrounding a cluster of epithelial cells with abundant pale cytoplasm (MGG, HP)

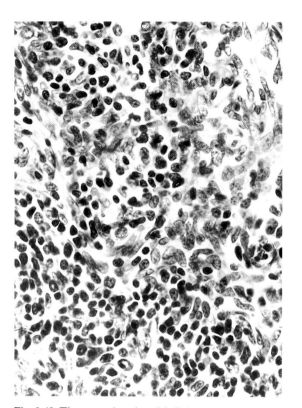

Fig. 8.63 Thymoma; lymphoepithelial
Tissue section; biphasic cell population (H & E, HP)

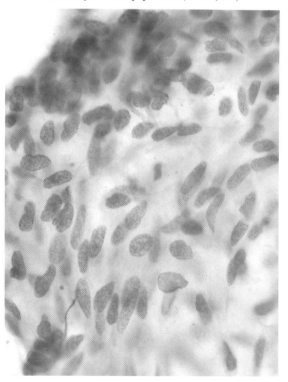

Fig. 8.64 Thymoma; spindle cell
Cohesive tissue fragment; elongated pale, regular nuclei; indistinct cell borders (H & E, HP Oil)

epithelial cells are oval or spindle shaped with slightly irregular nuclear outlines, and some cleaved or folded nuclei. Their nuclear chromatin is homogeneous, finely distributed and pale and, occasionally, small nucleoli are seen. Cytoplasmic borders are indistinct, but nuclei are separated by moderate amounts of pale cytoplasm (Figs 8.61, 8.62 and 8.64). In one case of thymoma metastatic to lung, Hassall's corpuscles were evident in the clumps of tumour cells (Fig. 8.61); this is an unusual manifestation, however, and will not be present in most thymomas. When there is a lymphoid population, the bimodal pattern enables one to make a virtually certain diagnosis.[158,170,173] In pure epithelial or spindle-cell forms, definitive diagnosis is more difficult (Figs 8.64 and 8.68) although in Dahlgren's series[158] most thymomas were diagnosed, and in Tao's 37 cases[173] all FNA diagnoses of thymoma were verified histologically. Tao describes more variation in the degree of cohesion than we have seen.[170,173]

Problems in diagnosis

1. Other lymphoid lesions.
2. Other spindle cell neoplasms.
3. Malignant thymoma.

If an epithelial component cannot be recognised within a lymphoid lesion then other possibilities such as Hodgkin's or non-Hodgkin's lymphoma and angiofol-

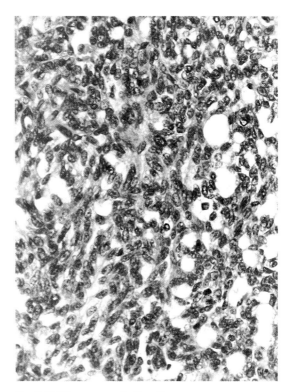

Fig. 8.65 Thymoma; spindle cell
Tissue section; same case as Fig. 8.64 (H & E, HP)

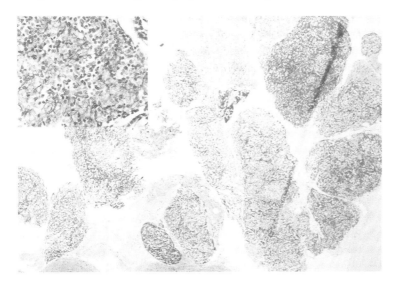

Fig. 8.66 Thymoma; lymphoepithelial
Cell block preparation
cohesive fragments of tumour tissue (H & E, LP). Inset: staining of epithelial cell cytoplasm with polyclonal antikeratin (IPOX, HP).

licular lymphoid hyperplasia must be contemplated. Ultrastructural or immunoperoxidase demonstration of an epithelial component will be particularly helpful in these cases. Cytological diagnosis of *angiofollicular lymphoid hyperplasia* and its differentiation from low grade lymphomas may not be possible (see Ch. 5, p. 86).

Other spindle cell tumours within the mediastinum include connective tissue neoplasms, mesothelioma,

spindle cell squamous carcinoma, and spindle cell carcinoid. Connective tissue neoplasms may be cohesive but generally (and especially in neural tumours) have a more abundant and more myxoid stroma than thymomas. Spindle cell squamous carcinoma shows cytological features of malignancy usually lacking in thymoma although cases of squamous carcinoma and small cell carcinoma arising in the thymus are described.

8 LUNG, MEDIASTINUM, CHEST WALL AND PLEURA

Malignant thymoma (Figs 8.67–8.69)[159]

Some thymomas without cytological evidence of malignancy will behave aggressively (invasive thymoma) and very occasionally metastasize. Clinical assessment, including open surgical biopsy, will usually be necessary for accurate assessment of their biological potential.[159]

Thymic carcinomas are very uncommon and have a wide variety of morphological apperances including squamous, large cell, basaloid, mucoepidermoid, and small cell types. We have seen two cases in which a cytological diagnosis of carcinoma could be made by FNA, including the suggestion of a biphasic epithelial and lymphoid pattern in one and a more anaplastic growth pattern in another. In both, the loosely cohesive large malignant cells were diagnostic of carcinoma and in one the rounded tumour cells with their prominent single nucleolus (Fig. 8.67) were reminiscent of epithelial cells of other thymomas we had seen. Thymic carcinoma was suggested in both by FNA but was confirmed by open biopsy and clinical evaluation to exclude other primary sites. Similar cases are reported in the literature.[159]

The distinction between thymic carcinoma and invasive thymoma is based on cytological characteristics of malignancy in the former; however, we have seen a biologically aggressive case of borderline cytological malignancy in which this distinction was difficult (Figs 8.68 and 8.69).[170]

Lymphoma in the mediastinum[12]

The presentation of lymphoma in the mediastinum as a primary event is not uncommon especially nodular sclerosing Hodgkin's disease. The mediastinum is also a characteristic site of presentation of T-lymphoblastic lymphoma and sclerosing large cell lymphoma in younger patients; however, all types of Hodgkin's and non-Hodgkin's lymphoma, angiofollicular lymphoid

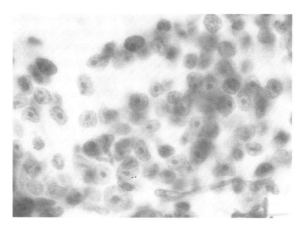

Fig. 8.67 Thymic carcinoma
Disorganised aggregate of pleomorphic malignant cells with macronucleoli (Pap, HP)

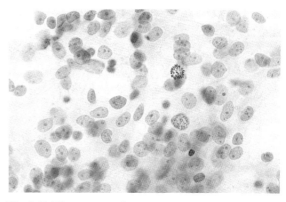

Fig. 8.68 Thymoma; malignant
Poorly cohesive cells with fragile cytoplasm, rounded or ovoid nuclei, bland chromatin and small but prominent nucleoli; note the mitosis (Pap, HP)

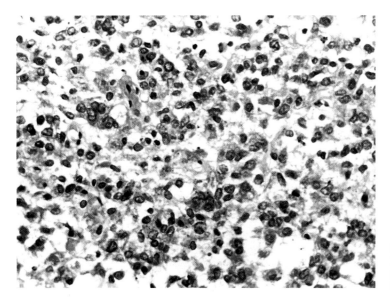

Fig. 8.69 Thymoma malignant
Tissue section; same case as Fig. 8.54; poorly cohesive undifferentiated tissue within superior vena cava (H & E, MP)

LUNG, MEDIASTINUM, CHEST WALL AND PLEURA 8

hyperplasia, and thymoma with a high proportion of lymphocytes, enter the differential diagnosis. Small cell anaplastic carcinoma presenting in the mediastinum may also be difficult to distinguish from lymphoma.

Discussion of the diagnosis of lymphoid lesions has been covered in Chapter 5.

Problems in diagnosis

1. Obtaining material.
2. Angiofollicular lymphoid hyperplasia (Castleman's Giant Lymph Node hyperplasia).
3. Lymphoepithelial thymoma (se p. 203).
4. Small cell anaplastic carcinoma (see p. 192).

Several authors comment on the difficulty of obtaining material from nodular sclerosing or other fibrotic forms of Hodgkin's lymphoma by simple FNA.[155] In one of our cases of sclerosing large cell lymphoma of the mediastinum, Rotex sampling gave adequate material for diagnosis. In our single case of angiofollicular lymphoid hyperplasia, small mature lymphoid cells predominated but a diagnosis was not possible; lymphoma could not be excluded.

Neural neoplasms
We have aspirated several neurofibromas and ganglioneuromas in the posterior mediastinum, but were unable to obtain diagnostic material from them, probably because of the small size of needles used (23 G). Dahlgren[157] achieved more success using larger needles (18G) (see also Ch. 11, p. 319).

Germ cell neoplasms
Germ cell neoplasms of all types occur in the mediastinum;[169] and confirmation of metastatic spread of germ cell neoplasms within the thorax will also be a problem occasionally confronting the pathologist. Evidence of elevated blood levels of human chorionic gonadotrophin (HCG) and alpha-fetoprotein (AFP) together with clinical findings may virtually establish the diagnosis in non-seminomatous tumour. In addition, because of the good therapeutic results achieved for all subtypes of non-seminomatous germ-cell tumours there is less need for exhaustive histological assessment, especially in advanced cases with widespread disease.

We have been faced with this problem on several occasions; the following case will serve as an example.

The patient was a young male with a mediastinal mass and numerous lung metastases; serum levels of HCG and AFP were markedly elevated. No testicular or abdominal lesion was evident. Needle aspiration of a lung lesion yielded abundant material consisting of an epithelial-like component resembling carcinoma together with a spindle-cell component. A bimodal growth pattern was also evident in cell block preparations. Seminoma and lymphoma could be excluded and the cytological findings were thought to be fully compatible with a malignant germ cell neoplasm. Treatment with CIS-platinum was begun without further diagnostic procedures.

We have seen several other germ cell neoplasms in the mediastinum; in one primary mature cystic teratoma, the aspirate consisted mainly of foreign body giant cells from the granulomatous reaction at the edge of the lesion; there was a small amount of very cohesive keratinising squamous epithelium, but its significance was not appreciated before the lesion was resected. In several embryonal carcinomas, the tumour cells were cohesive, highly pleomorphic and appeared epithelial or even 'squamoid'[170] (see also Ch. 10). One tumour had a prominent endodermal sinus growth pattern, recognisable in cell block prepartions.

Other biphasic tumours such as *carcinosarcoma*[40] or *blastoma* or *malignant* mesothelioma would also enter the differential diagnosis when teratoma was being considered.

Cysts
It is often possible to suggest the nature of a cyst in the mediastinum, based on FNA findings.[162,166] In pericardial cysts the location and injection of radiopaque dye into the lesion which outlines a thin, smooth, cyst wall helps confirm this diagnosis. We found that the cytological findings in a case of presumed pericardial cyst were inconclusive; no mesothelial cells could be identified; macrophages were the main cellular element, and there were some lymphocytes. It is worth recalling that many benign and malignant mediastinal lesions may present as largely cystic structures so that one should exercise caution in diagnosing a cyst as benign solely on the cytological contents. Developmental or degenerative thymic cysts or parathyroid cysts may be extremely large and contain lymphocytes and macrophages similar to pericardial cysts. Thymomas may occasionally be so cystic that they resemble non-neoplastic cysts, until sectioning of their wall reveals small areas of residual newgrowth. Hodgkin's lymphoma in young women, germinoma in young males, and teratoma may all be largely cystic, the neoplastic element forming only a small part of the cyst. Bronchogenic or gastro-enteric cysts are also well described in this site.[162] CT criteria for diagnosing benign cysts include a smooth oval mass with thin walls, homogeneous CT attenuation, near water density, no vascular enhancement or infiltration of nearby mediastinal structures; and these, when combined with cytological findings, may allow conservative management in selected cases.[162] Atypical fibroblastic cells in cysts have been reported as mimicking malignancy in this site.[164]

Retrosternal thyroid
We have seen several cases of large retrosternal or ectopic mediastinal multinodular goitres presenting as

8 *LUNG, MEDIASTINUM, CHEST WALL AND PLEURA*

superior mediastinal masses. The diagnosis is easily made if colloid and benign thyroid epithelial cells are recognised; this is not easy without MGG preparations and has been a source of error in our own and others experience,[156] leading to suspicion of neoplasm. Ectopic anterior mediastinal thyroid can also give rise to masses including neoplasms.[165]

CHEST WALL AND PLEURA

Malignant mesothelioma (Figs 8.70–8.76)[177,178,181,182]

Usual findings

1. Papillary processes; cell balls or cell clusters (tubulo-papillary tumours).
2. Flat sheets of epithelial cells with abundant dense cytoplasm and some cell separation (epithelial or biphasic tumours); cytoplasmic vacuolation; intracytoplasmic hyaluronic acid.
3. Polygonal cells, dispersed, with binucleation and multinucleation.
4. Spindled epithelial cells.
5. Spindle-cells with a fibroblastic appearance (biphasic or sarcomatous tumours).
6. Pleomorphic malignant cells with a multinucleated cell component (anaplastic tumours).

When the clinical findings indicate this diagnosis and there has been asbestos exposure, the cytological findings can offer a clearcut diagnosis of malignancy or strong supportive evidence. Tao was able to diagnose most cases of mesothelioma by FNA.[181] If material for cell block preparations, immunoperoxidase, and ultra-structural studies is available, definitive diagnosis as a basis for management may be obtained.[177] We have now seen FNA material from over 40 cases and find the technique particularly useful for lesions presenting without effusions (approximately 10–15% of pleural cases) or in unusual sites such as mediastinum or metastases.

In contrast to effusions in which the tumours are mainly epithelial the full range of growth patterns of malignant mesothelioma may be seen in FNA material including highly differentiated epithelial tumours, biphasic, sarcomatous, and anaplastic forms.[178,181,182] The most characteristic cytological pattern is a combination of sheets of cells, some dispersed polygonal cells with dense cytoplasm, spindled epithelial cells, and spindled fibroblastic cells (Figs 8.70–8.72); however, only a small proportion of cases present in this way. In our experience, and in Tao's, mesenchymal elements tend to be under represented in smears in comparison with histological sections.

Problems in diagnosis

1. Well differentiated adenocarcinoma.
2. Other carcinomas/sarcomas.
3. Reactive mesothelial proliferation.

A distinction from well differentiated adenocarcinoma is difficult; even with adequate histopathological material this problem may arise, particularly in peripheral lung lesions with a bronchiolo-alveolar growth pattern. Histochemical tests are of value; epithelial mucin excludes mesothelioma; positive staining for carcino-embryonic antigen (CEA) (Fig. 8.73)[183] or LeuM-1 and perhaps Mab 44-3A6 by the immunoperoxidase method also helps in achieving this purpose. The identification of hyaluronic acid within epithelial tumour cells (Fig.

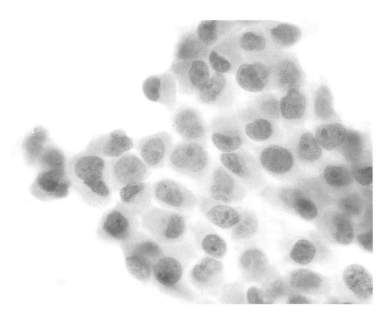

Fig. 8.70 Malignant mesothelioma
Flat sheet of tumour cells showing 'spongiotic' separation similar to benign mesothelium (H & E, HP Oil)

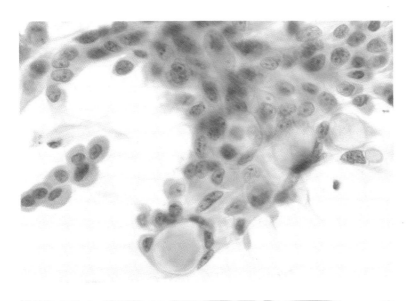

Fig. 8.71 Malignant mesothelioma
Flat sheet of cells with dense metaplastic cytoplasm, and foci of vacuolation (hyaluronic acid) (Pap, HP)

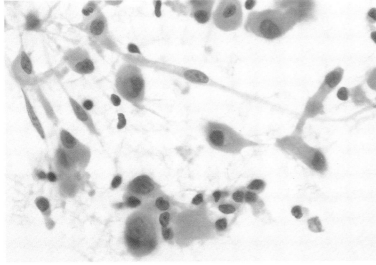

Fig. 8.72 Malignant mesothelioma
Dispersed polygonal cells with dense cytoplasm and fibroblastic tumour cells (biphasic tumour) (H & E, HP)

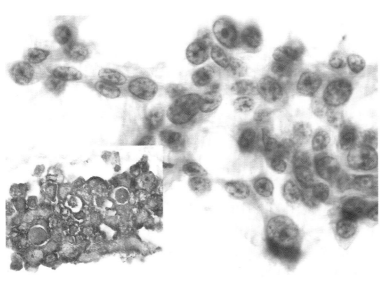

Fig. 8.73 Peripheral large cell carcinoma of lung
Disorganised sheet of tumour cells not readily distinguishable from malignant mesothelioma (Pap, HP). Inset: cell block preparation showing intense staining for CEA (polyclonal) (IPOX, HP).

8 LUNG, MEDIASTINUM, CHEST WALL AND PLEURA

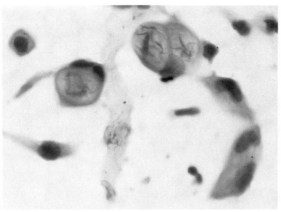

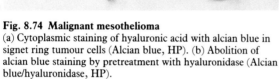

(a)

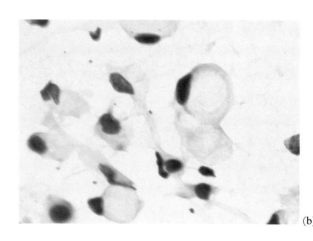

(b)

Hy. 5

Fig. 8.74 Malignant mesothelioma
(a) Cytoplasmic staining of hyaluronic acid with alcian blue in signet ring tumour cells (Alcian blue, HP). (b) Abolition of alcian blue staining by pretreatment with hyaluronidase (Alcian blue/hyaluronidase, HP).

8.74) indicates mesothelioma; this substance is water soluble and is better preserved in alcohol-fixed FNA smears than in smears from effusions or paraffin blocks, although it can occasionally be demonstrated in cell blocks. In one of our early cases, cytoplasmic vacuolation gave a strikingly adenocarcinomatous appearance; in several others, vacuoles containing hyaluronic acid displayed magenta staining material with MGG, a possible cause of confusion with mucin secreting adenocarcinoma (Fig. 8.75). The prominent finger-like microvilli of the surface mesothelioma cells, without a glycocalyceal coat, are the most distinctive element of ultrastructural diagnosis of mesothelioma, which can be extremely reliable (Fig. 8.76).

The wide variation in growth patterns and degree of differentiation in mesothelioma is well known, and particularly in the more poorly differentiated and the sarco-

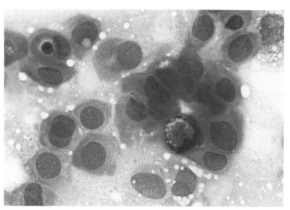

Fig. 8.75 Malignant mesothelioma
Magenta staining of intracytoplasmic lumena in tumour cells (MGG, HP)

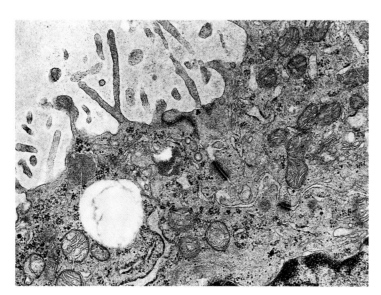

Fig. 8.76 Malignant mesothelioma
Long-branching finger-like microvilli (EM)

LUNG, MEDIASTINUM, CHEST WALL AND PLEURA 8

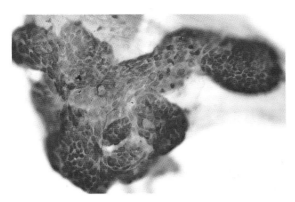

Fig. 8.77 Atypical reactive mesothelial proliferation
Finger-like papillae (H & E, MP)

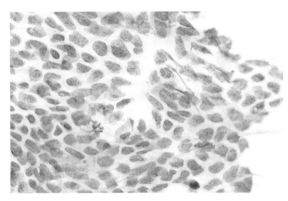

Fig. 8.78 Atypical reactive mesothelial proliferation
Sheet of slightly distorted but irregular cells (H & E, HP)

matous forms,[178,181,182] differentiation from anaplastic epithelial or mesenchymal neoplasms may be impossible with FNA, even with recourse to electron microscopy and immunostaining.

We have seen an isolated case in which a florid reactive mesothelial reaction occurred at the site of a previous hiatus hernia repair in a 70-year-old woman. A mass became evident at this site radiographically, giving rise to suspicion of neoplasm. The material aspirated consisted of papillary, three-dimensional aggregates of cells with irregular nuclei (Figs 8.77 and 8.78). Some calcific (psammoma) bodies were present within the cell clumps. Thoracotomy was performed; no neoplasm was evident either in the lung or pleura. The 'mass' was a fat pad, herniating through the diaphragm at the site of earlier operation. Johnston[59] mentions a similar case.

Strong positive staining for epithelial membrane antigen (EMA) has featured, in our experience, in most malignant mesotheliomas in cell blocks of effusions and pleural biopsy, and we have not seen strong widespread mesothelial decoration in reactive conditions. This finding may be a useful adjunct where distinction between reactive and malignant meosthelioma is a problem in FNA.

Submesothelial fibrous tumours (Benign; malignant; pleural fibroma) (Figs 8.79–8.81)

We have aspirated four submesothelial fibrous tumours including two histologically malignant metastasising tumours. Smears were surprisingly cellular in all, including the benign lesions. Many spindle-shaped fibroblastic cells were present; nuclei were moderately pleomorphic and some chromatin was clumped, leading to a suspicion of low grade malignancy in one benign case, a situation encountered by others.[23] Fibres of

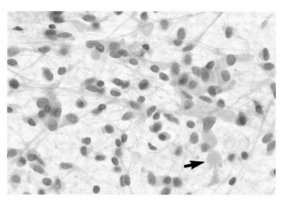

Fig. 8.79 Benign pleural fibroma
Dispersed fibroblastoid cells; some plump epithelial-like cells; collagen bundles (arrow) (H & E, HP)

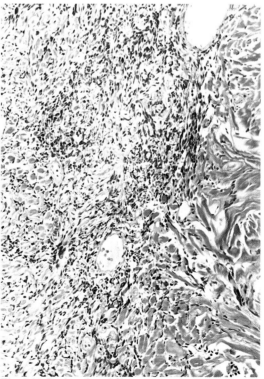

Fig. 8.80 Benign pleural fibroma
Tissue section; same case as Fig. 8.59 (H & E, MP)

8 *LUNG, MEDIASTINUM, CHEST WALL AND PLEURA*

collagen with adherent spindle cells were included in several cases, some more epithelial-like cells probably representing bronchiolar epithelium entrapped within the growing edge of the lesion were seen in one case.

In one of the histologically malignant lesions, only material from more benign appearing areas was aspirated (Fig. 8.81). In the other, the tumour was an overtly malignant mesenchymal tumour with areas of immature cartilage. We recognised only one of these four cases as being of submesothelial fibrous origin, but believe the combination of a localised, rounded pleural mass yielding dispersed small fibroblastic cells with dark spindled nuclei and background collagen should allow the lesion to be recognised and differentiated from mesothelioma.[131,178] Even in histologically malignant forms, the biologial behaviour is much less aggressive than malignant tumours of mesothelial origin and surgical management may be curative; a distinction from mesothelioma or sarcoma of other types is crucial.

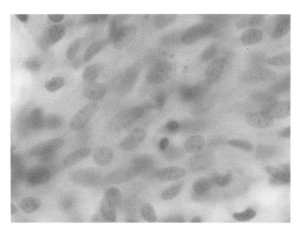

Fig. 8.81 Malignant submesothelial fibrous tumour
Aggregate of monomorphic fibroblastoid cells; in the resected specimen there were areas of pleomorphic mitotically active tissue (H & E, HP)

REFERENCES AND SUGGESTED FURTHER READING

Lung

1. Aberle D R, Gamsu G, Golden J A: Fatal systemic arterial air embolism following lung needle aspiration. Radiology 165: 351–353, 1987.
2. Akhtar M, Ashraf Ali M, Huq M, Faulkner C: Fine needle biopsy: Comparison of cellular yield with and without aspiration. Diagn Cytopathol 5: 162–165, 1989.
3. Alonso P, Sanchez S, Ramirez E, Cicero R: Transthoracic needle biopsy in neoplastic and non-neoplastic pathology: experience in a general hospital. Diagn Cytopathol 2: 284–289, 1986.
4. Anderson R J, Johnston W W, Szpak C A: Fine needle aspiration of adenoid cystic carcinoma metastatic to the lung. Acta Cytol 29: 527–532, 1985.
5. Andriole J G, Haaga J R, Adams R B, Nunez C: Biopsy needle characteristics assessed in the laboratory. Radiology 148: 659–662, 1983.
6. Bailey T M, Akhtar M, Ashraf Ali M: Fine needle aspiration biopsy in the diagnosis of tuberculosis. Acta Cytol 29: 732–736, 1985.
7. Banner B F, Gould V E, Radosevich J A, Ma Yixing, Lee Inchul, Rosen S T: Application of Monoclonal Antibody 44–3A6 in the Cytodiagnosis and Classification of Pulmonary Carcinomas. Diagn Cytopathol 1: 300–307, 1985.
8. Batra P, Wallace J M, Ovenfors C O: Efficacy and complications of transthoracic needle biopsy of lung in patients with *Pneumocystis carinii* pneumonia and AIDS. J Thorac Imaging 2: 79–80, 1987.
9. Berquist T H, Bailey P B, Cortese D A, Miller W E: Transthoracic needle biopsy. Accuracy and complications in relation to location and type of lesion. *Mayo Clin Proc* 55: 475–481, 1980.
10. Boe J, Arve J, Johansson S: Fine needle and screw needle samples in CT-assisted biopsies of chest lesions. Eur J Respir Dis 71: 108–112, 1987.
11. Bonfiglio TA: Cytopathologic interpretation of transthoracic fine needle biopsies. Masson, New York, 1983.
12. Bonfiglio T A, Dvoretsky P M, Piscioli F, dePapp E W, Patten S F: Fine needle aspiration biopsy in the evaluation of lymphoreticular tumors of the thorax. Acta Cytol 29: 548–553, 1985.
13. Bourgouin P M, Shepard J A, McLoud T C, Spizarny D L, Dedrick C G: Transthoracic needle aspiration biopsy: evaluation of the blood patch technique. Radiology 166: 93–95, 1988.
14. Buchanan A J, Gupta R K: Cytomegalovirus infection of the lung: Cytomorphologic diagnosis by fine needle aspiration cytology. Diagn Cytopathol 2: 341–342, 1986.
15. Calhoun P, Feldman P S, Armstrong P, Black W C, Pope T L, Minor G R, Daniel T M: The clinical outcome of needle aspirations of the lung when cancer is not diagnosed. Ann Thorac Surg 41: 592–596, 1986.
16. Carter D, Yesner R. Carcinomas of the lung with neuroendocrine differentiation. Semin Diagn Pathol 2: 235–254, 1985.
17. Carter R R, Wilson J P, Turner H R, Chapman S W: Cutaneous blastomycosis as a complication of transthoracic needle aspiration. Chest 91: 917–918, 1987.
18. Caya J G, Clowry L J, Wollenberg N J, Tieu T M: Transthoracic fine needle aspiration cytology. Analysis of 82 patients with detailed verification criteria and evaluation of false-negative cases. Am J Clin Pathol 82: 100–103, 1984.
19. Chen K T K: Megakaryocytes in a fine needle aspirate of the lung. Acta Cytol 31: 81–82, 1987.
20. Chretien M F, Chassevent A, Malkani K, Rebel A: Flow cytometric DNA analysis in the diagnosis of lung tumors. A comparison with conventional methods. Anal Quant Cytol Histol 10: 251–255, 1988.
21. Christ M L, Fry W A: Intraoperative fine needle aspiration and rapid diagnosis of thoracic lesions. Appl Pathol 4: 125–131,1986.
22. Cianci P, Posin J P, Shimshak R R, Singzon J: Air embolism complicating percutaneous thin needle biopsy of lung. Chest 92: 749–751, 1987.
23. Conces D J Jr, Schwenk G R Jr, Doering P R, Glant

M D: Thoracic needle biopsy. Improved results utilizing a team approach. Chest 91: 813–816, 1987.

24. Costello P, Onik G, Cosman E: Computed tomographic-guided stereotaxic biopsy of thoracic lesions. J Thorac Imaging 2: 27–32, 1987.

25. Craig I D, Finley R J: Spindle cell carcinoid tumour of lung. Cytologic, histopathologic and ultrastructural features. Acta Cytol 26: 495–498, 1982.

26. Craig I D, Desrosiers P, Lefcoe M S: Giant-cell carcinoma of the lung. A cytologic study. Acta Cytol 27: 293–298, 1983.

27. Cropp A J, DiMarco A F, Lankerani M: False-positive transbronchial needle aspiration in bronchogenic carcinoma. Chest 85: 696–697, 1984.

28. Crosby J H, Hoeg K, Hager B: Transthoracic fine needle aspiration of primary and metastatic sarcomas. Diagn Cytopathol 1: 221–227, 1985.

29. Cummings S R, Lillington G A, Richard R J: Managing solitary pulmonary nodules. The choice of strategy is a 'close call'. Am Rev Respir Dis 134: 453–460, 1986.

30. Curtin C T, Proux J, Davis E: Cartilaginous hamartoma of the lung: A potential pitfall in pulmonary fine needle aspiration. Acta Cytol 32: 764, 1988.

31. Dahlgren S E: Needle biopsy of intrapulmonary hamartoma. Scand J Respir Dis 47: 187–194, 1966.

32. Dahlgren S E: Aspiration biopsy of intrathoracic tumours. Acta Pathol Microbiol Scand 70: 566–576, 1967.

33. Dahlgren S E, Ekstrom P: Aspiration cytology in the diagnosis of pulmonary tuberculosis. Scand J Resp Dis 53: 196–201, 1972.

34. Davies D C, Russell A J, Tayar R, Cooke N T, Levene M M: Transmission electron microscopy of percutaneous fine needle aspirates from lung: a study of 70 cases. Thorax 42: 296–301, 1987.

35. DeCaro L F, Pak H Y, Yokota S, Teplitz R L, Benfield J R: Intraoperative cytodiagnosis of lung tumors by needle aspiration. J Thorac Cardiovasc Surg 85: 404–408, 1983.

36. de Rooij P D, Meijer S, Calame J, Golding R P, van Mourik J C, Stam J: Solitary hamartoma of the lung: is thoracotomy still mandatory? Neth J Surg 40: 145–148, 1988.

37. di Sant'Agnese P A, de Mesy Jensen K L, Bonfiglio T A, King D E, Patten S F Jr: Plastic-embedded semi-thin sections of fine needle aspiration biopsies with dibasic staining. Acta Cytol 29: 477–483, 1985.

38. Dunbar F, Leiman G: The aspiration cytology of pulmonary hamartomas. Diagn Cytopathol 5: 174–180, 1989.

39. Farley M L, Mabry L, Munoz L A, Diserens H W: Crystals occurring in pulmonary cytology specimens. Association with aspergillus infection. Acta Cytol 29: 737–744, 1985.

40. Finley J L, Silverman J F, Dabbs D J: Fine needle aspiration cytology of pulmonary carcinosarcoma with immunocytochemical and ultrastructural observations. Diagn Cytopathol 14: 239–243, 1988.

41. Fish G D, Stanley J H, Miller K S, Schabel S I, Sutherland S E: Post-biopsy pneumothorax: estimating the risk by chest radiography and pulmonary function tests. AJR 150: 71–74, 1988.

42. Flint A, Kumar N B, Naylor B: Pulmonary Hodgkin's disease. Diagnosis by fine needle aspiration. Acta Cytol 32: 221–225, 1988.

43. Freedman S I, Ang E P, Haley R S: Identification of Coccidioidomycosis of the lung by fine needle aspiration biopsy. Acta Cytol 30: 420–424, 1986.

44. Friedman M, Shimaoka K, Fox S, Panahon A M: Second malignant tumors detected by needle aspiration cytology. Cancer 52: 699–706, 1983.

45. Frierson, H F, Covell J L, Mills S E: Fine needle

aspiration cytology of atypical carcinoid of the lung. Acta Cytol 31: 471–475, 1987.

46. Gephardt G N, Belovich D M: Cytology of pulmonary carcinoid tumours. Acta Cytol 26: 434–438, 1982.

47. Gobien R P, Bouchard E A, Gobien B S, Valicenti J F, Vujic I: Thin needle aspiration biopsy of thoracic lesions: Impact on hospital charges and patterns of patient care. Radiology 148: 65–67, 1983.

48. Green R, Szyfelbein W M, Isler R J, Stark P, Janstsch H: Supplementary tissue-core histology from fine needle transthoracic aspiration biopsy. AJR 144: 787–792, 1985.

49. Hajdu S I: Cytology and pathology of acquired immune deficiency syndrome. Acta Cytol 30: 599–602, 1986.

50. Hamper U M, Khouri N F, Stitik F P, Siegelman S S: Pulmonary hamartoma: diagnosis by transthoracic needle-aspiration biopsy. Radiology 155: 15–18, 1985.

51. Hawkins A G, Hsiu J G, Smith III R M, Stitik F P, Siddiky M A, Edwards O E: Pulmonary dirofilariasis diagnosed by fine needle aspiration biopsy. A case report. Acta Cytol 29: 19–22, 1985.

52. Henderson D W, Papadimitriou J: The ultrastructural appearances of tumours. A diagnostic atlas. 2nd edition. Churchill Livingstone Edinburgh, 1987.

53. Herman P G, Hessel S J: The diagnostic accuracy and complications of closed lung biopsies. Radiology 125: 11–14, 1977.

54. Horan D C, Bonfiglio T A, Patten S F: Fine needle aspiration cytopathology of bronchial carcinoid tumours. An analytical study of the cells. Anal Quant Cytol 4: 105–109, 1982.

55. Horsley J R, Miller R E, Amy R W M, King E G: Bronchial submucosal needle aspiration performed through the fiberoptic bronchoscope. Acta Cytol 28: 211–217, 1984.

56. Hsiu J G, Stitik F P, D'Amato N A, Kaplan A S, Burger R L, Hawkins A G: Primary amyloidosis presenting as a unilateral hilar mass. Report of a case diagnosed by fine needle aspiration biopsy. Acta Cytol 30: 55–58, 1986.

57. Jarrett D D, Betsill W L: A problem oriented approach regarding the fine needle aspiration cytologic diagnosis of bronchioloalveolar carcinoma of the lung: A comparison of diagnostic criteria with benign lesions mimicking carcinoma. Acta Cytol 31: 684, 1987.

58. Johnsrude I S, Silverman J F, Weaver M D, McConnell R W: Rapid cytology to decrease pneumothorax incidence after percutaneous biopsy. AJR 144: 793–794, 1985.

59. Johnston W W: Percutaneous fine needle aspiration biopsy of the lung. A study of 1,015 patients. Acta Cytol 28: 218–224, 1984.

60. Johnston W W: Fine needle aspiration biopsy versus sputum and bronchial material in the diagnosis of lung cancer. A comparative study of 168 patients. Acta Cytol 32: 661–666, 1988.

61. Jordan A G, Predmore L, Sullivan M M, Memoli V A: The cytodiagnosis of well-differentiated neuroendocrine carcinoma. A distinct clinicopathologic entity. Acta Cytol 31: 465–470, 1987.

62. Kato H, Konaka C, Kawate N, Yoneyama K, Nishimiya K, Saito M, Sakai H, Kinoshita K, Hayata Y: Percutaneous fine needle cytology for lung cancer diagnosis. Diagn Cytopathol 2: 277–283, 1986.

63. Kawahara E, Nakanishi I, Kuroda Y, Morishita T: Fine needle aspiration biopsy of primary malignant fibrous histiocytoma of the lung. Acta Cytol 32: 226–230, 1988.

64. Khouri N F, Stitik F P, Erozan Y S, Gupta P K, Kim W S, Scott W W Jr, Hamper U M, Mann R B, Eggleston J C, Baker R R: Transthoracic needle aspiration biopsy of benign and malignant lung lesions.

8 LUNG, MEDIASTINUM, CHEST WALL AND PLEURA

AJR 144: 281–288, 1985.

65. Kim K, Mah C, Dominquez J: Carcinoid tumours of the lung. Cytologic differential diagnosis in fine needle aspirates. Diagn Cytopathol 2: 343–346, 1986.

66. Kim K, Naylor B, Han I H: Fine needle aspiration cytology of sarcomas metastatic to the lung. Acta Cytol 30: 688–694, 1986.

67. Koprowska I, Zipfel S L: The potential usefulness of types of monoclonal antibodies in the determination of histologic types of lung cancer in cytologic preparations. Acta Cytol 32: 675–679, 1988.

68. Kucharczyk W, Weisbrod G L, Cooper J D: Cardiac tamponade as a complication of thin needle aspiration lung biopsy. Chest 82: 120–121, 1982.

69. Kunstaetter R, Wolkove N, Kreisman H, Cohen C, Frank H: The solitary pulmonary nodule. Decision analysis. Med Decis Making 5: 61–75, 1985.

70. Lee S H, Barnes W G, Schaetzel W P: Pulmonary Aspergillosis and the importance of oxalate crystal recognition in cytology specimens. Arch Pathol Lab Med 110: 1176–1179, 1986.

71. Leiman G: Asbestos bodies in pulmonary fine needle aspirates: A more sinister finding than in other cytologic specimens? Acta Cytol 30: 555–556, 1986.

72. Levine M S, Weiss J M, Harrell J H, Cameron T J, Moser K M: Transthoracic needle aspiration biopsy following negative fiberoptic bronchoscopy in solitary pulmonary nodules. Chest 93: 1152–1155, 1988.

73. Lorch D G Jr, John J F Jr, Tomlinson J R, Miller K S, Sahn S A: Protected transbronchial needle aspiration and protected specimen brush in the diagnosis of pneumonia. Am J Respir Dis 136: 565–569, 1987.

74. Lozowski W, Hajdu S I: Cytology and immunocytochemistry of bronchiolo-alveolar carcinoma. Acta Cytol 31: 717–725, 1987.

75. Machicao C N, Sorensen K L, Abdul-Karim F W, Somrak T M: Transthoracic fine needle aspiration in inflammatory pseudotumor of the lung. Diagn Cytopathol 5: 400–403,1989.

76. Menetrier P. Cancer primitif du poumon. Bull Soc Anat 61: 643–647, 1886.

77. Michel R P, Lushipan A, Ahmed M N: Pathologic findings of transthoracic needle aspiration in the diagnosis of localised pulmonary lesions. Cancer 51: 1563–1672, 1983.

78. Miller K S, Fish G B, Stanley J H, Schabel S I: Prediction of pneumothorax rate in percutaneous needle aspiration of the lung. Chest 93: 742–745, 1988.

79. Miller D A, Carrasco C H, Katz R L, Cramer F M, Wallace S, Charnsangavej C: Fine needle aspiration biopsy: the role of immediate cytologic assessment. AJR 147: 155–158, 1986.

80. Mitchell M L, King D E, Bonfiglio T A, Patten S Jr: Pulmonary fine needle aspiration cytopathology. A five year correlation study. Acta Cytol 28: 72–76, 1984.

81. Moloo Z, Finley R J, Lefcoe M S, Turner-Smith L, Craig I D: Possible spread of bronchogenic carcinoma to the chest wall after a transthoracic fine needle aspiration biopsy. A case report. Acta Cytol 29: 167–169, 1985.

82. Mrkve O, Skaarland E, Myking A, Stangeland L, Gulsvik A: Transthoracic fine needle aspiration guided by fluoroscopy: validity and complications with 19 operators. Respiration 53: 239–245, 1988.

83. Muller N L, Bergin C J, Miller R R, Ostrow D N: Seeding of malignant cells into the needle track after lung and pleural biopsy. J Can Assoc Radiol 37: 192–194, 1986.

84. Nguyen G K: Fine needle aspiration biopsy cytology of metastatic renal cell carcinoma. Acta Cytol 32: 409–414, 1988.

85. Nguyen G-K: Aspiration biopsy cytology of benign clear cell ('sugar') tumour of the lung. Acta Cytol 32: 409–414, 1988.

86. Nguyen G-K: Cytology of bronchial gland carcinoma. Acta Cytol 32: 235–239, 1988.

87. Nguyen G-K, Shnitka T K: Aspiration biopsy cytology of adenocarcinoid tumor of the bronchial tree. Acta Cytol 31: 726–730, 1986.

88. Pauli G, Pelletier A, Bohner C, Roeslin N, Warter A, Roegel E: Transbronchial needle aspiration in the diagnosis of sarcoidosis. Chest 85: 482–484, 1984.

89. Payne C R, Hadfield J W, Stovin P G, Barker V, Heard B E, Stark J E: Diagnostic accuracy of cytology and biopsy in primary bronchial carcinoma. J Clin Pathol 34: 773–778, 1981.

90. Penketh A R, Robinson A S, Barker V, Flower C D: Use of percutaneous needle biopsy in the investigation of solitary pulmonary nodules. Thorax 42: 967–71, 1987.

91. Perlmutt L M, Braun S D, Newman G E, Oke E J, Dunnick N R: Timing of chest film follow-up after transthoracic needle aspiration. AJR 146: 1049–1050, 1986.

92. Perry M D, Gore M, Seigler H F, Johnston W W: Fine needle aspiration biopsy of metastatic melanoma. A morphologic analysis of 174 cases. Acta Cytol 30: 385–397, 1986.

93. Perry M D, Floyd P B, Johnston W W: Role of fine needle aspiration cytology in medical decision making for metastatic carcinoma of the lungs. Acta Cytol 28: 624, 1984.

94. Perry M D, Furlong J W, Johnston W W: Fine needle aspiration cytology of metastatic dermatofibrosarcoma protuberans. A case report. Acta Cytol 30: 507–512, 1986.

95. Philips J, Goodman B, Kelly V J: Percutaneous transthoracic needle biopsy. Pathology 14: 211–213, 1982.

96. Pilotti S, Rilke F, Gribaudi G, Damascelli B, Ravasi G: Transthoracic fine needle aspiration biopsy in pulmonary lesions. Updated results. Acta Cytol 28: 225–232, 1984.

97. Pilotti S, Rilke F, Lombardi L: Pulmonary carcinoid with glandular features. Report of two cases with positive fine needle aspiration biopsy cytology. Acta Cytol 27: 511–514, 1983.

98. Poe R H, Kallay M C: Transthoracic needle biopsy of lung in nonhospitalised patients. Chest 92: 676–678, 1987.

99. Poe R H, Kallay M C, Wicks C M, Odoroff C L: Predicting risk of pneumothorax in needle biopsy of the lung. Chest 85: 232–235, 1984.

100. Ramzy I: Pulmonary hamartomas: Cytologic appearances of fine needle aspiration biopsy. Acta Cytol 20: 15–19, 1976.

101. Rajwanshi A, Bhambbhani S, Das D K: Fine needle aspiration cytology diagnosis of tuberculosis. Diagn Cytopathol 3: 13–16, 1987.

102. Reyes C V, Walloch J, Tosoc L: The role of electron microscopy in fine needle aspiration cytology. Acta Cytol 31: 667, 1987.

103. Robicheaux G, Moinuddin S M, Lee L H: The role of aspiration biopsy cytology in the diagnosis of pulmonary tuberculosis. Am J Clin Pathol 83: 719–722, 1985.

104. Roggli V L, Johnston W W, Kaminsky D B: Asbestos bodies in fine needle aspirates of the lung. Acta Cytol 28: 493–498, 1984.

105. Roggli V L, Vollmer R T, Greenberg S D, McGavran M H, Spjut H J, Yesner R: Lung cancer heterogeneity: A blinded and randomized study of 100 consecutive cases. Hum Pathol 16: 569–579, 1985.

106. Rohwedder J J: The solitary pulmonary nodule. A new diagnostic agenda. Chest 93: 1124–1125, 1988.

107. Rollins S D, Genack L J, Schumann G B: Primary cytodiagnosis of dually differentiated lung cancer by

LUNG, MEDIASTINUM, CHEST WALL AND PLEURA 8

transthoracic fine needle aspiration. Acta Cytol 32: 231–234, 1988.

108. Rosenthal D L, Wallace J M: Fine needle aspiration of pulmonary lesions via fiberoptic bronchoscopy. Acta Cytol 28: 203–210, 1984.

109. Sagel S S, Ferguson T B, Forrest J V, Roper C L, Weldon C S, Clark R E: Percutaneous transthoracic aspiration needle biopsy. Ann Thorac Surg 26: 399–404, 1978.

110. Schantz H D, Ramzy I, Tio F O, Buhaug J: Metastatic spindle cell carcinoma. Cytologic features and differential diagnosis. Acta Cytol 29: 435–441, 1985.

111. Schenk D A, Bower J H, Bryan C L, Currie R B, Spence T H, Duncan C A, Myers D L, Sullivan W T: Transbronchial needle aspiration staging of bronchogenic carcinoma. Am Rev Respir Dis 134: 146–148, 1986.

112. Schenk D A, Bryan C L, Bower J H, Myers D L: Transbronchial needle aspiration in the diagnosis of bronchogenic carcinoma. Chest 92: 83–85, 1987.

113. Schwartz A R, Fishman E K, Wang K P: Diagnosis and treatment of bronchogenic cyst using transbronchial needle aspiration. Thorax 41: 326–327, 1986.

114. Sider L, Davis T M Jr: Hilar masses: evaluation with CT-guided biopsy after negative bronchoscopic examination. Radiology 164: 107–109, 1987.

115. Silverman J F, Finley J L, Park H K, Strausbauch P, Unverfeth M, Carney M: Fine needle aspiration cytology of bronchioloalveolar cell carcinoma of the lung. Acta Cytol 29: 887–894, 1985.

116. Silverman J F, Finley J L, Park H K, Norris H T, Strausbauch P H: Psammoma bodies and optically clear nuclei in bronchiolo-alveolar cell carcinoma. Diagnosis by fine needle aspiration biopsy with histologic and ultrastructural confirmation. Diagn Cytopathol 1: 205–215, 1985.

117. Silverman J F, Johnsrude I S: Fine needle aspiration cytology of granulomatous cryptococcosis of the lung. Acta Cytol 29: 157–161, 1985.

118. Silverman J F, Marrow H G: Fine needle aspiration cytology of granulomatous diseases of the lung, including nontuberculous mycobacterium infection. Acta Cytol 29: 535–541, 1985.

119. Silverman J, Weaver M D, Gardner N, Larkin E W, Park H R: Aspiration biopsy cytology of malignant schwannoma metastatic to the lung. Acta Cytol 29: 15–19, 1985.

120. Silverman J F, Weaver M D, Shaw R, Newman W J: Fine needle aspiration cytology of pulmonary infarct. Acta Cytol 29: 162–166, 1985.

121. Sinner W N: Complications of percutaneous transthoracic needle aspiration biopsy. Acta Radiol Diagn (Stockh) 17: 813–828, 1976.

122. Sinner W N: Importance and value of a preoperative diagnosis in oat cell carcinoma by radiography and its verification by fine needle biopsy (FNB). Eur J Radiol 5: 94–98, 1985.

123. Sinner W N: Pulmonary neoplasms diagnosed with transthoracic needle biopsy. Cancer 43: 1533–1540, 1979.

124. Sinner W N. Fine needle biopsy of hamartomas of the lung. AJR 138: 65–69, 1982.

125. Sinner W N, Zajicek J: Implantation metastasis after percutaneous transthoracic needle aspiration biopsy. Acta Radiol Diagn (Stockh) 17: 473–480, 1976.

126. Stanley J H, Fish G D, Andriole J G, Gobien R P, Betsill W l, Laden S A, Schabel S I: Lung lesions; cytologic diagnosis by fine needle biopsy. Radiology 162: 389–391, 1987.

127. Strobel S L, Keyhani-Rofagha S, O'Toole R V, Nahman B J: Non-aspiration needle smear preparations of

pulmonary lesions. A comparison of cytology and histology. Acta Cytol 29: 1047–1052, 1985.

128. Sterrett G, Whitaker D, Glancy J: Fine needle aspiration of lung mediastinum and chest wall. Pathol Annu Part 2 17: 197–228, 1982.

129. Szyfelbein W M, Ross J S: Carcinoids, atypical carcinoids, and small-cell carcinomas of the lung: differential diagnosis of fine needle aspiration biopsy specimens. Diagn Cytopathol 4: 1–8, 1988.

130. Tabatowski K, Vollmer R, Tello J W, Iglehart J D, Shelburne J D: The use of a panel of monoclonal antibodies in ultrastructually characterised small cell carcinomas of the lung. Acta Cytol 32: 667–674, 1988.

131. Tao L C: Guides to Clinical Aspiration Biopsy. Lung, Pleura and Mediastinum. Igaku-Shoin, New York, 1988.

132. Tao L C, Sanders D E, Weisbrod G L, Ho C S, Wilson S: Value and limitations of transthoracic and transabdominal fine needle aspiration cytology in clinical practice. Diagn Cytopathol 2: 271–276, 1986.

133. Tao L C, Weisbrod G, Ritcey E L, Ilves R: False 'false-positive' results in diagnostic cytology. Acta Cytol 28: 450–455, 1984.

134. Tao L C, Weisbrod G L, Pearson F G, Sanders D E, Donet E E, Tilipetto L: Cytologic diagnosis of bronchiolo-alveolar carcinoma by fine needle aspiration biopsy. Cancer 57: 1565–1570, 1986.

135. Thunnissen F B J M, Arends J W, Buchholtz R T F, ten Velde G: Fine needle aspiration cytology of inflammatory pseudotumour of the lung (plasma cell granuloma) Report of 4 cases. Acta Cytol 33: 917–921, 1989.

136. Tolly T L, Feldmeier J E, Czarnecki D: Air embolism complicating percutaneous lung biopsy. AJR 150: 555–556, 1988.

137. Tsumuraya M, Kodama T, Kameya T, Shimosato Y, Koketsu H, Uei Y: Light and electron microscopic analysis of intranuclear inclusions in papillary adenocarcinoma of the lung. Acta Cytol 25: 523–532, 1981.

138. Valicenti J, Daniell C, Gobian R D: Thin needle aspiration of benign intrathoracic lesions. Acta Cytol 25: 659–664, 1981.

139. van Sonnenberg E, Casola G, Ho M, Neff C C, Varney R R, Wittich G R, Christensen R, Friedman P J: Difficult thoracic lesions: CT-guided biopsy experience in 150 cases. Radiology 167: 457–461, 1988.

140. Veale D, Gilmartin J J, Sumerling M D, Wadehra V, Gibson G J: Prospective evaluation of fine needle aspiration in the diagnosis of lung cancer. Thorax 43: 540–544, 1988.

141. Walker A N, Feldman P S, Walker G K: Fine needle aspiration of thoracic extramedullary hematopoiesis. Acta Cytol 27: 170–172, 1983.

142. Wallace J M, Batra P, Gong H Jr, Ovenfors C O: Percutaneous needle lung aspiration for diagnosing pneumonitis in the patient with acquired immunodeficiency syndrome (AIDS). Am Rev Respir Dis 131: 389–392, 1985.

143. Walts A E: Localised pulmonary cryptococcosis: diagnosis by fine needle aspiration. Acta Cytol 27: 457–459, 1983.

144. Wang K P: Flexible transbronchial needle aspiration biopsy for histologic specimens. Chest 88: 860–863, 1985.

145. Wang K P, Marsh B R, Summer W R, Terry P B, Erozan Y, Robinson Baker R: Transbronchial needle aspiration for diagnosis of lung cancer. Chest 80: 48–50, 1981.

146. Wang S E, Nieberg R K: Fine needle aspiration cytology of sclerosing hemangioma of the lung, a mimicker of bronchioloalveolar carcinoma. Acta Cytol 30: 51–54, 1986

8

LUNG, MEDIASTINUM, CHEST WALL AND PLEURA

147. Watts, W J, Green R A: Bacteremia following transbronchial fine needle aspiration. A case report. Chest 85: 295, 1984.
148. Weisbrod G L, Cunningham I, Tao L C, Chamberlain D W: Small cell anaplastic carcinoma: cytological-histologic correlations from percutaneous fine needle aspiration biopsy. J Can Assoc Radiol 38: 204–208, 1987.
149. Weisbrod G L, Herman S J, Tao L C: Preliminary experience with a dual cutting edge needle in thoracic percutaneous fine needle aspiration biopsy. Radiology 163: 75–78, 1987.
150. Whitaker D, Sterrett G F: Cryptococcus neoformans diagnosed by fine needle aspiration cytology of the lung. Acta Cytol 20: 105–107, 1976.
151. Winning A J, McIvor J, Seed W A, Husain O A, Metaxas N: Interpretation of negative results in fine needle aspiration of discrete pulmonary lesions. Thorax 41: 875–879, 1986.
152. Yazdi M Y, Dardick I: What is the value of electron microscopy in fine needle aspiration biopsy? Diagn Cytopathol 4: 177–179, 1988.
153. Yazdi H M, MacDonald L L, Hickey N M: Thoracic fine needle aspiration biopsy versus fine needle cutting biopsy. A comparative study of 40 patients. Acta Cytol 32: 635–640, 1988.

Mediastinum

154. Adler O, Rosenberger A: Invasive radiology in the diagnosis of mediastinal masses. Use of fine needle for aspiration biposy. Radiology 19: 169–172, 1979.
155. Adler O B, Rosenberger A, Peleg H: Fine needle aspiration biopsy of mediastinal masses: evaluation of 136 experiences. AJR 140: 393–396, 1983
156. Bartholdy N J, Andersen M J, Thommesen P: Clinical value of percutaneous fine needle aspiration biopsy of mediastinal masses. Analysis of 132 cases. Scand J Thorac Cardiovasc Surg 18: 81–83, 1984.
157. Dahlgren S E, Ovenfors C-O: Aspiration biopsy diagnosis of neurogenous mediastinal tumours. Acta Radiol Diagn (Stockh) 10: 408–421, 1970.
158. Dahlgren S, Sandstedt B, Sunstrom C: Fine needle aspiration cytology of thymic tumors. Acta Cytol 27: 1–6, 1983.
159. Finley J L, Silverman J F, Strausbauch P, Dabbs D J, West R L, Weaver M D, Norris H T: Malignant thymic neoplasms: Diagnosis by fine needle aspiration biopsy with histologic, immunocytochemical, and ultrastructural confirmation. Diagn Cytopathol 2: 118–125, 1986.
160. Heimann A, Sneige N, Shirkhoda A, DeCaro L F: Fine needle aspiration cytology of thymolipoma. A case report. Acta Cytol 31: 335–339, 1987.
161. Jereb M, Us-Krasovec M: Transthoracic needle biopsy of mediastinal and hilar lesions. Cancer 40: 1354–1357, 1977.
162. Kuhlman J E, Fishman E K, Wang K P, Zerhouni E A, Siegelman S S: Mediastinal Cysts: Diagnosis by CT and needle aspiration. AJR 150: 75–78, 1988.
163. Linder J, Olsen G A, Johnston W W: Fine needle aspiration biopsy of the mediastinum. Am J Med 81: 1005–1008, 1986.
164. Marco V, Carrasco M A, Marco C, Bauza A: Cytomorphology of a mediastinal parathyroid cyst. Report of a case mimicking malignancy. Acta Cytol 27: 688–692, 1983.
165. Mishriki Y Y, Lane B P, Lozowski M S, Epstein H: Hurthle-cell tumor arising in the mediastinal ectopic thyroid and diagnosed by fine needle aspiration. Light

microscopic and ultrastructural features. Acta Cytol 27: 188–192, 1983.
166. Nath P H, Sanders C, Holley H C, McElvein R B: Percutaneous fine needle aspiration in the diagnosis and management of mediastinal cysts in adults. South Med J 81: 1225–1228, 1988.
167. Pak H Y, Yokota S B, Friedberg H A: Thymoma diagnosed by transthoracic fine needle aspiration. Acta Cytol 26: 210–216, 1982.
168. Sajjid S M, Lukeman J M, Thomas et al: Needle biopsy diagnosis of thymoma. Acta Cytol 26: 503–506, 1982.
169. Sangalli G, Livraghi T, Giosano F, Tavani E, Schiaffino E: Primary mediastinal embryonal carcinoma and choriocarcinoma. A case report. Acta Cytol 30: 543–546, 1986.
170. Sterrett G F, Whitaker D, Shilkin K B, Walters M N-I: Fine needle aspiration cytology of mediastinal lesions. Cancer 51: 127–135, 1983.
171. Suen K, Quenville N: Fine needle aspiration cytology of uncommon thoracic lesions. Am J Clin Pathol 75: 803–809, 1981.
172. Taccagni G, Cantaboni A, Dell'Antonio G, Vanzulli A, Del Maschio A. Electron microscopy of fine needle aspiration biopsies of mediastinal and paramediastinal lesions. Acta Cytol 32: 868–879, 1988.
173. Tao L C, Griffith Pearson F, Coper J D, Sanders D E, Weisbrod G, Donat E E: Cytopathology of thymoma. Acta Cytol 28: 165–170, 1984.
174. van Sonnenberg E, Lin A S, Deutsch A L, Mattrey R F: Percutaneous biopsy of difficult mediastinal, hilar, and pulmonary lesions by computed tomographic guidance and modified coaxial technique. Radiology 148: 300–302, 1983.
175. Weisbrod G L. Percutaneous fine-needle aspiration biopsy of the mediastinum. Clin Chest Med 8: 27–41, 1987.
176. Weisbrod G L, Lyons D J, Tao L C, Chamberlain D W: Percutaneous fine needle aspiration biopsy of mediastinal lesions. AJR 143: 525–529, 1984.

Chest Wall and Pleura

177. Kwee W, Utama I: Malignant pleural mesothelioma and thoracic needle biopsy. Chest 93: 1115–1116, 1988.
178. Obers V J, Leiman G, Girdwood R W, Spiro F I: Primary chest wall and pleura, malignant pleural tumors (mesotheliomas) presenting as localised masses. Fine needle aspiration cytologic findings, clinical and radiologic features and review of the literature. Acta Cytol 32: 567–575, 1988.
179. Pang J A, Tsang V, Hom B L, Metreweli C: Ultrasound-guided tissue-core biopsy of thoracic lesions with Trucut and Surecut needles. Chest 91: 823–828, 1987.
180. Pedersen O M, Aasen T B, Gulsvik A: Fine needle aspiration biopsy of mediastinal and peripheral pulmonary masses guided by real-time sonography. Chest 89: 504–508, 1986.
181. Tao L C: Aspiration biopsy cytology of mesothelioma. Diagn Cytopathol 5: 14–21, 1989.
182. Sterrett G F, Whitaker D, Shilkin K B, Walters M N-I: Fine needle aspiration cytology of malignant mesothelioma. Acta Cytol 31: 185–193, 1987.
182a. Whitaker D, Shilkin K B, Sterrett G F: Cytological appearances of malignant mesothelioma. Malignant mesothelioma, Hemisphere, New York, 1992, pp. 167–182.
183. Whitaker D, Sterrett G F, Shilkin K B: Detection of tissue CEA-like substance as an aid in the differential diagnosis of malignant mesothelioma. Pathology 14: 255–258, 1982.

9

RETROPERITONEUM, LIVER AND SPLEEN

RETROPERITONEUM, LIVER AND SPLEEN

CLINICAL ASPECTS

Modern organ imaging techniques, mainly ultrasonography and computerised tomography, have made deep organs and tissues of the abdominal cavity and the retroperitoneum readily accessible to fine needle aspiration (FNA) biopsy as described in Chapter 3. This has become one of the most important applications of diagnostic cytology. The reason is obvious, for there is hardly an alternative way of obtaining a tissue diagnosis other than explorative laparotomy. The cytological diagnosis of retroperitoneal disease is difficult in view of the wide range of neoplasms and other processes occurring in this region. The pathologist must therefore have extensive background experience of tumour histopathology to accept this challenge. It is sometimes impossible to make a confident, specific diagnosis, but even then, the cytological pattern usually gives some clue to the nature of the lesion to guide further investigations and management.

Teams in Sweden and Denmark were the first to use FNA biopsy guided by angiography or ultrasonography to investigate renal and pancreatic masses.[32,55,111] The introduction of computerised tomography gave needle biopsy of deep abdominal organs a further boost, and it has now become part of the diagnostic routines in most major hospitals all over the world. Publications on the subject confirming a satisfactory level of diagnostic accuracy are too numerous to list.

As the confidence in cytological diagnosis has increased in recent years, there is an increasing pressure on the cytologist to provide specific information on tumour type, malignancy grade, etc. as a basis for therapeutic decisions. An explorative laparotomy is a major procedure which has a significant morbidity and which is not entirely free from mortality. Thus, in the investigation of deep processes in the abdomen and the retroperitoneum, there is a greater need for precise FNA diagnoses than in superficial lesions, and this has led to more extensive use of supplementary techniques such as cell blocks, EM and immunocytochemistry, and also of core needles in conjunction with or instead of the plain fine needle.[44]

This chapter will deal with the cytological investigation not only of retroperitoneal tissues in a narrow sense, but also with the pancreas and extrahepatic bile ducts, the gastrointestinal tract, the para-aortic and iliac lymph nodes, the adrenals, and the kidneys together with liver and spleen.

RETROPERITONEUM

The place of FNA in the investigative sequence

It is certainly possible and relatively easy to do a FNA biopsy of a palpable abdominal or retroperitoneal mass at the time of the initial examination. This approach is tempting; however, interposition of normal tissue of similar consistency to the mass can give a false impression of the depth, and cystic degeneration and haemor-

rhage may be extensive. If the mass is within the liver or the spleen, the thrombocyte count and prothrombin time should be checked. It is preferable therefore to have more precise information about the site and size of the lesion, its structure in respect of solid and cystic components, and particularly about its anatomical relationships, before proceeding to biopsy. This information, important not only for the biopsy procedure but also for the subsequent interpretation of the smears, is provided by various organ imaging techniques used also to guide the needle with necessary precision. Consequently, the biopsy should be performed by the radiologist and the pathologist in close co-operation.

Any lesion which can be exactly located by palpation or by radiological methods is a potential indication for percutaneous FNA (excluding arterial aneurysms and a few other conditions listed under 'Contraindications'). More specifically, in tumours of the *pancreas*, percutaneous FNA is mainly used to confirm inoperable malignancy so that the patient may be spared a merely explorative laparotomy. Sometimes, cytological examination unexpectedly shows an islet cell tumour, a metastatic malignancy or a lymphoma instead of the presumed pancreatic adenocarcinoma, and benign pancreatic tumours, although rare, do occur. Some patients are subjected to a laparotomy in the hope that the tumour may be resectable or for a by-pass palliative procedure. Unless the surgeon requires a preoperative diagnosis to help him plan in advance the extent of the operation, the biopsy can be taken more easily and with higher precision intraoperatively than percutaneously. Since a tumour must have reached a certain size before it becomes accessible to biopsy, FNA does not contribute significantly to early diagnosis. Neither is it suited, generally speaking, to the diagnosis of pancreatitis. However, in pancreatic pseudocyst, FNA can be both diagnostic and therapeutic. Decompression of an acutely developed cyst may relieve symptoms and facilitate surgical treatment.[31]

In tumours of the *retroperitoneum proper*, percutaneous FNA is a valuable supplement to preoperative radiological investigations.[42] In advanced inoperable disease, a cytological diagnosis is often a sufficient basis for palliative radiotherapy or chemotherapy, without the need for a formal surgical biopsy. The cytological diagnosis of primary soft tissue tumours of the retroperitoneum is difficult and a type specific diagnosis may not be possible, but the exclusion of metastatic malignancy or lymphoma is already of clinical value. Close co-operation between radiologist and pathologist is important not only to obtain a representative biopsy, but also in arriving at a diagnosis. One application of practical importance is the distinction between tumour recurrence and retroperitoneal fibrosis as the cause of ureteric obstruction in patients treated for cancer of this region.[94,100,102] The application of the technique to abdominal and retroperitoneal lesions in infants and children has been

RETROPERITONEUM, LIVER AND SPLEEN 9

discussed by Valkov and Bojikin.[75] In massive retroperitoneal *lymphadenopathy*, FNA is a convenient method to differentiate between metastatic malignancy and malignant lymphoma. In the former case, it often reveals the nature of the primary. FNA has also been used as a supplement to lymphangiography or computerised tomography in the preoperative staging of urogenital cancers.[78–90]

In the *adrenal*, FNA has been mainly applied to masses suspected clinically and/or radiologically to be metastatic. In particular, preoperative investigation by CT of potentially operable lung tumours sometimes reveals adrenal lesions. In such a case, further management obviously depends on whether the lesion is metastatic cancer or something else. This distinction is best made by CT-directed FNA biopsy which also allows the diagnosis of cysts and primary tumours in the adrenal.[109,126,135]

Puncture and aspiration through a thin needle has been a standard procedure for confirming the nature of simple cysts in the *kidney*. Today, the diagnostic accuracy of ultrasound investigation has rendered cytological confirmation of simple cysts unnecessary. The value of FNA in the investigation of solid renal tumours is somewhat controversial, mainly because the accuracy of angiography and CT is such that a preoperative tissue diagnosis may seem unnecessary. The contribution of FNA cytology to diagnosis may not be significant enough to justify its use as a separate procedure in addition to the radiological investigations. However, FNA biopsy is indicated in some situations, namely when the radiological findings are atypical or doubtful, when CT examination is not available, when preoperative embolisation or irradiation is considered, and in advanced, inoperable tumours. Also, if FNA is done as an integrated part of the ultrasonographic or CT scan examination preceding surgery, in many cases a precise tissue diagnosis can be obtained with little additional time and costs and without profound risks to the patient. In case of renal abscess, material for microbiological investigation can be obtained in this way.

Intraoperative diagnosis of abdominal and retroperitoneal processes is an important application of FNA. In the pancreas, it has the advantage over the traditional wedge biopsy for frozen section of being virtually free of complications such as haemorrhage and fistula formation. It can be repeated to sample many different parts of a large mass, thereby increasing the probability of obtaining representative material. For example, a pancreatic carcinoma may be surrounded by a wide zone of oedema and inflammation and a wedge biopsy may not be deep enough to include neoplastic tissue. A thin needle can pass through the stomach or duodenum without risk. With experience, interpretation of technically satisfactory smears is often easier than of a frozen section because of better preservation of cell detail.[27] Staining and mounting of smears is as quick or quicker

than cutting and staining frozen sections. We believe the potential of FNA cytology as a method of intraoperative tissue diagnosis, not only in pancreatic disease but of any abdominal mass lesions, is not sufficiently appreciated by most surgeons.

Accuracy of diagnosis

The diagnostic accuracy is related first and foremost to the adequacy and the representativeness of the biopsy, which in turn depends on the site, size and nature of the lesion and on the method used to guide the biopsy needle into it. The relative merits of available radiological techniques in guiding the biopsy are discussed in Chapter 3. Although technical progress continues to improve the quality of radiological tumour imaging, there is still a minimum size below which a lesion cannot be clearly demonstrated and precise needling is not possible. Intraoperatively, under the control of direct palpation, lesions measuring only a few millimetres in diameter can be biopsied successfully. Very large tumours present another problem: the difficulty of finding well-preserved cells on which to base a diagnosis in the presence of extensive necrosis or haemorrhage.

Not only must the sample contain an adequate number of well preserved cells representative of the basic disease process, but it must also be smeared, fixed and stained expertly. Even when all of these conditions are fulfilled, diagnostic accuracy still varies with the nature of the disease. For example, although diagnostic criteria are well established for the common carcinomas, experience with the cytological diagnosis of many mesenchymal tumours is still limited. With some of these a precise diagnosis cannot be given with confidence, merely a suggestion and a differential diagnosis which must be further investigated by other means. However, if it is possible to decide if the disease is inflammatory or neoplastic — and, if neoplastic, if it is epithelial, lymphoid or mesenchymal, whether it is benign, low grade or high grade malignant, and whether it is likely to be primary or metastatic — FNA is still of considerable value in clinical management. To improve accuracy by increasing experience, every opportunity should be taken to obtain smears from all kinds of tumours preoperatively or from fresh, unfixed tissue removed at operation. Histochemical, immunohistochemical and ultrastructural examination have the potential to improve diagnostic accuracy by providing more precise information of the histogenesis and differentiation of the tumour cells. However, expensive supplementary techniques should be used selectively in order to avoid non-productive increase in costs.

An estimate of diagnostic accuracy can be obtained by collating results from the numerous series of FNA biopsies of abdominal and retroperitoneal masses reported in the literature. Diagnostic specificity for malignant *pancreatic lesions* is 100% in nearly all published

9 RETROPERITONEUM, LIVER AND SPLEEN

series. However, occasional false positive diagnoses have been reported in cases of chronic pancreatitis.[33] Diagnostic sensitivity is much more variable. It is usually around 90% in intraoperative FNA biopsies,[2,16,25,34,43,60] generally lower and more variable — 50% to over 90% — in US- or CT-directed percutaneous biopsies.[7,9,13,17,19,21,26,29,31,36,48–50,61,62,77] Diagnostic accuracy tends to be lower for *biliary* tumours.[30,40] These figures would be more meaningful if they could be related to the size of the tumours, but this is rarely stated in the reports. FNA of lymphangiographically abnormal retroperitoneal *lymph nodes* has an average success rate of 70% in obtaining a representative sample from an individual node.[89] In a series of 100 cases in which lymphangiography and FNA were applied to the staging of urogenital cancer, there were no false positive diagnoses and the overall accuracy was 83%.[90] Even if the nodes are radiologically normal, FNA can reveal metastatic involvement in a significant proportion of cases.[84] In a total of 1585 *renal and adrenal masses* (both cystic and solid) from a review of the literature,[128] the false positive rate was 2.3% if cases reported as cytologically atypical or as suspicious of malignancy were included. The diagnostic sensitivity was 86% for 603 malignant tumours, specificity was 98% and the predictive value of a positive result was 96%. The main factor which limits diagnostic sensitivity is the difficulty to obtain preserved neoplastic cells from large tumours with extensive necrosis and haemorrhage.

Complications

Significant complications are rare if thin needles of less than 21 gauge are used. Such needles pass through stomach or bowel without causing peritonitis, although caution is recommended in cases of bowel obstruction or distension. A few examples of severe pancreatitis or exacerbation of pancreatitis have been recorded following FNA of the pancreas.[15,20,49,51] FNA is therefore not recommended for the investigation of pancreatitis but should be reserved for cases with a radiological mass lesion.[20] A single case of septicaemia following pancreatic biopsy has been reported.[74] Major haemorrhage is very rare. Tearing of blood vessels is prevented if the needle is advanced during apnoea, if the peritoneum is anaesthesised to prevent uncontrolled movements, and if rigid inflexible needle systems are not used. The coagulation status should be noted but a full investigation is unnecessary unless the spleen or the liver are involved. We usually keep patient under observation for a couple of hours following transperitoneal needle biopsy.

Lang[113] studied the complications of puncture of renal cysts in many cases accumulated from several institutions in the USA. Haemorrhage, infection, and pneumothorax did occur after puncture, but the rate was low and was reduced by experience and by technical modifications. In solid renal masses, complications were recorded in 0.4% of cases.[106,128,131,137] Six cases of tumour implantation in the needle-track following FNA of pancreatic carcinoma have been reported.[5,10,22,24,63,69] Four cases of needle-track implantation after aspiration of renal cell cancers have also occurred.[93,101,136,140] In one instance the biopsy was performed with an 18 gauge needle. Considering the large number of aspirations which have been performed, this event is extremely rare.

Contraindications

An aortic or other arterial aneurysm must obviously be excluded before needling an abdominal/retroperitoneal mass. An aneurysm may be largely filled by organising blood clot, it may not pulsate, and it may appear solid on ultrasonographic examination. This is one good reason never to use larger needles than 21 gauge. Hydatid cysts and adrenal phaeochromocytomas have also been regarded as contraindications for needle biopsy in view of possible serious complications. However, this risk seems to have been exaggerated. FNA biopsies have been performed successfully and without complications in several such cases; also in our own institutions.

Technical considerations

Transperitoneal deep FNA biopsy is not quite as simple as that of superficial lesions. It is best done as a hospital procedure and performed in the radiology department where all the facilities for tumour imaging are available. In some suitable cases, distinctly palpable masses can be biopsied in the clinic to save time and expense, provided the simple safety rules mentioned above are observed.

Preparation for the biopsy procedure is simple. Mild sedation is occasionally justified in the very anxious patient. Theatre sterility is not required, only routine skin disinfection is necessary. It is recommended to use local anaesthetic in the skin and in the parietal peritoneum to facilitate patient co-operation. The patient should be instructed before the procedure is commenced to hold his breath when the needle is advanced, and to breath quietly while the position of the needle is checked and during the aspiration.

A 22 gauge, 90 mm lumbar puncture needle with trocar is suitable for most deep biopsies. Longer Chiba needles of the same calibre are sometimes required. A 22 gauge Rotex screw needle is recommended for fibrous lesions and mesenchymal tumours if insufficient material is obtained with the usual needles. The choice of transducers for ultrasonically guided biopsies is discussed in Chapter 3. In CT guided biopsy, a haematoma sometimes forms around the tip of the needle while further scans are taken to check the position of the needle. As this can have an adverse effect on the sample, the needle is preferably placed at the periphery of the lesion so that it can be advanced into fresh tissue when the sample is taken. Smears should be prepared and stained immediately so that the adequacy of the specimen can be checked and the aspiration repeated if necessary. Multiple smears, both air-dried and wet-fixed, should be made whenever possible to allow histochemical and immunocytochemical staining if necessary. In selected cases, a cell block can be of great value, or biopsy material can be fixed in glutaraldehyde for EM, particularly if preliminary smears suggest a small round cell or other anaplastic tumour, sarcoma, etc.[35,66]

INTRA-ABDOMINAL ORGANS

Lesions of the gastrointestinal tract are as a rule investigated by radiological methods and by endoscopy. However, FNA is sometimes used as the first investigation of a palpable abdominal mass which may prove to be a neoplasm arising from the large bowel or from the stomach.[57] In our limited experience of FNA of such lesions, there is no risk of complications, although we feel that puncture of obstructed and distended bowel should be avoided. FNA can also be performed through a fibreoptic endoscope.[39] The diagnosis of adenocarcinoma, carcinoid tumours, lymphoma, etc. offers no particular difficulties specific to site.

LIVER

Single or multiple focal abnormalities demonstrated by palpation, by nuclear scan, by CT scan or by ultrasonography constitute the main indication for FNA biopsy of the liver. In western countries, metastatic tumour deposits are by far the commonest cause of such focal abnormalities.[186] A recent review of our material showed that 3–5% of all FNA biopsies were of the liver, and in nearly 90% of these it was a question of metastatic malignancy. The differential diagnosis is primary liver carcinoma — much more common in Asian and African populations, but important also in western countries in view of recent advances in hepatic surgery — as well as other primary liver tumours, congenital and acquired cysts, abscess and haemangioma. Single echogenic spots or holes in the liver are not infrequently found at ultrasonic scanning of asymptomatic patients, for example in the follow up of treated colo-rectal carcinoma. The question is then is it metastatic cancer or is it a benign lesion such as haemangioma. Haemangioma is the commonest solid benign lesion in the liver. The ultrasonic picture is diagnostic in well over 50% of cases, but sometimes FNA is necessary to exclude adenoma or metastasis.

Some Scandinavian workers[180,188,218] have advocated the use of FNA biopsy in diffuse parenchymal liver disease. Although we agree that in some acute situations FNA may be considered as a preliminary test to indicate the presence and severity of disease, we feel that cytological methods lack the precision necessary to be of real diagnostic value.[195] The pathologist must nevertheless be familiar with the cytological patterns of diffuse liver disease. For example, mild hepatitic changes may be present as a local reaction next to a tumour, and primary or metastatic disease may occur in a setting of severe parenchymal abnormality such as cirrhosis. FNA biopsy is definitely of value in the diagnosis of haemosiderosis, amyloidosis, and myeloid metaplasia. One should also remember that metastatic carcinoma, particularly of breast and lung, and malignant lymphoma can cause diffuse hepatomegaly without demonstrable focal abnormalities. FNA has also been used for monitoring liver transplants.[178,182]

FNA biopsy has now largely replaced conventional large needle core biopsy (Vim-Silverman, Menghini, Tru-cut needles) in the diagnosis of focal lesions. It has the advantage of causing significantly less discomfort and a very low risk of complications. Hospitalisation of the patient is not necessary. Focal abnormalities can be missed by either method. The accuracy of large needle biopsy as reported in the literature is quite variable (60–82%).[177] Most studies comparing core needle biopsy and FNA favour fine needle biopsy for focal liver disease.[145,168,179] The main advantage of using fine needles and cytological techniques is that smears can be stained and checked immediately and the biopsy repeated from different sites in the liver until a satisfactory sample has been obtained, without undue risks to the patient. In this way, diagnostic sensitivity is increased, usually to around 90% and in some series even higher.[153,158,166,173,177,183,206,207,221] Although diagnostic sensitivity is high for malignant lesions, type specific diagnosis can be difficult in smears. Many workers therefore advocate the parallel use of smears and cell blocks for histological sections.[148,174,200,215] However, the accuracy of FNA cytology in the specific diagnosis of primary hepatocellular carcinoma has been around 85% in reported series.[143,157,185,197,214] In one series, the combined use of smears and cell blocks increased the accuracy to 93.7%.[204]

Whenever possible, the biopsy should be directed rather than blind. If a mass cannot be clearly felt, the biopsy must be guided by some form of radiological tumour imaging. In large lesions, a nuclear scan may give sufficient indication of the best biopsy site. Ultrasonography or CT scan obviously provide much greater precision in guiding the needle and are indispensable for biopsy of small, deep-sited lesions. Ultrasound is the most commonly used modality, CT scan, being more expensive and time consuming, is reserved for small, deeply situated lesions, while about one-third of the biopsies are still done by free hand. The site of entry of the needle through the lower thoracic or upper abdo-

9 *RETROPERITONEUM, LIVER AND SPLEEN*

minal wall is chosen to provide the easiest possible access to the target. The pleural sinus should be avoided in view of the risk of pneumothorax, and whenever possible, the needle should pass through normal liver tissue separating the lesion from the capsule to reduce the risk of haemorrhage into the peritoneal cavity (particularly if haemangioma is a possibility). Sometimes, a defect shown on a scan appears larger than the true size of the tumour, and this may be the cause of non-representative samples. That even a correctly performed biopsy can result in misleading information is illustrated by Figure 9.61. It shows an abscess situated immediately beside a congenital cyst from which the aspirate was obtained. The abscess and the cyst appeared as one lesion on both nuclear scan and on ultrasonography.

For liver biopsies, a 22 gauge, 90 mm lumbar puncture needle with trocar is the most suitable. A local anaesthetic injected into the skin and into the parietal peritoneum practically eliminates any discomfort. When the needle is correctly positioned within the liver, the trocar is removed and negative pressure is applied. The needle is advanced steadily for 1–2 cm without any rapid to-and-fro movement, whereupon the pressure is released and the needle withdrawn. The whole procedure should be carried out quickly to avoid excessive admixture with blood. If this is still a problem, needle biopsy without aspiration may be tried. Haemorrhagic diathesis is a contraindication, and the prothrombin time and the platelet count should be checked before the biopsy. We like to keep the patient under observation for a few hours after biopsy. Lundqvist[187] had no deaths and only one significant complication, an intrahepatic haematoma, in 2600 FNA biopsies of the liver. A few cases of severe or fatal haemorrhage[175,201,216,219] and of bile peritonitis,[205] and a single case of seeding in the needle tract[193] have been reported. Other rare complications have been carcinoid crisis[151] and lymphorrhoea.[162] Hydatid cyst is considered to be a relative contraindication in view of the risk of an anaphylactic reaction. The risk of causing haemorrhage by needling haemangiomata has been shown to be very low if the correct techniques are used and this is no longer considered a contraindication.[159,190,209]

As in most other tissues, the parallel use of MGG and Pap staining is recommended for smears of liver aspirates. Special stains may be needed to demonstrate bile pigment, haemosiderin, amyloid, etc. Immunoperoxidase staining can be helpful in deciding the origin of primary or metastatic malignancy.[147] Several workers recommend paraffin embedding of cell blocks claiming that the demonstration of architectural patterns in sections of even minute tissue fragments, increase diagnostic accuracy significantly.[174,200,204] This is certainly helpful in the diagnosis of primary liver tumours. In fact, liver tissue and the better differentiated primary tumours have a high degree of cohesiveness, and tissue fragments or cores can often be obtained using standard

22 gauge needles (see Fig. 2.10). Electron microscopy may also contribute to type specific diagnosis.[146]

SPLEEN

FNA of the spleen is not a commonly performed procedure judging from the sparsity of reports in the cytological literature.[224,225,226,228,229,234] Probably most workers feel that needle biopsy of the spleen has little to contribute, except in cases of isolated splenomegaly, and this is an uncommon situation. In a review of splenic aspirations during a 5-year period (FMC, unpublished), we found only 18 cases performed in patients with isolated splenomegaly. The results from this small series suggest that cytology can contribute to diagnosis. Its main importance is as a means to confirm malignancy. Malignancy is unlikely if cytology is negative, particularly if the cause of splenomegaly can be explained, but it can not be confidently excluded.

The number of conditions which can be diagnosed by FNA is not great. The cause of splenic enlargement should first be sought by clinical and haematological investigations. Non-neoplastic disorders which can be diagnosed by FNA are abscesses,[231] myeloid metaplasia, granulomatous processes[232,236] and amyloidosis.[230] Large foamy macrophages raise a suspicion of lipid storage disease, but biochemical investigations are necessary to establish a specific diagnosis. The cytology is 'normal' in a proportion of cases of isolated splenomegaly and gives no clue to the aetiology (congestion, portal hypertension, etc.).

Malignant lymphoma most often involves the spleen diffusely, but can also occur as massive deposits. A nuclear or CT scan, or ultrasonography can thus be helpful in selecting the best site for a biopsy.[235] Splenic metastases are not uncommon in disseminated carcinoma, but rarely constitute a clinical problem. Splenoma, haemangioma and angiosarcoma are examples of the rare primary tumours of the spleen.

The risk of a needle biopsy causing rupture and major haemorrhage appears to be minimal, provided that the size of the needle is no greater than 22 gauge, the patient's coagulation status is satisfactory, and that the procedure is carried out quickly during apnoea. Söderström had no complications in over 1000 FNAs of the spleen[234] and Selroos et al had none in 557 cases.[232] Nevertheless, we feel that FNA of the spleen should not be undertaken as an office procedure and that the patient should be observed for 4 hours after biopsy. Haemorrhagic diathesis is a contraindication; we require a platelet count to be no less than 80 000. Söderström regarded glandular fever and polycythemia as relative contraindications.[234] Core needle biopsy of the spleen using the Biopty gun has been advocated by some, but has shown a significant rate of complications.[227]

The puncture is made below the costal margin in the

RETROPERITONEUM, LIVER AND SPLEEN 9

centre of the palpable part of the spleen, or in the 9th interspace in the mid-axillary line if the spleen is not palpable. A local anaesthetic is injected into the skin and into the parietal peritoneum to ensure that the patient co-operates during the biopsy. The biopsy should be carried out quickly. Negative pressure is only applied during the rapid advance of the needle within the spleen. We rarely perform more than one or two punctures in one session. Aspirates may appear to consist mainly of blood, but are, nevertheless, usually quite rich in cells. The material should be smeared thinly, and air-dried MGG-stained smears are essential to allow comparison with blood films and bone marrow aspirates. Spare slides should be kept if possible for special stains, which are sometimes helpful.

9 *RETROPERITONEUM, LIVER AND SPLEEN*

CYTOLOGICAL FINDINGS

THE PANCREAS

Normal structures (Figs 9.1 and 9.2)

1. Exocrine epithelial cells in rounded acinar clusters.
2. Ductal epithelial cells in monolayered sheets.
3. Naked single nuclei resembling nuclei of small lymphocytes.

FNA smears from normal pancreatic tissue are most often poor in cells but can occasionally be surprisingly cellular. Most of the cells are acinar unless the needle passes through a major duct. Acinar cells have indistinct cell borders, but their acinar arrangement suggests a triangular shape, the nuclei being disposed in a circle at the periphery of small, round clusters of cells. Larger aggregates are composed of several acini held together by sparse fibrovascular stroma. The nuclei are uniformly small, round, and of similar size and shape to those of small lymphocytes. Many cells are represented by single, naked nuclei. The nuclear chromatin is densely

granular and evenly distributed. There may be a single, relatively large nucleolus or multiple small nucleoli. The cytoplasm is dense and granular (Fig. 9.1). The ductal epithelial cells form monolayered sheets (Fig. 9.2). Cell borders are usually visible, the cytoplasm is pale and the nuclei are regularly distributed within the sheets. The nuclei are slightly larger than those of the acinar epithelial cells and are more ovoid. They are paler and have finely granular chromatin and small nucleoli. Palisading may be seen along the edge of sheets. Ductal epithelial cells from major bile ducts and surface epithelial cells from the duodenal mucosa look similar and cannot be clearly distinguished from those of the major pancreatic ducts in smears.

Pancreatitis (Figs 9.3–9.6)

Usual findings

1. Normal acinar and ductal epithelial cells.
2. Variable acute and chronic inflammatory cells.
3. Foamy macrophages, some multinucleated.
4. Abundant mucus, degenerating epithelial cells and debris.

Problems in diagnosis

1. Paucity of inflammatory cells.
2. Regenerative epithelial atypia.

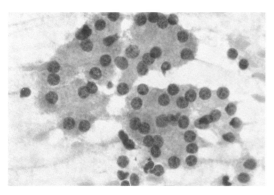

Fig. 9.1 Pancreatic acinar cells
Cohesive clusters of acinar epithelium; note granular cytoplasm and small round uniform nuclei, some of which are bare; intra-operative aspirate of mass of ectopic pancreatic tissue in gastric wall (H & E, HP)

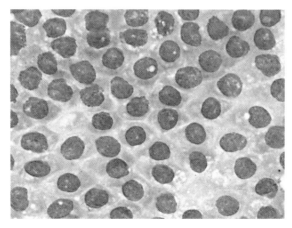

Fig. 9.2 Pancreatic ductal cells
Monolayered sheet of uniform ductal epithelial cells (MGG, HP)

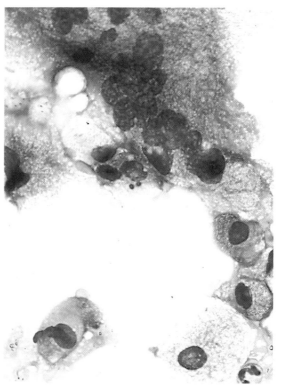

Fig. 9.3 Pancreatic fat necrosis
Foamy mononuclear and multinucleate macrophages (MGG, HP)

RETROPERITONEUM, LIVER AND SPLEEN 9

Acute haemorrhagic pancreatitis is unlikely to be subjected to FNA biopsy. Percutaneous FNA is not a suitable method to confirm clinically suspected chronic pancreatitis, partly because the inflammatory cells found in smears are often too sparse to be diagnostic, partly because of the risk of the biopsy causing exacerbation of pre-existing pancreatitis.[20] However, if, on surgical exploration, the gland is felt to be increased in size and/or consistency, whether diffusely, focally or multifocally, intraoperative FNA can help to differentiate between chronic pancreatitis and malignancy. Since oedema and inflammation peripheral to a carcinoma can simulate true pancreatitis, multiple biopsies should be taken from different parts of the abnormal area to exclude malignancy. This can be done without significant risk of local complications.

In severe chronic pancreatitis most of the exocrine parenchyma may be destroyed and be replaced by fibrous tissue. In such cases, remaining ductal and acinar epithelium can show prominent regenerative atypia which can be difficult to distinguish from well differentiated adenocarcinoma. Figures 9.4–9.6 from a case of severe chronic pancreatitis illustrate this problem. The epithelial atypia shown in Figure 9.4 is quite severe. Not only is there nuclear enlargement and variation in nuclear size and shape, but also crowding of nuclei and microglandular arrangement of cells, as in carcinoma. Such severe atypia was shown by only a few cell groups while most of the epithelial cells were only mildly atypical (Fig. 9.5). The overall findings in combination with the clinical presentation made chronic pancreatitis with regenerative atypia the favoured diagnosis, but malignancy could not be excluded cytologically. Pancreatectomy was performed to relieve severe symptoms, regardless of the cytological report. Histological examination revealed nearly total loss of exocrine

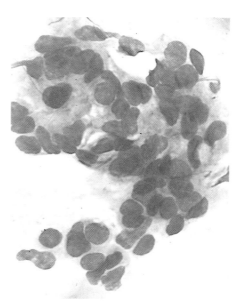

Fig. 9.4 Chronic pancreatitis; epithelial atypia
Aggregate of glandular cells showing acinar pattern and prominent nuclear atypia (MGG, HP)

glandular tissue, massive fibrosis and focally marked regenerative epithelial atypia of residual small ducts and acini (Fig. 9.6).

Regenerative epithelial atypia severe enough to cause diagnostic difficulties is uncommon in the pancreas in our experience, but this possibility must be kept in mind when a diagnosis of well differentiated pancreatic adenocarcinoma is considered.[33,70] It is more commonly seen in extrahepatic bile ducts where it can cause problems also for the histopathologist.

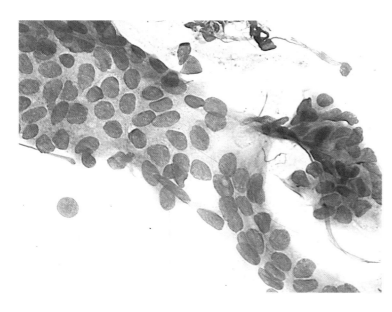

Fig. 9.5 Chronic pancreatitis; epithelial atypia
Monolayered sheet of ductal epithelial cells with mild nuclear atypia (MGG, HP)

9 *RETROPERITONEUM, LIVER AND SPLEEN*

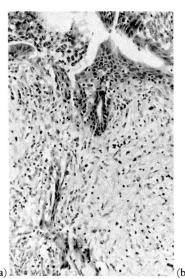 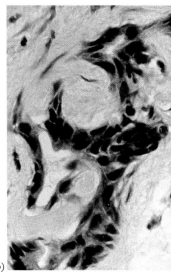

(a)   (b)

Fig. 9.6 Chronic pancreatitis
Tissue section; same case as Figures 9.4 and 9.5. (a) Total exocrine atrophy and fibrosis (H & E, LP); (b) severe regenerative epithelial atypia (H & E, HP).

Cysts (Fig. 9.7)

Cysts in the pancreas can be congenital, post-pancreatitic pseudocysts, abscesses, or neoplastic. An aspirate from a pseudocyst consists of mucinous fluid containing variable amounts of debris, inflammatory cells, macrophages, and sometimes groups of preserved epithelial or mesothelial cells which may show some degree of atypia (Fig. 9.7). An amylase assay of the fluid will confirm the pancreatic origin of the cyst. Purulent cyst contents suggest an abscess and should be submitted for microbiological examination.

Cystadenoma and other benign neoplasms

We have no personal experience of these rare lesions but several case reports have appeared in the literature.[41] One would expect an aspirate from a *mucinous cystadenoma* to resemble that of well differentiated adenocarcinoma. The distinction is difficult even in histological sections and total excision has therefore been recommended for these tumours.[12]

In a case of *glycogen rich (microcystic) cystadenoma* smears from the aspirated fluid showed normal pancreatic epithelium and a small number of small, bland, mesothelial-like cells. A number of case reports have been published describing the cytological findings in the rare *solid and papillary neoplasm of the pancreas.*[6,11,23,71]

Adenocarcinoma (Figs 9.8–9.12)

Criteria for diagnosis

1. Cellular smears.
2. Microglandular patterns, nuclear crowding; loss of cell cohesion.
3. Nuclear criteria of malignancy.

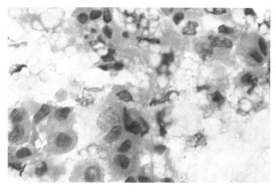

Fig. 9.7 Pancreatic pseudocyst
Degenerating atypical ductal epithelial cells; background of debris and inflammatory cells (Pap, HP)

4. Moderate amount of cytoplasm, often mucin vacuoles, indistinct cell borders.
5. Evidence of necrosis.

Most pancreatic adenocarcinomas are of ductal type. The neoplastic cells may have a columnar or cuboidal shape but the nuclei are more often rounded or ovoid than elongated. Focal palisading may be seen and microglandular patterns are often present (Figs 9.8 and 9.9). Carcinoma of acinar epithelial type is uncommon. In this type, the cells have smaller, rounded nuclei with prominent nucleoli, cell aggregates lack architectural patterns, and cell dissociation is prominent. Mixed patterns occur. Squamous differentiation is not uncommon in pancreatic adenocarcinoma and may be a prominent feature (adenosquamous carcinoma). Anaplastic pan-

RETROPERITONEUM, LIVER AND SPLEEN 9

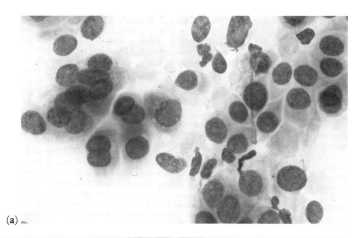

(a)

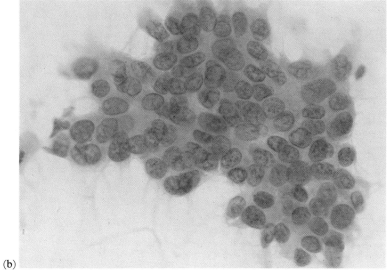

(b)

Fig. 9.8 Adenocarcinoma (pancreas)
Well-differentiated adenocarcinoma;
relatively mild nuclear atypia, but nuclear
crowding and some dissociation, and in
(b) a tendency to microacinar
arrangement. (a) MGG, HP. (b) H & E,
HP.

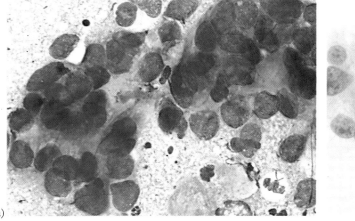

(a)

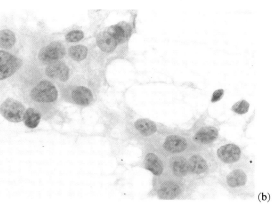

(b)

Fig. 9.9 Adenocarcinoma (pancreas)
Moderately differentiated adenocarcinoma; poorly cohesive clusters with some acinar arrangements; background of necrotic debris.
(a) MGG, HP. (b) H & E, HP.

9 *RETROPERITONEUM, LIVER AND SPLEEN*

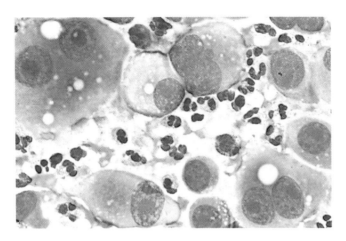

Fig. 9.10 Adenocarcinoma (pancreas)
Anaplastic giant cell carcinoma; dispersed large
pleomorphic cells; some multinucleate forms with
macronucleoli (MGG, HP)

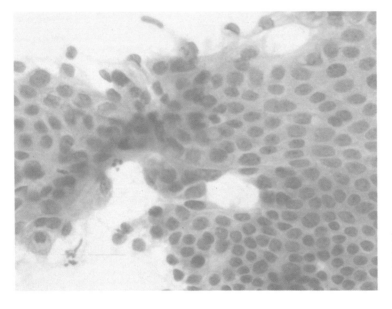

Fig. 9.11 Adenocarcinoma (pancreas)
A very well differentiated adenocarcinoma
presenting as cohesive, monolayered
sheets of moderately atypical cells
(Pap, HP).

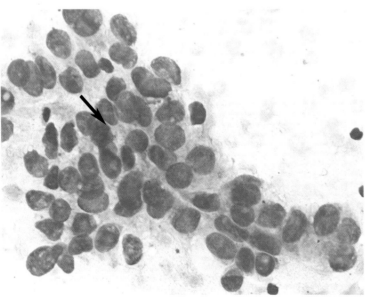

Fig. 9.12 Adenocarcinoma (bile duct)
Moderately differentiated
adenocarcinoma; loose aggregate of
malignant cells; some acinar-like
structures (arrow) (MGG, HP)

creatic carcinomas may have very large, pleomorphic, even bizarre and multinucleated giant cells which are largely dissociated (Fig. 9.10). Such tumours are difficult to distinguish from other anaplastic carcinomas, particularly from large cell anaplastic carcinoma of lung.[67]

Problems in diagnosis

1. Well differentiated adenocarcinoma.
2. Regenerative atypia.
3. Metastatic carcinoma.
4. Lymphoma.

Cohesive, monolayered sheets of glandular epithelial cells with a low nuclear/cytoplasmic ratio from a very well differentiated adenocarcinoma can look deceptively bland (Fig. 9.11). However, if there is nuclear and nucleolar enlargement, a few bizarre nuclei are usually found and the nuclear chromatin is abnormal compared to benign epithelial cells. Regenerative epithelial atypia in chronic pancreatitis and inflammatory bile duct disease may be severe enough to cause diagnostic difficulties as described above under pancreatitis (Fig. 9.4).[33,70] Regular, cohesive, monolayered sheets of cells favour a benign process, a microglandular pattern, nuclear crowding, dissociation of cells and evidence of necrosis favour carcinoma. Irregularities of nuclear chromatin

and of nuclear contours are important indicators of malignancy. Anisokaryosis, prominent nucleoli and mitotic figures may be seen in both. The cytological findings in *mucinous cystadenocarcinoma* of the pancreas have been described in several reports.[18,28,76]

Deposits of metastatic cancer within the pancreas or adjacent lymph nodes are common. This possibility should be considered whenever the cytological pattern deviates from that of typical adenocarcinoma. Whether an anaplastic carcinoma is most likely primary or metastatic depends mainly on the clinical findings. The pancreas is not an uncommon site for metastases from small cell undifferentiated carcinoma of lung, but this type of tumour can, although rarely, also be primary in the pancreas. The differential diagnosis between anaplastic carcinoma and lymphoma is discussed in Chapter 5.

A pancreatic adenocarcinoma of ductal type is cytologically indistinguishable from adenocarcinoma of extrahepatic bile duct origin (Fig. 9.12).

Islet cell tumours (Figs 9.13 and 9.14)[4,37,52]

Criteria for diagnosis

1. Many single and loosely grouped cells in rows or poorly formed follicles.

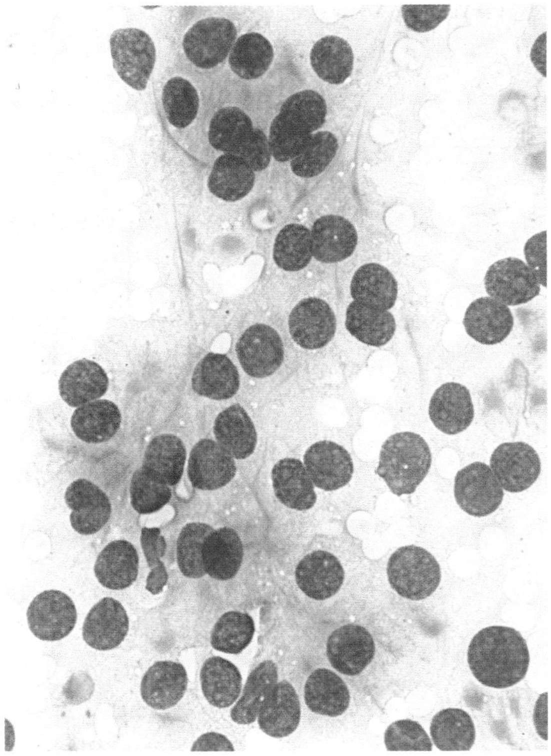

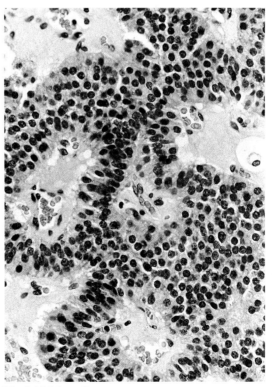

Fig. 9.13 Islet cell tumour
Mainly dispersed cells with uniformly round nuclei, moderate anisokaryosis; delicate cytoplasm; a suggestion of follicular pattern (MGG, HP)

Fig. 9.14 Islet cell tumour
Tissue section; same case as Figure 9.13; trabecular and solid pattern (H & E, IP)

9 *RETROPERITONEUM, LIVER AND SPLEEN*

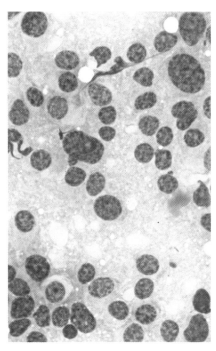

Fig. 9.15 Carcinoid tumour
Dispersed population of cells with round nuclei; moderate anisokaryosis; speckled chromatin; fragile cytoplasm (MGG, HP)

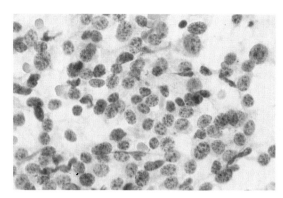

Fig. 9.16 Carcinoid tumour
Dispersed cells; round nuclei and speckled chromatin; fragile cytoplasm (H & E, HP)

plastic cells can be identified by immunocytochemical methods, a more specific diagnosis can be made with confidence. Another difficult problem is to decide if a tumour in this group is benign or malignant. In general, nuclear atypia and pleomorphism cannot be relied on as cytological criteria of malignancy in endocrine tumours.[47]

2. Anisokaryosis but a 'bland' or speckled nuclear chromatin.
3. 1–3 small nucleoli.
4. Poorly defined, finely granular cytoplasm, often dispersed in the background.

The neoplastic cells are mainly dissociated, but also tend to form loose acinar or follicular clusters and curved or circular rows. Nuclear anisokaryosis may be prominent, but the nuclear chromatin pattern varies little between cells. The chromatin is evenly distributed, coarsely granular or 'speckled'. The small nucleoli are not easily seen in Giemsa-stained smears. Due to its fragility the cytoplasm is often dispersed in the background, and where it is preserved around nuclei, cell borders are indistinct. A very fine, red granularity is often discernible in MGG smears under high magnification (Fig. 9.13). Clumps of amyloid may occasionally be seen.

The cytological pattern of most islet cell tumours is characteristic enough to be easily distinguished from that of pancreatic adenocarcinoma; however, the many variants within this group of tumours, for example, insulin-producing tumours, gastrinomas, non-functioning islet cell tumours, and *carcinoids*[46,47] (Figs 9.15–9.17) cannot be separated on the basis of routine cytological smears. If the secretory products of the neo-

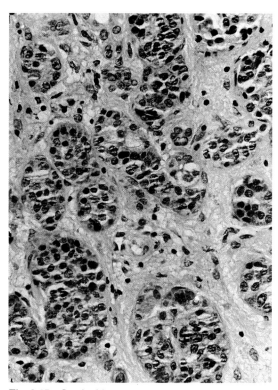

Fig. 9.17 Carcinoid tumour
Tissue section; same case as Figures 9.15 and 9.16; solid nests of uniform tumour cells (H & E, IP)

RETROPERITONEUM, LIVER AND SPLEEN 9

INTRA-ABDOMINAL TUMOURS

Most tumours of the gastrointestinal tract are adenocarcinomas of a variable degree of differentiation without specific cytological characteristics. The origin of the tumour is usually indicated by clinical and radiological findings but cytological features may be helpful. For example, a poorly differentiated adenocarcinoma of signet ring cells with intracytoplasmic mucin vacuoles is most likely of gastric origin, a well differentiated adenocarcinoma of columnar cells showing a palisaded arrangement, and with a tendency to necrosis has probably arisen from the large bowel. However, distinction from adenocarcinoma of pancreas, biliary tract or the female genital tract is often not possible.

The cytological characteristics of carcinoid tumours are described on page 193, those of lymphoma in Chapter 5, and those of benign and malignant smooth muscle tumours in Chapter 11. The following case is an example of an uncommon neural tumour arising from small bowel wall, diagnosed by FNA.

A 60-year-old man presented with an abdominal mass shown on CT to arise within mesentery. Percutaneous FNA revealed a spindle cell tumour of mesenchymal appearance thought to be either of smooth muscle, fibroblastic or neural origin. Ultrastructural assessment of aspirated material suggested a neural tumour of the type recently described as 'gastrointestinal autonomic nerve tumour' (GANT), a biologically aggressive neoplasm with metastatic potential. At laparotomy, the lesion was 9 cm in diameter, well-circumscribed, invading through bowel wall to mucosa. Immunohistochemistry and EM confirmed the diagnosis of GANT. Neurosecretory granules were frequent, and staining with antibodies to synaptophysin, S-100 and NSE was observed. There was vimentin positivity but no desmin staining (Figs 9.18–19).

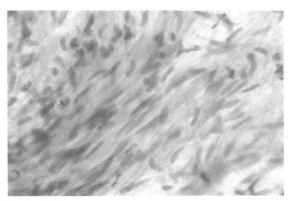

Fig. 9.18 Gastrointestinal autonomic nerve tumour
Cohesive tissue fragment of bland-looking spindle cells resembling Schwannoma. Re. result of immunohistochemistry, see text (Pap, HP).

RETROPERITONEAL LYMPH NODES

The cytological presentation of different types of metastatic carcinomas in lymph nodes and of malignant lymphoma are described in Chapter 5. Cancers of the urogenital tract, of the large bowel, and of the pancreas are the most frequent sources of metastases in retroperitoneal nodes. The possibility of a germ cell tumour should be considered in cases without a known primary.[38,73] These tumours have a fairly characteristic presentation in FNA smears (see Ch. 10), although we have seen examples of primary germ cell tumours in the retroperitoneum and mediastinum with a distinctly squamoid appearance in smears causing diagnostic difficulties. Metastatic renal cell carcinoma, transitional cell carcinoma, and prostatic adenocarcinoma can also be recognised if the cancer is not too poorly differenti-

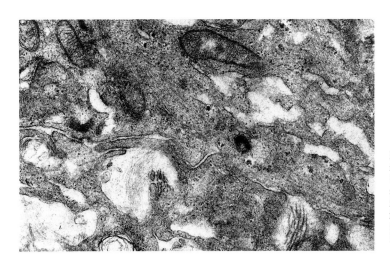

Fig. 9.19 Gastrointestinal autonomic nerve tumour
Several interleaving tumour cell processes showing numerous microtubules and irregularly arranged cytoplasmic filaments. EM of fine needle aspirate × 34 100, same case as Fig. 9.18 (courtesy of Dr D. V. Spagnolo).

9 *RETROPERITONEUM, LIVER AND SPLEEN*

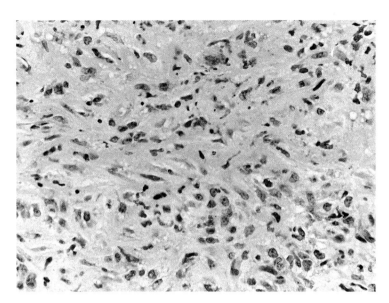

Fig. 9.20 Sclerosing lymphoma
Tissue section; non-Hodgkin's lymphoma with extensive sclerosis (H & E, IP)

ated. Squamous cell carcinoma usually originates from the uterine cervix, or, occasionally, from the bladder. Ovarian, endometrial, pancreatic and colorectal adenocarcinomas are more difficult to separate cytologically.

The tendency to fibrosis shown by some malignant lymphomas of retroperitoneal nodes can cause diagnostic problems, mainly due to the difficulty in obtaining a sufficient number of cells with a fine needle (Fig. 9.20). One may have to resort to a Rotex screw needle or a 22 gauge core biopsy needle in such cases. The criteria for diagnosis of retroperitoneal lymphoma are the same as those given for peripheral lymph nodes.

RETROPERITONEUM PROPER

The soft tissues of the retroperitoneum can give rise to a great variety of neoplasms, both benign and malignant. Criteria for cytological diagnosis of some of these tumours have yet to be clearly defined. Of malignant soft tissue tumours occurring in the retroperitoneum, liposarcoma, leiomyosarcoma, and malignant fibrous histiocytoma are the most common. Rhabdomyosarcoma is seen mainly in children. Fibrosarcoma and neurogenic sarcoma are rare in this site. Among benign soft tissue tumours, the fibromatoses, xanthogranuloma, lipoma, leiomyoma, neurinoma, neurofibroma, and angiomatous tumours should be mentioned. The cytological findings in soft tissue tumours in general are described and illustrated in Chapter 11. However, a few uncommon lesions which we have only encountered in the retroperitoneum will be presented in this section.

Aneurysm
Arterial aneurysm is a contraindication to needle biopsy. However, an aneurysm which is filled with old throm-

bus can be mistaken for a solid tumour clinically and radiologically and thus be subjected to FNA. Smears show mainly altered blood, amorphous debris, and a few macrophages with intracytoplasmic lipid droplets and blood pigment. There may be some degenerating cells and nuclei the nature of which cannot be identified and which may raise a suspicion of necrotic tumour. An aspirate of this appearance from an appropriate site should make one aware of the possibility of an aneurysm so that further non-invasive investigations are undertaken.

Cystic lymphangioma[65]
Smears of fluid aspirated from a cystic lymphangioma show only lymphoid cells, mainly small lymphocytes, in variable numbers. Its presentation is illustrated by the following case.

A 66-year-old man was investigated for suspected abdominal aortic aneurysm. A CT scan demonstrated a round mass below the left kidney between the aorta and the psoas muscle which was clearly separated from the aorta. The mass appeared to be cystic on ultrasonography. FNA yielded several millilitres of milky fluid and the mass decreased considerably in size. Smears of the fluid showed numerous normal lymphocytes. A diagnosis of cystic lymphangioma was made and follow up was uneventful.

Haemangiopericytoma (Figs 9.21–9.25)[53,54]
We have seen aspirates from a few cases of haemangiopericytoma. In one of these the cytological findings allowed us to suggest the correct diagnosis.

A 62-year-old man had some months history of increasing pelvic pain on defaecation. A firm mass was felt between the sacrum and the posterior rectal wall. FNA performed per rectum yielded abundant blood but also many tumour cells in closely packed aggregates (Fig. 9.21). The cells were elongated

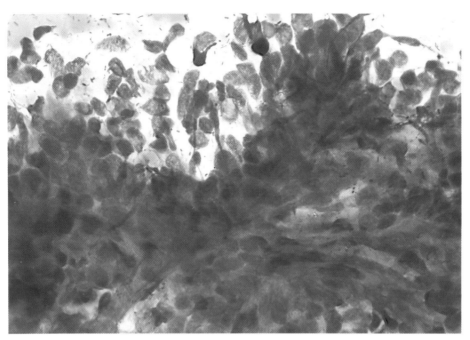

Fig. 9.21 Malignant haemangiopericytoma
Cohesive fragment of mesenchymal tissue; spindle cells fanning out from a vascular core (MGG, HP)

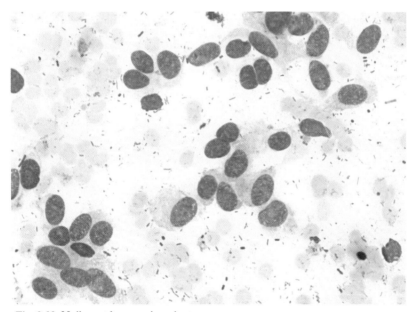

Fig. 9.22 Malignant haemangiopericytoma
Dispersed endothelial-like spindle cells; uniform ovoid nuclei and indistinct cytoplasm (MGG, HP)

or spindle-shaped and appeared to radiate out from a central core of red-pink (MGG) basement membrane-like material. Many single cells were also seen which resembled endothelial cells. The nuclei were ovoid or elongated and measured on average 10 × 30 μm. They were relatively uniform and had an evenly distributed granular nuclear chromatin and inconspicuous nucleoli. Many nuclei were bare, others had a moderate amount of pale, fragile cytoplasm and indistinct cell borders (Fig. 9.22). Mitoses were not seen, but the high cellularity of the tumour tissue raised a suspicion of a low-grade malignancy.

9 *RETROPERITONEUM, LIVER AND SPLEEN*

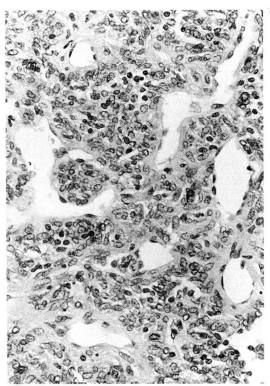

Fig. 9.23 Malignant haemangiopericytoma
Tissue section; same case as Figures 9.21 and 9.22; classical
pattern (H & E, IP)

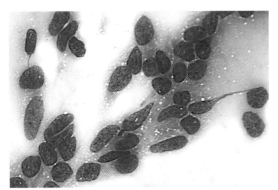

Fig. 9.24 Malignant haemangiopericytoma
Loose aggregate of cells with dark ovoid or elongated nuclei,
scant cytoplasm and some nuclear moulding (MGG, HP)

Histologically, the tumour was regarded as probably malignant
on the basis of its large size, the presence of necrosis and its
focally infiltrating borders (Fig. 9.23). Some months after the
tumour was excised, a solitary lung metastasis was found.

Predominantly solid variants of haemangiopericytoma
may be difficult to recognise cytologically as a vasoformative tumour (Figs 9.24 and 9.25). Variants with
larger cells may simulate epithelial papillary tumours.
The diagnosis can be supported by EM of the aspirate.

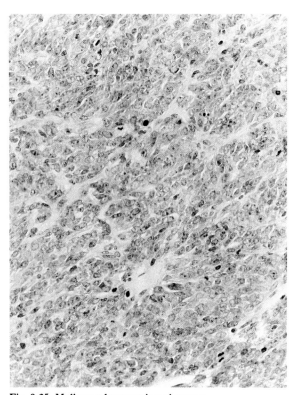

Fig. 9.25 Malignant haemangiopericytoma
Tissue section; same case as Figure 9.24; predominantly solid
pattern (H & E, IP)

Non-chromaffin paraganglioma (Figs 9.26 and 9.27)[64]
We have only seen one example of this tumour in the
retroperitoneum, in which the correct diagnosis was
suggested on FNA smears (see also p. 43).

A 40-year-old man presented with a large palpable retroperitoneal mass. A FNA biopsy done as one of the initial investigations raised the possibility of paraganglioma. The differential

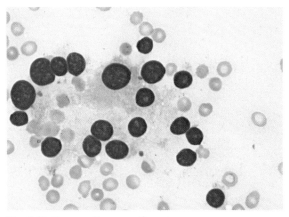

Fig. 9.26 Paraganglioma; malignant
Loose follicular cluster of cells with small round dark nuclei
resembling thyroid epithelium and with indistinct very finely
granular cytoplasm (MGG, HP)

RETROPERITONEUM, LIVER AND SPLEEN

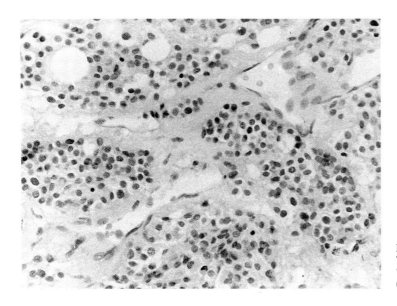

Fig. 9.27 Paraganglioma; malignant
Tissue section; same case as Figure 9.26;
'Zellballen' in a vascular stroma
(H & E, IP)

diagnosis included other APUD tumours such as carcinoid and phaeochromocytoma, but also metastasis of follicular thyroid carcinoma and of renal cell carcinoma. The diagnosis was confirmed by surgical biopsy at laparotomy. The tumour metastasised widely and the patient died 4 months later. The tumour apparently arose from the organ of Zuckerkandl. Smears showed a moderate number of cells, single and in loose acinar/follicular clusters resembling thyroid follicular epithelial cells. Nuclei were uniformly round and small, about the size of lymphocytes, but there was a moderate degree of anisokaryosis. The nuclear chromatin was granular and evenly distributed, the nucleoli were indistinct. The cytoplasm was abundant, pale, without distinct cell borders. Many cells showed a fine, distinct red cytoplasmic granularity (MGG), which together with cell dispersal and absence of pleomorphism suggested an APUD tumour (Fig. 9.26). Serum catecholamines were not significantly raised, but abundant neurosecretory granules were demonstrated by EM.

A case of follicular carcinoma of the thyroid metastasising to para-aortic lymph nodes allowed us to compare smears of thyroid carcinoma and of paraganglioma in the same site. The similarity was striking, except that the cells from the thyroid carcinoma lacked cytoplasmic granulation.

ADRENALS

Non-neoplastic lesions
Haemorrhage within the adrenal is not always symptomatic and an *old haematoma* is sometimes discovered incidentally by CT examination. It is of course difficult or impossible to decide by FNA biopsy if an old haematoma is spontaneous or if it represents a centrally necrotic tumour. Smears must be screened carefully for identifiable tumour cells.

Fluid aspirated from adrenal *cysts* is, like cyst fluid from other sites, usually acellular or contains only a few macrophages.[135] Smears from *myelolipoma* show a mixture of fat droplets, fat cells and haematopoetic cells.[108,121,132]

Metastatic carcinoma
The confirmation or exclusion of metastatic carcinoma is the main indication for FNA biopsy. The primary is most commonly in the lung. The cytological findings are the same as in metastatic cancers in any other site and will not be further discussed here.

Adrenal cortical adenoma (Fig. 9.28)

Criteria for diagnosis

1. Large number of epithelial cells, single and in loose monolayered sheets.
2. Many stripped nuclei; background of lipid droplets.
3. Some cells with abundant vacuolated cytoplasm and indistinct cell borders.
4. Uniformly round, small, dark nuclei; anisokaryosis may be prominent.

The cortical adenomas which become subjected to FNA are usually asymptomatic tumours detected by abdominal CT in the preoperative investigation of patients with potentially resectable lung tumours. The indication for biopsy is the need to exclude metastatic cancer. Smears are quite cellular. The cells are not very cohesive and are seen single, in groups, and in loose

9 RETROPERITONEUM, LIVER AND SPLEEN

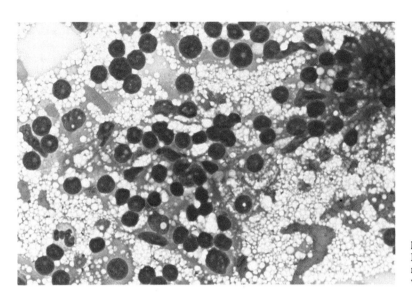

Fig. 9.28 Adrenal cortical adenoma
Poorly cohesive cells, mainly small, round
nuclei, prominent cytoplasmic lipid
vacuoles (MGG, HP)

monolayered sheets without a distinct architectural pattern. A large proportion of the cells appear as stripped nuclei with a background of lipid droplets, but some have an abundant cytoplasm containing many relatively large lipid vacuoles. Lipofuscin pigment may be seen. The nuclei are generally small and uniformly round and have one or several prominent nucleoli. Anisokaryosis may be prominent. Nuclear chromatin is granular and evenly distributed. As with other endocrine tumours, the cytological pattern does not allow a confident prediction of biological behaviour. Nuclear pleomorphism is not an indicator of malignancy; irregularity of nuclear chromatin and evidence of tumour necrosis carry more weight. Distinction between adrenal cortical adenoma and low grade renal cell tumour can also be a problem.

Both are composed of cells with abundant, vacuolated cytoplasm, a low nuclear/cytoplasmic ratio, and small, round, bland nuclei. However, the architectural pattern of cells adhering to vascular structures is more typical of renal cell tumour, and the cytoplasmic lipid vacuoles appear larger and more discrete in adrenal cortical adenoma. The radiological appearances are helpful in most cases.

Adrenal cortical carcinoma (Fig. 9.29)[115]
As has already been stated, the cytological pattern is not a reliable indicator of clinical behaviour of adrenal cortical tumours. At one end of the spectrum are the adenomas showing a bland, clearly benign cytology, at the other, poorly differentiated carcinomas with severe

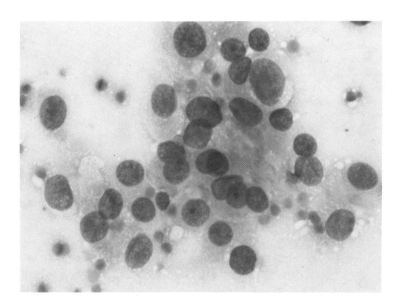

Fig. 9.29 Adrenal cortical carcinoma
Cluster of pleomorphic cells with an
acinar pattern; abundant fragile, finely
vacuolated cytoplasm (compare Fig. 9.43)
(MGG, HP)

RETROPERITONEUM, LIVER AND SPLEEN 9

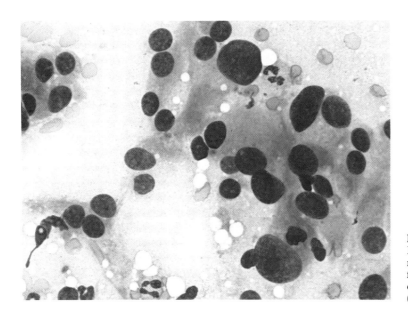

Fig. 9.30 Phaeochromocytoma
Loose cluster of cells with pleomorphic nuclei, some large nucleoli, and fragile finely granular cytoplasm; nuclear chromatin uniformly granular (MGG, HP)

pleomorphism, nuclear chromatin abnormalities and very large nucleoli. Tumours which have a cytological pattern intermediate to these cannot be confidently classified as benign or malignant on cytology alone. In addition, the cytological pattern of adrenal cortical carcinoma is similar, sometimes indistinguishable from that of renal cell carcinoma (see p. 241). Clinical findings, including any evidence of hormone secretion by the tumour, and angiography usually establish the correct diagnosis. Histochemical and ultrastructural examination may be of some help.

Phaeochromocytoma (Fig. 9.30)[122]

Criteria for diagnosis

1. Many dispersed and loosely clustered neoplastic cells.
2. Prominent anisokaryosis, bland nuclear chromatin.
3. Abundant, poorly defined cytoplasm; fine red granularity (MGG).
4. Prominent nucleoli.

FNA biopsy of suspected phaeochromocytoma has been regarded as contraindicated in view of the risk of precipitating a hypertensive crisis. This risk may have been exaggerated; no complications were recorded in the cases reported in the literature, nor in the few cases we have biopsied. The only hypertensive reaction we have observed in relation to FNA biopsy was in a case of adrenal cortical adenoma. Also, since phaeochromocytoma may be an unexpected finding and may occur in extra-adrenal sites, the cytopathologist should be familiar with its cytological pattern.

Smears tend to be rich in cells which are to a large extent dissociated, but which may form loose, some-

times acinar clusters. Anisokaryosis is quite marked and some very large nuclei may be seen. Binucleate cells occur. The nuclear chromatin is uniformly dense, granular and evenly distributed. The nuclei have single large or multiple smaller nucleoli; intranuclear inclusions can also be seen. The cytoplasm is abundant and fragile and shows a red granularity (MGG); some granules may be quite coarse. Cell borders are indistinct. Due to fragmentation of the cytoplasm, the red granules are also seen diffusely in the background (Fig. 9.30). The pattern closely resembles that of medullary carcinoma of the thyroid, non-chromaffin paraganglioma, and other APUD tumours. Chromaffin tests can be carried out on FNA smears.

Neuroblastoma (Fig. 9.31)[119]

Smears from a neuroblastoma basically show the pattern of a malignant small round cell tumour similar to that of small cell anaplastic carcinoma, Wilms' tumour,

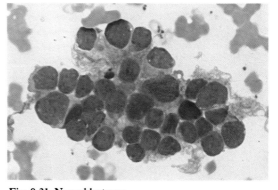

Fig. 9.31 Neuroblastoma
Cell aggregate; irregular hyperchromatic nuclei; note the small amount of fibrillar intercellular material (MGG, HP)

9 RETROPERITONEUM, LIVER AND SPLEEN

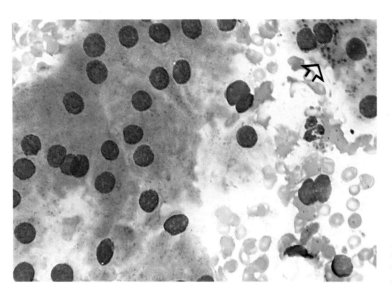

Fig. 9.32 Kidney; proximal tubule
Monolayered sheet of large cells with abundant granular cytoplasm and small dark nuclei; note coarse cytoplasmic granules in some cells (arrow) (MGG, HP)

embryonal rhabdomyosarcoma, etc. Characteristic rosettes of tumour cells in the centre of which there is finely fibrillar, pink staining (MGG) material, are sometimes found (Fig. 9.31). However, rosette-like structures may also be seen in Ewing's sarcoma (p. 331). Nuclear pleomorphism is less prominent than in small cell anaplastic carcinoma. Whenever possible, the diagnosis should be confirmed by ultrastructural studies of the aspirate.

We have no personal experience of FNA of *ganglioneuroblastoma* and *ganglioneuroma*. The diagnosis rests with the recognition of ganglion cells amongst neuroblasts or Schwann cells and fibroblasts.[56,58,59]

THE KIDNEY

Normal structures; cortical pseudotumour
(Figs 9.32–9.34)[142]

1. Tubular epithelial cells — large, intermediate and small — from different levels of the nephron.
2. Whole glomeruli or fragments of glomeruli.
3. Absence of necrosis or haemorrhage.

In FNA biopsy of renal tumours, the mass is sometimes missed by the needle and the adjacent renal tissue is sampled. Such smears must be recognised as representing normal tissue and must not be mistaken for low-grade renal cell tumour. Furthermore, focal hyperplasia of renal cortical tissue, either as a mass at the convexity of the kidney (cortical pseudotumour) or as a rounded expansion of a medullary pyramid (inversion of renal lobule or lobular dysmorphism), may simulate an avascular solid tumour radiologically. FNA smears from such lesions contain only normal cells. The hallmark of renal cortical tissue — normal or pseudotumour — is

the co-existence of epithelial cells from different parts of the nephron, and the presence of glomeruli (not always found).

The predominant cell type, large epithelial cells from the proximal convoluted tubules, can be mistaken for cells from a well-differentiated renal cell tumour of granular cell type. The cells have abundant, pale eosinophilic (grey-blue in MGG), finely granular cytoplasm, indistinct cell borders, relatively small, uniform, round nuclei, and one or two small nucleoli (Fig. 9.32). Intracytoplasmic vacuoles do not occur in normal tubular epithelial cells. Single cells and stripped nuclei may be seen but most of the cells form monolayered sheets with some alveolar arrangement. Cells of intermediate size, from the distal convoluted tubules, also lack distinct cell borders. The small tubular epithelial cells from the loop

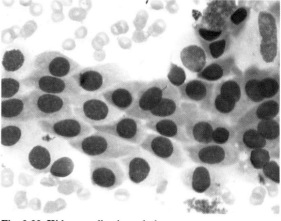

Fig. 9.33 Kidney; collecting tubule
Cast-like sheet of epithelial cells of moderate size; dense cytoplasm; uniform nuclei (MGG, HP)

RETROPERITONEUM, LIVER AND SPLEEN 9

of Henle and from the collecting tubules do have distinct cell borders and are seen in sheets with a roof-tile pattern or as short tubular segments (Fig. 9.33). These cells may contain coarse, dark, cytoplasmic granules, which are probably lipofuscin. Aggregates of tubular epithelial cells may include strands of hyaline material staining pink with MGG, probably representing basement membrane. This is a feature shared with renal cell tumours. Glomeruli appear in smears as tight clusters of small, spindly endothelial cells with indistinct cytoplasm and intervening strands of pink (MGG) basement membrane material. The clusters have a lobulated shape similar to glomerular tufts in histological sections, but may of course be rather distorted by the smear action (Fig. 9.34).[129]

Cysts (Figs . 9.35–9.37)

Criteria for diagnosis

1. A large volume of thin, clear fluid.
2. Few degenerating epithelial cells and cyst macrophages.
3. Absence of necrotic debris or old blood.

The diagnosis of a simple renal cyst can now be made so confidently by ultrasonographic examination that cytological confirmation is rarely necessary.

Occasionally the number of cells in the cyst fluid may be surprisingly large and macrophages may appear moderately pleomorphic and atypical (Fig. 9.35). This may

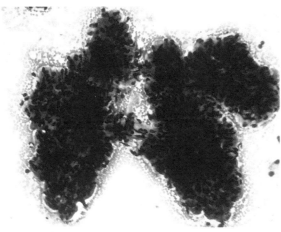

Fig. 9.34 Glomerulus
Glomerular tuft with some separation of lobules (MGG, LP)

raise the suspicion of a cystic tumour, but if the radiological appearances are typical of a cyst and if the aspirated fluid is clear, there is no reason to suspect malignancy. On the other hand, if the fluid contains old blood and/or necrotic debris, a neoplasm must be strongly suspected even if tumour cells cannot be identified in the smears. The biopsy procedure can of course cause fresh bleeding which can make it difficult to confidently exclude a neoplasm. The presence of a carcinoma within the wall of an apparently solitary simple cyst is a rare but well-recognised event in which the malignant component risks to be missed by needle biopsy.[107,110]

We have seen one case in consultation of a *solitary multiloculated cyst* of the kidney in which the aspirate contained quite atypical cells, single and in clusters (Fig. 9.36). Most of the cells were probably macro-

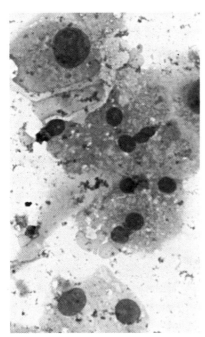

Fig. 9.35 Renal cyst macrophages
Atypical macrophages in a simple renal cyst (MGG, HP)

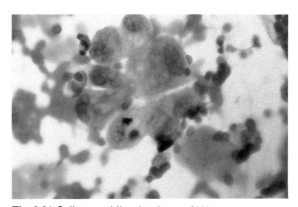

Fig. 9.36 Solitary multiloculated cyst of kidney
Clusters of histiocyte-like cells with large, excentric, atypical nuclei (Pap, HP) (courtesy of Dr B. H. Coombes, Southport, Queensland)

RETROPERITONEUM, LIVER AND SPLEEN

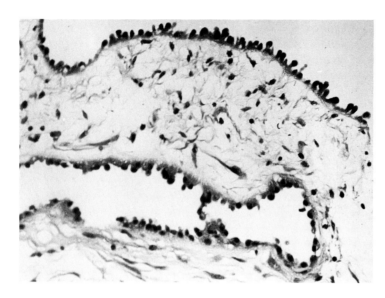

Fig. 9.37 Solitary multiloculated cyst of kidney
Tissue section, same case as Fig. 9.36; hob nail-type cells with similarly atypical nuclei lining some of the cyst wall
(H & E, IP)

phages, but some could represent the hobnail type of epithelial cells lining some of the cystic spaces (Fig. 9.37).

Abscess
The aspirate is purulent and smears show mainly degenerating polymorphs and macrophages. A few normal or degenerating tubular epithelial cells may be present. Part of the aspirate should be submitted for culture.

Xanthogranulomatous pyelonephritis[138]
Zajicek has pointed out that macrophages from xanthogranulomatous pyelonephritis with finely vacuolated cytoplasm may look quite atypical, particularly in air-dried, MGG-stained smears, and may suggest renal cell carcinoma.[142] We have not yet seen such a case, but we have seen chronic inflammatory processes involving adipose tissue in other sites with a similar cytologic pattern (Fig. 9.38). The overall inflammatory pattern of the smear should be appreciated, and the histiocytic nature of the atypical cells recognised, perhaps more easily in alcohol-fixed smears.

Angiomyolipoma of kidney (Figs 9.39–9.41)[125,128]

Criteria for diagnosis

1. Spindle cells with features of smooth muscle cells.
2. Syncytial aggregates.
3. A background of blood and prominent fat droplets.

The nuclei are elongated or spindle-shaped and often have characteristically truncated ends. Their size and shape is moderately variable. The nuclear chromatin is finely granular, the granules sometimes form parallel rows. The eosinophilic cytoplasm (grey-blue in MGG)

forms a syncytial background to the nuclei; cell borders are not visible. Large fat vacuoles are intimately associated with the spindle cells (Fig. 9.39).

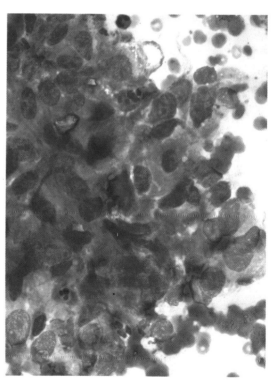

Fig. 9.38 Xanthogranulomatous inflammation
Cluster of somewhat foamy reactive macrophages (MGG, HP)

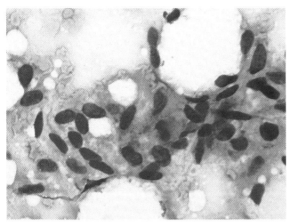

Fig. 9.39 Angiomyolipoma
Spindle cells of benign appearance; large fat vacuoles
(MGG, HP)

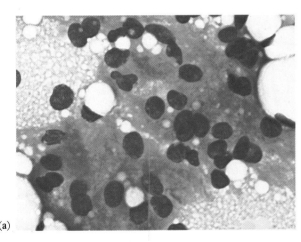

(a)

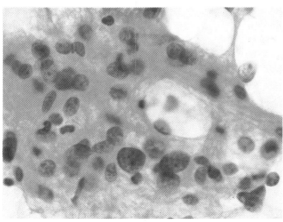

(b)

Fig. 9.40 Angiomyolipoma (atypical)
(a) Unusual round cell pattern; note syncytial, relatively dense
cytoplasm and prominent fat vacuoles (MGG, HP). (b) Note
the cytoplasmic eosinophilia and some spindle-shaped nuclei
(H & E, HP).

Problems in diagnosis

Highly cellular areas in an angiomyolipoma may have a
predominantly round cell, epithelioid pattern (Figs 9.40
and 9.41). In cytological preparations this appearance
can be mistaken for a low-grade renal cell tumour of
granular cell type. However, the cytoplasm of smooth
muscle cells is not granular or vacuolated, it is eosinophilic and relatively dense. Some typical spindle-
shaped nuclei can usually be found also in predominantly round cell areas. Background fat droplets are more
prominent than in smears from a renal cell tumour.
Strands of basement membrane material intimately
associated with tumour cells are a characteristic feature
of renal cell tumours, but not of angiomyolipoma.

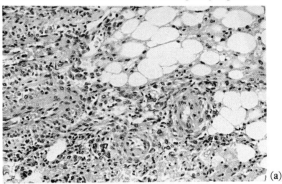

(a)

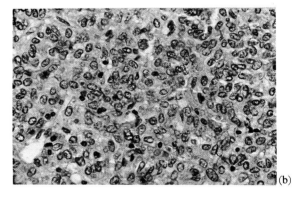

(b)

Fig. 9.41 Angiomyolipoma (atypical)
Tissue section; same case as Figure 9.40. (a) Typical pattern
(H & E, IP). (b) Round cell pattern (H & E, HP).

Renal cell tumour (Figs 9.42–9.48)[99,105,116,123]

Criteria for diagnosis

1. Smears either rich in cells or showing mainly
   necrosis or haemorrhage.
2. Single cells and sheet-like, alveolar or papillary
   aggregates.
3. Abundant cytoplasm — pale (but not clear) with
   lipid droplets or finely granular.
4. Anisokaryosis; low nuclear/cytoplasmic ratio.

9 *RETROPERITONEUM, LIVER AND SPLEEN*

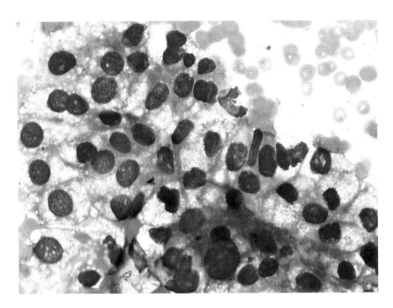

Fig. 9.42 Renal cell carcinoma; grade I tumour
Cohesive cluster of cells with small nuclei and abundant vacuolated cytoplasm (MGG, HP)

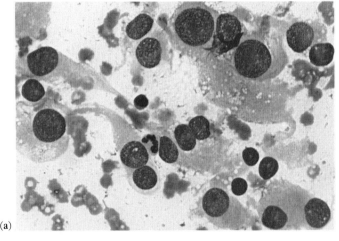

(a)

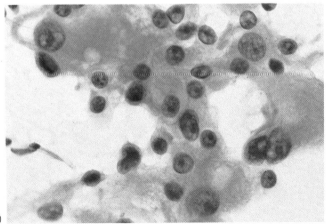

(b)

Fig. 9.43 Renal cell carcinoma; grade II tumour
Poorly cohesive cells; pleomorphic nuclei with some prominent nucleoli; abundant vacuolated cytoplasm. (a) MGG, HP. (b) H & E, HP.

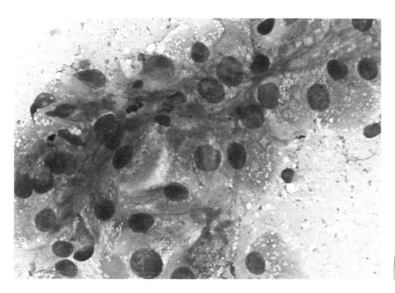

Fig. 9.44 Renal cell carcinoma; grade II tumour
Moderately cohesive large cells adhering to a strand of pink basement membrane material (MGG, HP)

5. Bland nuclear chromatin (low-grade tumours); macronucleoli (high-grade tumours).
6. Intranuclear vacuoles common.
7. Tumour cells adhering to strands of basement membrane material.

Since one cannot distinguish between adenoma and well-differentiated carcinoma on the cytological pattern alone, renal cell tumours are best reported as low-, intermediate-, or high-grade. The management of these cases is based also on clinical and radiological findings and on tumour size. Histological grading appears to be a useful indicator of prognosis. In spite of the variability of patterns within a given tumour which is often seen in histological sections, von Schreeb demonstrated good agreement between cytological and histological grading in a series of 47 renal cell tumours.[137] In our own experience, there is a tendency for the cytological grade to be lower than the histological grade because of limited sampling.[128] Selective sampling has been shown to diminish the value of DNA measurements on fine needle aspirates of renal cell cancers in some series.[117]

The tumour cells are often arranged along or around strands of hyaline or fibrillary material staining a characteristic pink colour with MGG (Fig. 9.44). This material probably represents the basement membrane or wall of sinusoidal blood vessels. Cytological grading is based on an evaluation of nuclear size, nuclear pleomorphism, chromatin pattern, N/C ratio, degree of cell cohesion, and mitotic activity. Cell cohesion is high in low-grade tumours, poor in high-grade tumours. Prominent nuclear pleomorphism, macronucleoli and an increasing N/C ratio also indicate a high-grade tumour (Fig. 9.45). In low-grade tumours, the nuclear morphology does not meet the usual criteria of malignancy, the chromatin

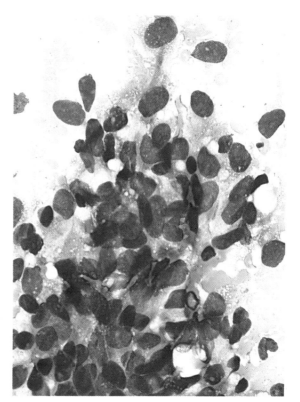

Fig. 9.45 Renal cell carcinoma; grade III tumour
Poorly cohesive pleomorphic malignant cells; high N/C ratio but finely vacuolated cytoplasm still discernible (MGG, HP)

pattern is bland (Fig. 9.42). Intranuclear cytoplasmic inclusions are seen in about one-third of renal cell tumours.

9 *RETROPERITONEUM, LIVER AND SPLEEN*

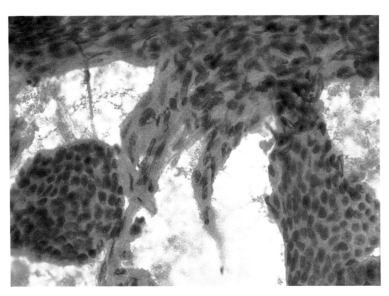

Fig. 9.46 Renal cell carcinoma; papillary type
Papillary fragments of bland epithelial cells; prominent, cellular stroma (H & E, HP)

Problems in diagnosis

1. Normal tubular epithelial cells.
2. Xanthogranulomatous pyelonephritis (p. 240).
3. Angiomyolipoma (p. 240).
4. Massive necrosis and haemorrhage.
5. Anaplastic malignancy of other types.
6. Papillary variant of renal cell carcinoma.
7. Renal oncocytoma.

Epithelial cells of proximal convoluted tubules may be mistaken for granular tumour cells. This problem has been mentioned in relation to cortical pseudotumours (p. 238). Smears of non-neoplastic renal cortical tissue are best recognised by the presence, side by side, of tubular epithelial cells of distinctly different types and of occasional glomeruli. Some non-neoplastic tubular epithelial cells may be found in an aspirate from a tumour, but in this situation their presence may in fact be helpful in bringing out the contrast between normal and neoplastic cells. Some cells with intracytoplasmic lipid droplets are usually seen also in predominantly granular cell tumours.

Massive necrosis or haemorrhage is a common problem, particularly in very large tumours. From a practical point of view, necrotic material aspirated from a solid renal mass is highly suggestive of carcinoma even in the absence of preserved neoplastic cells.

Anaplastic renal cell carcinoma with a sarcoma-like pattern can present diagnostic problems also in histopathology. The cytopathologist can only report the presence of anaplastic malignant tumour cells and exact typing has to be deferred. Renal cell carcinoma can also be indistinguishable from adrenal cortical carcinoma in routine smears (Fig. 9.29).

The cytological presentation of the *papillary variant* of *renal cell carcinoma* (Fig. 9.46) has been described.[98]

The neoplastic cells have small, bland, uniform nuclei which look cytologically benign. Papillary fragments occur. There are numerous macrophages in the background.

Renal oncocytoma (Figs 9.47 and 9.48) is an increasingly recognised neoplasm in which the neoplastic cells are fairly uniform and have abundant, granular, eosinophilic cytoplasm and small blond nuclei. Absence of necrosis and monotonous pattern of cells of oncocytic type might alert one to this diagnosis.[92,97,124,134] However, caution in making the diagnosis on the basis of a FNA biopsy is warranted, as some renal cell carcinomas may contain areas identical to oncocytoma which may have been selectively sampled.[95]

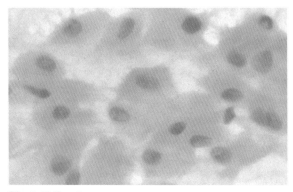

Fig. 9.47 Renal oncocytoma
Only tumour cells with small bland nuclei and abundant, eosinophilic, finely granular cytoplasm seen in multiple smears (H & E, HP)

RETROPERITONEUM, LIVER AND SPLEEN 9

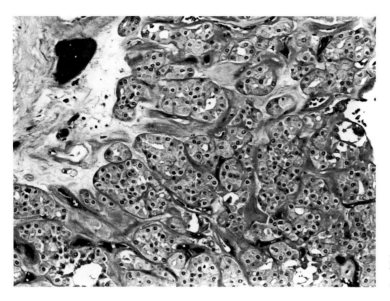

Fig. 9.48 Renal oncocytoma
Tissue section, same case as Fig. 9.47 (H & E, IP)

Wilms' tumour (Figs 9.49–9.51)[133,141]

Usual findings

1. Numerous small cells, single and in tight clusters.
2. Small, round or ovoid, hyperchromatic nuclei; multiple small nucleoli.
3. Scanty blue cytoplasm (MGG).
4. A bimodal cell population.
5. Tubular structures, palisades or cords (epithelial cells).
6. Clusters of spindle cells (mesenchymal cells).

To make a confident diagnosis of Wilms' tumour one would like to see a mixture of malignant, poorly differentiated epithelial and mesenchymal cells, the former forming tubular patterns (Figs 9.49 and 9.50). How-

ever, it is difficult to distinguish between epithelial and mesenchymal cells in FNA smears other than by their arrangement, and tubular patterns may be poorly formed in poorly differentiated tumours. Clinical and radiological findings must of course be taken into account when smears are evaluated.

The differential diagnosis of malignant small round cell tumours such as small cell anaplastic carcinoma, malignant lymphoma, neuroblastoma, embryonal rhabdomyosarcoma, Ewing's sarcoma, Merkel cell carcinoma and Wilms' tumour, is a difficult problem. Distinguishing features in routine smears are rather subtle. Nuclear moulding is particularly prominent in small cell anaplastic carcinoma, cytoplasm is minimal and nucleoli are absent in the classical type. Tight cell clusters are rarely a feature in lymphoma, lymphoid glo-

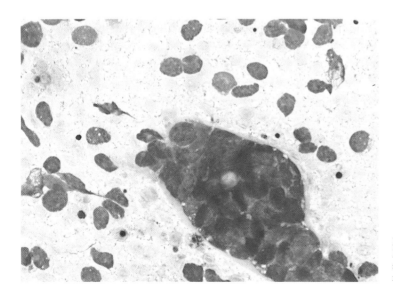

Fig. 9.49 Wilms' tumour
Biphasic tumour; cohesive tubular structure, and undifferentiated mesenchymal cells (MGG, HP)

9 *RETROPERITONEUM, LIVER AND SPLEEN*

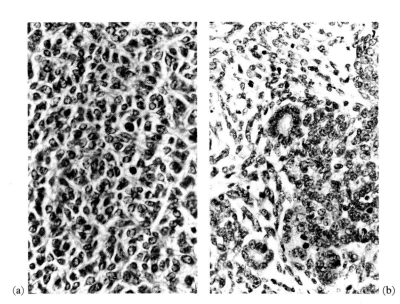

Fig. 9.50 Wilms' tumour
Tissue section; same case as Figure 9.49.
(a) Undifferentiated pattern. (b) Biphasic
pattern with tubular structures
(H & E, IP).

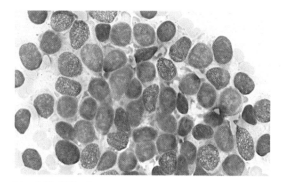

Fig. 9.51 Wilms' tumour
Undifferentiated tumour, cytologically indistinguishable from
other small round cell tumours (MGG, HP)

bules are present in the background, and some cells are usually seen with more abundant pale blue cytoplasm and a perinuclear pale zone. Some rhabdomyoblasts which have eccentric nuclei and a 'tail' of dense eosinophilic cytoplasm, are usually identifiable in smears of rhabdomyosarcoma. In neuroblastoma, one may find the characteristic tumour cell rosettes which have finely fibrillar material in the centre. Glycogen may be demonstrable in the cells of Ewing's sarcoma. Merkel cell carcinoma can be mistaken for small cell anaplastic carcinoma in smears and a full knowledge of the clinical presentation is essential. The cytological findings are described in detail in Chapter 11. A bimodal cell population suggests Wilms' tumour, but is only recognisable in the better differentiated tumours. Ultrastructural characteristics are particularly distinctive in this group of tumours and EM examination is necessary to allow a confident, type-specific diagnosis in most cases.[35] Sufficient cell material for electron microscopy

is relatively easy to obtain with a standard needle due to the high cellularity of these tumours.

Transitional cell carcinoma (Figs 9.52–9.54)

Criteria for diagnosis

1. Relatively large cells — single and in multilayered clusters, rarely papillary structures.
2. Obvious nuclear criteria of malignancy; markedly variable hyperchromasia.
3. Eccentric nuclei within a dense cytoplasm.
4. Prominent nucleoli.

Transitional cell carcinoma developing from the epithelial lining of the renal pelvis involves the parenchyma by invasion and this is why smears often show the malignant cells mixed with normal tubular epithelial cells (Figs 9.52 and 9.53). Most of the tumours are solid and poorly differentiated and true papillary structures are therefore not often found. A tendency to squamous differentiation is not uncommon, some tumours show a spindle cell pattern, and some are highly anaplastic and can not be recognised as of renal pelvic origin.

Metastatic carcinoma and malignant lymphoma
Metastatic carcinoma is not uncommon in the kidneys. Clinical and radiological data usually indicate if one is dealing with a metastatic or with a primary tumour. As mentioned above, adrenal cortical carcinoma or hepatocellular carcinoma directly encroaching upon the kidney may be cytologically indistinguishable from primary renal cell carcinoma, and the correct diagnosis depends on clinical and radiological investigations.

In the reverse situation, a patient presenting with metastases, for example in lungs or bone, without a known primary, renal cell carcinoma is usually not dif-

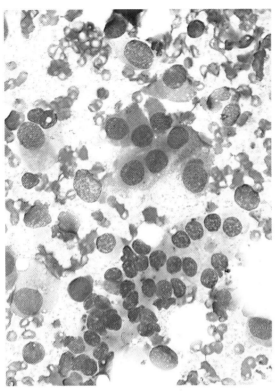

Fig. 9.52 Transitional cell carcinoma
Mixture of normal tubular epithelium and malignant cells with dense cytoplasm and eccentric nuclei (MGG, HP)

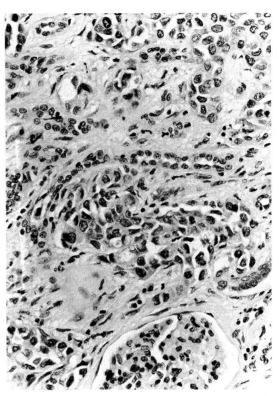

Fig. 9.53 Transitional cell carcinoma
Tissue section; same case as Figure 9.52; carcinoma cells infiltrating between normal renal structures (H & E, IP)

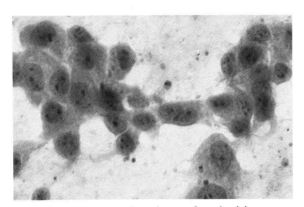

Fig. 9.54 Transitional cell carcinoma of renal pelvis
Irregular clusters of cells with excentric, pleomorphic nuclei, prominent nucleoli, abundant eosinophilic cytoplasm and distinct cell borders (H & E, HP)

ficult to recognise in a FNA smear from the metastasis. This is of some clinical importance since a metastasis of renal cell carcinoma is often solitary and may be considered for surgical excision. Tumours which can closely resemble renal cell carcinoma are adrenal cortical carcinoma and hepatocellular carcinoma. Follicular carcinoma of thyroid of oncocytic type, and breast carcinoma

with apocrine differentiation can occasionally cause problems. High grade renal cell cancers may resemble large cell anaplastic carcinoma of lung or of pancreas. Malignant lymphoma may involve the kidneys, and may cause bilateral diffuse enlargement. Rarely, this can be the first manifestation of systemic lymphoma and thus be subjected to investigation by FNA.

The cytology of *clear cell sarcoma* of the kidney has recently been described.[91]

LIVER

Normal structures (Fig. 9.55)

1. Cohesive sheets of hepatocytes.
2. Kupffer cells.
3. Bile duct epithelium.

Although the aspirate may appear to consist of blood only, it usually contains plenty of liver cells. Cell cohesion is particularly strong, and when the blood is spread on a slide or on a watch glass one easily sees small, firm, semi-translucent tissue fragments which are difficult to smear. In comparison, tumour tissue fragments are usually soft, fragile and easily smeared. Sometimes, a thin tissue core is obtained which can be fixed and embedded for histological sectioning (see Fig. 2.11).

9 *RETROPERITONEUM, LIVER AND SPLEEN*

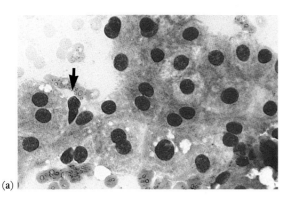

(a)

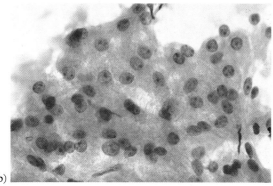

(b)

Fig. 9.55 Hepatocytes
Cohesive cells with dense cytoplasm, indistinct cell borders, mild anisokaryosis and prominent nucleoli; note the small wedge-shaped Kupffer cell in (a) (arrow). (a) MGG, HP. (b) H & E, HP.

In smears, normal hepatocytes form cohesive sheets, and single cells are infrequent. The hepatocytes have a dense eosinophilic (grey-blue with MGG) cytoplasm which is finely granular and sometimes vacuolated. The cell membrane is indistinct (Fig. 9.55). Normal hepatocytes display anisokaryosis, mild to moderate depending on the patient's age. Occasional nuclei may be very large in non-neoplastic liver tissue. Nucleoli are small but prominent. Coarse, granular intracytoplasmic pigment is commonly present in hepatocytes. It stains green-black with MGG, brown with H & E, and is probably lipofuscin. A few Kupffer cells can usually be found and appear as single, bare, comma-shaped nuclei between the hepatocytes. A few lymphocytes may be present. Bile duct epithelial cells form small, mono-layered sheets. These are few in numbers in smears from normal liver tissue.

If information about the architectural pattern of the liver is essential, the embedding of any tissue fragments obtained with the thin needle for paraffin sections may be worthwhile.

Diffuse parenchymal disease (Figs 9.56–9.59)[180,188,218]

Usual findings

1. Decreased cohesion of hepatocytes.
2. Degenerative changes in hepatocytes.

3. Hepatocytic regeneration.
4. Increased lymphocytes and Kupffer cells.
5. Increase of bile duct epithelial cells (cirrhosis).
6. Cholestasis (variable).

As already stated, we do not attempt to make specific diagnoses cytologically in diffuse liver disease. We only report the presence of parenchymal disease and try to assess its severity as suggested by the cytological pattern.

The presence of parenchymal disease is indicated by decreased cohesion of hepatocytes and the finding of many single cells. The hepatocytes are swollen to a variable degree, the cytoplasm is paler than usual and it stains less uniformly, paler at the periphery of the cell. Cell membranes which are indistinct in normal hepatocytes become more clearly visible (Fig. 9.56). Fatty change is commonly seen as intracytoplasmic vacuoles of variable size. Liver cell necrosis may be obvious in severe disease. Acidophilic bodies and alcoholic hyaline are difficult to identify in cytological preparations. Although anisokaryosis, binucleation, and enlarged nucleoli indicate liver cell regeneration, this should be interpreted with caution as these features normally increase with age. The number of lymphocytes and of Kupffer cells is increased. The Kupffer cells often appear swollen, and may form granuloma-like clusters. The number of sheets of bile duct epithelium is often increased, particularly in cirrhosis (Fig. 9. 57).

The degree of abnormality as described varies over a wide range. The reactive hepatitis commonly seen adjacent to a neoplasm is an example of mild change including moderate increase of lymphocytes and of Kupffer cells, some dissociation and swelling of hepatocytes and mild to moderate anisokaryosis (Fig. 9.56). In cirrhosis, there is a marked increase in the number of Kupffer cells and of bile duct epithelial cells, fatty change, dissociation of hepatocytes, and a tendency for the cells to appear in single files and acini. Anisokaryosis and nucleolar enlargment may be quite prominent (Fig. 9.58). Bile stasis is easily recognised as casts of dense material between hepatocytes, staining black-green with MGG (Fig. 9.59), yellow-green with Pap or HE. *Haemosiderosis* is recognised by the demonstration of golden yellow to brown haemosiderin pigment in the Kupffer cells and in the hepatocytes (Fig. 9.58). It is not always easy to distinguish haemosiderin from lipofuscin in routinely stained smears, and a suitable special stain should be used if haemosiderosis is suspected. Increased copper content of hepatocytes has been demonstrated using FNA in primary biliary cirrhosis and in Wilson's disease.[208] *Amyloid* appears in smears as a dense amorphous, vaguely fibrillar material, which stains from pink to purple with MGG. Its presence should be confirmed with special stains such as Congo red (see Fig. 4.3).[154]

The findings in *myeloid metaplasia* are described on page 257.

RETROPERITONEUM, LIVER AND SPLEEN 9

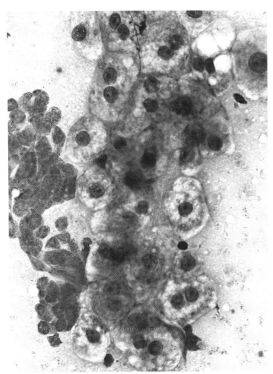

Fig. 9.56 Hepatocyte degeneration
Swollen hepatocytes with pale non-uniformly stained cytoplasm and distinct cell borders; the material is from a case of metastatic oat cell carcinoma to liver; note the cluster of small malignant cells adjacent to the hepatocytes (MGG, HP)

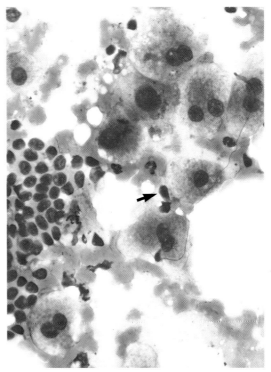

Fig. 9.57 Cirrhosis
Poorly cohesive hepatocytes with degenerative/regenerative features; sheet of small cohesive bile ductal cells; note several Kupffer cells (arrow) (MGG, HP)

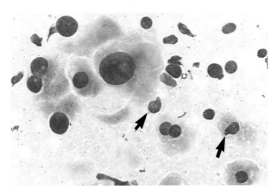

Fig. 9.58 Haemochromatosis and cirrhosis
Dissociated hepatocytes showing moderate anisokaryosis; intracytoplasmic pigment is evident in several cells; several Kupffer cells (arrows) and lymphocytes (MGG, HP)

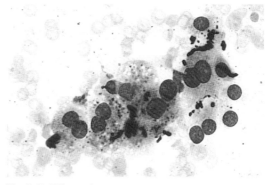

Fig. 9.59 Bile stasis
Cords of inspissated bile in canaliculi between hepatocytes (MGG, HP)

The finding of histiocytic/epithelioid *granulomata* in fine-needle aspirates of liver does not permit a specific diagnosis. Poorly formed granulomata can be seen in cirrhosis, drug-induced hepatitis, mononucleosis, etc. Well-formed epithelioid granulomata, sometimes with Langhans' giant cells, occur in tuberculosis, sarcoid, some fungal and parasitic diseases, Hodgkin's disease, and primary biliary cirrhosis. Their demonstration in fine-needle aspirates thus requires further investigation to determine their exact aetiology.[211]

Non-neoplastic focal lesions

Cysts

An aspirate from a *congenital cyst* consists of thin, clear fluid. A few uniform, cuboidal epithelial cells, single or

9 RETROPERITONEUM, LIVER AND SPLEEN

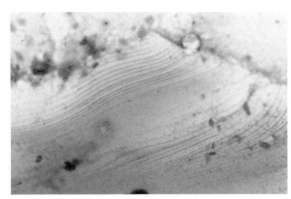

Fig. 9.60 Hydatid cyst, liver
Fragments of laminar membrane, background debris
(MGG, HP)

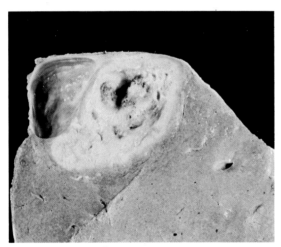

Fig. 9.61 Abscess adjacent to cyst
Macrophotograph of liver tissue containing an abscess adjacent
to a congenital cyst; only the cyst contents were aspirated.

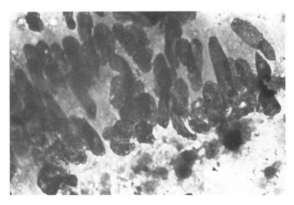

Fig. 9.62 Liver metastasis of colonic adenocarcinoma
Columnar cells with palisaded nuclei, necrotic debris (MGG,
HP)

in monolayered sheets, and some macrophages with vacuolated cytoplasm may be found in the smears. Fluid from a *hydatid cyst* is turbid or thick and creamy. Fragments of the hyaline, laminated membrane, best demonstrated with a PAS stain, are a characteristic finding (Fig. 9.60), and the diagnosis is confirmed by the demonstration of scolices and/or hooklets.[217]

Abscess (Fig. 9.61)
Purulent material aspirated from a focal lesion should, of course, be subjected to microbiological investigation. Routine smears should also be prepared and searched for neoplastic cells, as tumour metastases, for example from a primary in the bowel, can become secondarily infected or undergo cystic degeneration. CEA assay has been found helpful in the distinction between benign and malignant cystic lesions in the liver.[198] The diagnosis of hepatic *actinomycosis* by CT and FNA has been reported.[202]

Figure 9.61 illustrates an abscess adjacent to a congenital cyst. Only the cyst was sampled by ultrasound-guided needle biopsy, which emphasises the occasional failure to obtain a representative specimen in spite of modern imaging techniques.

Focal fatty change in the liver can simulate neoplasia on ultrasound and diagnosis by FNA is of practical importance.[160]

Neoplasms

Metastatic carcinoma (Figs 9.62 and 9.63)
The macroscopical appearance of the aspirate is usually quite different from that of normal liver tissue. There is less admixture with blood; there is often a high cell content and the aspirate is easily smeared into a greyish film. Necrosis may be pre-eminent, sometimes to the extent that preserved, diagnostic cancer cells are hard to find. A metastatic tumour deposit may present as a cyst.[198] If hepatocytes are found amongst the neoplastic cells, they provide a useful baseline for the evaluation of cell and nuclear size. Hepatocytes are more numerous and evenly dispersed in aspirates from diffusely infiltrating metastatic carcinoma. This uncommon pattern is mainly seen in carcinoma of the breast and in anaplastic small cell carcinoma of lung (Fig. 9.56).

The cytological patterns of metastatic carcinoma and clues to the indentification of the primary tumour are described in Chapter 5 and will not be repeated here. Colonic adenocarcinoma is probably the most common source of liver metastases. The cytological pattern is characteristic: columnar malignant epithelial cells in palisaded rows or acini with a background of necrotic debris (Fig. 9.62).[152] Carcinoids are usually distinguishable from metastatic adenocarcinoma by their endocrine appearance (p. 230). The nuclei have a uniformly rounded shape and 'speckled' chromatin (Fig. 9.63a), and a red (MGG) cytoplasmic granularity may be prominent (Fig. 9.63b). If spare smears are available, the

RETROPERITONEUM, LIVER AND SPLEEN 9

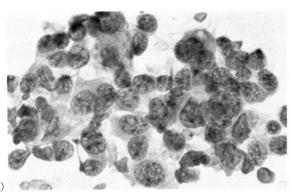
(a)

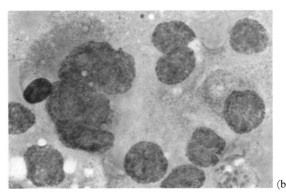
(b)

Fig. 9.63 Liver metastasis of carcinoid tumour
(a) Loose clusters of tumour cells, some follicular grouping, uniformly 'speckled' nuclear chromatin (Pap, HP). (b) Rounded tumour cells with striking red cytoplasmic granularity and indistinct cell borders (MGG, HP).

diagnosis can be confirmed with a Grimelius stain, or by immunoperoxidase staining for NSE or chromogranin. The differential diagnosis between metastatic carcinoma and primary hepatocellular carcinoma and cholangiocarcinoma will be discussed in the following paragraphs. A type specific cytological diagnosis of some unusual metastatic tumours may be possible.[181,199]

Liver cell adenoma (Figs 9.64 and 9.65)

Criteria for diagnosis

1. Highly cellular smears from a clearly defined focal lesion.
2. Cells resembling normal hepatocytes.
3. Absence of bile duct epithelium.

This diagnosis can hardly be made with confidence by cytology alone since distinction from well differentiated hepatocellular carcinoma on one hand, and focal nodu-

lar hyperplasia and regenerative nodules on the other, may be impossible in FNA smears. The cytological pattern must be correlated with clinical presentation and radiological findings. A solitary liver mass found in a young woman who has been taking oral contraceptives is most likely a liver cell adenoma whereas a mass in an older patient with cirrhosis is more likely either a regenerative nodule or a primary liver cell cancer.

Problems in diagnosis

1. Well differentiated hepatocellular carcinoma.
2. Focal nodular hyperplasia and regenerative nodules.[203]

The differences in cytological patterns between adenoma and well differentiated carcinoma can be subtle. The cytoplasm is less fragile and better defined with more distinct cell borders in adenoma, the nuclear/cytoplasmic ratio is consistently low, and single, bare

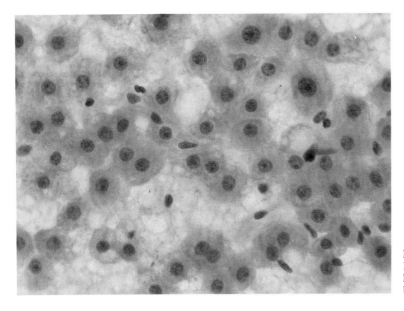

Fig. 9.64 Liver cell adenoma
Dissociated epithelial cells resembling hepatocytes, bland nuclei, Kupffer cells but no bile duct epithelium (H & E, HP).

251

9 RETROPERITONEUM, LIVER AND SPLEEN

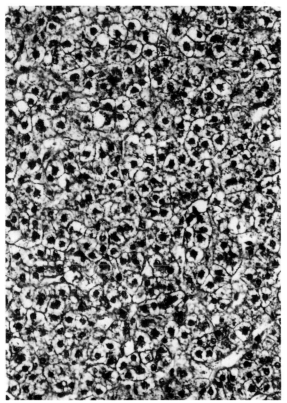

Fig. 9.65 Liver cell adenoma
Tissue section, same case as Fig. 9.64 (H & E, IP)

neoplastic nuclei (see below) are less apparent (Fig. 9.64).

In the distinction between adenoma and *focal nodular hyperplasia*, absence of bile duct epithelium favours the former, but bile duct epithelium is sometimes absent in smears from the latter. Marked anisokaryosis is more a feature of regenerative nodules than of adenoma. In liver cell dysplasia, there is a dominant background of normal hepatocytes among which are scattered atypical cells with pleomorphic nuclei (Fig. 9.66).[149]

Hepatocellular carcinoma
(Figs 2.11, 9.67–9.73)[144,155,169,170,172,192]

Criteria for diagnosis

1. Neoplastic cells forming trabecules, acini or sheets.
2. Polygonal cells with central nuclei and abundant, fragile cytoplasm.
3. Cytoplasm eosinophilic, granular and/or vacuolated.
4. Nuclei round with large central nucleoli.
5. Many atypical stripped nuclei.
6. Intranuclear cytoplasmic inclusions.
7. Intracytoplasmic eosinophilic inclusions.
8. Intracytoplasmic bile pigment and/or bile plugs between cells.
9. Bile duct epithelium absent.

The most consistent and characteristic features in FNA smears are: an abundant eosinophilic, granular and/or vacuolated cytoplasm, nuclear roundness, the presence of many stripped, malignant nuclei[194] (Figs 9.70 and 9.71), and large central nucleoli. Tumour cells are often adherent to strands of pink (MGG) fibrillar material representing vascular structures similar to that seen in renal carcinoma. A lining of endothelial cells at the periphery of clusters or cords of tumour cells is particularly characteristic of hepatocellular carcinoma.[164] Intranuclear cytoplasmic inclusions are seen in over 50% of cases. Bile pigment in and between tumour cells is a diagnostic finding, but is demonstrable in only about 25% of cases. Small amounts of bile pigment are beautifully demonstrated by Fouchet's reagent counterstained with haematoxylin/Sirius red, staining intensely green (see Fig. 2.16). Positive immunocytochemical staining of neoplastic cells for alphafetoprotein and/or alpha-1-antitrypsin is supportive evidence but is not demonstrable in all cases. The cells are said to stain negatively for EMA.

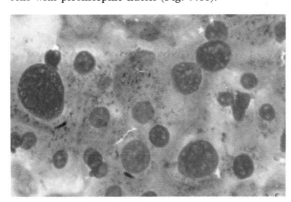

Fig. 9.66 Liver cell dysplasia
Cluster of hepatocytes, the majority normal but some very large nuclei and large nucleoli; from a case of cirrhosis (MGG, HP)

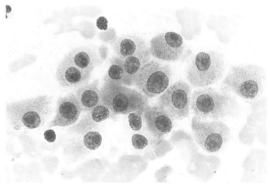

Fig. 9.67 Hepatocellular carcinoma
Well-differentiated tumour composed of poorly cohesive hepatocytic cells with some anisokaryosis and very large nucleoli; differentiation from adenoma difficult or impossible (MGG, HP)

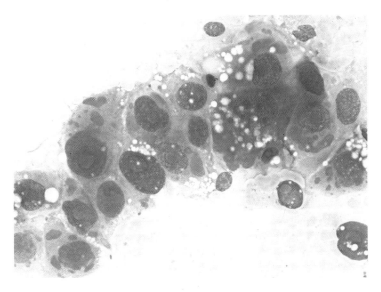

Fig. 9.68 Hepatocellular carcinoma
Moderately differentiated tumour with
severe anisokaryosis; note the large
intracytoplasmic inclusions (MGG, HP)

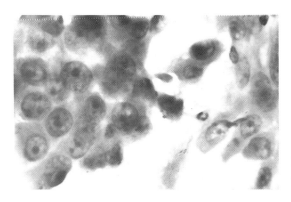

Fig. 9.69 Hepatocellular carcinoma
Moderately differentiated tumour; dense cytoplasm; large
nucleoli (H & E, HP)

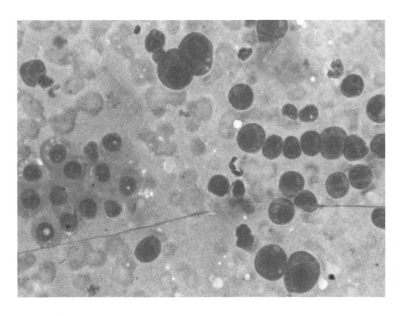

Fig. 9.70 Hepatocellular carcinoma
Mainly naked nuclei; nuclei round,
macronucleoli; note cluster of normal
hepatocytes (MGG, HP)

9 *RETROPERITONEUM, LIVER AND SPLEEN*

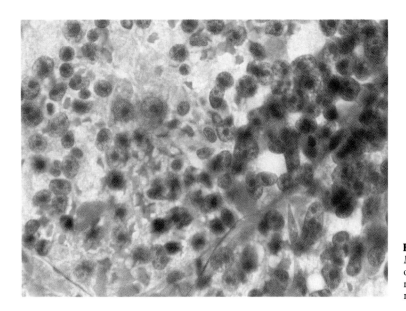

Fig. 9.71 Hepatocellular carcinoma
Malignant cells loosely adhering to strand of endothelium; round nuclei, central macronucleoli, many naked malignant nuclei (Pap, HP)

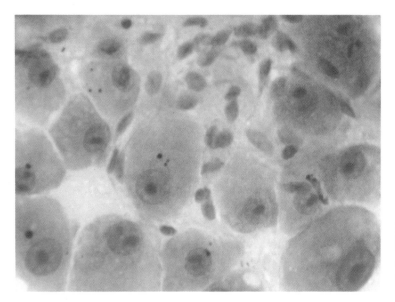

Fig. 9.72 Hepatocellular carcinoma, fibrolamellar type
Very large, malignant hepatocytes with well differentiated cytoplasm, clusters of stromal spindle cells (MGG, HP)

Large, sometimes very large, hyaline cytoplasmic inclusions staining red with MGG (Fig. 9.68) are seen in about 25% of liver cell cancers.[171,186] They have been claimed to be pathognomonic for this tumour, but can be seen in poorly differentiated, large cell carcinomas of other sites such as lung, kidney and ovary. Their presence in smears is nevertheless very suggestive of hepatocellular carcinoma. Ultrastructurally, the inclusions are mainly giant lysosomes or autophagic vacuoles, but some are aggregates of filaments (Mallory bodies), a few are giant mitochondria, and some remain unclassified.

The *fibrolamellar subtype* of hepatocellular carcinoma should be distinguished from the common type since it has a better prognosis following resection. The tumour cells, readily recognised as of hepatocellular origin, are very large, they have a polygonal, sometimes bizarre shape, abundant, dense eosinophilic, granular cytoplasm, large nuclei and large, single, central nucleoli. The neoplastic cells are intermingled with bundles of spindle-shaped fibrocytes (Figs 9.72 and 9.73).[212,213]

Problems in diagnosis

1. Liver cell adenoma and regenerative nodules.
2. Metastatic carcinoma.

The problem of distinguishing well-differentiated hepatocellular carcinoma from a benign regenerative nodule or an adenoma has been mentioned. There is a considerable risk of overdiagnosing malignancy because nuclear enlargement, anisokaryosis, macronucleoli, and

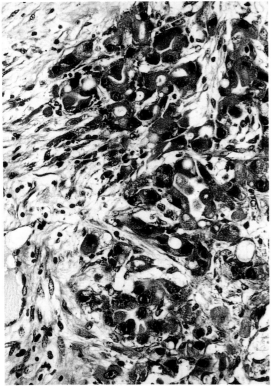

Fig. 9.73 Hepatocellular carcinoma, fibrolamellar type
Tissue section, same case as Fig. 9.72 (H & E, IP)

dissociation may be prominent in regenerative nodules (Fig. 9.66). Total absence of bile duct epithelium in a cellular smear favours a neoplasm, and if there is nuclear enlargement and pleomorphism, loss of cell cohesion, many naked neoplastic nuclei and poorly defined

cell borders, the lesion is probably carcinoma. Clinical data such as age and sex, presence or absence of cirrhosis, exposure to steroidal hormones, and radiological appearances must be known and may help to distinguish between these entities.

Poorly differentiated hepatocellular carcinoma is difficult to distinguish from metastatic adenocarcinoma or large cell undifferentiated carcinoma, for example from the pancreas or from the lung. A positive immunoperoxidase staining for alphafetoprotein favours primary cancer. Bile pigment in or between tumour cells is diagnostic of liver cell cancer but is often not present. Naphthylamidase staining of bile canaliculi or fragments thereof has been used to confirm hepatocellular origin.[165] Demonstration of intracellular mucin would exclude a hepatocellular tumour.

Cholangiocarcinoma (Fig. 9.74)[212]

Criteria for diagnosis

1. Sheets and clusters of cells resembling normal bile duct epithelium.
2. Microglandular arrangement and nuclear crowding.
3. Decreased cell cohesion — some single cells.
4. Nuclear enlargement and pleomorphism not prominent.

Problems in diagnosis

Cholangiocarcinomas often have abundant, desmoplastic stroma and it may prove difficult to aspirate enough tumour cells to allow a diagnosis. In one of our cases, multiple biopsies yielded only clear fluid which either contained no cells at all or only a few cells closely resembling normal bile duct epithelium. Conventional core needle biopsies were equally unsuccessful. The diagnosis was only made on a wedge biopsy taken from

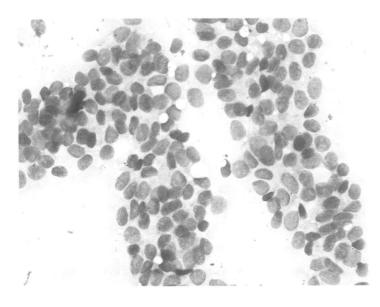

Fig. 9.74 Cholangiocarcinoma
Disorganised clusters of irregular but not very pleomorphic tumour cells with pale cytoplasm and relatively small nuclei (MGG, HP)

9 RETROPERITONEUM, LIVER AND SPLEEN

the visible tumour at laparotomy. Although cells from a cholangiocarcinoma may not appear very different from normal bile duct epithelium, hepatocytes are absent and the number and size of epithelial sheets is much larger than is ever obtained from non-neoplastic liver tissue (Fig. 9.74). Less well differentiated carcinomas are indistinguishable from metastatic adenocarcinoma, particularly from those of pancreatic origin. Staining for AFP is also often positive in cholangiocarcinoma.

Hepatoblastoma

We have not seen any examples of this tumour in our FNA practise. The reader is referred to a couple of reports in the literature.[150,163]

Malignant lymphoma[161]

The diagnosis is based on the demonstration in smears of abnormal lymphoid cells, Reed-Sternberg giant cells, etc. The criteria are the same as for malignant lymphoma in other tissues (see Ch. 5). Liver involvement by malignant lymphoma is commonly in the form of microscopical foci. These can be widely separated and can easily be missed also by multiple needle biopsies. In our limited experience, FNA of the liver does not, therefore, appear to be of great value in the staging of lymphoma.

Vascular tumours

Cavernous haemangioma is the commonest benign solid lesion in the liver, and is not infrequently found by US or by CT in the routine investigation of cancer patients. The diagnosis can usually be made by ultrasonography alone, but in some cases, a needle biopsy is necessary to confidently exclude metastatic tumour or adenoma.[156,159,190,209,210,220] In our experience, clusters

of benign spindle cells recognisable as endothelial cells are not often found. The diagnosis is based on the aspiration of profuse blood as from a venopuncture, provided the correct positioning of the needle can be ascertained. The cytological findings in *angiosarcoma*[191] are described in the section on the spleen below.

SPLEEN

Non-specific findings in splenomegaly (Fig. 9.75)

1. Abundant blood and platelet aggregates.
2. Tissue fragments (lymphoid cells and endothelial cells).
3. Numerous lymphoid cells.
4. Endothelial cells and histiocytes.

It is unlikely that normal spleens are ever subjected to FNA and the normal cytological pattern is, therefore, not well known. The above features are seen in cases of splenomegaly in which cytological examination does not contribute to a specific diagnosis, for example in portal hypertension, haemolytic anaemia, etc.

Lymphoid cells predominate in smears from the spleen as in smears from reactive lymph nodes. There is invariably a background of abundant blood and platelet aggregates. The lymphoid cells are more often seen in tissue fragments, trapped in a meshwork of endothelial cells, than as evenly spread, isolated cells. Blast cells constitute a relatively higher proportion of the cell population than in smears from reactive lymph nodes. Diagnostic criteria applied in lymph node cytology must therefore be used with caution when smears from the spleen are examined.

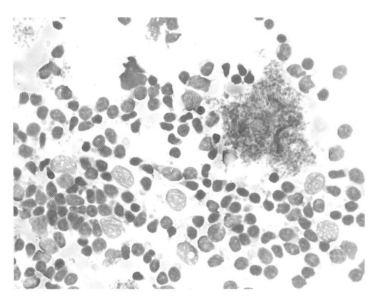

Fig. 9.75 Spleen
Mixed population of small and transformed lymphoid cells and a platelet aggregate (MGG, HP)

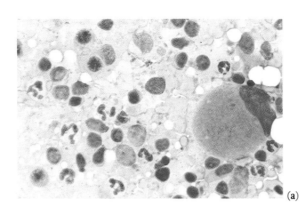

(a)

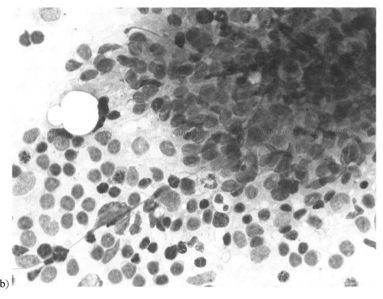

(b)

Fig. 9.76 Myeloid metaplasia
(a) Megakaryocyte and several erythroblasts adjacent to smeared lymphoid cells. (b) The appearance of a tissue fragment with a vascular core and many lymphocytes and macrophages is characteristic of white pulp origin (MGG, HP).

Non-neoplastic processes[228,234]

Myeloid metaplasia (Fig. 9.76)

The findings in myeloid metaplasia include normoblasts, myelocytes and megakaryocytes intermingled with the cells of normal splenic tissue. Normoblasts are easily recognised by their relatively small, round, hyperchromatic nuclei and their homogenous, dense eosinophilic or amphophilic cytoplasm. Megakaryocytes may be mistaken for malignant neoplastic cells but should be recognisable by the giant, lobulated nucleus and the abundant, granular cytoplasm. Myelocytes have specific cytoplasmic granules. All these features are of course best seen in Giemsa-stained smears.

Granulomatous processes

Histiocytes in granulomatous clusters may be found in several unrelated conditions and do not permit a specific diagnosis when found in splenic aspirates. Well-formed granulomata of epithelioid histiocytes, with or without

Langhans' giant cells, are seen in sarcoidosis.[232,236] If caseation is present, miliary tuberculosis must be suspected. Whenever non-caseating granulomas are found in splenic aspirates, malignant lymphoma, particularly Hodgkin's disease, must be considered and the lymphoid cells need to be studied closely.

Others

Conspicuous large histiocytes with foamy cytoplasm indicate *lipid storage disease*. Histiocytes in Gaucher's disease have a characteristic striated cytoplasmic appearance (Fig. 9.77). The foamy histiocytes seen in Niemann-Pick disease are less characteristic and the specific diagnosis rests on biochemical analyses. The cytology of *histiocytosis X* is described in Chapter 11 and *amyloidosis*[230] in Chapter 4 (see also Fig. 4.3). Other examples of non-neoplastic lesions in the spleen diagnosed by FNAC are splenic abscesses[231] and splenic epidermoid cyst.[223]

9 *RETROPERITONEUM, LIVER AND SPLEEN*

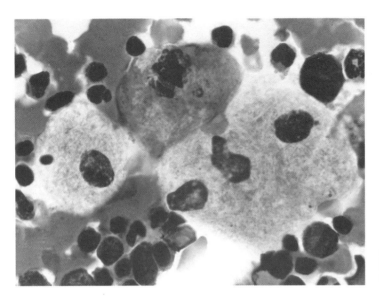

Fig. 9.77 Gaucher's disease
Bone marrow smear with large
characteristic histiocytes (MGG, HP Oil)

Neoplasms

Malignant lymphoma

The findings in malignant lymphoma in splenic aspirates are the same as in other tissues (see Ch. 5). The
abnormal lymphoid cells are more dispersed, distributed
as single cells, and tissue fragments are less conspicuous
than in smears of non-neoplastic splenic tissue. Non-
Hodgkin's lymphoma of mixed cell type is particularly
difficult to diagnose with confidence in splenic aspirates,
and immune marker studies are often indispensable. In
Hodgkin's disease, the diagnosis rests on the demonstration of Reed-Sternberg giant cells.

Hairy cell leukaemia (Fig. 9.78)

Criteria for diagnosis

1. A monotonous population of abnormal lymphoid
   cells.
2. Nuclei ovoid or kidney-shaped; larger and paler than
   those of small lymphocytes.
3. Pale basophilic cytoplasm; fine, hair-like cytoplasmic
   projections (EM).
4. Positive staining for tartrate-resistant acid
   phosphatase and for acid non-specific esterase.

Splenomegaly is one of the main symptoms in hairy
cell leukemia, whereas lymph node involvement appears
late in the disease and is less conspicuous. The diagnosis
is usually made on examination of a bone marrow
aspirate or of peripheral blood but can also be made on
a splenic aspirate.

Vascular tumours

Splenoma (Figs 9.79 and 9.80) is a hamartomatous
tumour of the spleen consisting exclusively of red pulp

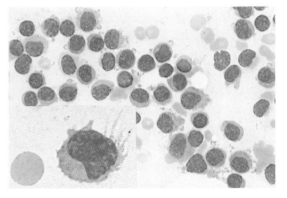

Fig. 9.78 Hairy cell leukaemia
Uniform lymphoid cells, larger and paler than small
lymphocytes and with slightly reniform nuclei (MGG, HP).
Inset: fine hair-like cytoplasmic processes which may
however be artefactually produced in other lymphoid cells.
(MGG, HP Oil).

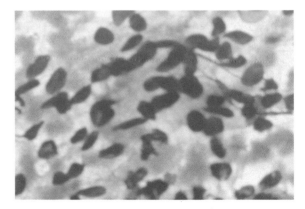

Fig. 9.79 Splenoma
Numerous uniform spindle cells of endothelial type with bland
nuclei (MGG, HP)

tissue. We have seen one example in which the smears were dominated by numerous spindle cells of endothelial type. The nuclei were elongated, uniform, with a bland, finely granular chromatin. The FNA biopsy was reported as an angiomatous tumour. It seems unlikely that a distinction between splenoma and *haemangioma* would be possible cytologically.

Angiosarcoma (Figs 9.81 and 9.82)[191] occasionally presents as a primary tumour of the spleen. We have seen one case in which the diagnosis was correctly made on FNA biopsy.

The patient was an elderly woman admitted to hospital for a cardiovascular problem. On examination, a very large spleen was felt for which there was no obvious cause. FNA biopsy was performed without complications. Smears were very rich in cells. These were spindly and had elongated, mildly pleomorphic, hyperchromatic nuclei. Most of the cells formed highly cellular tissue fragments which showed a distinctly vasoformative pattern with bunches of spindle cells radiating from a vascular core (Fig. 9.81; see also Fig. 7.68).

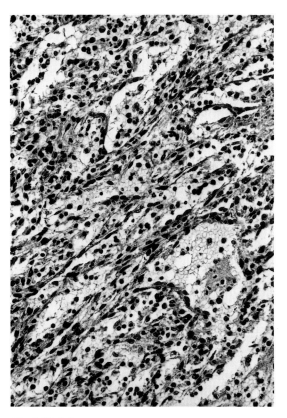

Fig. 9.80 Splenoma
Tissue section, same case as Fig. 9.79 (H & E, IP)

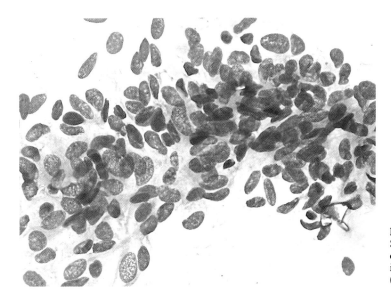

Fig. 9.81 Angiosarcoma
Spindle cells radiating from the centre of a loose cluster; irregular nuclei; pale ill-defined cytoplasm; moderately cohesive (MGG, HP)

9 RETROPERITONEUM, LIVER AND SPLEEN

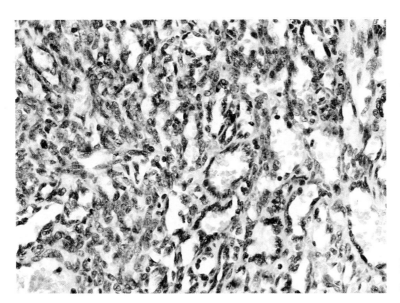

Fig. 9.82 Angiosarcoma
Tissue section; same case as Figure 9.81
(H & E, IP)

REFERENCES AND SUGGESTED FURTHER READING

Pancreas, Abdomen and Retroperitoneum

1. An-Foraker S H, Fong-Mui K K: Cytodiagnosis of lesions of the pancreas and related areas. Acta Cytol 26: 814–818, 1982.
2. Arnesjö B, Stormby N, Åkerman M: Cytodiagnosis of pancreatic lesions by means of fine-needle biopsy during operation. Acta Chir Scand 138: 363–369, 1972.
3. Beazley R M: Needle biopsy diagnosis of pancreatic cancer. Cancer 47: 1685–1687, 1981.
4. Bell D A: Cytologic features of islet-cell tumours. Acta Cytol 31: 485–492, 1987.
5. Bergenfeldt M, Genell S, Lindholm K, Ekberg O, Aspelin P: Needle-tract seeding after percutaneous fine-needle biopsy of pancreatic carcinoma. Case report. Acta Chir Scand 154: 77–79, 1988.
6. Bondeson L, Bondeson A-G, Genell S, Lindholm K, Thorstenson S: Aspiration cytology of a rare solid and papillary neoplasm of the pancreas. Acta Cytol 28: 605–509, 1984.
7. Bognel C, Rougier P, Leclare J, Duvillard P, Charpentier P, Prade M: Fine needle aspiration of the liver and pancreas with ultrasound guidance. Acta Cytol 32: 22–26, 1988.
8. Bret P M, Nicolet V, Labadie M: Percutaneous fine-needle aspiration biopsy of the pancreas. Diagn Cytopathol 2: 221–227, 1986.
9. Bret P M, Fond A, Bretagnolle M, Barral F, Labadie M: Percutaneous fine needle biopsy of intra-abdominal lesions. Eur J Radiol 4: 322–328, 1982.
10. Caturelli E, Rappaccini GL, Anti M, Fabiano A, Fedeli G: Malignant seeding after fine-needle aspiration biopsy of the pancreas. Diagn Imaging Clin Med 54: 88–91, 1985.
11. Chen K T K, Workman R D, Efird T A, Cheng A C: Fine needle aspiration cytology diagnosis of papillary tumour of the pancreas. Acta Cytol 30: 523–527, 1986.
12. Compagno J, Oertel J E: Mucinous cystic neoplasms of the pancreas with overt and latent malignancy (cystadenocarcinoma and cystadenoma): a clinicopathologic study of 41 cases. Am J Clin Pathol 69: 573–580, 1978.
13. Droese M, Altmannsberger M, Kehl A, Lankisch P G, Weiss N, Weber K, Osborn M: Ultrasound-guided percutaneous fine needle aspiration biopsy of abdominal and retroperitoneal masses. Acta Cytol 28: 368–384, 1984.
14. Duston M A, Skinner M, Shirahama T, Cohen A S: Diagnosis of amyloidosis by abdominal fat aspiration. Analysis of four years' experience. Am J Med 82: 412–414, 1987.
15. Dzieniszewski G P, Neher M, Linhart P, Frank K: Nekrotisierende Pankreatitis nach ultraschallgezielter Feinnadelpunktion. Dtsch Med Wschr 107: 1438–1440, 1982.
16. Eggert A, Lattmann E, Kopf R, Pfeiffer M, Klloppel G: Intraoperative pancreas puncture cytology. Zentralbl Chir 109: 540–544, 1984.
17. Ekberg O, Bergenfeldt M, Aspelin P, Genell S, Lindholm K, Nilsson P, Sigurjonsson S: Reliability of ultrasound-guided fine-needle biopsy of pancreatic masses. Acta Radiol 29: 535–539, 1988.
18. Emmert G M, Bewtra C: Fine-needle aspiration biopsy of mucinous cystic neoplasm of the pancreas: a case study. Union Med Can 115: 258–262, 1986.
19. Evander A, Ihse I, Lunderquist A, Tylen U, Åkerman M: Percutaneous cytodiagnosis of carcinoma of the pancreas and bile duct. Ann Surg 188: 90–92, 1978.
20. Evans W K, Ho C S, McLoughlin M J, Tao L C: Fatal necrotizing pancreatitis following fine-needle aspiration biopsy of the pancreas. Radiology 141: 61–62, 1981.
21. Fekete P S, Nunez C, Pitlik D A: Fine-needle aspiration biopsy of the pancreas: a study of 61 cases. Diagn Cytopathol 2: 301–306, 1986.
22. Ferrucci J T, Wittenberg J, Margolies M N, Carey R W: Malignant seeding of the tract after thin-needle aspiration biopsy. Radiology 130: 345–346, 1979.
23. Foote A, Simpson J S, Stewart R J, Wakefield J S,

RETROPERITONEUM, LIVER AND SPLEEN 9

Buchanan A, Gupta R K: Diagnosis of the rare solid and papillary epithelial neoplasm of the pancreas by fine needle aspiration cytology. Light and electron microscopic study of a case. Acta Cytol 30: 519–522, 1986.

24. Fornari F, Civardi G, Cavanna L, Di Stasi M, Rossi S, Sbolli G, Buscarini L: Complications of ultrasonically guided fine-needle abdominal biopsy. Results of a multicenter Italian study and review of the literature. The cooperative Italian Study Group. Scand J Gastroenterol 24: 949–955, 1989.

25. Forsgren L, Orell S: Aspiration cytology in carcinoma of the pancreas. Surgery 73: 38–42, 1973.

26. Fröhlich E, Wehrmann K, Seeliger H, Vierling P, Frühmorgen P. Ultrasound controlled fine needle cytology and fine needle histology in circumscribed pancreatic processes. Leber Magen Darm 236: 239–244, 1988.

27. Godwin J T: Rapid cytologic diagnosis of surgical specimens. Acta Cytol 20: 111–115, 1976.

28. Gupta R K, Scally J, Stewart R J: Mucinous cystadenocarcinoma of the pancreas: diagnosis by fine-needle aspiration cytology. Diagn Cytopathol 5: 408–411, 1989.

29. Hajdu E O, Kumari-Subaiya S, Phillips G: Ultrasonically guided percutaneous aspiration biopsy of the pancreas. Semin Diagn Pathol 3: 166–175, 1986.

30. Hall-Craggs M A, Lees W R: Fine-needle aspiration biopsy: pancreatic and biliary tumours. Am J Roentgenol 147: 399–403, 1986.

31. Hancke S: Biopsy of the pancreas under echographic guidance. In: Percutaneous biopsy and therapeutic vascular occlusion. Anacher H, Gulotta U, Rupp N. (eds), George Thieme, Stuttgart, 1980.

32. Hancke S, Holm H H, Koch F: Ultrasonically guided percutaneous fine needle biopsy of the pancreas. Surg Gynecol Obstet 140: 361–364, 1975.

33. Hancke S, Holm H H, Koch F: Ultrasonically guided puncture of solid pancreatic mass lesions. Ultrasound Med Biol 10: 613–615, 1984.

34. Hastrup J, Thommesen P, Frederiksen P: Pancreatitis and pancreatic carcinoma diagnosed by peroperative fine needle aspiration biposy. Acta Cytol 21: 731–734, 1977.

35. Henderson D W, Papadimitriou J M, Coleman M: Ultrastructural appearances of tumours. A diagnostic atlas. 2nd edn. Churchill Livingstone, Edinburgh, 1986.

36. Hewett P J, Le P Langlois S, Orell S R: The diagnosis of mass lesions in the pancreas by fine needle aspiration biopsy. J Gastroenterol Hepatol 3: 71–76, 1988.

37. Hsiu J G, D'Amato N A, Sperling M H, Greenspan M, Jaffe A H, Smith R 3rd, DeLaTorre R: Malignant islet-cell tumor of the pancreas diagnosed by fine needle aspiration biopsy. A case report. Acta Cytol 29: 576–579, 1985.

38. Hoover L A, Hafiz M A: Fine-needle aspiration diagnosis of extragonadal choriocarcinoma with immunoperoxidase studies. Diagn Cytopathol 3: 84–87, 1989.

39. Iishi H, Yamamoto R, Tatsuta M, Okuda S: Evaluation of fine-needle aspiration biopsy under direct vision gastrofiberscopy in diagnosis of diffusely infiltrative carcinoma of the stomach. Cancer 57: 1365–1369, 1986.

40. Jan G M, Mahajan R: Ultrasound guided percutaneous fine needle aspiration biopsy (FNAB) of intra-abdominal and retroperitoneal masses. Indian J Gastroenterol 8: 99–100, 1989.

41. Jones E C, Suen K C, Grant D R, Chan N H: Fine-needle aspiration cytology of neoplastic cysts of pancreas. Diagn Cytopathol 3: 238–243, 1987.

42. Juul N, Torp-Pedersen S, Holm H H: Ultrasonically guided fine needle aspiration biopsy of retroperitoneal mass lesions. Br J Radiol 57: 43–46, 1984.

43. Kline T S, Abramson J, Goldstein F, Neal H S: Needle aspiration biopsy of the pancreas at laparotomy. Am J Gastroenterol 68: 30–33, 1977.

44. Knelson M, Haaga J, Lazarus H, Ghosh C, Abdul-Karim F, Sorenson K: Computed tomography-guided retroperitoneal biopsies. J Clin Oncol 7: 1169–1173, 1989.

45. Lee Y T: Tissue diagnosis for carcinoma of the pancreas and periampullary structures. Cancer 49: 1035–1039, 1982.

46. Leiman G, Mair S: Aspiration cytology of neuroendocrine tumors below the diaphragm. Diagn Cytopathol 5: 263–268, 1989.

47. Lozowski W, Hajdu S I, Melamed M R: Cytomorphology of carcinoid tumours. Acta Cytol 23: 360–365, 1979.

48. Lüning M, Kursawe R, Schlopke W, Lorenz D, Menzel A, Hoppe E, Meyer R: CT guided percutaneous fine-needle biopsy of the pancreas. Eur J Radiol 5: 104–108, 1985.

49. McLoughlin M J, Ho C S, Langer B, McHattie J, Tao L C: Fine needle aspiration biopsy of malignant lesions in and around the pancreas. Cancer 41: 2413–2419, 1978.

50. Mitty H A, Efremidis S C, Yeh H C: Impact of fine-needle biopsy on management of patients with carcinoma of the pancreas. Am J Roentgenol 137: 1119–1121, 1981.

51. Mueller P R, Miketic L M, Simeone J F, Silverman S G, Saini S, Wittenberg J, Hahn P F, Steiner E, Forman B H: Severe acute pancreatitis after percutaneous biopsy of the pancreas. Am J Roentgenol 151: 493–494, 1988.

52. Nguyen G K, Rayani N A: Hyperplastic and neoplastic endocrine cells of the pancreas in aspiration biopsy. Diagn Cytopathol 2: 204–211, 1986.

53. Nguyen G K, Neifer R: The cells of benign and malignant hemangiopericytomas in aspiration biopsy: Diagn Cytopathol 1: 327–331, 1985.

54. Nickels J, Koivuniemi A: Cytology of malignant hemangiopericytoma. Acta Cytol 23: 119–125, 1979.

55. Oscarsson J, Stormby N, Sundgren R: Selective angiography in fine-needle aspiration cytodiagnosis of gastric and pancreatic tumours. Acta Radiol (Diagn) 12: 737–750, 1972.

56. Otal-Salaverri C, Gonjalez-Cjampora R, Hevia-Vazquez A, Lerma-Puertas E, Galera-Davidson H: Retroperitoneal ganglioneuroblastoma. Report of a case diagnosed by fine needle aspiration cytology and electron microscopy. Acta Cytol 33: 80–84, 1989.

57. Owman T, Idvall I: Percutaneous fine needle biopsy guided by barium examinations of the GI tract. Gastrointest Radiol 7: 327–333, 1982.

58. Palombini L, Vetrani A: Cytologic Diagnosis of ganglioneuroblastoma. Acta Cytol 20: 286–287, 1976.

59. Palombini L, Vetrani A, Vecchione R, Del Basso De Caro M L: The cytology of ganglioneuroma on fine needle aspiration smear. Acta Cytol 26: 259–260, 1982.

60. Parsons L Jr, Palmer C H: How accurate is fine-needle biopsy in malignant neoplasia of the pancreas. Arch Surg 124: 681–683, 1989.

61. Payan M J, Choux R, Raphael M, Tachon C, Agostini S, Sahel J: Fine-needle cyto-puncture. Apropos of 138 liver cytologies and 66 pancreas cytologies. Ann Pathol 7: 260–262, 1987.

62. Pilotti S, Rilke F, Claren R, Milella M, Lombardi L: Conclusive diagnosis of hepatic and pancreatic malignancies by fine needle aspiration. Acta Cytol 32: 27–38, 1988.

63. Rashleigh-Belcher H J, Russell R C, Lees W R: Cutaneous seeding of pancreatic carcinoma by fine-needle aspiration biopsy. Gastrointest Radiol 11: 81–84, 1986.

64. Rupp M, Ehya H: Fine needle aspiration cytology of retroperitoneal paraganglioma with lipofuscin

RETROPERITONEUM, LIVER AND SPLEEN

pigmentation. Acta Cytol 34: 84–88, 1990.

65. Sarno R C, Carter B L, Bankoff M S: Cystic lymphangiomas: CT diagnosis and thin needle aspiration. Br J Radiol 57: 424–426, 1984.
66. Sehested M, Juul N, Hainau B, Torp-Pedersen S: Electron microscopy of ultrasound-guided fine-needle biopsy specimens. Br J Radiol 60: 351–353, 1987.
67. Silverman J F, Dabbs D J, Finley J L, Geisinger K R: Fine-needle aspiration biopsy of pleomorphic (giant cell) carcinoma of the pancreas. Cytologic, immunocytochemical, and ultrastructural findings. Am J Clin Pathol 89: 714–720, 1988.
68. Silverman J F, Dabbs D J, Ganick D J, Holbrook C T, Geisinger K R: Fine needle aspiration cytology of neuroblastoma, including peripheral neuroectodermal tumor, with immunocytochemical and ultrastructural confirmation. Acta Cytol 32: 367–376, 1988.
69. Smith F P, Macdonald J S, Schein P S, Ornitz R D: Cutaneous seeding of pancreatic cancer by skinny-needle aspiration biopsy. Arch Int Med 140: 855, 1980.
70. Soudah B, Fritsch R S, Wittekind C, Hilka B, Spindler B: Value of the cytologic analysis of fine needle aspiration biopsy specimens in the diagnosis of pancreatic carcinomas. Acta Cytol 33: 875–880, 1989.
71. Stachura J, Popiela T, Pietron M, Tomaszewska R, Kulig J, Nowak K: Cytology of solid and papillary epithelial neoplasms of the pancreas: a case report. Diagn Cytopathol 4: 339–341, 1988.
72. Tao L C, Ho C S, McLoughlin M J, McHattie J: Percutaneous fine needle aspiration biopsy of the pancreas. Cytodiagnosis of pancreatic carcinoma. Acta Cytol 22: 215–220, 1978.
73. Tao L C, Negin M L, Donat E E: Primary retroperitoneal seminoma diagnosed by fine needle aspiration biopsy. A case report. Acta Cytol 28: 598–600, 1984.
74. Ulich T R, Layfield L J: Fatal septic shock after fine needle aspiration of a pancreatic pseudocyst. Acta Cytol 29: 879–881, 1985.
75. Valkov I, Bojikin B: Fine-needle aspiration biopsy of abdominal and retroperitoneal tumors in infants and children. Diagn Cytopathol 3: 129–133, 1987.
76. Vallet D, Leisman G, Mair S, Bilchik A: Fine needle aspiration cytology of mucinous cystadenocarcinoma of the pancreas. Further observations. Acta Cytol 32: 43–48, 1988.
77. Welch T J, Sheedy P F 2nd, Johnson C D, Johnson C M, Stephens D H: CT-guided biopsy: prospective analysis of 1,000 procedures. J Radiol 68: 35–38, 1987.

Retroperitoneal Lymph Nodes

78. Bandy L C, Clarke-Peassen D L, Silverman P M, Creasman W T: Computed tomography in evaluation of extrapelvic lymphadenopathy in carcinoma of the cervix. Obstet Gynaecol 65: 73–76, 1985.
79. Chagnon S, Cochand-Priollet B, Gzaeil M, Jacquenod, P, Roger B, Boccon-Gibod L, Blery M: Pelvic cancers: staging of 139 cases with lymphography and fine-needle aspiration biopsy. Radiology 173: 103–106, 1989.
80. Crosby J H, Bryan A B, Gallup D G, Talledo O E: Fine-needle aspiration of inguinal lymph nodes in gynecologic practice. Obstet Gynecol 73: 281–284, 1989.
81. Edeiken-Monroe B S, Zornoza J: Carcinoma of the cervix, percutaneous lymph node aspiration biopsy. Am J Roentgenol 138: 655–657, 1982.
82. von Eschenbach A C, Zornoza J: Fine-needle percutaneous biopsy. A useful evaluation of lymph node metastases from prostatic cancer. Urology 20: 589–590, 1982.
83. Fujioka T, Koike H, Aoki H, Ohhori T, Chiba R, Okamoto S: Significance of staging pelvic lymphadenectomy for prostatic cancer. Urol Int 42: 380–384, 1987.
84. Göthlin J H, Hoeim L: Percutaneous fine needle biopsy of radiographically normal lymph nodes in the staging of prostatic carcinoma. Radiology 141: 351–354, 1981.
85. Göthlin J H, Rupp N, Rothenberger K H, MacIntosh P K: Percutaneous biopsy of retroperitoneal lymph nodes. A multicentric study. Eur J Radiol 1: 46–50, 1981.
86. Kidd R, Crane R D, Dail D H: Lymphangiography and fine-needle aspiration biopsy: ineffective for staging early prostate cancer. Am J Roentgenol 142: 1007–1012, 1984.
87. Luciani L, Piscioli F: Aspiration Cytology in the staging of Urological cancer. Springer, Berlin, 1988.
88. Luciani L, Piscioli F, Pusiol T, Scappini P: The value of aspiration cytology in the definitive staging of bladder carcinoma. Br J Urol 58: 26–30, 1986.
89. Rupp N, Rothenberger K H: Transabdominal lymph node biopsy. In: Percutaneous biopsy and therapeutic vacular occlusion. Anacher H, Gulotta U, Rupp N. (eds) Georg Thieme, Stuttgart, 1980.
90. Wajsman Z, Gamarra M, Park J J, Beckley S, Pontes J E: Transabdominal fine needle aspiration of retroperitoneal lymph nodes in staging of genito-urinary tract cancer (correlation with lymphangiography and lymph node dissection findings). J Urol 128: 1238–1240, 1982.

Kidneys and Adrenals

91. Akhtar M, Ashraf Ali M, Sackey K, Burgess A: Fine-Needle aspiration biopsy of clear-cell sarcoma of the kidney: Light and electron microscopic features. Diagn Cytopathol 5: 181–187, 1989.
92. Alanen K A, Tyrkko J E S, Nurmi M J: Aspiration biopsy cytology of renal oncocytoma. Acta Cytol 29: 859–862, 1985.
93. Auvert J, Abbou C C, Lavarenne V: Needle tract seeding following puncture of renal oncocytoma. Prog Clin Biol Res 100: 597–598, 1982.
94. Barbaric Z L, MacIntosh P K: Periureteral thin-needle aspiration biopsy. Urol Radiol 2: 181–185, 1981.
95. Barnes C A, Beckman E N: Renal oncocytoma and its congeners. Am J Clin Pathol 79: 312–318, 1983.
96. Beyer D, Fiedler V: Ist die Nierenzystenpunktion eine brauchbare Methode zur Differentialdiagnostic gefässarmer raumfordernder Nierenprozesse? Urologe A 16: 339–345, 1977.
97. Cochand-Priollet B, Rothschild E, Chagnon S, Nezelof C, Debure A, Galian A: Renal oncocytoma diagnosed by fine-needle aspiration cytology Br J Urol 61: 534–535, 1988.
98. Flint A, Cookingham C: Cytologic diagnosis of the papillary variant of renal-cell carcinoma. Acta Cytol 31: 325–329, 1987.
99. Franzén S, Brehmer-Andersson E: Cytologic diagnosis of renal cell carcinoma. Prog Clin Biol Res 100: 425–432, 1982.
100. Freiman D B, Ring E J, Oleaga J A, Carpiniello V C, Wein A J: Thin needle biopsy in the diagnosis of ureteral obstruction with malignancy. Cancer 42: 714–716, 1978.
101. Gibbons R P, Bush W H, Burnett L L: Needle tract seeding following aspiration of renal cell carcinoma. J Urol 118: 865–867, 1977.
102. Göthlin J H, Barbaric Z L: Fluoroscopy-guided percutaneous transperitoneal fine needle biopsy of renal

RETROPERITONEUM, LIVER AND SPLEEN 9

masses. Urology 11: 300–302, 1978.
103. Heaston D K, Handel D B, Ashton P R, Korobkin M: Narrow gauge needle aspiration of solid adrenal masses. Am J Roentgenol 138: 1143–1148, 1982.
104. Heckemann R: Fine-needle biopsy of the kidneys. Radiology 28: 257–264, 1988.
105. Hidvegi D, DeMay R M, Nunez-Alonso C, Nieman H L: Percutaneous transperitoneal aspiration of renal adenocarcinoma guided by ultrasound. Morphologic appearance of normal and malignant cells. Acta Cytol 23: 467–470, 1979.
106. Holm H H, Pedersen J F, Kristensen J K, Rasmussen S N, Hancke S, Jensen F: Ultrasonically guided percutaneous puncture. Radiol Clin North Am 13: 493–503, 1975.
107. Jeans W D, Penry J B, Roylance J: Renal puncture. Clin Radiol 23: 298–311, 1972.
108. Katsuta K, Nakabayashi H, Kuroda Y, Liu P I: Adrenal myelolipoma: preoperative diagnosis by fine-needle aspiration cytology. Diagn Cytopathol 5: 298–300, 1989.
109. Katz R L, Patel S, Mackay B, Zornoza J: Fine needle aspiration cytology of the adrenal gland. Acta Cytol 28: 269–282, 1984.
110. Khorsand D: Carcinoma within solitary renal cysts. J Urol 93: 440–444, 1965.
111. Kristensen J K, Holm H H, Rasmussen S N, Barlebo H: Ultrasonically guided percutaneous puncture of renal masses. Scand J Urol Nephrol 6, Suppl 15: 49–56, 1972.
112. Lang EK: Roentgenographic assessment of asymptomatic renal lesions. Radiol 109: 257–269, 1973.
113. Lang E K: Renal cyst puncture and aspiration: a survey of complications. Am J Roentgenol 128: 723–727, 1977.
114. Leiman G: Audit of fine needle aspiration cytology of 120 renal lesions. Cytopathol 1: 65–72, 1990.
115. Levin N P: Fine needle aspiration and histology of adrenal cortical carcinoma. A case report. Acta Cytol 25: 421–424, 1981.
116. Linsk J A, Franzén S: Aspiration cytology of metastatic hypernephroma. Acta Cytol 28: 250–260, 1984.
117. Ljungberg B, Stenling R, Roos G: Flow cytometric DNA analysis of renal-cell carcinoma. A study of fine needle aspiration biopsies in comparison with multiple surgical samples. Surg Endosc 3: 42–45, 1989.
118. Malatskey A, Fields S, Shapiro A: Complete hemorrhagic necrosis of renal adenocarcinoma following percutaneous biopsy. Urology 33: 125–126, 1989.
119. Miller T R, Bottles K, Abele J S, Beckstead J H: Neuroblastoma diagnosed by fine needle aspiration biopsy. Acta Cytol 29: 461–468, 1985.
120. Nadel L, Baumgartner B R, Bernardino M E: Percutaneous renal biopsies: accuracy, safety, and indications. Urol Radiol 8: 67–71, 1986.
121. Neumann M P, Manivel C, Dehner L P: Adrenal myelolipoma: fine-needle aspiration of an asymptomatic retroperitoneal mass. Diagn Cytopathol 3: 82–84, 1987.
122. Nguyen G K: Cytopathologic aspects of adrenal pheochromocytoma in a fine needle aspiration biopsy. A case report. Acta Cytol 26: 354–358, 1982.
123. Nguyen G K: Fine needle aspiration biopsy cytology of metastatic renal cell carcinoma. Acta Cytol 32: 409–414, 1988.
124. Nguyen G K, Amy R W, Tsang S: Fine needle aspiration biopsy cytology of renal oncocytoma. Acta Cytol 29: 33–36, 1985.
125. Nguyen G K: Aspiration biopsy of renal angiomyolipoma. Acta Cytol 28: 261–264, 1984.
126. Nguyen G K: Percutaneous fine-needle aspiration biopsy cytology of the kidney and adrenal. Pathol Annu 22 (pt 1): 163–191, 1987.
127. Nosker J L, Amorosa J K, Leiman S, Plafker J: Fine

128. Orell S R: The diagnosis of solid renal and adrenal masses by aspiration cytology. In: Aspiration cytology in the staging of urological cancer. Luciani L, Piscioli F (eds) Springer, Berlin, pp 215–223, 1988.
129. Pasternack A, Helin H, Törnroth T, Rantala I, Vaisanen J, Rahka R: Aspiration biopsy of the kidney with a new fine needle: a way to obtain glomeruli for morphologic study. Clin Nephrol 10: 79–84, 1978.
130. Perrin P, Monsallier M, Delorme E, Labadie M: Contribution of cytological punctures to the diagnosis of kidney tumors. J Urol (Paris) 93: 179–182, 1987.
131. Pilotti S, Rilke F, Alasio L, Garbagnati F: The role of fine needle aspiration in the assessment of renal masses. Acta Cytol 32: 1–10, 1988.
132. Pinto M M: Fine needle aspiration of myelolipoma of adrenal gland. Acta Cytol 29: 863–866, 1985.
133. Quijano G, Drut R: Cytologic characteristics of Wilms' tumors in fine needle aspirates. A study of ten cases. Acta Cytol 33: 263–266, 1989.
134. Rodriguez C A, Buskop A, Johnson J, Fromowitz F, Koss L G: Renal oncocytoma. Preoperative diagnosis by aspiration biopsy. Acta Cytol 24: 355–359, 1980.
135. Scheible W, Coel M, Siemers P T, Siegel H: Percutaneous aspiration of adrenal cysts. Am J Roentgenol 128: 1013–1016, 1977.
136. von Schreeb T, Arner O, Skovsted G, Wikstad N: Renal adenocarcinoma. Is there a risk of spreading tumour cells in diagnostic puncture? Scand J Urol Neophrol 1: 270–276, 1967.
137. von Schreeb T, Franzén S, Ljungqvist A: Renal adenocarcinoma. Evaluation of malignancy on a cytologic basis: A comparative cytologic and histologic study. Scand J Urol Nephrol 1: 265–269, 1967.
138. Sease W C, Elyanderani M K, Belis J A: Ultrasonography and needle aspiration in diagnosis of xanthogranulomatous pyelonephritis. Urology 29: 231–235, 1987.
139. Thommesen P, Nielsen B: The value of fine needle aspiration biopsy and intravenous pyelography in the diagnosis of renal masses. Fortschr Roentgenstrahl 122: 248–251, 1975.
140. Wehle M J, Grabstald H: Contraindications to needle aspiration of a solid renal mass: tumor dissemination by renal needle aspiration. J Urol 136: 446–448, 1986.
141. Wong J Y, Zaharopoulos P: Cytologic features on needle aspiration of Wilms' tumour in an adult. A case report. Acta Cytol 27: 69–72, 1983.
142. Zajicek J: Aspiration biopsy cytology. Part 2. Cytology of infradiaphragmatic organs. Karger, Basel, 1979.

Liver

143. Ajdukiewicz A, Crowden A, Hudson E, Pyne C: Liver aspiration in the diagnosis of hepatocellular carcinoma in the Gambia. J Clin Pathol 38: 185–192, 1985.
144. Ali M A, Akhtar M, Mattingly R C: Morphologic spectrum of hepatocellular carcinoma in fine needle aspiration biopsies. Acta Cytol 30: 294–302, 1986.
145. Babb R R, Jackman R J: Needle biopsy of the liver. A critique of four currently available methods. West J Med 150: 39–42, 1989.
146. Barsu M, Ghiurca V, Porutiu D, Badea R: Ultrastructural aspects of human liver tumours collected by needle aspiration biopsy. Morphol Embryol (Bucur); 35: 279–283, 1989.
147. Bedrossian C W, Davila R M, Merenda G:

RETROPERITONEUM, LIVER AND SPLEEN

Immunocytochemical evaluation of liver fine-needle aspirations. Arch Pathol Lab Med 113: 1225–1230, 1989.

148. Bell D A, Carr C P, Szyfelbein W M: Fine-needle aspiration cytology of focal liver lesions results obtained with examination of both cytologic and histologic preparations. Acta Cytol 30: 397–402, 1986.

149. Bermad J J, McNeill R D: Cirrhosis with atypia. A potential pitfall in the interpretation of liver aspirates. Acta Cytol 32: 11–14, 1988.

150. Bhatia A, Mehrotra P: Fine-needle aspiration cytology in a case of hepatoblastoma. Acta Cytol 30: 439–441, 1986.

151. Bissonnette R T, Gibney R G, Berry B R, Buckley A R: Fatal carcinoid crisis after percutaneous fine-needle biopsy of hepatic metastasis: case report and literature review. Radiology 174: 751–752, 1990.

152. Bizjak-Schwarzbartl M: Fine-needle aspiration biopsy in the diagnosis of metastases in the liver. Diagn Cytopathol 3: 278–283, 1987.

153. Bognel C, Rougier P, Leclere J, Duvillard P, Charpentier P, Prade M: Fine needle aspiration of the liver and pancreas with ultrasound guidance. Acta Cytol 32: 22–26, 1988.

154. Bose S, Kapila K, Verma K: Amyloidosis of the liver diagnosed by fine-needle aspiration cytology (letter). Acta Cytol 33: 935–936, 1989.

155. Bottles K, Cohen M B, Holly E M, Chiu S H, Abele J S, Cello J P, Lim R C Jr, Miller T R: A step-wise logistic regression analysis of hepatocellular carcinoma. An aspiration biopsy study. Cancer 62: 558–563, 1988.

156. Brambs H J, Spamer C, Volk B, Wimmer B, Koch H: Histological diagnosis of liver hemangiomas using ultrasound-guided fine-needle biopsy. Hepatogastroenterology 32: 284–287, 1985.

157. Bret P M, Labadie M, Bretagnolle M, Palliard P, Fond A, Valette P J: Hepatocellular carcinoma: diagnosis by percutaneous fine-needle biopsy. Gastrointest Radiol 13: 253–255, 1988.

158. Bret P M, Sente J M, Bretagnolle M, Fond A, Labadie M, Paliard P: Ultrasonically guided fine-needle biopsy in focal intrahepatic lesions: six years' experience. Can Assoc Radiol J 37: 5–8, 1986.

159. Caturelli E, Rapaccini G L, Sabelli C, De Simone F, Fabiano A, Romagna-Manoja E, Anti M, Fedeli G: Ultrasound-guided fine-needle aspiration biopsy in the diagnosis of hepatic hemangioma. Liver 6: 326–330, 1986.

160. Caturelli E, Rapaccini G L, Sabelli C, de Simone F, Anti M, Savini E, Grattagliano A: Ultrasonography and echo-guided fine-needle biopsy in the diagnosis of focal fatty liver change. Hepatogastroenterology 34: 137–140, 1987.

161. Cavanna L, Di Stasi M, Fornari F, Civardi G, Sbolli G, Buscarini E, Buscarini L: Ultrasound and ultrasonically guided biopsy in hepatic lymphoma. Eur J Cancer Clin Oncol 23: 323–326, 1987.

162. Damascelli B, Spagnoli I, Garbagnati F, Ceglia E, Milella M, Masciadri N: Massive haemorrhoea after fine-needle biopsy of the cystic haemolymphangioma of the liver. Eur J Radiol 4: 107–109, 1984.

163. Dekmezian R, Sneige N, Popok S, Ordonez N G: Fine-needle aspiration cytology of pediatric patients with primary hepatic tumors: a comparative study of two hepatoblastomas and a liver-cell carcinoma. Diagn Cytopathol 4: 162–168, 1988.

164. Domagala W, Lasota J, Weber K, Osborn M: Endothelial cells help in the diagnosis of primary versus metastatic carcinoma of the liver in fine needle aspirates. An immunofluorescence study with vimentin and endothelial cell-specific antibodies. Anal Quant Cytol Histol 11: 8–14, 1989.

165. Ekelund P, Wasastjerna C: Cytologic identification of primary hepatic carcinoma cells. Acta Med Scand 189: 373–375, 1971.

166. Gebel M, Horstkotte H, Kloster C, Brunkhorst R, Brandt M, Atay Z: Ultrasound-guided fine needle puncture of the abdominal organs: indications, results, risks. Ultraschall Med 7: 198–202, 1986.

167. Glaser K S, Weger A R, Schmid K W, Bodner E: Is fine-needle aspiration of tumours harmless? (letter). Lancet 1: 620, 1989.

168. Glenthöj A, Sehested M: Histological and cytological fine-needle biopsies from focal liver lesions. Intra- and interobserver reproducibility of diagnoses. APMIS 97: 611–618, 1989.

169. Gondos B, Forouhar F: Fine-needle aspiration cytology of liver tumors. Ann Clin Lab Sci 14: 155–158, 1984.

170. Greene C A, Suen K C: Some cytological features of hepatocellular carcinoma as seen in fine-needle aspirates. Acta Cytol 28: 713–718, 1984.

171. Grimelius L, Stenram U, Westman J, Westman-Naeser S: Hyaline cytoplasmic inclusions in human hepatoma. A case report. Acta Cytol 21: 469–476, 1977.

172. Gupta S K, Das D K, Rajwanshi A, Bhusnurmath S R: Cytology of hepatocellular carcinoma. Diagn Cytopathol 2: 290–294, 1986.

173. Hajdu S I, D'Ambrosio F G, Fields V, Lightdale C J: Aspiration and brush cytology of the liver. Semin Diagn Pathol 3: 227–238, 1986.

174. Hall-Craggs M S, Lees W R: Fine needle biopsy: cytology, histology or both? Tumori 73: 507–512, 1987.

175. Hertzanu Y, Peiser J, Zirkin H: Massive bleeding after fine needle aspiration of liver angiosarcoma. Gastrointest Radiol 15: 43–46, 1990.

176. Hällén J, Nilsson G, Tedbrant A: Fine-needle aspiration compared with scintigraphy for detection of liver neoplasia. Acta Med Scand 215: 481–486, 1984

177. Ho C S, McLoughlin M J, Tao L C, Blendis L, Evans W K: Guided percutaneous fine-needle aspiration biopsy of the liver. Cancer 47: 1781–1785, 1981.

178. Hockerstedt K, Lautenschlager I: Fine-needle aspiration biopsy in liver transplants. Transplant Proc 21: 3625–3626, 1989.

179. Jacobsen G K, Gammelgaard J, Fugl M: Coarse needle biopsy versus fine-needle aspiration biopsy in the diagnosis of focal lesions of the liver. Ultrasonically guided needle biopsy in suspected hepatic malignancy. Acta Cytol 27: 152–156, 1983.

180. Johansen S, Myren J: Fine-needle aspiration biopsy smears in the diagnosis of liver diseases. Scand J. Gastroenterol 6: 583–588, 1971.

181. Lagrange W: Fine needle aspiration biopsy of myxoid variant of malignant leiomyoblastoma metastatic to the liver. Acta Cytol 32: 443–446, 1988.

182. Lautenschlager I: Fine-needle aspiration biopsy in liver transplants. Transplant Proc 21: 3618–3620, 1989.

183. Leiman G, Leibowitz C B, Dunbar F: Fine-needle aspiration of the liver; out of the ivory tower and into the community. Diagn Cytopathol 5: 35–39, 1989.

184. Livraghi T, Pilotti S, Ravetto C, Sangalli G, Solbiati L: Inclusion-cytology versus smear-cytology in fine needle abdominal biopsy. Eur J Radiol 5: 11–14, 1985.

185. Livraghi T, Sangalli G, Giordano F, Ravetto C, Solbiati L, Fornari F, Cavanna L, Matricardi L, Gaguano E. 240 hepatocellular carcinomas: ultrasound features, tumour size, cytologic and histologic patterns, serum alpha-fetoprotein and HbS Ag. Tumori 73: 507–512, 1987.

186. Lundqvist A: Fine-needle aspiration biopsy for cytodiagnosis of malignant tumours in the liver. Acta Med Scand 188: 465–470, 1970.

187. Lundqvist A: Liver biopsy with a needle of 0.7 mm outer diameter. Safety and quantitative yield. Acta Med Scand

RETROPERITONEUM, LIVER AND SPLEEN 9

188: 471–474, 1970.

188. Lundqvist A: Fine-needle aspiration biopsy of the liver. Acta Med Scand (Suppl) 520: 1–28, 1971.

189. Lupovitch A, Chen R, Mishra S: Inflammatory pseudotumor of the liver. Report of the fine needle aspiration cytologic findings in a case initially misdiagnosed as malignant. Acta Cytol 33: 259–262, 1989.

190. Nakaizumi A, Iishi H, Yamamoto R, Kasugai H, Tatsuta M, Okuda S, Kishigami Y, Kitamura T: Diagnosis of hepatic cavernous hemangioma by fine-needle aspiration biopsy under ultrasonic guidance. Gastrointest Radiol 15: 39–42, 1990.

191. Nguyen G K, McHattie J D, Jeannot A: Cytomorphologic aspects of hepatic angiosarcoma. Fine needle aspiration biopsy of a case. Acta Cytol 26: 527–531, 1982.

192. Noguchi S, Yamamoto R, Tatsuta M, Kasugai H, Okuda S, Wade A, Tamura H: Cell features and patterns in fine-needle aspirates of hepatocelluar carcinoma. Cancer 58: 321–328, 1986.

193. Onodera H, Oikawa M, Abe M, Chida N, Kimura S, Satake K, Motojima T, Goto Y: Cutaneous seeding of hepatocellular carcinoma after fine-needle aspiration biopsy. J Ultrasound Med 6: 273–275, 1987.

194. Pedio G, Landolt U, Zobeli L, Gut D: Fine needle aspiration of the liver. Significance of hepatocytic naked nuclei in the diagnosis of hepatocellular carcinoma. Acta Cytol 32: 437–442, 1988.

195. Perry M D, Johnston W W: Needle biopsy of the liver for the diagnosis of non-neoplastic liver diseases. Acta Cytol 29: 385–390, 1985.

196. Pieterse A S, Smith M, Smith L A, Smith P: Embryonal (undifferentiated) sarcoma of the liver. Fine-needle aspiration cytology and ultrastructural findings. Arch Pathol Lab Med 109: 677–680, 1985.

197. Pilotti S, Rilke F, Claren R, Milella M, Lombardi L: Conclusive diagnosis of hepatic and pancreatic malignancies by fine needle aspiration. Acta Cytol 32: 27–38, 1988.

198. Pinto M M, Kaye A D: Fine-needle aspiration of cystic liver lesions. Cytologic examination and carcinoembryonic antigen assay of cyst contents. Acta Cytol 33: 852–856, 1989.

199. Plafker J, Nosher J L: Fine-needle aspiration of liver with metastatic adenoid cystic carcinoma. Acta Cytol 27: 323–329, 1983.

200. Prior C, Kathrein H, Mikuz G, Judmaier G: Differential diagnosis of malignant intrahepatic tumors by ultrasonically guided fine needle aspiration biopsy and by laparoscopic/intraoperative biopsy. A comparative study. Acta Cytol 32: 892–895, 1988.

201. Riska H, Friman C: Fatality after fine-needle aspiration biopsy of liver. Br Med J 1: 517, 1975.

202. Roesler P J Jr, Wills J S: Hepatic actinomycosis: CT features. J Comput Assist Tomogr 10: 335–337, 1986.

203. Ruschenburg I, Droese M: Fine-needle aspiration cytology of focal nodular hyperplasia of the liver. Acta Cytol 33: 857–860, 1989.

204. Sangalli G, Livraghi T, Giordano F: Fine needle biopsy of hepatocellular carcinoma: improvement in diagnosis by microhistology. Gastroenterology 96: 524–526, 1989.

205. Schultz T B: Fine needle biopsy of the liver complicated with bile peritonitis. Acta Med Scand 199: 141–142, 1976.

206. Schwerk W B, Durr H K, Schmitz-Moormann P: Ultrasound guided fine-needle biopsies in pancreatic and hepatic neoplasms. Gastrointest Radiol 8: 219–225, 1983.

207. Servoll E, Viste A, Skaarland E, Larssen T B, Pedersen O M, Arnesjö B, Söreide O: Fine-needle aspiration cytology of focal liver lesions. Advantages and limitations. Acta Chir Scand 154: 61–63, 1988.

208. Sipponen P, Pikkarainen P, Vuori E, Salaspuro M: Copper deposits in fine needle aspiration biopsies in primary biliary cirrhosis. Acta Cytol 24: 203–207, 1980.

209. Solbiati L, Livraghi T, De Pra L, Ierace T, Masciadri N, Ravetto C: Fine-needle biopsy of hepatic hemangioma with sonographic guidance. Am J Roentgenol 144: 471–474, 1985.

210. Spamer C, Brambs H J, Koch H K, Gerok W: Benign circumscribed lesions of the liver diagnosed by ultrasonically guided fine-needle biopsy. JCV 14: 83–88, 1986.

211. Stormby N, Åkerman M: Aspiration cytology in the diagnosis of granulomatous liver lesions. Acta Cytol 17: 200–204, 1973.

212. Suen K C: Diagnosis of primary hepatic neoplasms by fine-needle aspiration cytology. Diagn Cytopathol 2: 99–109, 1986.

213. Suen K C, Magee J F, Halparin L S, Chan N H, Greene C A: Fine-needle aspiration cytology of fibrolamellar hepatocellular carcinoma. Acta Cytol 29: 867–872, 1985.

214. Tao L C, Ho C S, McLoughlin M J, Evans W K, Donat E E: Cytologic diagnosis of hepatocellular carcinoma by fine-needle aspiration biopsy. Cancer 53: 547–552, 1984.

215. Tatsuta M, Vamamoto R, Kasugai H, Okano Y, Noguchi S, Okuda S, Wada A, Tamura H: Cytohistologic diagnosis of neoplasms of the liver by ultrasonically guided fine-needle aspiration biopsy. Cancer 54: 1682–1686, 1984.

216. Terriff B A, Gibney R G, Scudamore CH: Fatality from fine-needle aspiration biopsy of a hepatic hemangioma (letter). Am J Roentgenol 154: 203–204, 1990.

217. Vercelli-Retta J, Manana G, Reissenweber N J: The cytologic diagnosis of hydatid disease. Acta Cytol 26: 159–164, 1982.

218. Wasastjerna C: Liver. In Zajicek J: Aspiration biopsy cytology. Part 2. Cytology of infradiaphragmatic organs. Zajicek J Karger, Basel, 1979.

219. Weiss H, Weiss A, Scholl A: Fatal complication of fine-needle biopsy of the liver. Dtsch Med Wochenschr 113: 139–142, 1988.

220. Wernecke K, Heckemann R, Rehwald U: Ultrasound-guided thin-needle biopsy in focal liver diseases. II. Benign focal liver disease. Ultraschall Med 5: 303–311, 1984.

221. Whitlatch S, Nurnez C, Pitlik D A: Fine-needle aspiration biopsy of the liver. A study of 102 consecutive cases. Acta Cytol 28: 719–725, 1984.

Spleen

222. Dagnini G, Cladironi M W, Marin G, Patella M: Laparoscopic splenic biopsy. Endoscopy 16: 55–58, 1984.

223. Goldfinger M, Cohen M M, Steinhardt M I, Rothberg R, Rother I: Sonography and percutaneous aspiration of splenic epidermoid cyst. JCU 14: 147–149, 1986.

224. Jansson S E, Bondestam S, Heinonen E, Gröhn P, Vuopio P: Value of liver and spleen aspiration biopsy in malignant diseases when these organs show no signs of involvement in sonography. Acta Med Scand 213: 279–281, 1983.

225. Kager P A, Rees P H: Splenic aspiration. Review of the literature. Trop Geogr Med 35: 111–124, 1983.

226. Kager P A, Rees P H, Manguyu F M, Bhatt K M, Bhatt S M: Splenic aspiration, experience in Kenya. Trop Geogr Med 35: 125–131, 1983.

227. Lindgren P G, Hagberg H, Eriksson B, Grimelius B,

RETROPERITONEUM, LIVER AND SPLEEN

Magnusson A, Sundström C: Excision biopsy of the spleen by ultrasonic guidance. Br J Radiol 58: 853–857, 1985.

228. Moeschlin S: Die Milzpunktion. Benno Schwabe, Basel, 1947.
229. Morrison M, Samwick A A, Rubinstein J, Morrison H, Loewe L: Splenic aspiration: clinical and haematological considerations based on observations in 105 cases. JAMA 146: 1575–1580, 1951.
230. Pasternack A: Fine-needle aspiration biopsy of the spleen in diagnosis of generalized amyloidosis. Br Med J 2: 20–22, 1974.
231. Schwerk W B, Maroske D, Roth S, Arnold R: Ultrasound-guided fine-needle puncture in the diagnosis and therapy of liver and spleen abscesses. Dtsch Med Wochenschr 111: 847–853, 1986.
232. Selroos O, Koivunen E: Usefulness of fine-needle aspiration biopsy of spleen in diagnosis of sarcoidosis. Chest 83: 193–195, 1983.
233. Söderström N: Fine-needle aspiration biopsy. Almqvist & Wiksell, Stockholm, 1966.
234. Söderström N: How to use cytodiagnostic spleen puncture. Acta Med Scand 199: 1–5, 1976.
235. Solbiati L, Bossi M C, Bellotti E, Ravetto C, Montali G: Focal lesions in the spleen: Sonographic patterns and guided biopsy. Am J Roentgenol 140: 59–65, 1983.
236. Taavitsainen M, Koivuniemi A, Helminen J, Bondestam S, Kivisaari L, Pamilo M, Tierala E, Tiitinen H: Aspiration biopsy of the spleen in patients with sarcoidosis. Acta Radiol 28: 723–725, 1987.

10

MALE AND FEMALE GENITAL ORGANS

10 *MALE AND FEMALE GENITAL ORGANS*

CLINICAL ASPECTS

The technique of fine-needle aspiration of the prostate was introduced by Franzén, Giertz and Zajicek in 1960.[15] The simple instruments designed by Franzén made transrectal biopsy of any palpable abnormality in the prostate or elsewhere in the pelvis relatively easy. The same technique can be used to biopsy lesions of the female genital tract palpable per vaginam or per rectum. The biopsy can be carried out as an office procedure. No preparation and no anaesthesia is necessary and complications are rare. These are the main advantages of FNA over transrectal or transperineal needle biopsy with a cutting needle of Vim-Silverman or Tru-cut type, the diagnostic accuracy being about equal for both methods.[9,10,28,50]

Preoperative incisional biopsy of testicular tumours is contra-indicated. Although some evidence has been presented that the use of a fine needle (22–23 gauge) does not carry a risk of tumour spread,[49,53] a cautious attitude to the biopsy of malignant testicular tumours is recommended until further experience has been critically evaluated.

PROSTATE

The place of FNA in the investigative sequence

Transurethral resection (TUR) is the standard treatment of outflow obstruction whether it is caused by cancer or by benign hyperplasia. Therefore, preoperative diagnosis by transrectal FNA may seem unnecessary since it will not alter the surgical management regardless of the result. In our opinion, preoperative FNA of the prostate is still of value, at least in patients with clinical suspicion of cancer, for the following reasons:

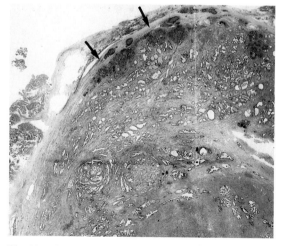

Fig. 10.1 Adenocarcinoma of prostate
Tissue section horizontally through prostatectomy specimen. Small, thin, subcapsular tumour (arrows) successfully biopsied by FNA (H & E)

1. A carcinoma may be missed by TUR which usually does not include subcapsular parts of the gland, the site of predilection for carcinoma (Fig. 10.1).

2. A preoperative tissue diagnosis allows staging procedures to be carried out before treatment and this may lead to a more rational approach to the management of patients with prostatic cancer.

3. In some cases, retropubic prostatectomy may be the preferred treatment for obstructive symptoms. Since the complication rate is considerably higher in cases of carcinoma than in cases of benign hyperplasia, preoperative FNA is an important means of excluding the former from this form of treatment. Also, some authors have suggested that TUR may adversely affect prognosis in locally advanced, poorly differentiated prostatic carcinoma, although others have found no evidence to support this.[31]

4. Younger patients with biopsy-proven, early stage cancers may be considered for radical prostatectomy.

In patients without outflow obstruction FNA is the least invasive method to diagnose carcinoma. Long term hormonal treatment (with its common and adverse side effects) should never be undertaken without a tissue diagnosis. A large needle biopsy, though as accurate as FNA, causes considerably greater patient discomfort and carries a greater risk of complications.

Radical prostatectomy is a potentially curative treatment of localised prostatic carcinoma. Radiotherapy has also been applied to localised disease with what appears to be significant rates of cure. Unfortunately, few cancers are diagnosed in stages I and II by conventional methods. So far, FNA has not made a significant contribution to early detection of prostatic cancer, stage I cancer being an uncommon chance finding in FNA of clinically benign prostatic enlargment.[45] However, recent advances in ultrasonographic techniques have made it possible to detect early stage, potentially curable cancer which can be confirmed by US-directed fine needle biopsy or by core needle biopsy using the Biopty device.[1,38] This is an interesting new development in the diagnosis of prostatic cancer.

Cytological grading of prostatic carcinoma correlates well with survival and is valuable in prognostication.[12] Grading may influence the choice of treatment. For example, asymptomatic, incidentally detected low-grade cancers are usually not treated, while high-grade tumours may receive early radiotherapy. More consistent and reproducible cytological predictions can be achieved by morphometric methods applied to FNA smears.[47,55] In addition, hormone receptors can now be studied at a cellular level using immunohistochemical techniques (see Ch. 7). The effect of hormonal treatment (and also of radiotherapy) on prostatic cancer is reflected by the cytological pattern. FNA can therefore be used to follow the response and to monitor dose levels.[25]

Accurate sampling can be a problem if the tumour is small and deeply situated in the testis, particularly if the consistency of the tumour tissue (for example seminoma) is not obviously different from that of normal testis. Ultrasonographic guidance is helpful to guide the biopsy and to select solid areas in tumours with a cystic component. Many germ cell tumours have a variable histological pattern. FNA does therefore not permit definitive typing which requires histological examination of the whole tumour.[49]

The capsule of the normal testis is quite sensitive, and local anaesthesia is recommended in FNA investigation of infertility. A testicle harbouring malignant or inflammatory disease is usually less sensitive. A 25 gauge needle and biopsy without aspiration is recommended as it allows optimal precision and minimal trauma. The site of biopsy should be recorded for future excision in cases of suspected malignancy. Air-dried and alcohol-fixed smears should be made in parallel and extra smears kept for immunocytochemistry if needed.

FEMALE GENITAL ORGANS

The place of FNA in the investigative sequence

FNA in gynaecological practice is mainly applied in the following three areas: the investigation of suspected pelvic recurrence in cases of known gynaecological cancer; the preoperative investigation of ovarian tumours; and the investigation of ovarian cysts and other abnormalities discovered at laparoscopy.[73,75]

1. Patients who have received surgical treatment and/or irradiation for cervical, endometrial or ovarian cancer are frequently re-examined in order to detect any recurrence at an early stage. A palpable nodule or mass in the vaginal vault, in the parametria or elsewhere in the pelvis usually signals recurrence, but this needs to be confirmed since post-treatment oedema, inflammation, suture granuloma or scarring can be the cause of the abnormality. If ureteric obstruction develops, this must be investigated and treated urgently (p. 218). The simplest and least invasive biopsy method under these circumstances is FNA, using the Franzén instrumentarium if the lesion is palpable per vaginam or per rectum, or percutaneously guided by ultrasound or by CT.[57,62,67,76,81,82]

2. FNA has not been widely used in the preoperative investigation of ovarian tumours. The possibility that puncture of a cystic carcinoma might cause intraperitoneal seeding of malignant cells has been a discouraging factor. It is also argued that preoperative biopsy is unnecessary since surgical exploration is mandatory. On the other hand, Kjellgren and Ångström[70] point out that a preoperative cytological assessment allows individualisation of treatment, particularly the preoperative irradiation of anaplastic carcinoma. Ramzy et al recom-

mend FNA biopsy of the contralateral ovary during laparotomy for ovarian tumour in premenopausal women in whom preservation of ovarian function is important.[79] We feel that needle biopsy of ovarian tumours should be restricted to patients who are poor surgical risks, who have evidence of disseminated cancer at the time of presentation, or who have suspected recurrence of previously diagnosed tumour. Indications can be widened if an extraperitoneal approach is possible, or if radiological tumour imaging proves the tumour to be solid.

3. Laparoscopy is a common investigative procedure in gynaecological practice. Small ovarian cysts detected at laparoscopy can be punctured and the contents aspirated for hormonal assay and for cytological examination. Most cysts detected in this way are of follicular origin, but there is always a possibility that a cyst may be neoplastic, and cytological examination of the cyst fluid is therefore important. However, the cytological distinction between a functional cyst which needs no treatment, and a benign epithelial cyst which should be removed, can be difficult. Hormonal assay of the fluid is helpful in distinguishing between functional and neoplastic cysts.[68,71]

Accuracy of diagnosis

The cytological diagnosis of recurrent or metastatic gynaecological cancer is usually not difficult, particularly if the histology of the primary is known. However, post-radiation atypia of epithelial or stromal cells can sometimes cause considerable problems. Detailed information of the nature and the sequence of any given treatment must be available to the pathologist.[75] Good quality aspirates are essential and abnormal cells which meet the appropriate criteria of malignancy must be present in significant numbers to allow confirmation of recurrence. If not, the biopsy must be repeated.

The diagnostic accuracy of preoperative FNA biopsy of ovarian tumours has been reported to be 90–95%.[70] The accuracy is lower in predominantly cystic tumours but can be improved by supplementing cytological examination with biochemical assays.[85] The clinical value of laparoscopic cyst aspiration has not yet been well documented. Correlation with ultrasonographic findings (size, multiloculation, solid areas) and with hormonal assay can reduce the need for surgery in carefully selected cases.[58,60]

Cytological typing of the common epithelial ovarian tumours is usually possible, although serous and endometrioid carcinomas are difficult to separate. Whether or not borderline cystadenoma can be distinguished cytologically from well differentiated cystadenocarcinoma has not been adequately studied, and this distinction must at present be left to histopathological examination.[66] A type specific diagnosis may not be possible in

10 *MALE AND FEMALE GENITAL ORGANS*

some stromal and other uncommon tumours. The exact nature of benign cysts can not be determined if the cyst fluid contains only cells of histiocytic type which is often the case. Finally, it should be remembered that, since the exact position of the needle is not always known, the aspirate may represent peritoneal fluid rather than the contents of an ovarian cyst.

Complications

Sepsis has been observed after transrectal biopsy of ovarian tumours, particularly cystic types. Biopsy per vaginam is therefore preferable. The question whether FNA of ovarian cystadenocarcinoma can cause peritoneal seeding of tumour cells is difficult to answer in view of the common tendency for ovarian cancer to spread transperitoneally. To our knowledge, no detailed study has yet been undertaken to examine this problem. Until the safety of the procedure has been clearly proven, we feel that transabdominal puncture should be avoided unless dissemination is already evident.[70] Significant complications have been recorded with core needle biopsy of pelvic lesions.[82,83]

Technical considerations

Any palpable pelvic mass can be biopsied per vaginam using the same instruments and the same technique as in FNA of the prostate. A rectal or transabdominal approach may appear preferable in some cases, but this involves a certain risk of complications as mentioned above. Also, one is more likely to sample a solid portion of a cystic ovarian tumour by transvaginal rather than by transabdominal puncture.[70] The biopsy can be performed as an office procedure without anaesthesia.[57] Whenever possible, it should, however, be co-ordinated with other procedures such as bimanual palpation, diagnostic curettage, or cystoscopy requiring general anaesthesia, so that any additional discomfort is avoided.

As a rule, alcohol-fixation and staining with Pap or with H & E is recommended for pelvic and ovarian aspirates. However, air dried smears and spares for special stains should also be made if possible. Cyst fluid is best processed by centrifugation with the Cytocentrifuge. Cell block preparations can be very useful in selected cases.

MALE AND FEMALE GENITAL ORGANS

CYTOLOGICAL FINDINGS

10

THE PROSTATE

Benign prostatic hyperplasia (Figs 10.3 and 10.4)[24,43]

Usual findings

1. A watery aspirate.
2. Monolayered sheets of glandular epithelial cells.
3. Uniformly distributed nuclei.
4. Distinct cell membranes; low N/C ratio.
5. Uniform, round or ovoid nuclei; finely granular chromatin; small nucleoli.
6. Coarse intracytoplasmic granules.

Cell cohesion is strong and the characteristically monolayered sheets of glandular epithelial cells can be quite large. Within the sheets, most cells are seen on end and appear polygonal with centrally placed nuclei. The abundant pale cytoplasm and the distinct cell membranes give the sheets a honeycomb pattern (Figs 10.3 and 10.4); only at their periphery are cells sometimes seen in profile as columnar. This appearance is similar to other columnar surface epithelia for example from the biliary and pancreatic ducts, gastrointestinal mucosa, and uterine cervix. The most important criteria of benignancy are the uniform distribution of nuclei within monolayered sheets of epithelium, distinct cell membranes, low N/C ratio and intracytoplasmic granules (Fig. 10.3). These granules stain dark purple with MGG but are less conspicuous in alcohol-fixed smears stained by H & E or Pap. Although granules are not seen in all benign epithelial cells, they are rarely present in carcinoma cells and never in epithelial cells from the rectal mucosa.

Other common findings in benign hyperplasia are various inflammatory cells, metaplastic squamous epithelial cells, clumps of condensed secretion, fragments of calculi, and corpora amylacea. Stromal smooth muscle cells are sometimes seen, mainly as tiny tissue fragments.

Prostatitis (Figs 10.5 and 10.6)

Usual findings

1. Many inflammatory cells: polymorphs, lymphocytes, and macrophages.
2. Mild epithelial atypia.

Mild epithelial atypia is acceptable in the presence of severe inflammation (Fig. 10.5). Degenerative changes such as cytoplasmic vacuolation are often seen. The distribution of cells within epithelial sheets may be less uniform than normal, and the cell membranes may be less distinct. Cytoplasmic granules are often absent. However, significant nuclear enlargement, pleomorphism, and chromatin abnormalities do not occur. There is little tendency to dissociation of epithelial sheets, and microglandular patterns are not seen. As inflammation

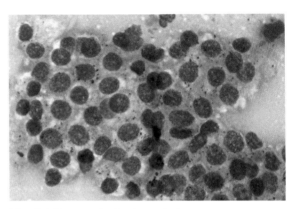

Fig. 10.3 Prostate; benign hyperplasia
Honeycomb-like sheet of uniform glandular epithelial cells; note visible cell borders and coarse cytoplasmic granules (MGG, HP)

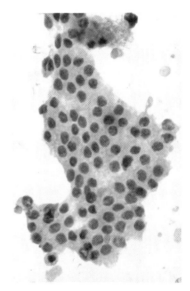

Fig. 10.4 Prostate; benign hyperplasia
Monolayered sheet of uniform glandular epithelial cells (Pap, HP)

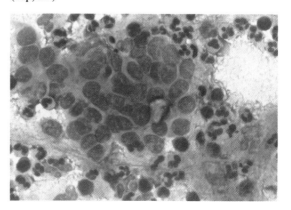

Fig. 10.5 Prostatitis (acute)
Irregular sheet of mildly atypical glandular cells; background of neutrophils (MGG, HP)

10 *MALE AND FEMALE GENITAL ORGANS*

may co-exist with carcinoma, the epithelial atypia must be carefully evaluated.

In *granulomatous prostatitis* histiocytes are prominent. These may be of epithelioid type and may occur in clusters. Multinucleated, histiocytic giant cells are plentiful, and are often seen in relation to inspissated secretion (Fig. 10.6). Epithelial cells are few relative to inflammatory cells and may be mildly atypical.

The cytological findings in *Malakoplakia* of the prostate diagnosed by FNA have been described. We have not seen any example of this condition and the reader is referred to the paper by Cazzaniga et al.[5]

Adenocarcinoma of prostate (Figs 10.7–10.9)[19,24,43]

Criteria for diagnosis

1. Cellular smears.
2. Decreased cell cohesion, variable numbers of single cells.
3. Nuclear crowding (multilayered clusters), microglandular pattern.
4. Indistinct cell membranes; high N/C ratio.
5. Variable nuclear and nucleolar enlargment.
6. Absence of intracytoplasmic granules (exceptions occur).

In FNA smears of prostatic carcinoma it is more common than in cancers of other sites to find sheets of benign glandular cells side-by-side with aggregates of malignant cells (Figs 10.7 and 10.8). This is due to the

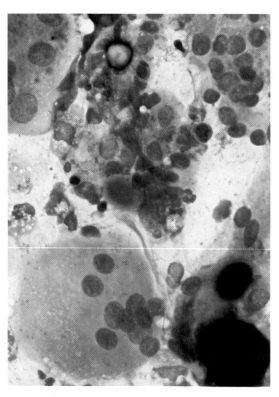

Fig. 10.6 Prostatitis (granulomatous)
Several multinucleate giant cells, one containing inspissated secretion; mildly atypical epithelial cells; some inflammatory cells (MGG, HP)

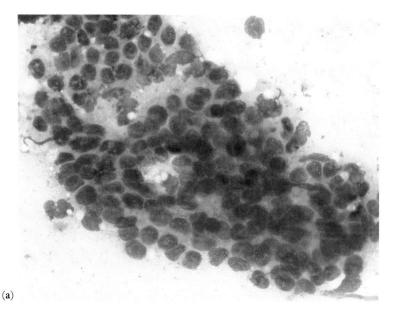

(a)

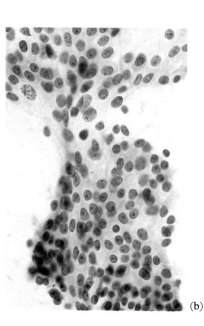

(b)

Fig. 10.7 Adenocarcinoma grade I
(a) Adjacent sheets of benign and malignant epithelium; mild nuclear enlargement, nuclear crowding and a microacinar pattern of malignant cells; absence of cytoplasmic granules (MGG, HP). (b) Large monolayered sheet of mildly atypical epthelial cells; note irregular distribution of nuclei with a tendency to microglandular arrangement, indistinct cell borders and prominent nucleoli; note mitotic figure (Pap, HP).

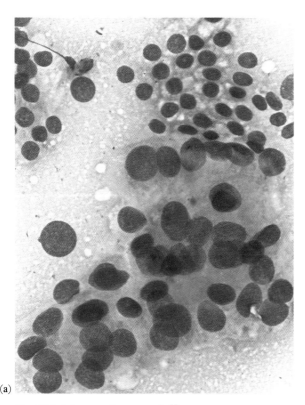
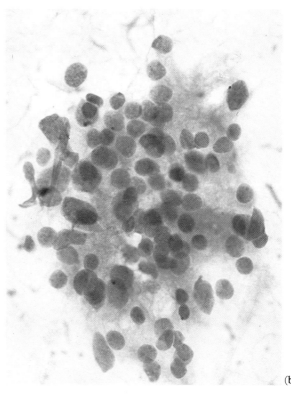

(a)   (b)

Fig. 10.8 Adenocarcinoma grade II
Aggregate of malignant cells; marked nuclear enlargement and nuclear pleomorphism; nuclear crowding; microacinar pattern: indistinct cell borders, note contrasting honeycomb sheet of benign epithelium in (a). (a) MGG, HP. (b) H & E, HP.

widely infiltrating growth pattern of prostatic cancer. It is very helpful to be able to compare benign and malignant cells directly in the same smear since this makes it easy to evaluate nuclear size, N/C ratio and nuclear crowding. Nuclear enlargement is perhaps the single most important criterion of malignancy (Fig. 10.7). Absence of visible cell membranes, nuclear crowding, and dissociation of cells are other important criteria (Fig. 10.8). The presence of the characteristic coarse intracytoplasmic granules is strong evidence against malignancy; however, it is not an infallible sign since granules are occasionally seen in cells from well differentiated adenocarcinoma. Numerous small intracytoplasmic vacuoles are striking in some well differentiated carcinomas but can also occur in epithelial cells of benign hyperplasia. Nuclear pleomorphism and chromatin abnormalities are obvious in less well differentiated cancers but are not very helpful in the sometimes difficult diagnosis of grade I carcinoma.

In addition to architectural and cytological criteria, a quantitative criterium should also be applied in the diagnosis of prostatic cancer. If only a small number of atypical cells are found in a predominantly benign cell population, a definitive diagnosis of cancer should not be made even if the cells are highly suspicious of malig-

nancy. The cells may represent atypical hyperplasia, carcinoma in situ or a microscopical focus of well differentiated carcinoma which does not require treatment. If clinically significant cancer is present, it should be possible to obtain a large number of malignant cells by repeat biopsies.

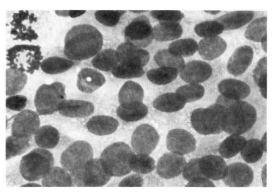

Fig. 10.9 Adenocarcinoma grade III
Dispersed population of malignant cells; several mitoses (MGG, HP)

10 *MALE AND FEMALE GENITAL ORGANS*

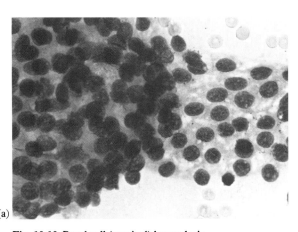

(a)

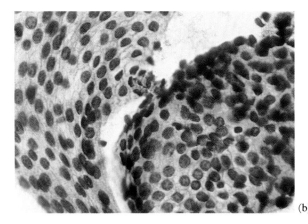

(b)

Fig. 10.10 Basal cell (atypical) hyperplasia
Sheets of glandular epithelial cells showing mild nuclear enlargement and nuclear crowding contrasting with normal epithelium.
(a) MGG, HP. (b) Pap, HP.

Problems in diagnosis

1. Basal cell and atypical hyperplasia.
2. Well-differentiated carcinoma.
3. Contamination from rectal mucosa.
4. Seminal vesicular epithelium.
5. Transitional cell carcinoma invading prostate.

Not infrequently smears from benign prostatic hyperplasia may contain a few cohesive aggregates of cells with increased N/C ratio, indistinct cell borders and crowding of dark nuclei. Such cells which represent basal cell or atypical hyperplasia can be mistaken for malignancy (Figs 10.10 and 10.11). However, nuclear enlargement is not prominent, the chromatin pattern is bland, nucleoli are inconspicuous and dissociation of cells does not occur. There is little tendency to form acini or microglandular structures which are so characteristic of well differentiated carcinoma.[7] Very importantly, the clusters of atypical cells constitute only a minor proportion of the cell population of the smear. Atypical hyperplasia/dysplasia of severe degree is probably indistinguishable from well differentiated carcinoma, but is almost always associated with carcinoma anyway.

Cytological features of malignancy may be subtle in well differentiated carcinoma, especially if normal epithelial cells are not present for comparison. Dissociation can be minimal, nuclei relatively uniform and the nuclear chromatin bland. The diagnosis is then based on moderate but definite nuclear enlargment (which is more easily appreciated in air-dried than in wet-fixed smears), nuclear crowding, indistinct cell membranes, and a microglandular pattern. Prominent nucleoli are a helpful feature in Pap-stained smears (Fig. 10.7). The number of cells aspirated is often much greater than in smears of benign hyperplasia and the amount of background secretion is less. Occasionally, the very high cell content of smears may be the only finding that could

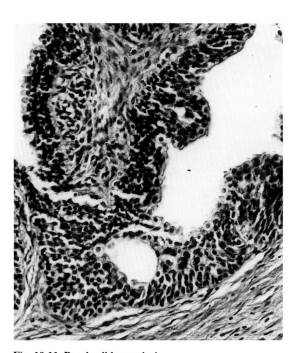

Fig. 10.11 Basal cell hyperplasia
Tissue section. Glandular epithelium multilayered showing mild nuclear atypia (H & E, IP).

raise a suspicion of malignancy in a very well differentiated carcinoma.

Epithelial cells from the *rectal mucosa* aspirated en passant are less regular than normal prostatic epithelial cells. They often form microglandular structures which represent the crypts, and they lack intracytoplasmic coarse granules. Under low power, they may be mistaken for well differentiated carcinoma. On closer examination, the presence of mucin, goblet cells, tall columnar cells with elongated nuclei, and the background of amorphous rectal contents reveals their true nature (Fig. 10.12).[10]

Epithelial cells from the *seminal vesicles* may have strikingly pleomorphic nuclei which can be hyperchromatic, very large, lobulated, even bizarre, features which are also commonly observed in histological sections. Such cells can easily be misdiagnosed as malignant by the inexperienced viewer. Spermatozoa in the background indicate that the smear may have been aspirated from the seminal vesicle. In addition, seminal vesicular epithelial cells are recognised by the coarse intracytoplasmic granules of lipofuscin which stain a dark green-blue with MGG, brown with Pap or H & E (Figs 10.13 and 10.14).[8,22]

The important differential diagnosis between prostatic adenocarcinoma and transitional cell carcinoma is discussed in a later section.

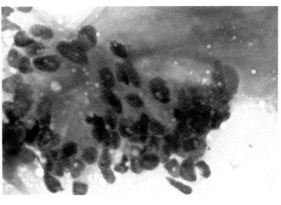

Fig. 10.12 Rectal epithelium
Aggregate of epithelial cells in relation to thick mucus; note columnar shape and abundant cytoplasm (MGG, HP)

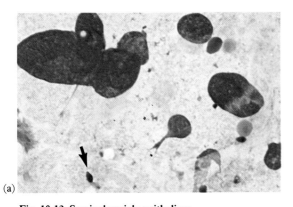

(a)

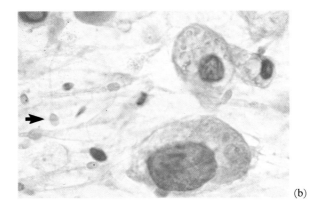

(b)

Fig. 10.13 Seminal vesicle epithelium
(a) Large bizarre nuclei; note occasional spermatozoa in the background (arrow) (MGG, HP). (b) Single epithelial cells with large pleomorphic nuclei; note coarse intracytoplasmic pigment and occasional spermatozoa (arrow) (Pap, HP Oil).

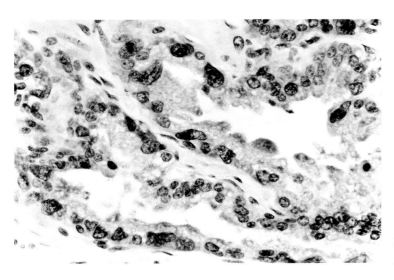

Fig. 10.14 Seminal vesicle
Tissue section; prominent nuclear pleomorphism (H & E, HP)

10 *MALE AND FEMALE GENITAL ORGANS*

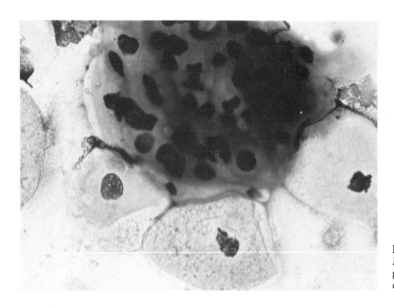

Fig. 10.15 Prostate; hormonal effect
Metaplastic squamous cells; large glycogenised cells and a cluster of smaller cells (MGG, HP)

Grading of adenocarcinoma[12]
Cytological grading follows a simple three point scale. The characteristics of grade I, well differentiated adenocarcinoma have already been described (Fig. 10.7). Grade III cancers show an almost total loss of cell cohesion and most of the cells in the smear are single. The cytoplasm is fragile and poorly defined and the nuclei are large and vesicular. Macronucleoli are common (Fig. 10.9). In grade II carcinoma, dissociation is moderate, a microglandular pattern is usually prominent, and the general cytological criteria of malignancy are obvious (Fig. 10.8). Differentiation is often variable within the same tumour. The cytological grade is decided by the most malignant pattern seen in available smears, which are, of course, not always representative of the whole neoplasm.

Effects of hormonal treatment/radiotherapy
Normal prostatic epithelial cells and cells from many of the better differentiated carcinomas respond to hormonal treatment in a similar way. The cells enlarge and appear pale due to increase in cytoplasmic glycogen (Fig. 10.15). Squamous metaplasia of normal epithelial cells becomes prominent, benign multinucleated giant cells and histiocytes occur. Nuclei of malignant cells shrink in size and may show other degenerative changes. After a few weeks, cells diagnostic of malignancy may no longer be found in smears from previously affected parts of the prostate. The response to radiotherapy is similarly reflected by the cytological pattern.[25,41]

Repeated FNA has been used to monitor the effect of conservative treatment of prostatic cancer. If a full cytological response is not seen, increasing the dosage or changing to a different type of treatment may achieve this, and, conversely, a malignant pattern may re-appear

if the dose is reduced. However, some authors have found clinical assessment superior to FNA in patient follow-up.[44]

Transitional-cell carcinoma (Figs 10.16–10.18)

Criteria for diagnosis

1. Cells single and in loose clusters with no distinct architectural pattern.
2. Moderate amount of dense cytoplasm with well defined borders; eccentric nuclei.
3. Pleomorphic, hyperchromatic, often large nuclei.
4. Nuclear chromatin coarse and irregular, varies from cell to cell.

Transitional cell carcinoma may invade the prostate from the urinary bladder, or it may arise from periurethral prostatic ducts within the prostate itself. Co-existence of transitional cell carcinoma and adenocarcinoma of the prostate is not rare (Figs 10.17 and

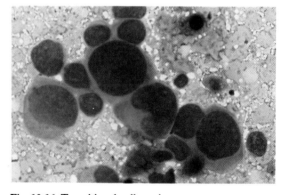

Fig. 10.16 Transitional-cell carcinoma
Pleomorphic malignant cells; hyperchromatic eccentric nuclei; dense cytoplasm (MGG, HP)

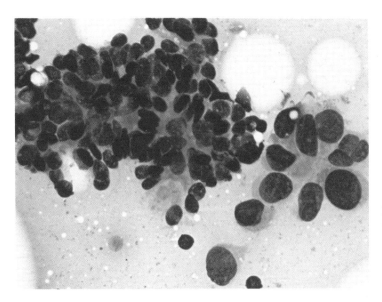

Fig. 10.17 Combined transitional/ adenocarcinoma
Aggregate of well-differentiated adenocarcinoma with nuclear crowding and microacinar pattern; adjacent group of larger more pleomorphic malignant transitional cells (MGG, HP)

10.18). It is important to distinguish transitional cell carcinoma from adenocarcinoma, since no response to hormonal treatment can be expected with the former tumour.

Transitional cell carcinoma involving the prostate is usually a deeply invasive tumour and is usually high grade. The cells clearly fulfil cytological criteria of malignancy. Variation in nuclear size, shape and staining is prominent (Figs 9.54, 10.16 and 10.17). Squamous differentiation is seen in some tumours, whereas papillary structures are rarely found.

Problems in diagnosis
The main problem is the distinction from prostatic adenocarcinoma. Cells from an adenocarcinoma of comparable differentiation show a lesser degree of nuclear pleomorphism, the nuclei are paler and the cytoplasm is indistinct and fragile, nuclei are also fragile and some are smudged. Microglandular groupings can always be found in adenocarcinoma except in truly anaplastic ones. Palisading at the periphery of cell aggregates from a transitional cell carcinoma should not be mistaken for glandular differentiation. Immunoperoxidase staining for prostatic specific antigen (PSA) and prostatic acid phosphatase is helpful in difficult cases.[20] However, there is a problem in interpreting the results in air-dried smears. The fragile cytoplasm of the neoplastic cells, particularly those of poorly differentiated adenocarcinoma, is largely dispersed in the background and any positive staining can be difficult to relate clearly to the tumour cells. In the interpretation of immunoperoxidase smears, one should therefore look closely at cell aggregates, in the centre of which cytoplasm is preserved around the nuclei.

Rare tumours of the prostate
Squamous metaplasia is common in the prostate, particularly in relation to infarcted adenomatous nodules and following hormonal treatment. The metaplastic cells may look atypical among the normal glandular epithelium and have been reported to cause diagnostic difficulties. The density and the staining properties of the cytoplasm point to their true nature. *Squamous cell carcinoma* of the prostate is rare. We have made this diagnosis by FNA in one patient who subsequently underwent surgery. On histological examination the prostate was widely infiltrated by squamous carcinoma. The origin of the cancer was difficult to decide but was most likely from the urethral mucosa. The poorly differentiated basaloid component of the tumour could have been mistaken for adenocarcinoma cytologically, but there were also better differentiated cells, some showing evidence of keratinisation and cytoplasmic orangeophilia (Pap).

Mucinous carcinoma and *endometrioid carcinoma* are uncommon variants of prostatic adenocarcinoma. The former can be of signet ring cell type and resemble a carcinoma invading the prostate from the bowel or the bladder. The latter has no cytologically distinguishing features. Cells of both variants stain positively for PSA, and the prognosis is not significantly different from that of ordinary adenocarcinoma. We have not seen examples of *small cell tumours*, carcinoid-like tumours, or of *adenoid cystic carcinoma*[65] in FNA smears of the prostate.

Rarely, *malignant lymphoma* may involve the prostate and cause enlargment. This can be difficult to differentiate cytologically from anaplastic carcinoma. Total lack of aggregation of cells, the presence of round fragments

10 *MALE AND FEMALE GENITAL ORGANS*

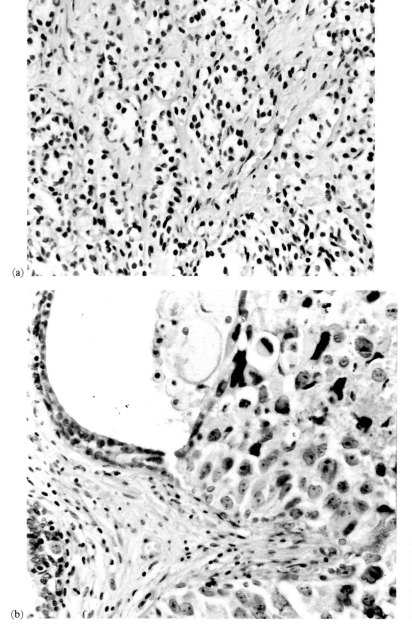

(a)

(b)

Fig. 10.18 Combined transitional/adenocarcinoma
Tissue section; same case as Figure 10.17.
(a) Well-differentiated prostatic adenocarcinoma (H & E, IP).
(b) Transitional cell carcinoma in a periurethral duct (H & E, IP).

of basophilic cytoplasm (lymphoid globules) in the absence of necrosis, and some cells with a rim of basophilic cytoplasm and a perinuclear pale zone raise a suspicion of lymphoma. The diagnosis can be confirmed by immune marker studies.

Sarcomas of the prostate are rare. These are mainly rhabdomyosarcomas in children, leiomyosarcomas or fibrosarcomas in adults (see Ch. 11).[6,33,52] A preoperative diagnosis was made by FNA in the following case.

A 45-year-old truck driver presented with pelvic pain and pain at defaecation. On examination his prostate was felt to be enlarged, firm and poorly delineated. FNA yielded malignant spindle cells consistent with a leiomyosarcoma. The diagnosis was confirmed by histological examination of a core needle biopsy. At explorative operation the tumour was found to be extensive within the pelvis and its exact origin could not be established.

MALE AND FEMALE GENITAL ORGANS 10

THE TESTIS

The non-neoplastic testis (Figs 10.19 and 10.20)[40,53]

Smears from normal testicular tissue contain cells which represent all stages of spermiogenesis, from spermatogonia to spermatozoa, in varying proportions. Spermatozoa and late spermatids are easily recognised from nuclear size, shape and hyperchromasia, whereas the less mature forms show a close resemblance to lymphoid cells of blastic type, particularly in air-dried Giemsa-stained smears (Fig. 10.19). Sertoli cells and Leydig cells are usually also present and may dominate the smears if the testicular tissue is atropic. Sertoli cells have pale, round nuclei, relatively large nucleoli and abundant, poorly defined, vacuolated cytoplasm (Fig. 10.20). Leydig cells have rather similar nuclei but a better defined, dense eosinophilic, granular cytoplasm and may contain Reinke's crystals. The principles of cytological evaluation of spermiogenesis in fine-needle aspirates have been presented by Persson et al.[35]

Chronic, non-specific *orchitis* is reflected in smears by the presence of lymphocytes and plasma cells and fewer spermiogenic cells. Sertoli cells are preserved and are relatively prominent.

Granulomatous orchitis is usually cryptogenic but may be caused by tuberculosis or other infection. Smears contain non-characteristic or epithelioid histiocytes, multinucleated histiocytic giant cells, and chronic inflammatory cells. Since lymphocytes and/or epithelioid cells may be prominent in smears of seminoma, a diagnosis of chronic or granulomatous orchitis should be made with care.[53]

Neoplasms

Seminoma (Figs 10.21 and 10.22)[2,46]

Criteria for diagnosis

1. Cellular smears.
2. Dispersed cells, little tendency to clustering.
3. Highly fragile cytoplasm and nuclei ('tigroid' background, nuclear smudging).
4. Large, vesicular nuclei, distinct nucleoli.
5. Pale cytoplasm, finely granular or vacuolated.
6. Lymphocyte-like cells.
7. Epithelioid histiocytes (variable).

The tumour cells are generally dispersed, but some loose clusters may be present. The fragile cytoplasm is characteristically spread over the slide and appears as a lace-like ('tigroid') background to the nuclei. The nuclei are also fragile and many are smudged. They are rounded or ovoid and relatively pale. The chromatin is coarse but is evenly distributed. Nucleoli may be multiple, prominent but of moderate size, and smaller than those of embryonal carcinoma cells. Mitotic figures may be found. Small, lymphocyte-like cells are scattered over

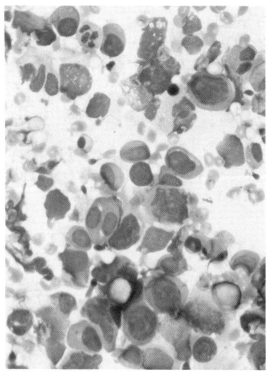

Fig. 10.19 Normal testis
Full range of spermatogenetic cells including some mature sperms (MGG, HP)

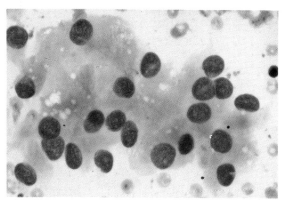

Fig. 10.20 Sertoli cells
Abundant finely vacuolar cytoplasm and indistinct cell borders (MGG, HP)

the smear, their number varies considerably (Fig. 10.21). Epithelioid histiocytes may be prominent enough to suggest a granulomatous process.

In *spermatocytic seminoma* the size range of the tumour cells is greater and there is not the striking contrast between large cells and lymphocyte-like cells.[29] In anaplastic seminoma, the cytological pattern approaches that of embryonal carcinoma; nuclei are larger and more pleomorphic, nucleoli are larger and there may be a tendency to microacinar grouping.

10

MALE AND FEMALE GENITAL ORGANS

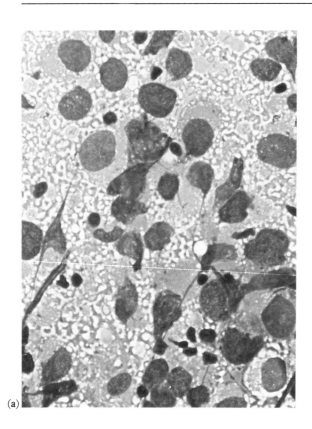

(a)

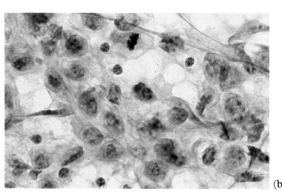

(b)

Fig. 10.21 Seminoma
(a) Dispersed cells with large pale nuclei and poorly defined cytoplasm; note 'tigroid' background, smudged nuclei and small lymphocytes (MGG, HP). (b) Dispersed cell pattern, and vesicular nuclei with multiple distinct nucleoli of moderate size (H & E, HP).

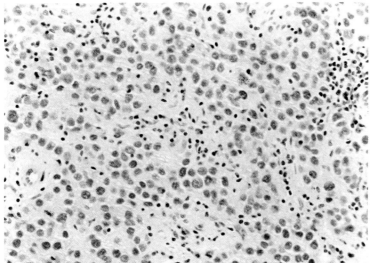

Fig. 10.22 Seminoma
Tissue section; same case as Figure 10.21 (H & E, IP)

Embryonal carcinoma (Figs 10.23–10.26)

Criteria for diagnosis

1. Cellular smear.
2. Cells single and in aggregates with a microacinar pattern.
3. Large vesicular nuclei, large nucleoli.
4. Indistinct, pale, often vacuolated cytoplasm.

5. Fragments of primitive mesenchymal tissue (variable).

The vesicular nuclei of an embryonal carcinoma are larger and more pleomorphic than those of seminoma, the nuclear chromatin is coarser and irregular, and nucleoli are large and eosinophilic. The cytoplasm is pale and is often vacuolated, cell borders are indistinct but the 'tigroid' background of seminoma is not seen.

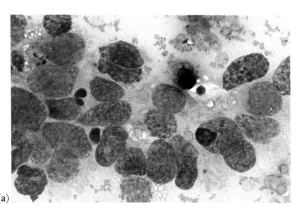

(a)

Fig. 10.23 Embryonal carcinoma
(a) Adenocarcinoma-like cluster of large malignant cells
with large nuclei and very coarse chromatin (MGG, HP).
(b) Fragment of undifferentiated mesenchymal tissue (above);
cluster of malignant epithelial cells; large vesicular nuclei,
prominent large nucleoli (below) (H & E, HP).

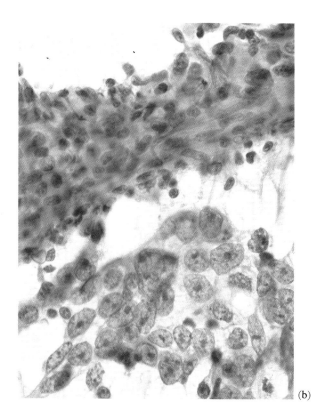

(b)

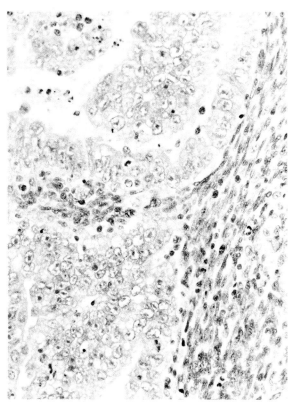

Fig. 10.24 Embryonal carcinoma
Tissue section; same case as Figure 10.23 (H & E, IP)

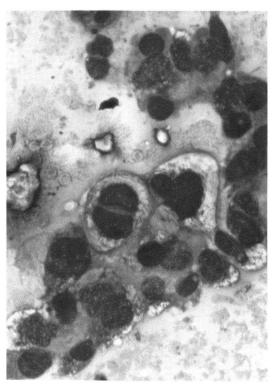

Fig. 10.25 Endodermal sinus tumour
Loose cluster of large malignant epithelial cells; prominent
cytoplasmic vacuolation (MGG, HP)

10 MALE AND FEMALE GENITAL ORGANS

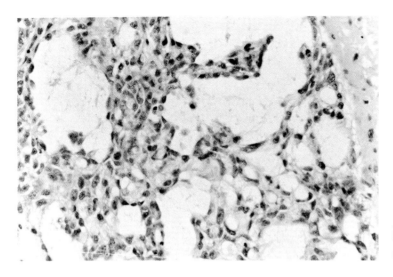

Fig. 10.26 Endodermal sinus tumour
Tissue section; same case as Figure 10.25
(H & E, IP)

Aggregates of tumour cells tend to show a microglandular pattern (Fig. 10.23a). Fragments of tissue composed of small, tightly packed spindle cells may be found, which represent primitive mesenchymal tissue (Fig. 10.23b).

Embryonal carcinoma of infantile type (endodermal sinus tumour) resembles the adult type cytologically, but the cells tend to form papillary clusters and cytoplasmic vacuolation is more prominent (Figs 10.25 and 10.26). Positive immunoperoxidase staining for alphafetoprotein supports the diagnosis.

Choriocarcinoma (Figs 10.27 and 10.28)

Choriocarcinoma is usually found as a minor component within other germ cell tumours and is rarely the pre-

dominant pattern. We have seen one case of almost pure choriocarcinoma of the testis which contained only a small focus of seminoma. Smears of this tumour showed syncytiotrophoblastic and cytotrophoblastic cells. The former are large and multinucleated with hyperchromatic nuclei of varying size and with abundant, dark, amphophilic cytoplasm. Cytotrophoblastic cells are either dissociated or form loose clusters. Cell borders are not as distinct in smears as they appear in tissue sections; the cytoplasm is pale and vacuolated, the nuclei are rounded, vesicular, of moderate size and are mildly pleomorphic; nucleoli are indistinct in air-dried smears (Fig. 10.27). Immunoperoxidase staining for HCG is helpful to identify syncytiotrophoblastic cells.

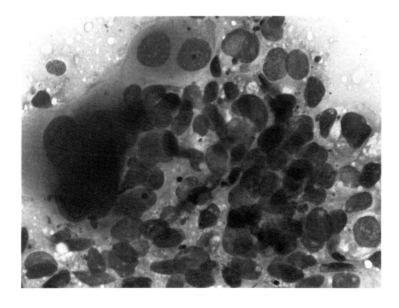

Fig. 10.27 Choriocarcinoma
Cluster of cytotrophoblastic cells with syncytiotrophoblastic cells at the periphery (MGG, HP)

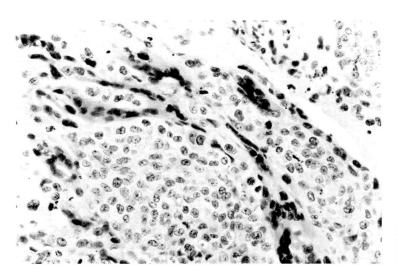

Fig. 10.28 Choriocarcinoma
Tissue section; same case as Figure 10.27
(H & E, IP)

Teratoma (Figs 10.29 and 10.30)
Teratomas contain a variety of epithelial and mesen-chymal tissues which may be mature or immature. Mature components are mainly represented in smears by epithelial sheets which may be squamous, ciliated, or intestinal (with goblet cells) in type. Immature epithelial cells are similar to those of embryonal carcinoma (Fig. 10.30). Fragments of cellular primitive or differentiating mesenchymal tissue may also be seen.[53] These tumours may contain extensive cystic or hyalinised, acellular areas making it difficult to obtain sufficient numbers of neoplastic cells (Fig. 10.29).

Other testicular tumours
We have not seen any case of *Leydig cell tumour* of the testis in FNA smears. The cytological features have been described by Linsk & Franzén.[27] The cytological findings in a *Sertoli cell tumour* of the testis have also been reported.[37] Other gonadal stromal tumours are rare.

Malignant lymphoma affects the testis not uncommon-ly and can present as a testicular mass, or more typically as bilateral testicular enlargment, without evidence of systemic disease. In fact, lymphoma is the commonest testicular tumour in males over the age of 60. Diagnostic criteria are the same as for lymphoma in other sites (see Ch. 5). Figure 10.31 is from a 14-year-old boy who had lymphoblastic leukaemia in remission for 1.5 years. Testicular swelling was the first evidence of recurrence. This is not uncommonly the case in childhood leukaemia, and FNA of the testes has therefore been recommended as a simple method for early detection of recurrence. Rarely, *metastatic carcinoma* may simulate a primary testicular tumour. The origin of the cancer is most often in the lung or in the prostate.

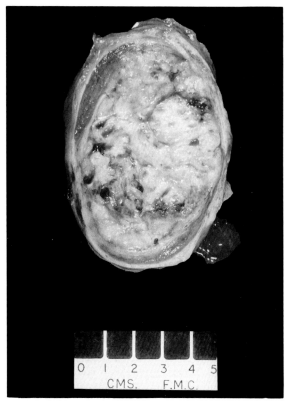

Fig. 10.29 Testicular teratoma (intermediate)
Large bisected tumour occupying most of the enlarged testicle in a male of 19. Note hyalinised and degenerate areas.

10 *MALE AND FEMALE GENITAL ORGANS*

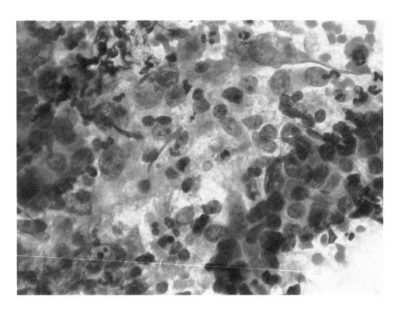

Fig. 10.30 Testicular teratoma (intermediate)
Well differentiated glandular epithelium to right, large malignant cells similar to embryonal carcinoma to left
(H & E, HP)

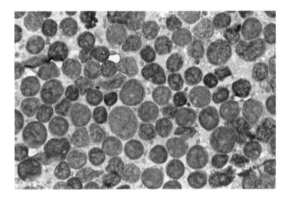

Fig. 10.31 Lymphoblastic leukaemia (ALL)
Testicular aspirate: uniform population of lymphoblasts
(MGG, HP)

EPIDIDYMIS

In acute and chronic *epididymitis*, FNA smears are dominated by inflammatory cells and there are few epithelial cells. Occasionally, quite atypical looking cells may be found probably representing regenerative atypia, and if the lesion cannot be clearly separated from the testicle clinically or radiologically, surgical exploration may be inevitable. Smears from a *spermatocoele* display spermatozoa against a proteinaceous background. In *tuberculous epididymitis* mainly caseous material may be aspirated which appears granular, eosinophilic and amorphous in smears. There may be clusters of epithelioid histiocytes which have characteristic pale, footprint-shaped nuclei, and some multinucleated Langhans' giant cells. The diagnosis rests on the demonstration of acid-fast bacilli in the smears or in cultures of the aspirate.

Adenomatoid tumour (Figs 10.32 and 10.33)[36]
Usually only the mesothelial-like component and not the stroma is represented in FNA smears. The cells form loose aggregates which may show a vaguely glandular pattern. The cells have ovoid, vesicular nuclei, a finely granular, evenly distributed chromatin, small nucleoli and abundant cytoplasm which may contain large vacuoles. The cells tend to be plump, spindly and they resemble mesothelial or endothelial cells (Figs 10.32 and 10.33). The diagnosis is not difficult in smears from a tumour in the epididymis, but can be more problematic in an atypical location such as the tunica of the testicle when it may appear to be intratesticular.

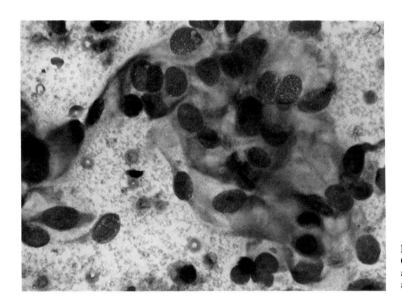

Fig. 10.32 Adenomatoid tumour
Cluster of plump spindle cells with
abundant pale cytoplasm; mild nuclear
atypia (MGG, HP)

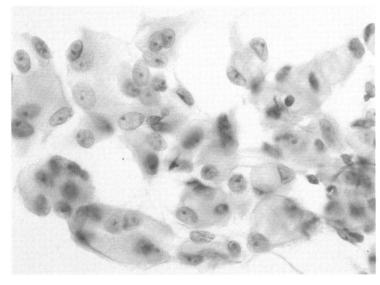

Fig. 10.33 Adenomatoid tumour
Clusters of cells with bland nuclei and
abundant, well defined cytoplasm,
resembling mesothelial cells (Pap, HP)

PENIS

Primary squamous cell carcinoma of the penis can be
diagnosed by scrape smears directly from the surface of
the lesion. We have seen a few cases of secondary carcinoma involving the deeper tissues of the shaft of the penis.
The primary tumours were adenocarcinoma of prostate or
transitional cell carcinoma of bladder. FNA of these
lesions with a 25 gauge needle was well tolerated by the
patients and caused no complications.

THE FEMALE GENITAL ORGANS

The cytology of squamous cell carcinoma, adenocarcinoma, foreign-body granuloma, etc. is described elsewhere
and will not be repeated here. Smears of aspirates from
suspected pelvic recurrence of previously diagnosed cancer should, of course, always be compared with histological sections of the original tumour if available. Great care
must be taken not to misinterpret post-radiation atypia
and repair as recurrence of cancer.

10 *MALE AND FEMALE GENITAL ORGANS*

Non-neoplastic ovarian cysts

Simple cysts[71,79]

Usual findings

1. Clear fluid; some erythrocytes and debris.
2. 'Cyst macrophages'.
3. A few bland, degenerate, often shrunk epithelial cells (epithelial cysts).

Under this heading are included a variety of cysts which cannot be confidently separated by cytological examination of cyst fluid. Surface epithelial inclusion cysts, parovarian cysts, regressing follicular cysts, and simple serous cysts fall into this category. The cysts contain clear fluid and are lined by a single layer of cuboidal or flattened, occasionally ciliated cells.

'Cyst macrophages' have small nuclei and abundant pale, vacuolated cytoplasm often containing haemosiderin pigment and with a distinct border. It is difficult to decide if they are true macrophages or degenerating epithelial cells. They are commonly found in all kinds of cystic lesions in many different sites, sometimes in large numbers. If well preserved epithelial cells are present, these may give a clue to the exact nature of the cyst.

Functional cysts (Figs 10.34 and 10.35)

Usual findings

1. Clear, cloudy or bloody fluid.
2. Erythrocytes and amorphous granular material.
3. Medium-sized, rounded cells, single or clustered (granulosa cells).
4. Rounded nuclei, anisokaryosis, some mitoses.
5. Scattered small naked, dark, lymphocyte-like nuclei.
6. Cytoplasm granular and vacuolated; poorly defined cell borders.

These cysts include cystic follicles and functioning follicular cysts (which are lined by multiple layers of granulosa and theca cells) and also cystic corpora lutea. Kovacic et al[71] have described the cytology of follicular cysts, corpus luteum and theca lutein cysts separately and in more detail.

Smears often have a surprisingly high cell content. Anisokaryosis is often prominent and nuclear diameter can vary from 10 to over 20 μm. The small, naked, hyperchromatic nuclei probably represent degenerating granulosa cells; the large nuclei are pale and have a finely granular, evenly distributed chromatin and multiple small nucleoli. Mitotic figures are frequently found. Single granulosa cells resemble macrophages (Fig. 10.34). Luteinised granulosa cells have a larger amount of more dense, but still granular and vacuolated cytoplasm and better defined cell borders (Fig. 10.35). Cells from a corpus luteum are quite cohesive and may form rounded, solid cords of cells with a well-defined surface, which can mimic papillary fragments without stromal cores. Blood and strands of fibrin are prominent

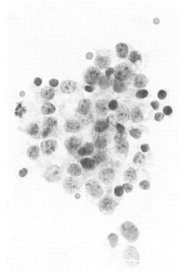

Fig. 10.34 Follicular cyst
Loose aggregate of small cells with pale nuclei, indistinct cytoplasm; the small hyperchromatic nuclei probably represent degenerate granulosa cells; note mitosis (H & E, HP)

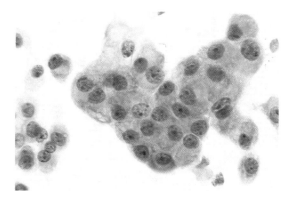

Fig. 10.35 Cystic corpus luteum
Cohesive luteinised cells with abundant well-defined cytoplasm (Pap, HP)

in the background of smears. Hormonal assay of cyst fluid may show a high oestrogen content.[68] Intracellular oestrogen may also be demonstrated in smears by the immunoperoxidase method.

Endometriotic cysts

Usual findings

1. Thick dark brown fluid or creamy material.
2. Smear background of altered blood.
3. Many haemosiderin-containing macrophages.
4. Occasional groups of columnar epithelial cells.

Endometrial epithelial cells do not show distinctive cytological features and cannot be confidently distinguished from columnar cells of other origin. A specific diagnosis of endometriosis must be based on the coexistence of epithelial and stromal cells. This is usually seen in aspirates from extra-ovarian endometriosis (see Fig. 11.3), but is rarely present in aspirates from endometriotic cysts. Old haemorrhage can also be the only finding in functional cysts and is not diagnostic of endometriosis.

Benign neoplasms

Uterine leiomyoma; ovarian fibroma/thecoma
(Figs 10.36 and 10.37)[75]

Usual findings

1. Smears poor in cells.
2. Mainly tissue fragments with intercellular collagen, few single cells.
3. Pale or eosinophilic syncytial cytoplasm.
4. Spindly, slender or plump, often bare nuclei.
5. Moderate nuclear pleomorphism; bland nuclear chromatin.

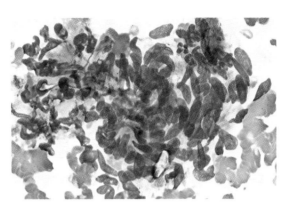

Fig. 10.36 Cellular leiomyoma
Cohesive cluster of spindle cells; high cell yield gave rise to suspicion of malignancy; the tumour was considered histologically to be of borderline malignancy (MGG, HP)

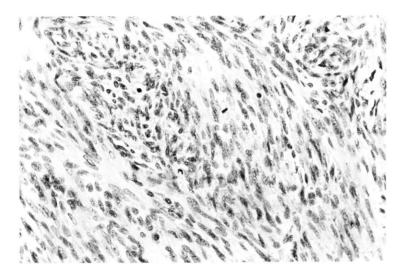

Fig. 10.37 Cellular leiomyoma
Tissue section; same case as Figure 10.34
(H & E, IP)

Uterine leiomyomas are not often subjected to FNA biopsy as the diagnosis is usually made clinically. The consistency felt through the needle is characteristically hard and tough and smears are poor in cells in contrast to benign leiomyomas in other sites. Low grade malignancy is difficult to rule out if tumours are highly cellular (Fig. 10.36). Smears of ovarian fibromas and thecomas are similar. Thecoma cells tend to have plumper and more irregular nuclei and a larger amount of indistinct, fragile cytoplasm. Intracytoplasmic fat droplets can be demonstrated by special stains in air-dried smears of thecoma.

Brenner tumour
We have no personal experience of the cytology of Brenner tumours. Ramzy *et al.*[79] described the cytological pattern as sheets of epithelial cells of benign appearance

which have ovoid nuclei with a 'coffee bean' groove. Extracellular, large, hyaline, eosinophilic globules are a characteristic finding in smears of this tumour. The cytology of a malignant Brenner tumour has not yet been described to our knowledge.

Benign cystic teratoma (dermoid cyst) (Fig. 10.38)

Criteria for diagnosis

1. Thick, greasy, yellowish aspirate.
2. Background of thick amorphous material.
3. Anucleate squames.
4. Some inflammatory cells, macrophages and foreign-body giant cells.
5. Fragments of hair shafts.
6. Cells from other differentiated tissues.

10 *MALE AND FEMALE GENITAL ORGANS*

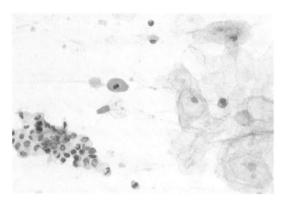

Fig. 10.38 Benign cystic teratoma
Anucleate squamous cells and a small sheet of benign glandular epithelial cells; hairshafts were present in the smear (Pap, IP)

If the aspirate consists entirely of cyst contents, smears show only thick amorphous debris with some anucleate squames. The finding of hair shaft fragments among the debris confirms the diagnosis.

Ovarian cystadenoma, serous and mucinous
(Figs 10.39 and 10.40)
In benign ovarian cystadenomas, the cyst fluid is poor in cells and any cells present are usually degenerating and show prominent shrinkage artefacts. A specific diagnosis beyond that of a benign cystic lesion is therefore often impossible. In serous cystadenomas, papillary aggregates of epithelial cells which have small, dark, bland nuclei, can sometimes be found. Papillary tufts of mesothelial cells from the lining of the pouch of Douglas may be indistinguishable from papillary clusters

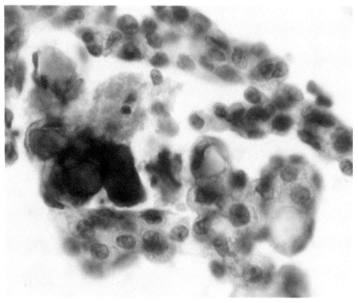

**Fig. 10.39 Serous cystadenoma
(borderline malignancy)**
Atypical cells forming papillary clusters. Moderate nuclear pleomorphism, some cytoplasmic vacuoles, psammoma bodies in centre left (Pap, HP)

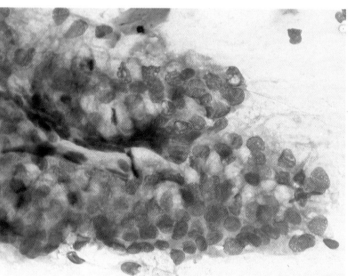

**Fig. 10.40 Mucinous cystadenoma
(borderline malignancy)**
Cohesive sheet of mildly atypical mucin-secreting columnar cells; there is an impression of multilayering; histology showed a tumour of borderline malignancy (MGG, HP)

MALE AND FEMALE GENITAL ORGANS 10

from a serous cystadenoma and may even appear atypical. This possibility must be kept in mind when examining ovarian aspirates since the exact position of the needle at biopsy can not always be demonstrated. Tall columnar cells with basally placed nuclei and empty looking cytoplasm characteristic of mucinous cystadenoma tend to be better preserved and are more easily recognised if at all present. The background of highly viscous mucus is of course suggestive of this diagnosis. Large numbers of well preserved epithelial cells of serous or of mucinous type showing cytological atypia but no definite malignant features suggest a *borderline cystadenoma* (Figs 10.39 and 10.40). Cytological criteria which clearly separate this category of tumour from well differentiated cystadenocarcinoma have not yet been defined.

Malignant neoplasms

Serous cystadenocarcinoma of ovary (Fig. 10.41)

Criteria for diagnosis

1. Mucoid, turbid fluid of variable viscosity.
2. Single cells and papillary, glandular, and/or solid multilayered aggregates.
3. Columnar cells, relatively high N/C ratio.
4. Cytological criteria of malignancy.
5. Psammoma bodies (some tumours).

The tumour cells generally have a small to moderate amount of cyanophilic (Pap) cytoplasm which may be vacuolated but does not stain positively for mucin. Psammoma bodies are a helpful sign when present. Differentiation from endometrioid carcinoma and

from metastatic adenocarcinoma can be difficult, since glandular aggregates can mimic papillary fragments in smears. True papillary fragments have a fibrovascular stromal core. Multilayered clusters of cells which have a distinct surface on three sides defined by a row of columnar or cuboidal cells can also be accepted as papillary structures. Psammoma bodies stain intensely dark blue/black with MGG and may be overlooked as artefacts. Their characteristic concentric structure is more evident in Pap-stained smears (Fig. 10.39).

Mucinous cystadenocarcinoma of ovary (Fig. 10.42)

Criteria for diagnosis

1. Mucinous, highly viscous, sticky fluid.
2. Smear background of stringy mucin.
3. Cohesive sheets and aggregates of cells.
4. Columnar, mucin-secreting cells.
5. Cytological criteria of malignancy.

Cells from a well differentiated, mucinous cystadenocarcinoma are similar to those of benign mucinous cystadenoma but usually occur in larger numbers. However, if the smears represent only cyst contents, cells may be few in numbers and most of them are mucinophages or bland-looking, spindly epithelial cells similar to the cells seen in pseudomyxoma peritonei. There is a background of thick, stringy mucus, staining violet with MGG. Cells lining the cystic spaces and from more solid areas show a variable degree of nuclear enlargement and crowding, and some cells have an increased N/C ratio. The usual cytological criteria of malignancy apply in less well differentiated cancers. Distinction from metastatic adenocarcinoma, particularly of colonic origin, may be impossible.

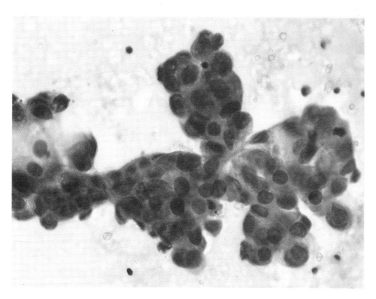

Fig. 10.41 Serous cystadenocarcinoma
Papillary aggregate of malignant glandular cells (H & E, HP)

10 MALE AND FEMALE GENITAL ORGANS

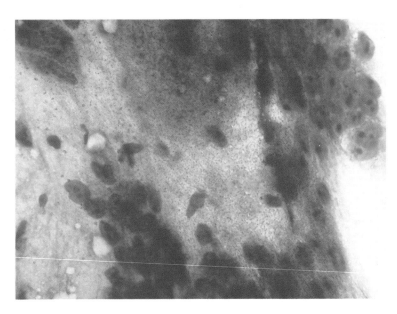

Fig. 10.42 Mucinous cystadenocarcinoma
Clusters of malignant cells with vesicular, moderately pleomorphic nuclei and large nucleoli, in background of stringy mucus (MGG, HP)

Endometrioid adenocarcinoma of uterus and of ovary
(Fig. 10.43)

Criteria for diagnosis

1. Cytological criteria of adenocarcinoma.
2. Microglandular and cribriform patterns.

Differentiation between endometrioid neoplasms and serous carcinoma of the ovary is difficult and may be impossible. An eosinophilic granular cytoplasm and a microglandular pattern favours endometrioid carcinoma; papillary structures favour serous tumours. Evidence of mucin secretion suggests mucinous ovarian carcinoma or colorectal cancer. The poorer the differentiation, the greater the diagnostic difficulties.

Clear cell carcinoma (Fig. 10.44)
Clear cell carcinoma occurs in the cervix, the endometrium, and the ovary. The cytological presentation is that of adenocarcinoma in which the cells have abundant, pale, finely vacuolated cytoplasm. Cell borders are indistinct and nuclear pleomorphism may not be prominent. Air-dried smears allow staining for glycogen.

Anaplastic carcinoma of ovary

Criteria for diagnosis

1. Cellular smears.
2. Dispersed cell population with little aggregation.
3. Undifferentiated malignant cells.
4. Fragile cytoplasm, bare nuclei, prominent nucleoli.

Anaplastic carcinoma is usually bilateral. It has a very poor prognosis. Preoperative radiotherapy has been recommended for this category, and this has been one of the arguments for diagnosis by FNA. The tumours are

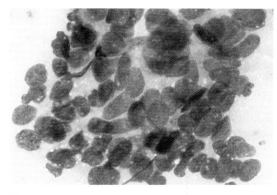

Fig. 10.43 Endometrioid carcinoma
Loose cluster of malignant glandular cells with an acinar pattern and some nuclear palisading (MGG, HP)

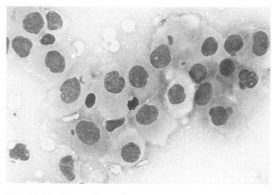

Fig. 10.44 Clear cell carcinoma
Tumour cells with abundant, pale, finely vacuolated cytoplasm (MGG, HP)

predominantly solid and aspirates tend to be thick due to the high cell content. Some evidence of glandular differentiation may be seen. The malignant cells have large, pleomorphic nuclei and sometimes large, intra-cytoplasmic, hyaline, eosinophilic inclusions similar to those seen in hepatocellular carcinoma. Distinction from anaplastic tumours of mesenchymal or lymphatic origin may require immunoperoxidase staining for EMA, CEA, etc.

Confident distinction from *metastatic carcinoma* is not possible. If the cells are relatively small and uniform, and if they tend to form small, solid aggregates and single files, metastatic breast cancer should be considered. Smears from *Krukenberg tumours* contain signet-ring cells with intracytoplasmic mucin. The cells are single or form small clusters. It may prove difficult to obtain a satisfactory sample with a standard needle due to the fibrous stroma, and a Rotex screw needle or other core needles may have to be used. *Malignant melanoma* not uncommonly metastasises to the ovary. The criteria for diagnosis have been described elsewhere (p. 305).

Granulosa cell tumour (Figs 10.45–10.47)[61,63]

Criteria for diagnosis

1. Smears rich in cells.
2. Cells in loose aggregates with a tendency to follicular grouping, some dispersed.
3. Moderate amount of pale cytoplasm; indistinct cell borders.
4. Nuclei monomorphous, round or ovoid, many with a longitudinal groove (coffee bean), finely granular chromatin.
5. Call-Exner bodies in some tumours.

We have examined a few granulosa cell tumours of follicular type by FNA. The findings were similar to those described by others. The smears were rich in cells. There were both single cells and cells in loose aggregates, often with a discernible follicular pattern. In one of the cases, there were many rounded bodies, 30–100 μm in diameter, which were bright purple and had a fibrillar structure in MGG-stained smears (Fig. 10.45), pale eosinophilic and structureless in H & E. These globules, surrounded by neoplastic cells, represented Call-Exner bodies, described in previous case reports. Nuclei were uniformly rounded and did not vary much in size. Nuclear grooves ('coffee bean') were seen in many nuclei, particularly in alcohol-fixed Pap smears, and these caused some nuclei to appear lobated. Nuclear chromatin was granular and evenly distributed. Nucleoli were small and indistinct. The amount of cytoplasm was quite variable between cases, it was pale, finely granular or vacuolated. The cytoplasm appeared syncytial without discernible cell borders.

Granulosa cell tumours with a diffuse pattern histolo-

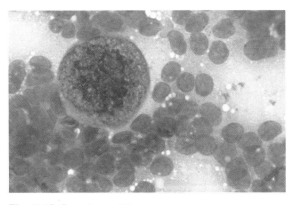

Fig. 10.45 Granulosa cell tumour
Clusters of cells with uniformly small round nuclei and a tendency to microfollicular groupings. Scanty, poorly defined cytoplasm, Call-Exner body in centre (MGG, HP)

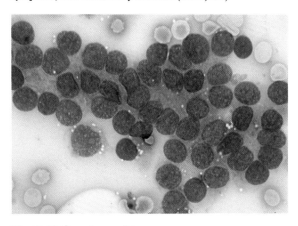

Fig. 10.46 Granulosa cell tumour
Loose aggregate of small cells with uniform round nuclei and a bland nuclear chromatin; indistinct cell borders and a tendency to microacinar formations (MGG, HP)

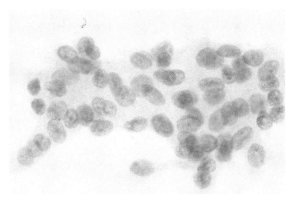

Fig. 10.47 Granulosa cell tumour, diffuse pattern
Loose cluster of cells with uniform, ovoid nuclei, some with grooves (Pap, HP)

gically have a less characteristic cytological presentation. Spindle cells predominate, nuclear grooves are present, but the cells show no characteristic architectural arrangement (Fig. 10.47). Other *gonadal stromal tumours*

10 *MALE AND FEMALE GENITAL ORGANS*

are rare and their cytological appearances are little known. The less well differentiated variants cannot be specifically typed.

Dysgerminoma[2]

The cytological pattern of dysgerminoma of ovary is identical to that of testicular seminoma (p. 281, Fig. 10.21).

Endometrial stromal sarcoma

(Figs 10.48 and 10.49)[69,77,87]

Our experience is limited to a few cases, one of which was a low grade tumour (endolymphatic stromal myosis). Smears showed many cells both single and in loose clusters without any specific pattern. The nuclei were plump ovoid, vesicular, relatively large, and varied moderately in size and in shape. The chromatin pattern was bland, finely

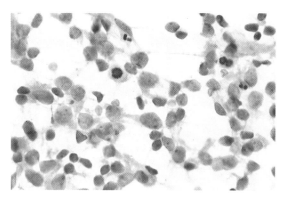

Fig. 10.48 Endometrial stromal sarcoma
Dispersed cell population of plump spindle cells with pale ovoid nuclei and small nucleoli; note anastomosing strands of eosinophilic cytoplasm and scattered mitoses (H & E, IP)

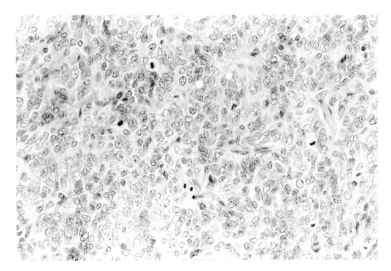

Fig. 10.49 Endometrial stromal sarcoma
Tissue section; same case as Figure 10.48
(H & E, IP)

granular, and there were one to two small nucleoli. The cytoplasm was eosinophilic and formed either a 'tail' on the eccentric nucleus, or thin anastomosing strands, or a syncytial background to crowded nuclei. Mitotic figures were frequently observed in the high-grade tumours. Co-existence of malignant glandular epithelial cells and malignant mesenchymal cells in smears from an ovarian tumour suggests a *malignant mixed Mullerian tumour*.

Leiomyosarcoma of uterus

The cytological pattern is that of a spindle-cell sarcoma. Smooth muscle differentiation reflected by a dense, eosinophilic cytoplasm and truncated nuclei may not be obvious and the appearances are then similar to tumours of fibroblastic origin (see Ch. 11). In one of our cases, the tumour had a prominent round cell pattern and was misdiagnosed as a carcinoma by FNA (Fig. 10.50).

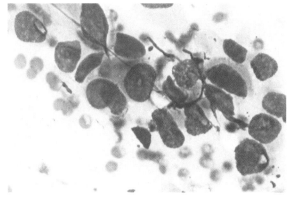

Fig. 10.50 Leiomyosarcoma, round cell pattern
Dispersed, pleomorphic malignant cells of predominantly rounded shape, abundant pale cytoplasm (MGG, HP)

REFERENCES AND SUGGESTED FURTHER READING

Male Genital Organs

1. Abe M, Hashimoto T, Matsuda T, Saitoh M, Watanabe H: Prostatic biopsy guided by transrectal ultrasonography using real-time linear scanner. Urology 29: 567–569, 1987.
2. Akhtar M, Ashraf Ali M, Huq M, Bakry M: Fine-needle aspiration biopsy of seminoma and dysgerminoma: Cytologic, histologic and electron microscopic correlations. Diagn Cytopathol 6: 99–105, 1990.
3. Benson M C: Fine-needle aspiration of the prostate. NCI Monogr 7: 19–24, 1988.
4. Carlton C E Jr.: The risk of distant metastases after transurethral resection of the prostate versus needle biopsy in patients with localized prostate cancer. J Urol 142: 320–325, 1989.
5. Cazzaniga M G, Tommasini-Degna A, Negri R, Pioselli F: Cytologic diagnosis of prostatic malakoplakia. Report of three cases. Acta Cytol 31: 48–52, 1987.
6. Cookingham C L, Kumen N B: Diagnosis of prostatic leiomyosarcoma with fine needle aspiration cytology. Acta Cytol 29: 170–173, 1985.
7. De Gaetani C F, Trentini G P: Atypical hyperplasia of the prostate. A pitfall in the cytologic diagnosis of carcinoma. Acta Cytol 22: 483–486, 1978.
8. Droese M, Voeth C: Cytologic features of seminal vesicle epithelium in aspiration biopsy smears of the prostate. Acta Cytol 20: 120–125, 1976.
9. Ekman H, Hedberg K, Persson P S: Cytological versus histological examination of needle biopsy specimens in the diagnosis of prostatic cancer. Br J Urol 39: 544–548, 1967.
10. Epstein N A: Prostatic biopsy: a morphologic correlation of aspiration cytology with needle biopsy histology. Cancer 38: 2078–2087, 1976.
11. Esposti P L: A cytologic diagnosis of prostatic tumours with the aid of transrectal aspiration biopsy: a critical review of 1110 cases and a report of morphologic and cytochemical studies. Acta Cytol 10: 182–186, 1966.
12. Esposti P L: Cytologic malignancy grading of prostatic carcinoma by transrectal aspiration biopsy. Scand J Urol Nephrol 5: 199–209, 1971.
13. Esposti P L, Elman A, Norlen H: Complications of transrectal aspiration biopsy of the prostate. Scand J Urol Nephrol 9: 208–213, 1975.
14. Esposti P L, Franzén S: Transrectal aspiration biopsy of the prostate. A re-evaluation of the method in the diagnosis of prostatic carcinoma. Scand J Urol Nephrol Suppl 55: 49–52, 1980.
15. Franzén S, Giertz G, Zajicek J: Cytological diagnosis of prostatic tumours by transrectal aspiration biopsy: a preliminary report. Br J Urol 32: 193–196, 1960.
16. Graham J B, Ignatoff J M, Holland J M, Christ M L: Prostatic aspiration biopsy: an assessment of accuracy based on long-term observations. J Urol 139: 971–974, 1988.
17. Hillyard J W: Bacteraemia following perineal prostatic biopsy. Br J Urol 60: 252–254, 1987.
18. Jocham D, Schmiedt E, Gottinger H, Faul P, Schmeller N, Laible V: Prostate cytology. 12 years' experience with transrectal fine needle biopsy. Urologe 22: 120–126, 1983.
19. Kaufman J J, Ljung B M, Walther P, Waisman J: Aspiration biopsy of prostate. Urology 19: 587–591, 1982.
20. Keshgegian A A, Kline T S: Immunoperoxidase demonstration of prostatic acid phosphatase in aspiration biopsy cytology (ABC). Am J Clin Pathol 82: 586–589, 1984.
21. Kline T S, Kohler P, Kelsey D M: Aspiration biopsy cytology (ABC). Its use in diagnosis of lesions of the prostate gland. Arch Pathol Lab Med 106: 136–139, 1982.
22. Koivuniemi A, Tyrkko J: Seminal vesicle epithelium in fine needle aspiration biopsies of the prostate as a pitfall in the cytologic diagnosis of carcinoma. Acta Cytol 20: 116–119, 1976.
23. Lange P H, Naryan P: Understaging and undergrading of prostatic cancer. Argument for post-operative radiation as adjuvant therapy. Urology 21: 113–118, 1983.
24. Leistenschneider W, Nagel R: Atlas of prostatic cytology. Springer, Berlin, 1984.
25. Leistenschneider W, Nagel R: Cytological and DNA-cytophotometric monitoring of the effect of therapy in conservatively treated prostatic carcinomas. Scand J Urol Nephrol Suppl 55: 197–204, 1980.
26. Lin B P C, Davies W E L, Harmata P A: Prostatic aspiration cytology. Pathology 11: 607–614, 1979.
27. Linsk J A, Franzén S: Clinical aspiration cytology, 2nd edn. Lippincott, Philadelphia, 1989.
28. Ljung B M, Cherrie R, Kaufman J J. Fine needle aspiration biopsy of the prostate gland: a study of 103 cases with histological follow up. J Urol 135: 955–959, 1986.
29. Lopez J I, Aranda F I: Fine needle aspiration cytology of spermatocytic seminoma. Report of a case. Acta Cytol 33: 627–630, 1989.
30. Maksem J A, Johenning P W: Is cytology capable of adequately grading prostate carcinoma? Matched series of 50 cases comparing cytologic and histologic pattern diagnoses. Urology 31: 437–444, 1988.
31. Meacham R B, Scardino P T, Hoffman G S, Easley J D, Wilbanks J H, Carlton C E Jr: The risk of distant metastases after transurethral resection of the prostate versus needle biopsy in patients with localized prostate cancer. J Urol 142: 320–325, 1989.
32. Moul J W, Miles B J, Skoog S J, McLeod D G: Risk factors for perineal seeding of prostate cancer after needle biopsy. J Urol 142: 86–88, 1989.
33. Muller H A, Wunsch P H: Features of prostatic sarcomas in combined aspiration and punch biopsies. Acta Cytol 25: 480–484, 1981.
34. Ostrzega N, Cheng L, Layfield L J: Keratin immunoreactivity in fine-needle aspiration of the prostate: an aid in the differentiation of benign epithelium from well-differentiated adenocarcinoma. Diagn Cytopathol 4: 38–41, 1988.
35. Persson P S, Ahren C, Obrant K O: Aspiration biopsy smear of testis in azoospermia: cytological versus histological examination. Scand J Urol Nephrol 5: 22–26, 1971.
36. Perez-Guillermo M, Thor A, Löwhagen T: Paratesticular adenomatoid tumours. The cytologic presentation in fine needle aspiration biopsies. Acta Cytol 33: 6–10, 1989.
37. Pettinato G, Insabato L, DeChiara A, Latella R: Fine needle aspiration cytology of a large cell calcifying Sertoli cell tumour of the testis. Acta Cytol 31: 578–582, 1987.
38. Ragde H, Aldape, Bagley C M Jr. Ultrasound-guided prostate biopsy. Biopty gun superior to aspiration. Urology 32: 503–506, 1988.
39. Ryan P G, Peeling W B: Perineal prostatic tumor seedling after 'Tru-Cut' needle biopsy: case report and review of the literature. Eur Urol 17: 189–192, 1990.
40. Schenk U, Schill W-B: Cytology of the human seminiferous epithelium. Acta Cytol 32: 689–696, 1988.
41. Spieler P, Gloor F, Egle N, Bandhauer K: Cytological findings in transrectal aspiration biopsy of hormone- and radio-therapy treated carcinoma of the prostate. Virchow's Arch (Pathol Anat) 372: 149–159, 1976.

10 *MALE AND FEMALE GENITAL ORGANS*

42. Sprenger E, Michaelis W E, Vogt-Schader M, Otto C: The significance of DNA flow-through fluorescence cytophotometry for the diagnosis of prostate carcinioma. Beitr Pathol 159: 292–298, 1976.
43. Staehler W, Ziegler H, Volter D, Schubert G E: Zytodiagnostik der prostata — Grundriss und Atlas. Schattauer, Stuttgart, 1975.
44. Studer U, Kraft R, Wiemer-Bridel J: Fine needle puncture of prostatic cancer. Schweiz Med Wochenschr 112: 810–816, 1982.
45. Suhrland M J, Deitch D, Schreiber K, Freed S, Koss L G. Assessment of fine needle aspiration as a screening test for occult prostatic carcinoma. Acta Cytol 32: 495–498, 1988.
46. Tao L-C, Negin M L, Donat E E: Primary retroperitoneal seminoma diagnosed by fine needle aspiration biopsy. A case report. Acta Cytol 28: 598–600, 1984.
47. Tribukait B, Esposti P L, Rönström L: Tumour ploidy for characterization of prostatic carcinoma: Flow cytofluorometric DNA studies using aspiration biopsy material. Scand J Urol Nephrol Suppl 55: 59–64, 1980.
48. Volter D, Siegler H: Die Frühdiagnose des Prostatakarzinoms. Dtsch Med Wschr 100: 1573–1575, 1975.
49. Verma K, Ram T R, Kapila K: Value of fine needle aspiration cytology in the diagnosis of testicular neoplasms. Acta Cytol 33: 631–634, 1989.
50. Wajsman Z, Klimberg I: Needle aspiration and needle biopsy procedures. Urol Clin North Am 14: 103–113, 1987.
51. Willems J S, Löwhagen T: Transrectal fine-needle aspiration biopsy for cytologic diagnosis and grading of prostatic carcinoma. Prostate 2: 381–395, 1981.
52. Yao J C, Wang W C, Tseng H H, Hwang W S: Primary rhabdomyosarcoma of the prostate. Diagnosis by needle biopsy and immunocytochemistry. Acta Cytol 32: 509–512, 1988.
53. Zajicek J: Aspiration biopsy cytology. Part 2. Cytology of infradiaphragmatic organs. Karger, Basel, 1979.
54. Zattoni F, Pagano F, Rebuffi A, Costantin G: Transrectal thin-needle aspiration biopsy of prostate: four years' experience. Urology 22: 69–72, 1983.
55. Zetterberg A, Esposti P L: Prognostic significance of nuclear DNA levels in prostatic carcinoma. Scand J Urol Nephrol Suppl 55: 53–58, 1980.

Female Genital Organs

56. Bandy L C, Clarke-Pearson D L, Silverman P M, Creasman W T: Computed tomography in evaluation of extrapelvic lymphadenopathy in carcinoma of the cervix. Obstet Gynecol 65: 73–76, 1975.
57. Belinson J L, Lynn J M, Papillo J L, Lee K, Korson R: Fine-needle aspiration cytology in the management of gynecologic cancer. Am J Obstet Gynecol 139: 148–153, 1981.
58. Buckley C H: Is needle aspiraton of ovarian cysts adequate for diagnosis? Br J Obstet Gynaecol 96: 1021–1023, 1989.
59. Crosby J H, Bryan A B, Gallup D G, Talledo O E: Fine-needle aspiration of inguinal lymph nodes in gynaecologic practice. Obstet Gynecol 73: 281–284, 1989.
60. DeCrespigny L Ch, Robinson H P, Davoren R A M, Fortune D: The 'simple' ovarian cyst: aspirate or operate? Br J Obstet Gynecol 96: 1035–1039, 1989.
61. Ehya H, Lang W R: Cytology of granulosa cell tumor of ovary. Am J Clin Pathol 85: 402–405, 1986.
62. Einhorn N, Zajicek J: Aspiration biopsy of intrapelvic metastases of cervical carcinoma. Acta Radiol (Ther) 17: 257–262, 1978.
63. Fidler W J: Recurrent granulosa-cell tumour. Aspiration cytology findings. Acta Cytol 26: 688–690, 1982.
64. Flint A, Terhart K, Murad T M, Taylor P T: Confirmation of metastases by fine needle aspiration biopsy in patients with gynecologic malignancies. Gynecol Oncol 14: 382–391, 1982.
65. Frable W J, Goplerud D R: Adenoid cystic carcinoma of Bartholin's gland. Diagnosis by aspiration biopsy. Acta Cytol 19: 152–153, 1975.
66. Ganjei P, Nadji M: Aspiration cytology of ovarian neoplasms. A review. Acta Cytol 28: 329–332, 1984.
67. Geier G: Aspirationszytologie am Parametrium. Geburtsh Frauenheilk 37: 423–428, 1977.
68. Geier G R, Strecker J R: Aspiration cytology and E_2 content in ovarian tumours. Acta Cytol 25: 400–406, 1981.
69. Hsiu J G, Stawicki M E: The cytologic findings in two cases of stromal sarcoma of the uterus. Acta Cytol 23: 487–489, 1979.
70. Kjellgren O, Ångström T: Transvaginal and transrectal aspiration biopsy in diagnosis and classification of ovarian tumours. In: Aspiration biopsy cytology. Part 2. Cytology of infradiaphragmatic organs, Zajicek J (ed) Karger, Basel, 1979.
71. Kovacic J, Rainer S, Levicnik A, Cizelj T: Cytology of benign ovarian lesions in connection with laparoscopy. In: Aspiration biopsy cytology. Part 2. Cytology of infradiaphragmatic organs, Zajicek J (ed) Karger, Basel, 1979.
72. Lurain J R: Newer diagnostic approaches to the evaluation of gynecologic malignancies. Obstet Gynecol Surv 37: 437–448, 1982.
73. Moriarty A T, Glant M D, Stehman F B: The role of fine needle aspiration cytology in the management of gynaecologic malignancies. Acta Cytol 30: 59–64, 1986.
74. McDonald T W, Shepherd J H, Morley G W, Naylor B, Ruffolo E H, Cavanagh D: Role of needle biopsy in the investigation of gynaecologic malignancy. J Reprod Med 32: 287–292, 1987.
75. Nadji M, Greening S E, Sevin B U, Averett H E, Nordqvist S R B, Ng A B P: Fine needle aspiration cytology in gynecologic oncology. II. Morphologic aspects. Acta Cytol 23: 380–388, 1979.
76. Nash J D, Burke T W, Woodward J E, Hall K L, Weiser E B, Heller P B: Diagnosis of recurrent gynaecologic malignancy with fine-needle aspiration cytology. Obstet Gynaecol 71: 333–337, 1988.
77. Nguyen G K, Berendt R C: Aspiration biopsy cytology of metastatic endometrial stromal sarcoma and extragenital mixed mesodermal tumor. Diagn Cytopathol 2: 256–260, 1986.
78. Ramzy I, Delaney M: Signet-ring cell stromal tumour of ovary. Cytologic appearances of fine needle aspiration biopsy. Acta Cytol 21: 14–17, 1977.
79. Ramzy I, Delaney M: Fine needle aspiration of ovarian masses. I. Correlative cytologic and histologic study of coelomic epithelial neoplasms. Acta Cytol 23: 97–104, 1979.
80. Ramzy I, Delaney M, Rose P: Fine needle aspiration of ovarian masses. II. Correlative cytologic and histologic study of non-neoplastic cysts and non-celoemic epithelial neoplasms. Acta Cytol 23: 185–193, 1979.
81. Selim M A, Beck D: Parametrial needle biopsy; follow-up of pelvic malignancies. Cancer Detect Prev 7: 269–273, 1984.
82. Sevin B U, Greening S E, Nadji M, Ng A B P, Averette H E, Nordqvist S R B: Fine needle aspiration cytology in gynecologic oncology. I. Clinical aspects. Acta Cytol 23: 277–281, 1979.
83. Shepherd J H, Cavanagh D, Ruffolo E, Praphat H: The value of needle biopsy in the diagnosis of gynecologic

cancer. Gynecol Oncol 11: 309–320, 1981.
84. Triller J, Schneekloth G, Marincek B, Kraft R: Computertomographisch gezielte Feinnadelaspirationspunktion pelviner Raumforderungen. Radiologe 22: 484–492, 1982.
85. Trope C: The preoperative diagnosis of malignancy of ovarian cysts. Neoplasma 28: 117–121, 1981.
86. Wajsman Z, Klimberg I: Needle aspiration and needle biopsy procedures. Urol Clin North Am 14: 103–113, 1987.
87. Zaharopoulos P, Wong J Y, Lamke C R: Endometrial stromal sarcoma. Cytology of pulmonary metastasis including ultrastructural study. Acta Cytol 26: 49–54, 1982.

11

SUPPORTING TISSUES

with Måns Åkerman

11 SUPPORTING TISSUES

CLINICAL ASPECTS

SKIN AND SOFT TISSUES

There are two main indications for FNA biopsy of tumours and tumour-like lesions of the skin, subcutis and soft tissues: a primary lesion, and a clinical suspicion of recurrent tumour or metastasis. In primary lesions, the indication for FNA is relative and should be considered individually in each case. A preoperative cytologic diagnosis offers several advantages. Patient anxiety can be relieved by providing an instant diagnosis followed by discussion of therapeutic options. Surgery can be avoided if the lesion proves to be non-neoplastic, or delayed for convenience if it is benign. A diagnosis of malignancy allows preoperative staging and planning of the extent of surgery.

As a general rule, all easily palpable lesions greater than 5 mm in size are suitable targets for fine needle biopsy. For soft tissue tumours it is recommended that the needle passes through the same point on the skin each time; the direction of the needle into the tumour may differ with each pass in order to cover as much of the abnormal tissue as possible. A single point of entry through the skin facilitates the inclusion of the needle track with the surgical excision. This is particularly important in deep-seated, intra- or intermuscular sarcomas in view of the hypothetical risk of causing tumour spread through seeding in the needle track.

FNA is of undisputed clinical value in the investigation of suspected recurrencies or metastases of previously diagnosed malignancies.[2,29,59] Diagnosis is usually easy since, in most cases, histological slides of the original tumour are available for comparison; however, as has been repeatedly emphasised, diagnosis may be difficult in irradiated tissues, not only because radiation may cause considerable cytologic atypia in non-neoplastic cells, but also because recurrences may be poorly defined and difficult to pinpoint in areas of post-radiation oedema and fibrosis. The diagnosis of a recurrence in a surgical scar is less of a problem, although at times tumour can be masked by surrounding firm scar tissue.

Diagnosis and classification of soft tissue tumours is one of the most difficult areas in surgical pathology. The relative absence of recognisable tissue architectural pattern in cytological preparations makes diagnosis by FNA even more difficult than by surgical biopsy. However, experience shows that open biopsy or inadequate surgical excision of a primary malignant mesenchymal tumour may jeopardise chances of cure, and, by opening up fascial planes, may lead to more extensive surgery with more subsequent loss of function than would otherwise have been necessary, especially in deep-seated, intra- or intermuscular tumours.[53]

A broad categorisation of a soft tissue tumour as being of primary soft tissue origin, benign, low- or high-grade malignant respectively, is possible in the majority of cases by a combined evaluation of clinical data, cytological features and radiological investigations, and definitive surgery may be planned without prior open biopsy.[38,47] In view of the low incidence of sarcomas in the population, such cases should preferably be referred to centres specialising in this field. The results of FNA cytology of soft tissue tumours reported by Åkerman et al[21] are promising. In their series of 349 cases the aspirated material was insufficient for diagnosis in 5.7%, and a false cytologic diagnosis was rendered in 5.8% of adequate smears; 51 out of 59 primary sarcomas were correctly diagnosed as such.

Although most pathologists would be reluctant to attempt cytological subclassification of primary soft tissue tumours and tumour-like lesions, some knowledge of the cytological pattern of the most common tumours is important. The following case may serve as an example:

A 68-year-old woman presented with a mass in the left axilla. 20 years previously she underwent left mastectomy for breast cancer followed by post-operative irradiation. Clinically, the mass was thought to represent recurrent breast cancer, but a diagnosis of a malignant fibrous histiocytoma could be made with confidence by FNA cytology. A radical surgical excision was performed and histology confirmed the diagnosis. It was felt that the sarcoma had probably been induced by radiation. Obviously, the cytological diagnosis radically altered the management of this patient.

During recent years a number of benign tumours as well as sarcomas have been characterised cytologically by comparative studies of aspirates from different cases of the same tumour type, and by correlative studies of FNA smears and histological sections.[19,20,22,26,27,28,40,50,51,55,56]

The biopsy technique is the same as for any superficial, palpable lesion. Local anaesthesia is rarely needed. Multiple aspirates are usually necessary to obtain sufficient and representative material. The site for the biopsy should, if possible, be choosen in consultation with the surgeon responsible for the definitive treatment. Tattooing of the needle insertion point on the skin is helpful if the needle track is to be included in the excision. Ultrasonography or computed tomography can be helpful in finding viable tissue in extensively necrotic or cystic tumours.[36,60]

As a rule, alcohol-fixed H & E or Pap stained smears and air-dried smears stained with MGG should be used in parallel. Wet-fixation gives excellent nuclear detail, particularly when cells occur mainly in microscopical solid tissue fragments as is often the case with several types of sarcoma. Air-dried MGG smears, however, provide important information about cytoplasmic and stromal components. If sufficient material can be aspirated, EM examination and/or immunocytochemical studies may give valuable information on histogenesis.[18,33,43,58]

BONE AND CARTILAGE

Needle aspiration of bone lesions has been performed ever since the technique was introduced. Martin and Ellis included several examples of primary and metastatic bone malignancies in their original paper.[67] The technique is now well established with some centres recording series of results from over 4000 biopsies;[82,83] however, not all biopsies are performed with fine needles and larger core-producing, 2 mm needles are frequently used by some groups.[79,80] Obviously the choice of needle depends on the character of the lesion. The usual 23–21 gauge needle can only be used for biopsy of tumours invading the surrounding soft tissue or when the cortical bone is destroyed or very thin. In deep sites, for example in vertebral bodies, the overlying cortex can be penetrated by an 18 gauge needle. Multiple aspirates can then be obtained at varying depths and angles with a 23 gauge needle passing through the heavier needle which remains in site during the procedure. Some workers believe that FNA should be restricted to the diagnosis of metastases and lesions such as myeloma or eosinophilic granuloma, leaving the diagnosis of primary bone lesions to histological examination of core biopsies or open biopsies.[69,79,82]

FNA has the advantage over open biopsy in being less disruptive to bone, leaving no scar, and permitting multiple sampling without complications. It is simple, cost-effective and rapid; its primary purpose is to obtain a morphologic or sometimes a bacteriologic diagnosis of an osteolytic lesion before treatment or formal biopsy. Its most common application is to confirm malignancy, but the technique can also be used to diagnose inflammatory conditions such as tuberculosis or other infections by providing material for culture, etc. The differential diagnosis between metastatic malignancy and osteomyelitis of the spine is an extremely important application of FNA. Threatening cord compression is a medical emergency, and, if successful, FNA can rapidly decide the correct treatment. The diagnosis of myeloma and eosinophilic granuloma is relatively easy, and the distinction between non-Hodgkin's lymphoma and other primary small cell malignant tumours is possible. FNA is well suited to the investigation of the cause of pathological fractures. Definitive diagnosis of primary bone neoplasms is possible as the cytomorphology of important primary bone tumours has been described in detail in correlative cytological/histological studies.[62,68,70,75,84,86,87]

The correct interpretation of smears from a bone lesion requires access to the full clinical and radiological assessment, the same as in histological diagnosis of a formal bone biopsy.

Adequate material is obtained from fine needles in up to 80% of cases,[63] and when using both thick and thin needles in up to 84% of cases.[79] The accuracy of the technique is very high in the diagnosis of metastases, being in the order of 90%.[61,76] Its value in diagnosing primary bone lesions is less well documented, but de Santos[69] records 93% diagnostic accuracy using thick and thin needles and Akerman et al[63] 90% in cases with satisfactory aspirates using only thin (21–22 gauge) needles.

FNA guided by fluoroscopy or computed tomography in non-palpable lytic lesions is a rapid and safe path to a morphologic diagnosis of lesions anywhere in the skeleton, particularly in the spine. Some pain is usually felt at aspiration. Local anaesthesia prevents periosteal pain and is recommended in conjunction with fluoroscopic or CT guidance as several passes with the needle may be necessary to obtain a representative specimen. Certain groups, however, do not use local anaesthesia,[61] maintaining that the local anaesthetic injection is as painful as the biopsy. Complications are very few; significant haemorrhage is unusual[79] as is pneumothorax after rib aspiration. Biopsy of spinal lesions carries the additional, albeit rare, complication of neurological damage.[77] Because of the increased likelihood of haemorrhage, needle biopsy of bone lesions is contraindicated in patients having a low platelet count or bleeding disorder.

Bone aspirates are often heavily bloodstained, and methods similar to those used for processing haematologic bone marrow aspirates are useful for concentrating material. In particular, the use of a watch glass to select cellular fragments and thrombin-clot preparations for histological assessment are valuable (see Ch. 2). Both air-dried MGG smears and wet-fixed smears for H & E or Pap should be made. MGG smears are particularly helpful in assessing bone-marrow elements and chondroid, myxoid or osteoid material; wet-fixed smears are superior for nuclear detail, particularly in tissue fragments.

11 SUPPORTING TISSUES

CYTOLOGICAL FINDINGS

SKIN AND SOFT TISSUES

Non-neoplastic lesions

Inflammatory processes

A purulent aspirate indicates an *abscess* and should be sent for microbiological study. It should be remembered that aspirates of necrotic malignant tumours may mimic pus. FNA smears from the wall of an abscess or from non-suppurating *chronic inflammatory processes* often contain fragments of inflammatory granulation tissue. The fragments consist of a framework of proliferating fibroblasts and of endothelial cells of capillary vessels with hyperplastic or swollen nuclei. Macrophages and inflammatory cells of all kinds are present. Macrophages often appear atypical and together with the proliferating fibroblasts may raise a suspicion of malignancy enhanced by the presence of mitoses; however, the very mixed population of cells in inflammatory granulation tissue is quite characteristic. In *suture granuloma* the granulation tissue includes multinucleated giant cells of foreign-body type which may contain birefringent particles. The *granulomatous inflammation* of TB, sarcoid, and some fungal infections, etc., is recognised by clusters of epithelioid histiocytes with poorly delimited cytoplasm and banana/bean-shaped or 'foot-print' nuclei. Langhans' giant cells cannot be distinguished with confidence from foreign-body giant cells in smears. The aetiology of granulomatous inflammation must be pursued by bacteriological and serological tests, etc.

Cysts and localised degenerative processes
(Figs 11.1 and 11.2)

FNA samples of *epidermal*, *pilar* or *dermoid cysts* consist of thick, greasy, foul-smelling material. Smears show debris with anucleate squames, some nucleated squamous epithelial cells and often inflammatory cells and foreign-body giant cells (Fig. 11.1). The three types of cysts cannot be separated cytologically. A postoperative *lymphocele* yields clear, yellowish, mucoid fluid on aspiration. Smears contain only a small number of normal lymphocytes. Smears of material aspirated from a *haematoma* contain altered red and white blood cells, haemosiderin-containing macrophages, amorphous material with cholesterol crystals, or fragments of reparative granulation tissue with haemosiderin pigment, depending on the age of the process.

The aspirate from a *rheumatoid nodule* is usually scanty, consisting of amorphous granular acidophilic material with a variable number of fibroblasts and/or histiocytes. Small multinucleated histiocytic giant cells may be seen. An aspirate from a *ganglion* consists of droplets of thick, colourless, myxoid or gelatinous material. Smears show a small number of single cells which have abundant pale cytoplasm and small ovoid nuclei, and a background of thick, myxoid material (Fig. 11.2).

Amyloidosis

FNA biopsy of periumbilical adipose tissue from the anterior abdominal wall has been found to be of value in the diagnosis of secondary systemic amyloidosis.[57] Rings of amyloid around fat cells and amyloid deposits in vessel walls can be demonstrated after Congo red staining and polarisation.

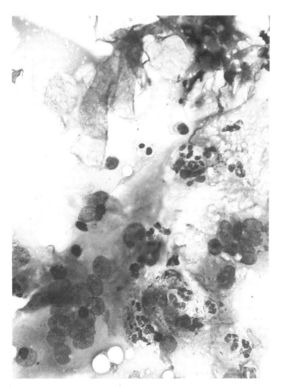

Fig. 11.1 Epidermal cyst
Keratinised squamous cells, multinucleate histiocytes, inflammatory cells and debris (MGG, HP)

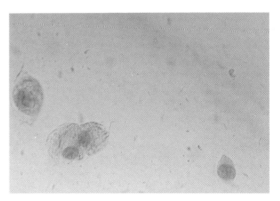

Fig. 11.2 Ganglion
A few pale histiocyte-like cells; background of amorphous mucoid material (Pap, HP)

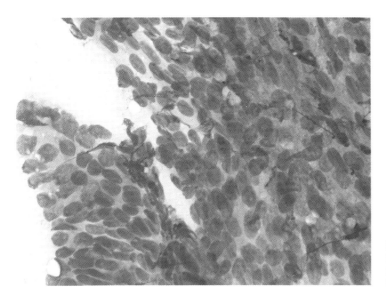

Fig. 11.3 Endometriosis
Biphasic tissue fragment; sheet of
palisading epithelial cells and cellular
stromal tissue (MGG, HP)

Endometriosis (Fig. 11.3)

Endometriosis may be the cause of tumour-like infiltrates, for example in surgical scars, in the abdominal
wall or in the umbilicus in young women. FNA may
yield mainly fresh or altered blood with haemosiderin-
containing macrophages. Sometimes smears contain
fragments of endometrial tissue including both glandular epithelium and endometrial stroma. The stroma
appears as syncytial clusters of cells with plump spindle
or ovoid nuclei; glandular epithelium appears as monolayered sheets of uniform cells with well-defined cell
borders. Single epithelial cells are distinctly columnar.
The nuclei of both stromal and epithelial cells are usually uniform and have a bland chromatin pattern and
are unlikely to be misinterpreted as malignant.[31] The
epithelial component can occasionally show nuclear
pleomorphism, but the coexistence of epithelium and
stroma together with the clinical presentation should
allow a correct diagnosis.

Metastatic malignancy

The cytological findings in recurrent and metastatic
malignancy have been described elsewhere, particularly
in Chapter 5. Access to histological slides of the primary
tumour for comparison with the smears is the most
important aid to diagnosis.

A mass in the skin or soft tissues may be the first
manifestation of *malignant lymphoma*, mainly non-
Hodgkin's lymphoma, or it may be the first sign of
recurrence of treated lymphoma. Cytological criteria for
the diagnosis of lymphoma are presented in Chapter 5.

Acute myeloid leukaemia can occasionally be preceded by a soft tissue mass, the so called *granulocytic
sarcoma* (Fig. 11.4). Smears reveal single, large cells
which have a moderate to scanty amount of basophilic
cytoplasm with perinuclear clearing, an eccentric, large,
slightly irregular nucleus, pale chromatin, and prominent nucleoli. Some cells may contain azurophilic cyto-

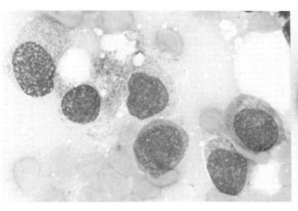
(a)

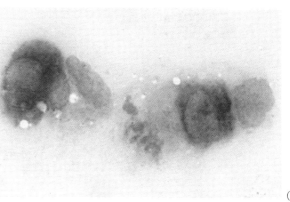
(b)

Fig. 11.4 Granulocytic sarcoma
(a) Myeloblasts and promyelocytes (azurophilic cytoplasmic granulation) (MGG, HP Oil). (b) Similar cells showing strong positive
staining for esterase

11

SUPPORTING TISSUES

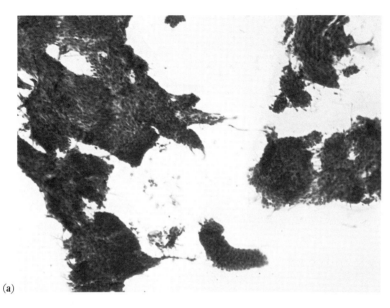

(a)

Fig. 11.5 Basal cell carcinoma
(a) Cohesive fragments with alternatingly sharp and irregular borders (H & E, IP).
(b) Tumour fragment of small closely packed cells resembling the tumour buds seen in histological sections (H & E, HP).

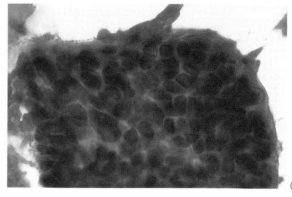

(b)

plasmic granules and are recognisable in MGG smears as promyelocytes. If granulated cells are not observed, the leukaemic cells may be misinterpreted as originating from a high grade non-Hodgkin's lymphoma. Histochemical stains for esterase and peroxidase, and immunocytochemical stains for muramidase and elastase may be helpful.

Primary neoplasms — skin

Squamous cell carcinoma
The cytological pattern has been described elsewhere (Ch. 8).

Basal cell carcinoma (Fig. 11.5)[5a,9]

Criteria for diagnosis

1. Tight aggregates with alternatingly smooth and very irregular outline.
2. Palisading of nuclei along the surface of aggregates.
3. Scanty cyanophilic cytoplasm (Pap); indistinct cell borders.
4. Small, dark, uniform, ovoid nuclei; no nuclear moulding; indistinct nucleoli.

Most basal cell carcinomas are diagnosed clinically. If rapid confirmation is desired, scrape smears from the skin surface are the simplest method. If the lesion is ulcerated, several scrapings are recommended as the first scrape smear often contains only debris and leucocytes.[5a] Non-ulcerated, deeply invasive tumours are suitable for FNA; a 25 gauge needle tends to give a better, less haemorrhagic yield than a thicker needle. The most characteristic feature of basal cell carcinoma in smears is the strong cohesiveness of the cells which remain in well-defined aggregates with palisading of nuclei similar to the tumour buds seen in histological sections.[9]

Adnexal tumours
The cytomorphology of these tumours has not yet been well described. Some benign adnexal tumours may be difficult to distinguish cytologically from basal cell carcinoma. FNA smears of cutaneous *cylindroma* may closely mimic adenoid cystic carcinoma. This is of practical importance if the tumour is related to the external auditory canal.[1] A case of *syringocystadenoma papilliferum* in which FNA smears were misinterpreted as metastatic breast cancer due to abundant cellularity, poor cell cohesion and mild nuclear atypia in combination with the clinical presentation, was briefly described in Chapter 7 (p. 166).

Pilomatrixoma (calcifying epithelioma of Malherbe) (Fig. 11.6)[15]

Criteria for diagnosis

1. Abundant aspirate.
2. Background of calcific debris including nuclear fragments.

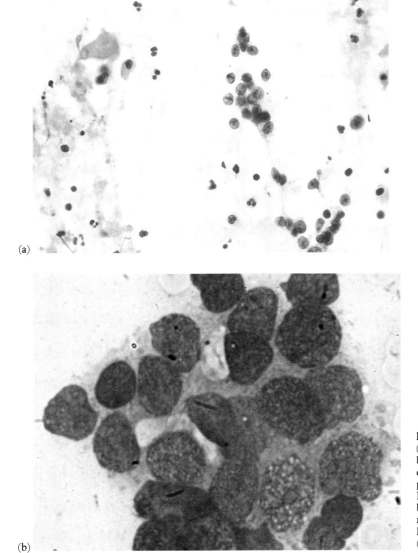

Fig. 11.6 Pilomatrixoma
(a) Anucleate squamous cells, pale basaloid cells, inflammatory cells and debris; note uniform nuclei and prominent nucleoli of basaloid cells (Pap, IP). (b) Cluster of small, tightly packed basaloid cells; may be mistaken for malignant if the complex smear pattern is lacking and basaloid cells dominate (MGG, HP Oil).

3. Inflammatory cells; foreign-body giant cells.
4. Clusters of degenerating squamous cells.
5. Solid aggregates of basaloid cells.

The basaloid cells superficially resemble those of basal cell carcinoma, but they have larger, more vesicular nuclei with prominent nucleoli and a larger amount of basophilic cytoplasm. Pilomatrixoma can be mistaken for necrotising squamous cell carcinoma in FNA smears. The very complex smear pattern of different cell types and the absence of clearly malignant cells point to the correct diagnosis. However, smears dominated by basaloid cells without the characteristic background may be misdiagnosed as carcinoma (Fig. 11.6b).

Malignant melanoma (Figs 11.7–11.11)[5,6,7,14]

Criteria for diagnosis

1. Highly cellular smears.
2. A predominantly dispersed cell population; aggregates or epithelial-like clusters may be encountered.
3. Abundant cytoplasm; eccentric nuclei.
4. Marked anisokaryosis; binucleate and multinucleate cells.
5. Uniformly hyperchromatic nuclei.
6. Intranuclear inclusions; prominent nucleoli.
7. Cytoplasmic pigment (variable).

11 SUPPORTING TISSUES

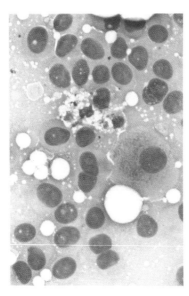

Fig. 11.7 Malignant melanoma
Dispersed population of relatively uniform cells, with indistinct cytoplasm; note the cell with abundant cytoplasm and dust-like pigment; some intranuclear vacuoles (MGG, HP)

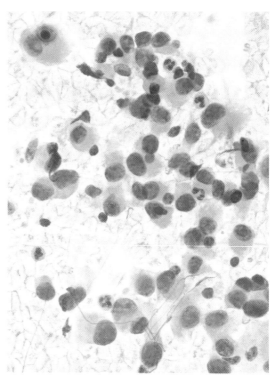

Fig. 11.8 Malignant melanoma
Dispersed population of pleomorphic cells with abundant eosinophilic cytoplasm, eccentric dark nuclei and some binucleate cells; no pigment seen in this field (H & E, HP)

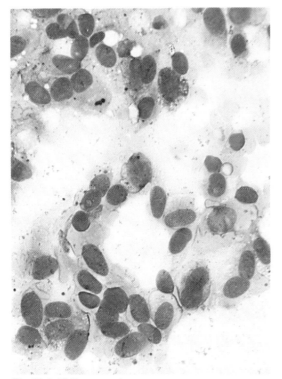

Fig. 11.9 Malignant melanoma
Poorly cohesive plump spindle cells; abundant pigment, both intracytoplasmic and dispersed in the background (MGG, HP)

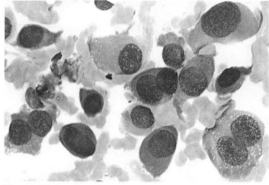

Fig. 11.10 Amelanotic melanoma
Dispersed large pleomorphic cells; some binucleate cells; abundant dense cytoplasm (MGG, HP)

The cytoplasm is usually abundant and dense but may be vacuolated and have a perinuclear pale zone. A characteristic feature noted in air-dried MGG smears is the uniformity of nuclear chromatin pattern between cells, strikingly different from the variation in chromatin pattern of the cells of most anaplastic carcinomas (Fig. 11.7). In alcohol-fixed smears the chromatin is often coarsely granular but is evenly distributed (Fig. 11.8). The staining properties of melanin pigment in routinely stained smears are similar to lipofuscin and haemosiderin; however, a fine dust-like distribution within the cytoplasm and its presence within well-preserved tumour cells identifies the pigment as melanin in most cases (Figs 11.7 and 11.9). Special stains may be necessary to determine the nature of the pigment in some cases. In amelanotic melanomas, demonstration of melanin precursors by formalin-induced fluorescence, of melanin by Masson-Fontana or of pre-melanosomes by EM may be necessary to confirm the diagnosis (Figs 11.10 and 11.11). Immunocytochemical staining with S-100 protein or monoclonal antibodies against melanoma-associated antigens is of considerable diagnostic value.

Problems in diagnosis

The criteria listed above apply mainly to the commonest melanoma — the epithelioid type. The cells of the spindle cell variant are smaller and have elongated, more uniform nuclei (Fig. 11.9). Cells of spindle cell melanoma may be more cohesive and can be mistaken for spindle cell sarcoma. The small cell type may mimic non-Hodgkin's lymphoma, especially if a lymph node metastasis is needled. The more pleomorphic variants may be difficult to distinguish from poorly differentiated carcinoma or pleomorphic sarcoma. FNA smears

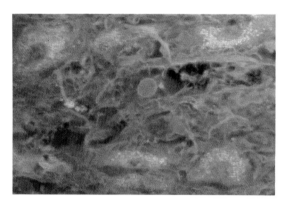

Fig. 11.11 Amelanotic melanoma
Granular yellow fluorescence of intracytoplasmic amines (HP)

from malignant melanoma with a myxoid stromal reaction may be misinterpreted as a myxomatous soft tissue tumour.[8,12]

Merkel cell carcinoma (Neuroendocrine carcinoma of the skin) (Fig. 11.12)[4,11,13]

Criteria for diagnosis

1. A smear population of small neoplastic cells.
2. Fragile cells; many stripped nuclei — cytoplasmic background.
3. Dispersed cells and small groups of cells; nuclear moulding, pseudorosettes or acinar structures.
4. Scanty cytoplasm; round or ovoid nuclei.
5. Mitoses.
6. Discrete cytoplasmic red granulation in a small number of cells (MGG).

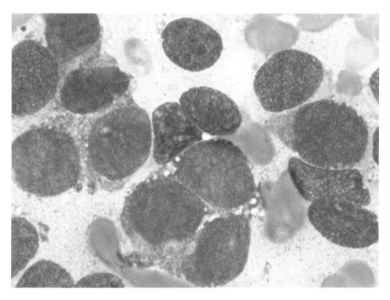

Fig. 11.12 Merkel cell carcinoma
Single cells and small groups of cells; nuclear moulding, discrete red cytoplasmic granules in some cells (MGG, HP Oil)

307

11 SUPPORTING TISSUES

Primary neuroendocrine carcinoma of the skin is a rare neoplasm, locally aggressive as well as metastasising, which usually arises in the dermis of elderly patients. Clinically, Merkel-cell carcinoma can be difficult to distinguish from non-Hodgkin's lymphoma, amelanotic melanoma, metastatic carcinoma, and primary carcinoma of the skin and epidermal appendages.

Smears are as a rule highly cellular. Clustered cells form indian files with nuclear moulding, curved rows or rosette-like structures. The most important differential diagnosis is metastasis of small cell bronchogenic carcinoma. The cells of Merkel cell carcinoma are less pleomorphic and the nuclei more uniformly rounded rather than irregular or spindle-shaped. Immunocytochemical demonstration of a globular keratin deposit or ultrastructural demonstration of cytoplasmic filaments arranged in a well demarcated whorl support the diagnosis.

Paget's disease[10]

Extramammary Paget's disease has similar cytologic features to Paget's disease of the nipple (see Ch. 7).

Histiocytoma (Fig. 11.13)

Criteria for diagnosis

1. Solid cell clusters.
2. Eosinophilic, finely granular or vacuolated cytoplasm; indistinct cell borders.
3. Ovoid, kidney-shaped or elongated nuclei; mild anisokaryosis; finely granular chromatin.
4. Nucleoli of moderate size.
5. Multinucleated giant cells of Touton type.

The spectrum of histological patterns from highly cellular histiocytoma to dermatofibroma is reflected in the number of cells and in the proportion of histiocytes, fibroblasts and collagen. A cellular histiocytoma can resemble a smooth muscle tumour in FNA smears; however, the cell population of a histiocytoma is more variable, the nuclei are larger, paler and plumper, and the cytoplasm is granular and vacuolated. Giant cells of Touton type are not seen in leiomyoma (Fig. 11.13). (Atypical fibroxanthoma, see p. 311).

Primary neoplasms — soft tissues

Reports of cytological patterns of different types of primary soft tissue tumours are mainly based on single case reports or on relatively small series of cases. Hajdu & Hajdu in their comprehensive *Cytopathology of Sarcomas*[32] describe the findings in exfoliative cytological smears such as pleural effusions and sputum samples, in imprints, and to a lesser extent in fine-needle aspirates. Diagnostic criteria applicable to FNA smears have been defined for some common benign tumours and sarcomas and also for a few more rare entities (Table 11.1). However, this is still not the case for the majority

Table 11.1 Tumours and tumour-like lesions the cytomorphological features of which have been defined through correlative histological and cytological studies

Nodular fasciitis
Intramuscular myxoma
Neurilemmoma
Malignant fibrous histiocytoma
Myxofibrosarcoma
Malignant giant cell tumour of soft tissues
Leiomyosarcoma
Lipomatous tumours
Embryonal rhabdomyosarcoma
Alveolar rhabdomyosarcoma

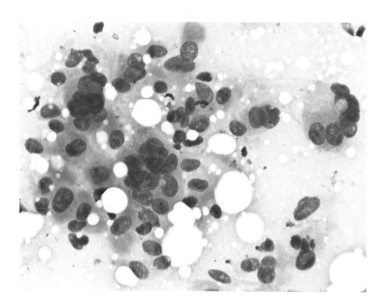

Fig. 11.13 Histiocytoma
Loose cell cluster; ovoid nuclei, abundant granular and vacuolated cytoplasm; indistinct cell borders; note multinucleated giant cells (MGG, HP)

of the large number of different types of tumours primary in soft tissues. Nevertheless, several cytological features are common to most mesenchymal tumours, and some general guidelines for grading malignancy can be applied in most cases.

Primary soft tissue tumours in general

Usual findings

1. A variable cell yield both in benign tumours and sarcomas; tumours rich in vessels or intercellular collagen generally yield smears poor in cells.
2. A mixture of single cells and more or less cohesive small tissue fragments; the proportion of single cells to fragments differ in different tumour types.
3. Myxoid ground substance or intercellular collagen.
4. Spindle-shaped nuclei.
5. Cytoplasmic projections and indistinct cell borders.
6. Multinucleated cells, giant cells and bizarre nuclei.
7. Malignant nuclear chromatin may be absent in high grade malignant sarcomas.
8. Benign tumours or tumour-like lesions may show prominent cellular pleomorphism.
9. Mitoses absent or rare in benign tumours and low grade malignant sarcomas.

FNA samples from high grade malignant sarcomas are usually abundant, whereas the yield from benign and low grade malignant tumours depends on the type of tumour. Collagen-rich intercellular stroma, areas of hyalinisation, fibrosis and prominent vascularity influence the yield. Single cells do not always dominate the smears of either benign or malignant tumours. Aggregates, cohesive bundles of cells or small tumour tissue fragments are a common finding in both benign tumours and sarcomas. The cells may not form any discernible architectural pattern, or they may be oriented in bundles. Bundles of spindle cells which seem to radiate out from a central basement membrane core suggest a vasoformative tumour (haemangiopericytoma, angiosarcoma, or haemangiopericytoma-like synovial sarcoma). Bundles of parallel spindle cells are common in smooth muscle tumours, tumours of Schwann cell origin and at times in fibroblastic tumours. Palisading of nuclei can be seen in Schwann cell tumours and smooth muscle tumours, and rosettes around a centre of finely fibrillar material in neuroblastoma.

Myxoid ground substance has a vaguely fibrillar structure and stains brightly blue-violet/red/purple in MGG. It is less conspicuous in wet-fixed H & E and Pap-stained smears. Collagen is also obvious in MGG smears as strands of pink material between cells. In some tumours, notably in myxoid liposarcoma, capillary vessels are prominent in tumour tissue fragments, and capillary fragments are often observed in the myxoid ground substance of myxofibrosarcoma or the myxoid

type of malignant fibrous histiocytoma. Inflammatory cells (nodular fasciitis) and mast cells (synovial sarcoma) should be looked for. Necrosis is suggestive of malignancy.

The cytoplasm of mesenchymal tumour cells is generally not as fragile as that of many epithelial tumour cells. Cell borders are usually indistinct, and the cytoplasm may be drawn out into thin strands which anastomose with adjacent cells. Aggregates of cells have a syncytial cytoplasm. Nuclei tend to be eccentric in rounded cells.

A significant proportion of nuclei are usually spindle-shaped even in highly pleomorphic tumours; however, nuclei may be quite plump, for example in synovial sarcoma and in uterine stromal sarcoma; irregularly ovoid, rounded, or kidney-shaped in histiocytic tumours, and mainly rounded in round cell liposarcoma, epithelioid cell sarcoma, clear cell sarcoma, alveolar soft part sarcoma, and in leiomyoblastoma. Round or ovoid nuclei are characteristic of a group of small cell malignant tumours which include alveolar rhabdomyosarcoma, neuroblastoma, and Ewing's sarcoma.

In general, nuclear pleomorphism is proportional to the grade of malignancy. Important exceptions occur, however. Anisokaryosis, multinucleation, and variation in nuclear shape can be prominent in benign, proliferating tumours, notably in the pseudosarcomatous lesions of soft tissue such as nodular fasciitis, proliferating myositis and pseudomalignant myositis ossificans. In such tumours, nuclear chromatin is invariably bland, granular and evenly distributed, but nucleoli may be large and prominent. Nuclear pleomorphism and chromatin clumping may be minimal in some low grade malignant sarcomas. Conversely, some high grade malignant tumours have deceptively uniform nuclei and bland chromatin. In such tumours, the malignant potential is mainly suggested by high cellularity as shown by a high cell yield, and by nuclear crowding in aggregates of cells and in tissue fragments, and also by the presence of necrosis. Bizarre nuclei with lobulation, budding, and nuclear satellites are common in high grade tumours. Mitoses are more difficult to find in smears than in sections, and mitotic counts are unreliable. Mitoses can be present in nodular fasciitis but are absent in most benign and low grade malignant tumours. Frequent and abnormal mitotic figures usually indicate a high grade sarcoma.

Fibroblastic and fibrohistiocytic tumours — benign

Criteria for diagnosis

1. Variable cellularity; a myxoid background, especially in nodular fasciitis and in intramuscular myxoma.
2. Both single cells and clusters of cells with intercellular collagen or myxoid ground substance.
3. Cells and nuclei predominantly spindly.
4. Pale cytoplasm.

11 SUPPORTING TISSUES

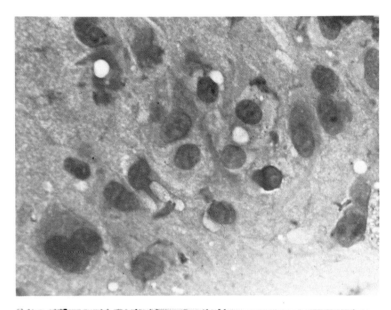

Fig. 11.14 Nodular fasciitis
Proliferating fibroblasts embedded in a myxoid background; note binucleate cell with abundant cytoplasm and eccentric nuclei (ganglion-cell-like) (MGG, Oil)

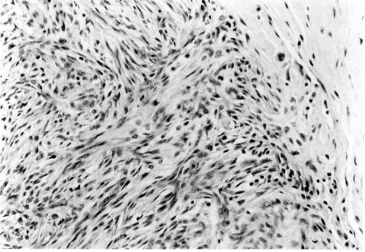

Fig. 11.15 Nodular fasciitis
Tissue section; same case as Figure 11.14 (H & E, IP)

5. Moderate nuclear pleomorphism, marked in the pseudosarcomatous processes.
6. Pale, granular, evenly distributed chromatin; prominent nucleoli; mitoses.
7. Lymphocytes and plasma cells (nodular fasciitis).

Nodular fasciitis (Figs 11.14 and 11.15) is among the commonest of these lesions. Dahl & Åkerman[26] reported 13 cases with cytology; at present our material comprises more than 30 cases, all with remarkably similar cytomorphology. Nuclei are predominantly spindle but a proportion of cells have plump, ovoid or kidney-shaped nuclei. Bi- or multinucleate forms are always present and, if looked for carefully, ganglion cell-like binucleate cells with triangular shape and eccentrically placed nuclei are found. A high cell content, nuclear pleomorphism, prominent nucleoli and the presence of

mitoses may suggest malignancy, but the pale, bland nuclear chromatin is a clear indication of the benign nature of the lesion (Fig. 11.15). The correct diagnosis depends on the recognition of the neoplastic cell as an actively proliferating fibroblast, a myxoid background, and the presence of inflammatory cells, the anatomical site and the clinical presentation.

Other fibromatoses such as *desmoid fibromatosis* (Figs 11.16 and 11.17) and *palmar and plantar fibromatosis* may resemble nodular fasciitis in FNA smears; however, the number of cells tend to be smaller, the nuclei are more consistently spindle, and nuclear pleomorphism, sometimes prominent in nodular fasciitis, is lacking. Also, collagen fragments are more common than myxoid ground substance and inflammatory cells are absent. Fragments of striated muscle including regenerating multinucleated muscle fibres are commonly seen in

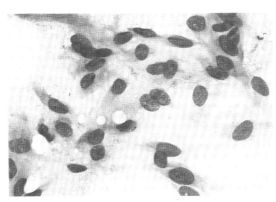

Fig. 11.16 Fibromatosis (desmoid)
Loose cluster of spindle cells with bland nuclei and indistinct attenuated cytoplasm (MGG, HP)

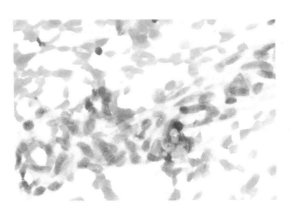

Fig. 11.17 Fibromatosis (desmoid)
Syncytial aggregate of spindle cells with bland spindle-shaped nuclei (H & E, HP)

smears from abdominal desmoids. FNA smears from *extra-abdominal desmoid* (aggressive fibromatosis) may be quite cellular and contain both single spindle cells and clusters of cells showing moderate anisokaryosis. Cytologically, the most important differential diagnoses are low grade malignant fibrosarcoma and monophasic synovial sarcoma.

Smears from *intramuscular myxoma* are quite characteristic.[20] Macroscopically, the aspirate consists of droplets of colourless, mucoid, stringy and semiliquid material resembling the aspirate from a ganglion. Smears show small tissue fragments and single cells in an abundance of myxoid background material. The cells are spindle-shaped or stellate and have elongated nuclei and often very long cytoplasmic processes. The chromatin is regularly dispersed and finely granular, and nucleoli, if present, are small. Some histiocyte-like cells with abundant vacuolated cytoplasm, sometimes containing a large cytoplasmic globule of bluish-violet material (MGG), are also present. Fragments of capillary vessels are very rare or totally absent, and this is important in distinguishing intramuscular myxoma from myxoid liposarcoma and low grade malignant myxofibrosarcoma[20] (see p. 316). *Fibrous histiocytoma* and *atypical fibroxanthoma* are mentioned on pages 308 and below.

Fibroblastic and fibrohistiocytic tumours — malignant

Criteria for diagnosis

1. Cellular smears; necrosis common.
2. Single cells and clusters; often small fragments of tumour tissue; intercellular collagen.
3. Spindle cells with elongated nuclei (fibroblastic cells).
4. Cells with abundant pale, vacuolated cytoplasm and often evidence of phagocytosis; nuclei ovoid, reniform or irregular, eccentrically placed (histiocytic cells).

5. Marked (variable) nuclear pleomorphism.
6. Multinucleated tumour giant cells and bizarre nuclei.
7. Coarse, irregular chromatin; nucleoli variable; mitoses.

Malignant fibrous histiocytoma (MFH) (Figs 11.18–11.20) is the commonest primary malignant soft tissue tumour. The criteria listed above are mainly based on the comprehensive study of MFH of pleomorphic type of Walaas et al[55] and on more than 40 cases from our files. Atypical spindle cells may dominate the smears, but large histiocyte-like cells with abundant foamy or vacuolated cytoplasm and one or several, highly irregular nuclei are always found, and also cells with a moderate amount of cytoplasm and rounded or ovoid atypical nuclei. It is not uncommon to find evidence of phagocytosis in the histiocyte-like cells (Fig. 11.20).[55] The histiocytic nature of these cells can be supported by a positive immunoperoxidase staining for alpha-1-antitrypsin, alpha-1-chymotrypsin, or for muramidase, or by EM examination of the aspirate. The anatomical site and the clinical presentation must be known since MFH and atypical fibroxanthoma of the skin may be cytologically indistinguishable. Smears from the predominantly subcutaneous myxoid variant of MFH, the *myxofibrosarcoma* (MFS)[40] often contain abundant myxoid ground substance (Fig. 11.22). The low grade malignant myxofibrosarcoma is dominated by spindle-shaped cells, the nuclear atypia of which may be slight. It may resemble intramuscular myxoma or myxoid liposarcoma cytologically; lipoblasts are, however, not present and the characteristic vascular component of myxoid liposarcoma is not seen although fragments of vessels are often noted embedded in the myxoid ground substance. High grade myxofibro-sarcoma resembles high grade malignant MFH. *Malignant giant cell tumour of soft tissues* is another variant in this group of tumours (Figs 11.23 and 11.24).[22] FNA smears from this growth contain many large multinucleated giant cells of benign

11

SUPPORTING TISSUES

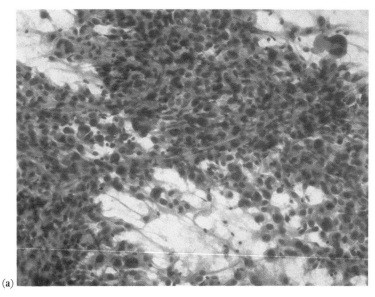

(a)

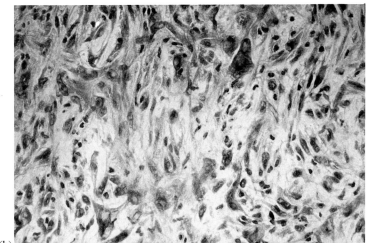

(b)

Fig. 11.18 Malignant fibrous histiocytoma
(a) Fragments of loosely cohesive pleomorphic cells: a mixture of fibroblast-like and histiocyte-like cells (H & E, IP).
(b) Tissue section; same case as (a) (H & E, IP).

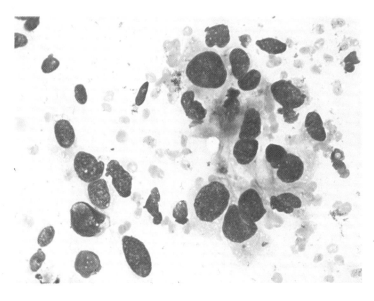

Fig. 11.19 Malignant fibrous histiocytoma
Poorly cohesive pleomorphic cells, most nuclei irregularly rounded; a few spindle forms; abundant pale granular and vacuolated cytoplasm (MGG, HP)

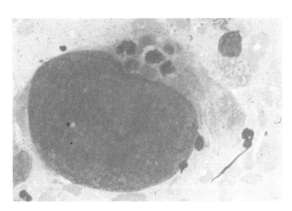

Fig. 11.20 Malignant fibrous histiocytoma
Histiocyte-like tumour cell with evidence of phagocytosis
(MGG, HP)

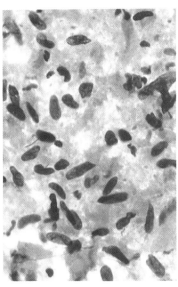

Fig. 11.21 Fibrosarcoma
Pure population of dispersed fibroblastic cells with moderately
pleomorphic spindle-shaped nuclei (H & E, HP)

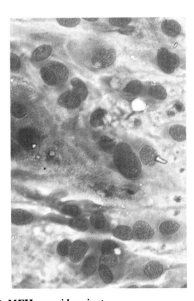

Fig. 11.22 MFH myxoid variant
Poorly cohesive plump spindle cells with pleomorphic nuclei;
myxoid background (MGG, HP)

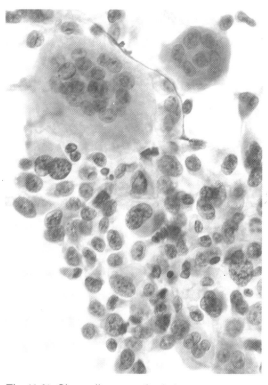

Fig. 11.23 Giant cell tumour of soft tissues
Poorly cohesive histiocyte-like cells with moderately
pleomorphic nuclei; irregular nuclear chromatin; multinucleate
giant cells of benign appearance (MGG, HP)

11

SUPPORTING TISSUES

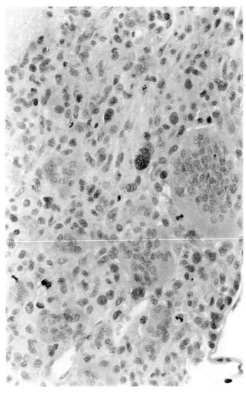

Fig. 11.24 Giant cell tumour of soft tissues
Tissue section; same case as Figure 11.23; note the occasional
malignant giant cells (H & E, IP)

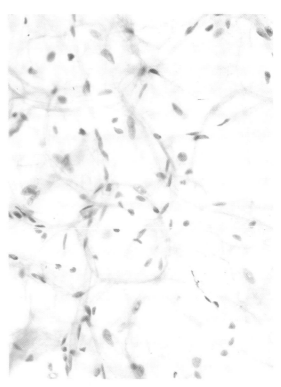

Fig. 11.25 Vascular lipoma
Mature adipose tissue with anastomosing capillaries
(H & E, HP)

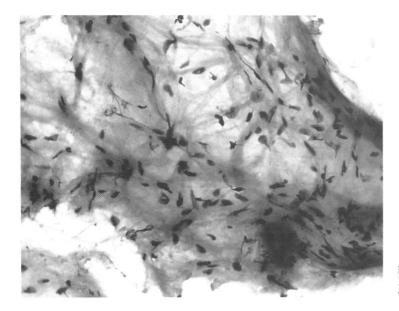

Fig. 11.26 Spindle cell lipoma
Fat cells trapped in fibromyxoid tissue
with spindle-shaped cells (H & E, HP)

SUPPORTING TISSUES

11

histiocytic type resembling osteoclasts. In addition, there are pleomorphic spindle cells, malignant histiocytic cells, and multinucleated malignant giant cells, as in smears of a high grade malignant MFH of the usual pleomorphic type.

The differential diagnosis of MFH is mainly the other pleomorphic, high grade malignant sarcomas such as pleomorphic liposarcoma and leiomyosarcoma. Anaplastic sarcomatoid carcinoma (e.g. of renal or bronchogenic origin), or anaplastic squamous cell carcinoma and pleomorphic melanoma may also resemble MFH. The identification of highly atypical lipoblasts, necessary for the confident diagnosis of pleomorphic liposarcoma can be difficult and may require EM examination. Immunocytochemical staining for keratin or S-100 protein

are of value in the differential diagnosis.

Tumours of adipose tissue — benign
(Figs 11.25–11.27)[19,56]

Lipoma is the commonest of all benign soft tissue tumours. Lipoma cannot be distinguished from normal adipose tissue cytologically — smears of both consist of fragments of mature fat tissue, a few single fat cells and fat droplets. The fat cells seen both single and in fragments are large and have abundant empty cytoplasm and a small, often eccentric dark nucleus. A few strands of branching capillary vessels may be seen in fragments of adipose tissue. It is important to make sure that the aspirate is representative of the suspected tumour. A needle with trocar is recommended for deep-seated

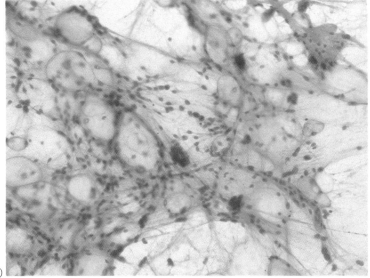

(a)

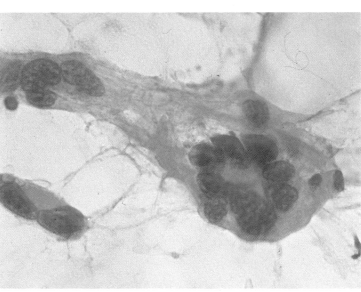

(b)

Fig. 11.27 Pleomorphic lipoma
(a) Mature adipose tissue; scattered large, dark, multinucleated cells (H & E, IP).
(b) Same case as (a); large multinucleated cell (floret-cell) (H & E, Oil).

11

SUPPORTING TISSUES

tumours to avoid contamination with normal subcutaneous fat. In *infiltrating intramuscular lipoma*, aspirated fragments of adipose tissue are intimately associated with muscle fibres. Skeletal muscle fibres appear in smears as large, strap-like structures which are strongly eosinophilic (navy-blue in MGG) and have rows of small, ovoid and elongated, pale nuclei. Cross striation is often evident. The vascularity of an *angiolipoma* can often be appreciated in FNA smears (Fig. 11.25). Smears of *spindle cell lipoma* may have a background of fibromyxoid ground substance and a variable number of spindle cells within tissue fragments (Fig. 11.26). In *atypical lipoma* large cells with abundant cytoplasm and atypical, often irregularly shaped nuclei are seen within and between tissue fragments. The yield is generally more cellular than that from a simple lipoma. Atypical lipoma cannot be distinguished from lipoma-like well-differentiated liposarcoma cytomorphologically, but mainly by the anatomical site and clinical presentation. So called floret cells are a typical feature of *pleomorphic lipoma* recognisable in FNA smears (Fig. 11.27).[19]

Tumours of adipose tissue — malignant
(Figs 11.28–11.31)[19,56]

Lipoma-like well-differentiated liposarcoma (Fig. 11.28) may closely resemble atypical and at times pleomorphic lipoma. The tumour usually has a fibrous-sclerotic component, and cells with moderately atypical, pleomorphic nuclei are seen both single and within fragments of adipose tumour tissue. There may be cells looking like atypical lipoblasts with vacuolated cytoplasm and scalloped nuclei. The cytological findings must be evaluated in relation to the anatomical site — superficial or deep. In *myxoid liposarcoma* the peculiar network of anastomosing capillary vessels is usually recognisable in FNA

smears and is one of the characteristic features. Smears consist mainly of small tumour tissue fragments with branching capillary vessels, and there is always an abundance of myxoid ground substance in the background. The tumour cells seen both in fragments and single between fragments have spindle or ovoid, relatively uniform nuclei and a thin cytoplasm. Typical lipoblasts are always found; uni- or multivacuolated with scalloped nuclei. The lipoblasts are best visualised in MGG, the cytoplasmic vacuoles are less prominent in H & E (Fig. 11.29). Differentiation from low-grade malignant MFS depends on the demonstration of the capillary network within tumour fragments and of lipoblasts. The vessel fragments seen in smears of MFS are usually thicker and are present in the myxoid ground substance. Smears of *round cell liposarcoma* show either numerous dissociated cells or tissue fragments containing closely packed tumour cells. The fragments are considerably more cellular than those of myxoid liposarcoma and a capillary network is less prominent. The tumour cells have irregular, rounded nuclei and a malignant chromatin pattern. The cytoplasm is fragile and many nuclei are stripped. Atypical lipoblasts are always found (Fig. 11.30). *Pleomorphic liposarcoma* resembles MFH cytologically. The diagnosis rests on the presence of highly atypical, sometimes multinucleated lipoblasts. Lipoblasts in liposarcoma smears may be univacuolated and resemble signet-ring cells or they may be multivacuolated containing small or large vacuoles or a mixture of both. The scalloped nucleus is an important cytological feature (Fig. 11.31). In FNA smears, superimposed fat vacuoles from adjacent fat tissue may produce artefacts in other cell-types causing a resemblance to lipoblasts, and macrophages in adipose tissue showing inflammatory or reactive change may have a vacuolated cytoplasm (lipophages).

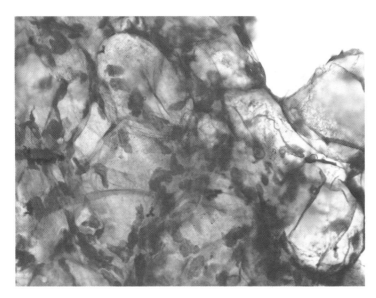

Fig. 11.28 Well-differentiated liposarcoma
Tissue fragment of fat cells and fibroblastic cells separated by fibromyxoid stroma; aspirate from large recurrent retroperitoneal tumour histologically diagnosed as well-differentiated liposarcoma (MGG, HP)

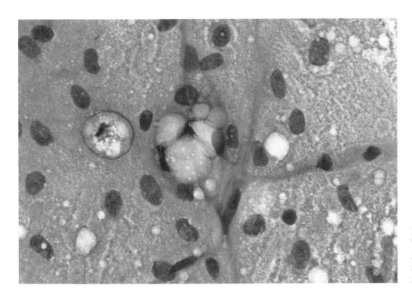

Fig. 11.29 Myxoid liposarcoma
Tissue fragment of cells embedded in myxoid background material; typical anastomosing vessels and scattered multivacuolated lipoblasts (MGG, HP)

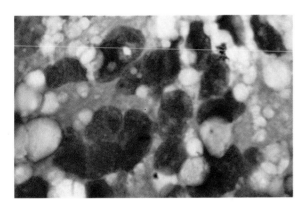

Fig. 11.30 Round cell liposarcoma
Tissue fragment of closely packed atypical lipoblasts (MGG, Oil)

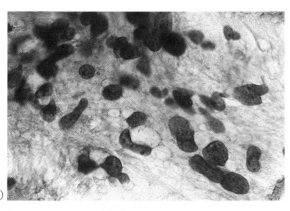

(a)

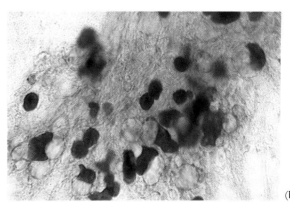

(b)

Fig. 11.31 Pleomorphic liposarcoma
Poorly cohesive cells with pleomorphic spindle or rounded nuclei and irregular nuclear chromatin; note several multivacuolate lipoblasts with scalloped nuclei. Multinucleate malignant giant cells were prominent in other fields. (a) and (b) show different fields of same tumour (H & E, HP).

317

11 *SUPPORTING TISSUES*

Tumours of smooth muscle — benign and malignant
(Figs 11.32 and 11.33)[27]

Criteria for diagnosis

1. Very variable degree of cellularity.
2. Cells more often in loose clusters and tissue fragments than single (single cells more common in benign tumours).
3. Cells in parallel bundles or in tandem.
4. Abundant, eosinophilic cytoplasm (grey-blue in MGG); indistinct cell borders.
5. Variable, predominantly cigar-shaped, sometimes truncated nuclei.
6. Finely granular barred chromatin.
7. One or more small, distinct nucleoli.
8. Many multinucleated giant tumour cells in high grade leiomyosarcoma.

The histological diagnosis of malignancy in well-differentiated tumours of smooth muscle origin is, to a large extent, dependant on mitotic counts, invasive growth and size, all of which are features which cannot be evaluated in FNA smears. The question of malignancy is therefore difficult to decide in aspirates from low-grade malignant leiomyosarcoma. In high grade tumours, however, malignancy is suggested by an abnormal nuclear chromatin, nuclear pleomorphism, and mitoses. The presence of necrosis also favours malignancy.[35]

Cell clusters or tissue fragments have a syncytial appearance due to the fairly abundant eosinophilic cytoplasm and lack of cell borders. The peculiar arrangement of the nuclear chromatin in a cross-striated pattern described by Hajdu and Hajdu is a helpful but also variable feature.[32] Low-grade malignant leiomyosarcoma can be difficult to distinguish from neurogenic and from fibroblastic tumours. The former tend to have more slender, elongated nuclei with pointed ends; the

Fig. 11.32 Leiomyoma
Poorly cohesive spindle cells; abundant eosinophilic cytoplasm forming interlacing strands; finely granular nuclear chromatin; small nucleoli (H & E, IIP)

latter have a smaller amount of pale cytoplasm. A leiomyoma with a predominantly round cell pattern can easily be mistaken for an epithelial tumour (see Fig. 10.50). The correct diagnosis is suggested by the presence of some slender, spindly nuclei and by the abundant syncytial, eosinophilic cytoplasm. The cytology of *leiomyoblastoma* has been described in a case report; the diagnostic criteria are still incomplete.[41] Poorly differentiated leiomyosarcoma may be impossible to differentiate cytologically from MFH or from high grade malignant neurogenic sarcoma.

Tumours of striated muscle
Benign *rhabdomyoma* is rare. We have seen smears from one such tumour in the neck of a 65-year-old man. The smears contained many fragments of muscle fibres which were paler, smaller and more irregular in shape than normal fibres of skeletal muscle. Nuclei were larger

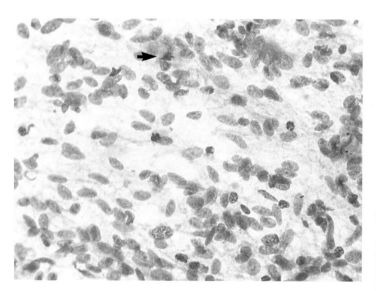

Fig. 11.33 Leiomyosarcoma
Loose clusters of cells and some single cells with indistinct cytoplasm and spindly, cigar-shaped nuclei of varying size; note mitotic figure (arrow) (H & E, HP)

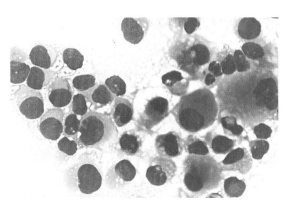

Fig. 11.34 Alveolar rhabdomyosarcoma
Loose arrangement of small cells with irregular eccentric nuclei; a few cells have abundant dense cytoplasm (rhabdomyoblasts) (MGG, HP)

and had prominent nucleoli. Cross-striation was difficult to distinguish. The fragments closely resembled regenerating myocytes. A few published case-reports describe similar findings.[23,24]

Embryonal rhabdomyosarcoma is the commonest soft tissue sarcoma in children. The cytological pattern has recently been described in a study of a relatively small material.[51] In FNA smears, although pleomorphic, the tumour has the general appearance of a small cell tumour. Cells with dense eosinophilic cytoplasm and an eccentric nucleus, triangular, strap-shaped or tadpole-like, may be recognised as rhabdomyoblasts and suggest the correct diagnosis. Giant cells with numerous small malignant nuclei are characteristic also in bone marrow aspirates. The cytological pattern of *alveolar rhabdomyosarcoma* has also been described (Fig. 11.34).[50] In FNA smears, alveolar rhabdomyosarcoma has a more consistent pattern of a small cell tumour. Alveolar or rosette-like structures may be seen. In our opinion, however, the diagnostic criteria are not specific enough to allow a confident, type-specific diagnosis in most cases. EM examination, or preferably immunocytochemical demonstration of desmin helps to confirm the diagnosis. The diagnosis of *pleomorphic rhabdomyosarcoma* has been challenged in a retrospective study; the great majority of re-evaluated tumours proved to be non-myogenic pleomorphic sarcomas of other types.[49]

Tumours of vascular origin

Aspiration of *haemangioma* of any type yields plenty of venous blood. Smears may contain a few strands of endothelial cells with pale, syncytial cytoplasm and pale, spindle nuclei. Macrophages, haemosiderin pigment and fibroblasts may be present if thrombosis has occurred. The cytological findings in *haemangiopericytoma*[42] have been described in Chapter 9 (Figs 9.21–25) and of *angiosarcoma*[16] in Chapter 7 (Fig. 7.68) and Chapter 9 (Fig. 9.81).

Neurogenic tumours (Figs 11.35–11.37)[28,44,46]

The needling of a *neurofibroma* or of a *neurilemmoma* may trigger a sharp pain radiating along the nerve, and this is a valuable diagnostic sign. The amount of material obtained by FNA varies from case to case; tissue fragments of cohesive cells are more commonly seen than single cells.[28] The cellularity of the fragments is variable. Intercellular collagen or a background of myxoid material may be present, but one of the most typical features is the fibrillar appearance of the background.[28] Nuclear palisading or less commonly Verocay bodies may be found.[44] Nuclei tend to be long and slender and have pointed ends. There may be a moderate degree of nuclear pleomorphism, but the chromatin pattern is uniformly bland (Figs 11.35 and 11.36). If cells with plump, spindle nuclei and more abundant cytoplasm predominate, a diagnosis of leiomyoma may be considered. The pleomorphic and bizarre cells in *ancient neurilemmoma* may be mistaken for malignant,[46] but the overall smear pattern is that of a benign tumour. Cells from a low grade *malignant Schwannoma* may be only moderately pleomorphic. In high grade malignant tumours, the smears are highly cellular and the cells have elongated, spindle, severely atypical and pleomorphic nuclei. Multinucleated tumour cells may be found. Nuclear chromatin is coarse and irregular and the cytoplasm is thin and fragile (Fig. 11.37). Cells occur singly and in clusters with intercellular collagen, and a background of myxoid material is occasionally present.

Other tumours and tumour-like lesions

We have recently described the cytological findings in a few cases of *pseudomalignant myositis ossificans*.[48] Smears showed a mixture of proliferating fibroblasts, osteoblast-like cells and multinucleated giant cells of osteoclast type. No osteoid was found, and the diagnosis was based on the cytological pattern in combination with the clinical and radiological presentation in all cases. If osteoid is found, osteogenic sarcoma may be considered; however, the absence of malignant nuclear characteristics and of highly atypical multinucleated cells helps to exclude this diagnosis.

We have seen FNA smears from four cases of *proliferative myositis*,[45] two of which were histologically confirmed. In the other two cases the mass resolved spontaneously in a relatively short time. These four cases illustrate the degree of atypia which reactive tissue can attain and which may well raise a suspicion of malignancy.

One of the cases without histology was a 70-year-old woman who spontaneously developed a firm mass some 2 cm in diameter within the body of the sternocleidomastoid. The lesion was slightly tender. Aspiration revealed skeletal muscle fibres, fibroblasts and some macrophages together with a dispersed population of highly atypical cells with large nuclei, prominent nucleoli and abundant cytoplasm. The nuclei were often eccentrically located (Fig. 11.38). In view of the cellular atypia,

11

SUPPORTING TISSUES

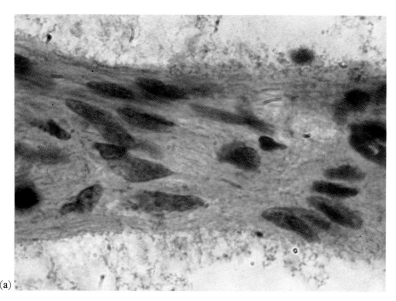

(a)

Fig. 11.35 Neurilemmoma
Cohesive tissue fragment; spindly, palisading nuclei with pointed ends; fibrillar background. (a) H & E, HP. (b) MGG, Oil (see also Fig. 2.14)

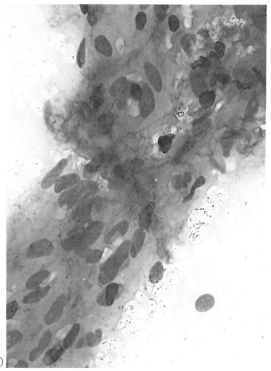

(b)

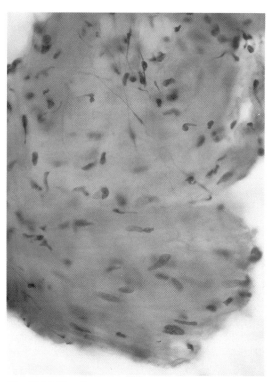

Fig. 11.36 Neurilemmoma
Fragment of mesenchymal tissue; widely separated, pale nuclei with pointed ends; abundance of intercellular collagen (Pap, HP)

biopsy was thought advisable but the lesion had virtually disappeared within a week, and the patient was followed without surgery. She remained well some months after FNA biopsy.

The atypical cells most probably represent the ganglion-like cells of proliferative myositis but may be regenerate muscle fibres or proliferating fibroblasts. The very large nucleoli of these cells is one of the features which could raise a suspicion of malignancy.

Granular cell tumour (Fig. 11.39)[30,37] is mainly found in the subcutaneous and submucosal tissues, most commonly in the head and neck region. In the breast, it can occasionally closely simulate cancer clinically. FNA

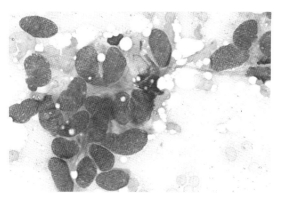

Fig. 11.37 Malignant schwannoma
Cohesive cluster of pleomorphic plump spindle cells; malignant chromatin pattern (MGG, HP)

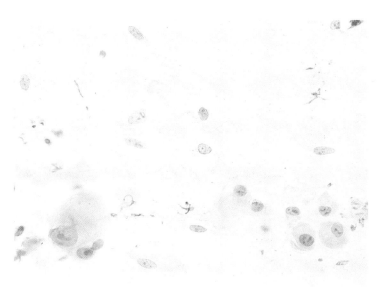

Fig. 11.38 Proliferative myositis
Large ganglion-like cells in a background of fibroblastic cells; note the irregular nuclei and huge nucleoli in the multinucleate cell (Pap, HP)

smears show many neoplastic cells most of which are in syncytial clusters. Within these, nuclei may be arranged in a vaguely follicular pattern, the cytoplasm is abundant and relatively dense, with a prominent granularity, eosinophilic in H & E and dark blue in MGG. The nuclei are small, round or ovoid, uniform and have a bland chromatin pattern and small nucleoli. The granules stain positively with PAS and variably for CEA with the immunoperoxidase method.[39,52] The cells are fragile and many nuclei are bare.

We have not seen smears of a primary *alveolar soft part sarcoma*, but we have seen material from a metastatic deposit in the lung (Figs 11.40 and 11.41). The tumour cells were very fragile, presenting mainly as bare nuclei. These were very large, rounded, and varied considerably in size. Large central nucleoli were evi-

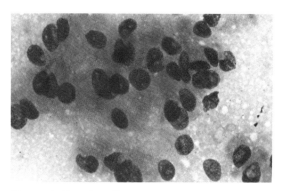

Fig. 11.39 Granular cell tumour
Acinar-like cluster of cells with small ovoid nuclei and abundant granular cytoplasm; indistinct cell borders (MGG, HP)

11 *SUPPORTING TISSUES*

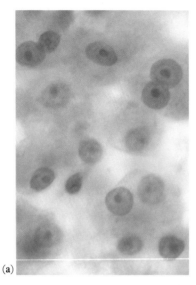

(a)

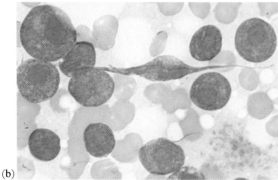

(b)

Fig. 11.40 Alveolar soft part sarcoma
(a) Loose aggregate of large cells with rounded vesicular nuclei, large nucleoli and abundant granular cytoplasm (H & E, HP Oil). (b) Pleomorphic nuclei and very large nucleoli (MGG, HP Oil).

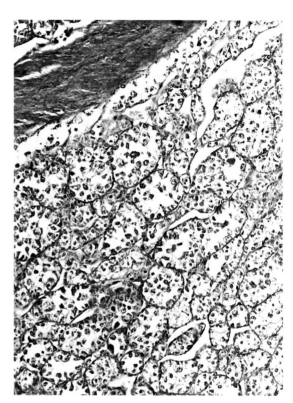

Fig. 11.41 Alveolar soft part sarcoma
Tissue section; same case as Figure 11.40 (H & E, IP)

dent. Loosely adherent intact cells could be seen in wet-fixed material; they possessed abundant rather granular cytoplasm and resembled macrophages apart from their prominent nucleoli. Some were binucleate.

FNA smears from a few cases we have seen of *clear cell* and *epithelioid sarcoma* contained cells with abundant cytoplasm and large, rounded or ovoid nuclei with prominent nucleoli. The neoplastic cells of epithelioid sarcoma were mixed with fibroblasts and histiocytes. The cytomorphology of these rare entities have not yet been defined although some case reports have been published.[17]

Smears from *synovial sarcoma*[32,34] are usually highly cellular. A specific diagnosis may be possible if the typical biphasic pattern is discernible, i.e. clusters of epithelial- or mesothelial-like cells with ovoid nuclei of medium size and indistinct, fragile cytoplasm, and

strands and bundles of spindle cells. Mast cells may be prominent. A number of recently aspirated cases of predominantly monophasic synovial sarcoma all showed a similar pattern: highly cellular smears dominated by clusters of tightly packed small to medium-sized cells with rounded or ovoid, uniform nuclei and indistinct cell borders. Single cells had a moderate amount of thin, uni- or bipolar cytoplasm. Acinar or rosette-like structures were seen in clusters of cells (Fig. 11.42a). The nuclear chromatin was finely granular, irregularly distributed, and the nucleoli were small. Mitoses were found in all cases. Myxoid or hyaline intercellular ground substance was not seen, but branching vessels were evident in clusters, the overall pattern resembling that of haemangiopericytoma. Purely monophasic synovial sarcoma may be extremely difficult to distinguish from fibrosarcoma (Fig. 11.42b).

We are only aware of a single case of *extraskeletal chondrosarcoma* reported in the cytological literature.[25] Smears from a case of *myxoid chondrosarcoma* which we have seen in consultation showed cords and solid groups of small, bland epithelial-like cells with a background of fibrillar, myxoid ground substance and a few single spindle cells. The overall pattern resembled to a degree that of pleomorphic adenoma of salivary gland.

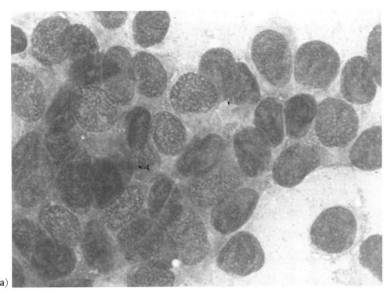

(a)

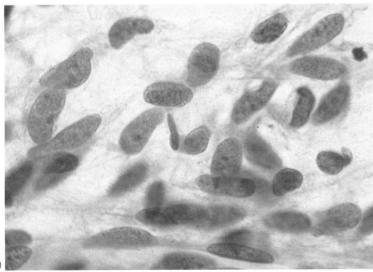

(b)

Fig. 11.42 Synovial sarcoma
(a) Cluster of tightly packed, plump spindle cells; rounded or ovoid uniform nuclei; acinar-like groupings within the cluster (MGG, Oil). (b) Monophasic type: fibroblast-like cells showing mild nuclear atypia (H & E, Oil).

BONE AND CARTILAGE

Our experience in the diagnosis of primary bone lesions is limited but covers the most common malignant tumours and a number of benign tumours and other lesions. Specialist texts and papers should be consulted for a more comprehensive review.[81]

Normal structures (Fig. 11.43)

1. Haematopoietic tissue.
2. Osteoblasts.
3. Osteoclasts.
4. Chondrocytes.
5. Cartilage.

The cytopathologist must be familiar with the appearance of cellular marrow. Taken individually, the nuclear

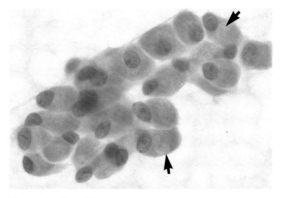

Fig. 11.43 Osteoblasts
Cluster of cells with a plasma cell-like appearance; abundant cytoplasm and eccentric nuclei; 'Hof' separated from nucleus (arrows); from an area of moderate osteoblastic activity and new bone formation (H & E, HP)

11 SUPPORTING TISSUES

features of immature marrow cells may be disturbingly similar to malignant cells, but the mixture of all types allows easy indentification. The irregular multilobed nucleus of the megakaryocyte in particular can also cause alarm if the site of origin is unsuspected. MGG-stained smears are much superior to wet-fixed H & E or Pap smears in identifying haemopoetic cells.

Osteoblasts are commonly seen in aspirates from all kinds of bone lesions. They present either as single cells or as small groups or runs. They have a characteristically eccentric nucleus which sometimes seem to protrude from the cytoplasm. The nucleus is rounded and often contains a central nucleolus. The cytoplasm is dense, amphophilic or basophilic with a central clear area or 'Hof' separated from the nucleus (Fig. 11.43). Osteoclasts are large cells which possess at least 10–15 uniform nuclei, and have an abundant cytoplasm with a similar texture to osteoblasts and well-defined borders. In MGG-stained smears there is a fine, pink granularity.

Normal cartilage does not smear well as it is very cohesive; flecks or clumps of cartilage may be removed from joint surfaces or costochondral junctions; these show bright red or magenta staining with MGG and are pale and translucent with Pap. Scalloped or fibrillar edges are a feature. Free chondrocytes are almost never seen, but the cells are visible within lacunae in the chondroid matrix. They have small, pale, rounded nuclei and poorly stained cytoplasm often presenting as a halo. They are best visualised in wet-fixed smears; the chondroid matrix stains heavily with MGG and obscures the fine structure of the cells.

Inflammatory processes

Osteomyelitis

Culture of the aspirated material is the most valuable part of the procedure if an infectious lesion is suspected. In bacterial osteomyelitis, the smears are dominated by abundant neutrophils but also contain other inflammatory cells and macrophages (Fig. 11.44). The aspirate

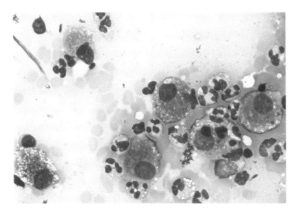

Fig. 11.44 Osteomyelitis
Histiocytes and neutrophils (H & E, HP)

may look like pus from any type of non-specific acute inflammatory process. Clusters of epithelioid cells with their characteristic banana- or beanshaped, pale nuclei and indistinct cell borders, Langhans'-type giant cells, and the amorphous, granular, eosinophilic material of caseous necrosis provoke a strong suspicion of tuberculosis; again, the need for cultural evidence is emphasised.

Neoplasms

Metastatic carcinoma

Criteria for diagnosis

1. Foreign cell population.
2. Cell clusters, acinar or gland-like structures.
3. Cells showing criteria of malignancy.

As with sites such as lymph nodes, diagnosis is usually easy, especially if the histological type of the primary tumour is known, and sections are available for comparison with smears. Descriptions of specific types of metastatic neoplasm are not included here; their cytological appearances have generally been discussed elsewhere.

Problems in diagnosis

1. Osteoblasts resembling mucin-secreting cells: the clear area of osteoblastic cytoplasm may resemble a mucin vacuole to the uninitiated; sometimes clustering or lining up of these cells may enhance this epithelial-like appearance (Fig. 11.43).
2. Smeared marrow elements resembling anaplastic carcinoma; caution should be exercised in reporting badly smeared or poorly preserved material. Marrow is composed of fragile cells and too forceful smearing can cause clumping which may resemble aggregates of small cell or other anaplastic carcinomas. As mentioned, megakaryocytes may also be misinterpreted as large, bizarre malignant cells. It should be remembered that metastatic carcinoma usually replaces marrow; therefore mixtures of marrow and new growth are uncommon.
3. A specific problem is the distinction between chordoma and metastatic renal cell carcinoma in wet-fixed smears (see under chordoma).
4. Excessive blood; this problem is very commonly met in metastatic malignancies as well as in primary bone tumours.

Myeloma; solitary plasmacytoma (Fig. 11.45)

Criteria for diagnosis

1. Many plasma cells.
2. Single cell presentation.
3. Variable cell differentiation.

If there is a uniform dispersed population of plasma cells including multinucleate and pleomorphic forms,

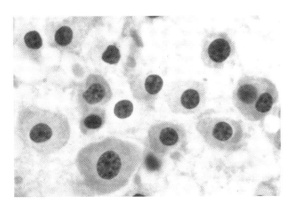

Fig. 11.45 Multiple myeloma
Pure population of atypical slightly pleomorphic plasma cells; the central position of the nuclei in most cells is an unusual feature (H & E, HP Oil)

the diagnosis is obvious. The eccentric nucleus with its speckled or clock-face chromatin pattern and abundant amphophilic cytoplasm makes recognition easy. A clear cytoplasmic zone near the nucleus is another distinctive cytological feature (see Fig. 5.32).

Problems in diagnosis

1. Excessive blood; aspirates from solitary plasmacytoma are often very haemorrhagic and plasma cells may be few in numbers.
2. Anaplastic forms: the more anaplastic forms are likely to cause confusion when a primary bone origin is unsuspected, for example, in lesions affecting the pleura and rib or other soft tissue/bone interfaces.
3. It may be impossible to distinguish between immunoblastic lymphoma with plasmacytoid features and poorly differentiated myeloma. The diagnosis will be decided by clinical, immunological and biochemical findings.
4. Mixtures of marrow elements: the dilemma of deciding whether the proportion of plasma cells in marrow is high enough to justify a diagnosis of myeloma is seldom a worry for the pathologist; usually only lytic lesions formed by solid tumours will be aspirated; mixtures with marrow are rarely seen in these cases.
5. Osteoblasts resembling plasma cells: if only small amounts of material are removed, osteoblasts may sometimes be mistaken for abnormal plasma cells. This will not occur if it is remembered that, unlike osteoblasts, the clear cytoplasmic zone in plasma cells is next to the nucleus.

Malignant lymphoma

Focal bone involvment, usually in the form of lytic lesions and most commonly involving the spine and pelvis, is relatively uncommon in non-Hodgkin's lymphoma and is even less common in Hodgkin's lympho-

ma. It can sometimes be the first manifestation of systemic disease. Primary malignant lymphoma of bone is rare. Cytological criteria for diagnosis are the same as in other sites (see Ch. 5). Primary non-Hodgkin's lymphoma of bone will be discussed in the differential diagnosis of Ewing's sarcoma (p. 332).

Eosinophilic granuloma (Histiocytosis X, Langerhans cell histiocytosis) (Fig. 11.46)[66,71,73,89]

Criteria for diagnosis

1. Large histiocytes with vesicular nuclei of irregular shape.
2. Variable numbers of eosinophils.
3. Giant cells of histiocytic type.

In contrast to most primary bone tumours, eosinophilic granuloma may present as a lytic lesion radiologically indistinguishable from metastatic malignancy. However, the cytological pattern may strongly suggest the correct diagnosis. The characteristic histiocytes have moderately larger and paler nuclei than those seen in common

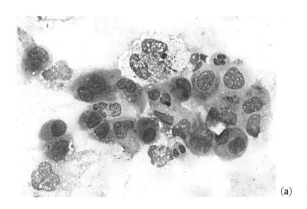

(a)

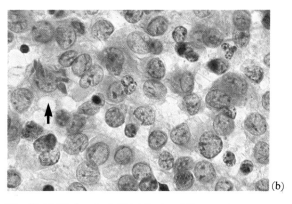

(b)

Fig. 11.46 Histiocytosis X (a) Eosinophilic granuloma
Lytic bone lesion cluster of large histiocytes with pale nuclei some with foamy cytoplasm; few scattered eosinophils (MGG, HP). **(b) Letterer-Siwe disease** Cervical lymph node from a child; numerous histiocytes with large, pale vesicular nuclei, rounded ovoid or reiniform with some deep clefts; small distinct nucleoli; fragile granular cytoplasm; note Charcot-Leyden crystals (arrow) (Pap, HP Oil).

11 *SUPPORTING TISSUES*

inflammatory processes. Although basically kidney-shaped, the nuclei have a distinctive irregular and folded outline. The chromatin is entirely bland and nucleoli are small. The cytoplasm is abundant and pale and has fairly well-defined borders. It is often vacuolated or foamy and may contain phagocytosed debris. Multinucleated cells of similar type are commonly present. These can be quite large and may resemble osteoclasts in wet-fixed smears. Large numbers of histiocytes can also occasionally be found in aspirates of chronic osteomyelitis, but these are of the common, smaller type seen in the usual inflammatory processes and are mixed with neutrophils, lymphocytes and plasma cells (compare Figs 11.44 and 11.46a). A definitive diagnosis is possible with the aid of ultrastructural assessment or by means of immunocytochemistry.[89] The soft tissue deposits of generalised Langerhans cell his-

tiocytosis (Letterer-Siwe's disease) generally consist of a more pure population of abnormal histiocytes and have a less inflammatory appearance as seen in Fig. 11.46b.

Vascular lesions

FNA of *haemangioma* or *aneurysmal bone cyst* is like a venipuncture — only blood is aspirated. A few cells may be present among the blood, such as strands of endothelial cells, haemosiderin-containing macrophages, osteoblasts, osteoclasts and fibroblasts.

Giant cell tumour (Fig. 11.47)[84]

Usual findings

1. Abundant material.
2. A double cell population: mononuclear spindle cells and giant cells of osteoclastic type.

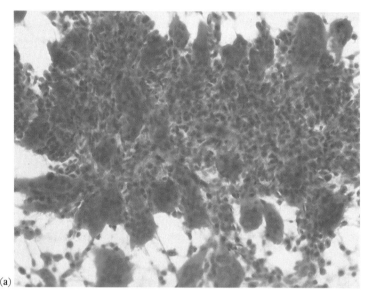

(a)

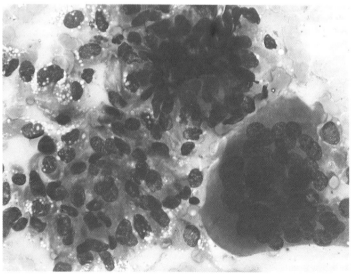

(b)

Fig. 11.47 Giant cell tumour of bone
(a) Tissue fragment of cohesive cells; multinucleated giant cells located peripherally (H & E, IP). (b) Multinucleate osteoclast-like giant cell and clusters of cohesive plump spindle cells some of which are vacuolated; some intercellular collagen; histological grade II (MGG, HP).

3. Cohesive cell clusters; giant cells attached to the periphery of clusters of spindle cells.

The giant cells have numerous (about 20–50) uniform ovoid or round nuclei. The spindle cells are strikingly cohesive and tend to remain in clusters and tissue fragments, but single cells are also always seen. The giant cells are often attached to the periphery of clusters of spindle cells (Fig. 11.47a). Strands of collagen or basement membrane material and endothelial cells are discernible in cell clusters and tissue fragments. The cells have a moderate amount of dense, amphophilic cytoplasm which is often vacuolated, and have well defined borders. The nuclei vary only moderately in size and shape. They are ovoid, have a bland chromatin structure and small nucleoli. Malignancy should be suspected if spindle and multinucleated cells show nuclear pleomorphism and if mitoses are plentiful. The differential diagnosis against other bone lesions (benign and malignant) with many osteoclastic giant cells may be difficult or impossible. As in the histological assessment of bone lesions, detailed knowledge of clinical and radiological data is essential. Stormby and Åkerman[85]

could not distinguish cytologically between true giant cell tumour, osteoblastoma, brown tumour of hyperparathyroidism and reparative granuloma of jaw.

Osteosarcoma (Figs 11.48 and 11.49)[86,87]

Criteria for diagnosis

1. Pleomorphic spindle and rounded cells.
2. Cells resembling osteoblasts and osteoclasts.
3. Multinucleated tumour cells.
4. Clumps of amorphous, eosinophilic (H & E) or red/ pink (MGG) material in the background or between cells (osteoid).
5. Mitotic figures.
6. Intensely positive alkaline phosphatase staining of tumour cells.

Smears contain a mixture of dissociated neoplastic cells and cell clusters. Osteoid is seen as clumps of eosinophilic (bright red or pink in MGG), amorphous or finely fibrillar material in the background or as thin intercellular strands within cell clusters. Both benign osteoclastic giant cells and malignant giant cells with

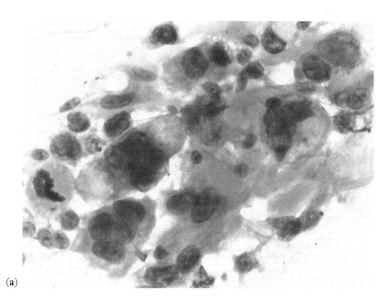

(a)

Fig. 11.48 Osteosarcoma
(a) Loose cluster of pleomorphic, often multinucleate cells; the fragments of pink amorphous material may represent osteoid; note mitotic figure (H & E, HP). (b) Small cluster of pleomorphic sarcoma cells; thin, branching strands of intercellular red/violet material, probably osteoid (MGG, Oil).

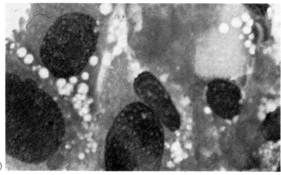

(b)

11 *SUPPORTING TISSUES*

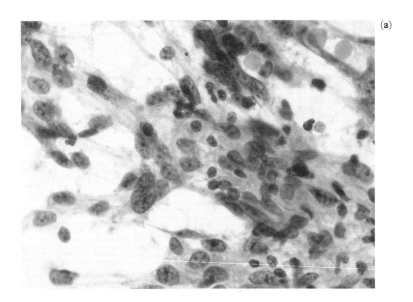

(a)

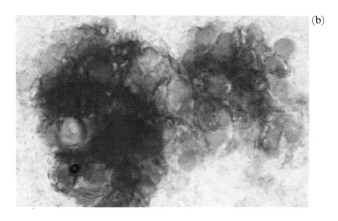

(b)

Fig. 11.49 Osteosarcoma (fibroblastic)
Smears from a patient with known Paget's disease who developed a large mass in the left hip region with extensive bone destruction. (a) Pleomorphic spindle cell sarcoma without distinctive features (H & E, HP). (b) Strong positive cytoplasmic staining for alkaline phosphatase in tumour cells (HP).

pleomorphic nuclei are commonly seen. Macronucleoli may be present.

The criteria listed above apply to osteoblastic osteosarcoma. The chondroblastic form may be difficult to distinguish from a high grade malignant chondrosarcoma, and in the fibroblastic type cellular pleomorphism is less marked. In all types of osteosarcoma, the tumour cells show a strong alkaline phosphatase activity; this histochemical characteristic would help to distinguish a primary bone lesion from metastatic pleomorphic malignancies such as spindle cell or anaplastic sarcoma-like carcinoma or melanoma (Fig. 11.49). In primary MFH of bone, however, the tumour cells also show an alkaline phosphatase activity. EM examination of aspirated material to confirm the presence of osteoid may help to establish the diagnosis.[86]

Chondroma and chondrosarcoma (Figs 11.50–11.53)[78]

Criteria for diagnosis

1. Predominantly tissue fragments in low grade tumours, single cells in high grade sarcomas.

2. Abundant eosinophilic, vacuolated cytoplasm.
3. Chondro-myxoid material.

The chondromyxoid ground substance is usually abundant in chondroma and low grade chondrosarcoma, and is very conspicuous in MGG-stained smears. It has a finely fibrillar texture and stains an intensely red-purple colour (Fig. 11.52). It is less obvious in wet-fixed smears where it is seen as a hyaline, pale violet material with H & E staining (Figs 11.50 and 11.51), and even paler with Pap. The neoplastic cells are best studied in wet-fixed preparations as they are obscured by the intensely stained ground substance in MGG smears. In benign chondroma, cartilaginous fragments dominate the smears; the tumour cells are relatively uniform and binucleate cells are almost never seen with the exception of enchondroma of small peripheral bones which may contain binucleate cells and show fairly marked pleomorphism. Cellularity is variable in low grade chondrosarcoma. The tumour cells have a well-defined cytoplasm and rounded nuclei with one or two nucleoli, binucleate cells are present and nuclear pleomorphism is

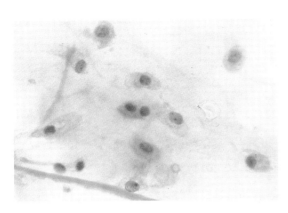

Fig. 11.50 Chondroma
Widely separated small chondrocytes; background of pale chondroid ground substance (H & E, HP)

of moderate degree. Single cells dominate in high grade malignant tumours, cellular and nuclear pleomorphism is prominent and mitoses are present. As can be expected from histopathological experience, it is difficult or impossible in FNA smears to distinguish between chondroma and some low grade chondrosarcomas. High grade sarcomas may be difficult to distinguish from osteosarcoma and from metastatic poorly differentiated epithelial tumours if cartilaginous fragments are absent.

Chordoma (Figs 11.54 and 11.55)[70,74,75]

Criteria for diagnosis

1. Abundant myxoid ground substance, encircling tumour cells.
2. Large cells with abundant bubbly cytoplasm (physaliphorous cells).

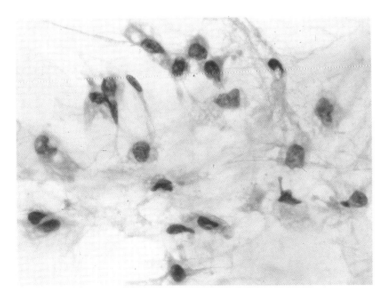

Fig. 11.51 Chondrosarcoma, well-differentiated
Increased numbers of larger, more irregular nuclei; some binucleate forms; background of pale chondroid matrix (H & E, HP)

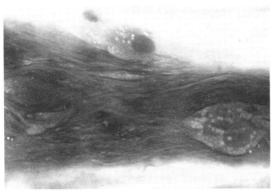

Fig. 11.52 Chondrosarcoma, well-differentiated
Same case as Figure 11.51; intensely purple chondroid ground substance obscuring tumour cells (MGG, HP)

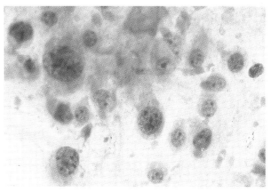

Fig. 11.53 Chondrosarcoma, poorly differentiated
Pleomorphic malignant cells in a background of chondroid matrix and collagen bundles (MGG, HP)

11 *SUPPORTING TISSUES*

3. Clusters of small epithelial-like cells.
4. Rounded nuclei, moderate anisokaryosis, bland chromatin.

The characteristic findings are the abundant background of myxoid ground substance and the large, physaliphorous cells which have abundant pale, vacuolated, bubbly cytoplasm with well defined cell borders. The cells have one, sometimes two, rounded nuclei of moderate size, a bland nuclear chromatin, and small nucleoli. Moderate anisokaryosis is common. The myxoid background material, often fibrillar, intensely purple in MGG smears, pale pink in H & E, forms a network encircling individual tumour cells, cell clusters or fragments. There are also clusters of small, non-characteristic or epithelial-like cells with rounded nuc-

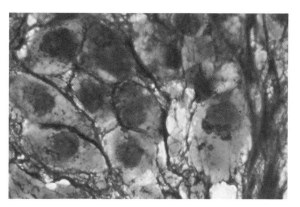

Fig. 11.54 Chordoma
A network of myxoid material staining strongly purple encircling individual tumour cells (MGG, HP)

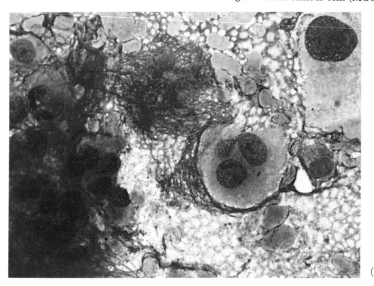

(a)

(b)

Fig. 11.55 Chordoma
(a) Large physaliphorous cells, and fragment with more epithelial-like cells in a chondromyxoid stroma (MGG, HP).
(b) The bubbly appearance of the cytoplasm of the physaliphorous cells is more obvious in an alcohol-fixed smear (H & E, HP Oil).

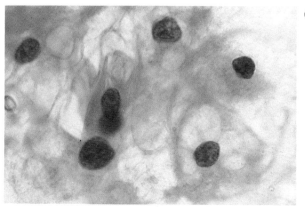

lei. The cytoplasm of these cells may be vacuolated; some cells may have one large vacuole pushing the nucleus to the periphery and may resemble signet-ring cells. The main differential diagnoses are chondrosarcoma and, if only wet-fixed smears are available, metasta-

tic clear cell carcinoma, especially renal cell carcinoma. The abundant ground substance may be inconspicuous in H & E or Pap-stained smears and the epithelial-like tumour cells may give a false impression of an epithelial neoplasm. Typical physaliphorous cells are never encountered in chondrosarcoma and the network of myxoid matrix encircling individual cells is not a feature of either chondrosarcoma or metastatic carcinoma.

Ewing's sarcoma (Figs 11.56 and 11.57)[62,68]

Criteria for diagnosis

1. Both dissociated cells and clusters of loosely cohesive cells.
2. Two cell types: large pale cells with abundant vacuolated cytoplasm and small dark cells with scanty cytoplasm.
3. Abundant cytoplasmic glycogen.
4. Occasionally rosette-like structures.

The cytological appearance of this lesion is distinctive. Smears are generally very cellular and are composed of a mixture of single cells and groups of loosely cohesive cells. The cells are fragile and naked nuclei are common. There is a characteristic mixture of two types of cells: one has abundant pale cytoplasm with vacuoles or clear spaces, rounded or ovoid nuclei with finely granular chromatin, and one to three small nucleoli; the other has scanty cytoplasm and irregular nuclei with a dense chromatin. The two types of cells are most clearly distinguished within groups and clusters of cells, the small dark cells are seen interspersed between the large pale cells. Rosette-like structures without a fibrillar centre are sometimes present. The cytoplasmic vacuoles or

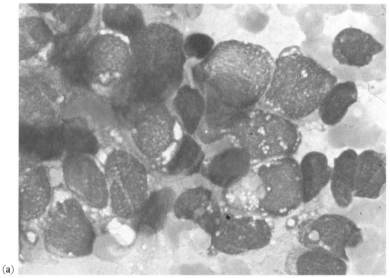
(a)

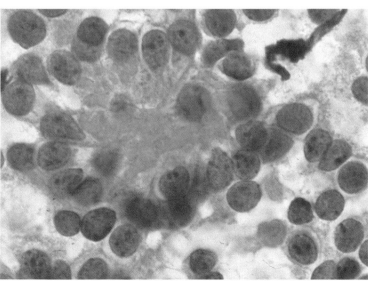
(b)

Fig. 11.56 Ewing's sarcoma
(a) A mixture of large light and small dark cells; note the cytoplasmic vacuoles and clear spaces in the light cells (MGG, Oil).
(b) Rosette-like structure; nuclear chromatin and nucleoli more clearly seen than in MGG (H & E, Oil).

11

SUPPORTING TISSUES

clear spaces correspond to large deposits of glycogen. Distinction from other malignant small cell tumours is easy in typical cases. Non-Hodgkin's lymphoma lymphoblastic is an important differential diagnosis. In the B-lymphoblastic (Burkitt) type, nuclei are round with multiple rather prominent nucleoli and the cytoplasm is scanty containing small vacuoles. In T-lymphoblastic lymphoma, nuclei are of variable size with irregular, lobulated or folded contours (convoluted) and the cytoplasm is narrow. Primitive neuroblastoma and rhabdomyosarcoma may be difficult to distinguish from Ewing's sarcoma cytologically. Ultrastructural study of aspirated cells and immunocytochemical stains are of considerable value in the differential diagnosis (Fig. 11.57).[18]

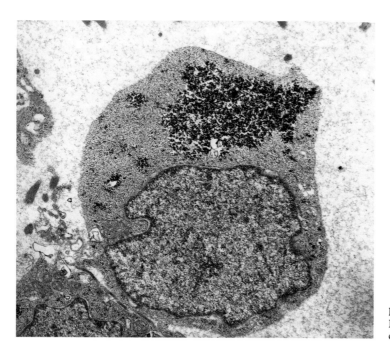

Fig. 11.57 Ewing's sarcoma
Electron micrograph of aspirated tumour cell; large cytoplasmic deposit of glycogen

REFERENCES AND SUGGESTED FURTHER READING

Skin

1. Bondeson L, Lindholm K, Thorstenson S: Benign dermal eccrine cylindroma. A pitfall in the diagnosis of adenoid cystic carcinoma. Acta Cytol 27: 326–328, 1983.
2. Brifford M, Gentile A, Hebert H: Cytopuncture in the follow-up of breast carcinoma. Acta Cytol 26: 195–200, 1982.
3. Canti G: Skin cytology and its value for rapid diagnosis: Acta Cytol 23: 516–517, 1979.
4. Domagala W, Lubinski J, Lasota J, Giryn I, Weber I, Osborn M: Neuroendocrine (Merkel cell) carcinomas of the skin: Cytology, intermediate filament typing and ultrastructure of tumor cells in fine needle aspirates. Acta Cytol 31: 267–275, 1987.
5. Friedman M, Forgione H, Shanbhag V: Needle aspiration of metastatic melanoma. Acta Cytol 24: 7–15, 1980.
5a. Gordon L A, Orell S R: Evaluation of cytodiagnosis of cutaneous basal cell carcinoma. J Am Acad Dermatol 11: 1082–1086, 1984.
6. Hajdu S I, Savino A: Cytologic diagnosis of malignant melanoma. Acta Cytol 17: 320–327, 1973.

7. Kline T S, Kannan V: Aspiration biopsy cytology and melanoma: Am J Clin Pathol 77: 597–601, 1982.
8. Lindholm K, de la Torre M: Fine needle aspiration cytology of myxoid metastatic malignant melanoma: Acta Cytol 32: 719–721, 1988.
9. Malberger E, Tillinger R, Lichtig Ch: Diagnosis of basal-cell carcinoma with aspiration cytology. Acta Cytol 23: 301–305, 1984.
10. Masukawa T, Friedrich E G Jr: Cytopathology of Paget's disease of the vulva. Diagnostic abrasive cytology. Acta Cytol 22: 476–478, 1978.
11. Mellblom L, Åkerman M, Carlén B: Aspiration cytology of neuroendocrine (Merkel cell) carcinoma of the skin: report of a case. Acta Cytol 28: 297–300, 1984.
12. Rocamora A, Carillo R, Vives R, Solera J C: Fine needle biopsy of myxoid metastasis of malignant melanoma. Acta Cytol 32: 94–100, 1988.
13. Skoog L, Schmitt F, Tani E: Neuroendocrine (Merkel cell) carcinoma of the skin: immunocytochemical and cytomorphologic analysis on fine needle aspirates. Diagn Cytopath 6: 53–57, 1990.
14. Woyke S, Domagala W, Czerniak B, Strokowska M: Fine

needle aspiration cytology of malignant melanomas of the skin. Acta Cytol 24: 529–538, 1980.

15. Woyke S, Olszewski W, Eichelkraut A: Pilomatrixoma. A pitfall in the aspiration cytology of skin tumors. Acta Cytol 26: 189–194, 1982.

Soft tissues

16. Abele J S, Miller T: Cytology of well-differentiated and poorly differentiated angiosarcoma in fine needle aspirates. Acta Cytol 26: 341–348, 1982.

17. Ahmed M N, Feldman M, Seemayer T A : Cytology of epithelioid sarcoma. Acta Cytol 18: 459–461, 1974.

18. Akhtar M, Ali M, Sabbah R, Bakry M, Nash J: Fine needle aspiration biopsy diagnosis of round cell malignant tumors of childhood. A combined light and electron microscopic approach. Cancer 55: 1805–1817, 1985.

19. Åkerman M, Rydholm A: Aspiration cytology of lipomatous tumors. A ten year experience at an Orthopedic Oncology Center. Diagn Cytopath 3: 295–302, 1987.

20. Åkerman M, Rydholm A: Aspiration cytology of intramuscular myxoma. A comparative clinical cytologic and histologic study of ten cases. Acta Cytol 27: 505–510, 1983.

21. Åkerman M, Rydholm A, Persson B M: Aspiration cytology of soft tissue tumors. The ten years experience at an Orthopedic Oncology Group. Acta Orthop Scand 56: 407–412, 1985.

22. Angervall L, Hagmar B, Kindblom L-G: Malignant giant cell tumor of soft tissues. A clinicopathologic, cytologic, ultrastructural, angiographic and microangiographic study. Cancer 47: 736–747, 1981.

23. Bertholf M F, Frierson H F, Feldman P S: Fine needle aspiration cytology of an adult rhabdomyoma of the head and neck. Diagn Cytopath 4: 152–155, 1988.

24. Bondeson L, Andreasson L: Aspiration cytology of adult rhabdomyoma. Acta Cytol 30: 679–682, 1986.

25. Calafati S A, Wright A L, Rosen S E, Walowitz A, Koprowska I: Fine needle aspiration cytology of extraskeletal chondrosarcoma. Acta Cytol 28: 81–85, 1984.

26. Dahl I, Åkerman M: Nodular fasciitis. A correlative cytologic and histologic study of 13 cases. Acta Cytol 25: 215–222, 1981.

27. Dahl I, Hagmar B, Angervall L: Leiomyosarcoma of the soft tissue. A correlative cytologic and histologic study of 11 cases. Acta Pathol Microbiol Immunol Scand (A) 89: 285–291, 1981.

28. Dahl I, Hagmar B, Idvall I: Benign solitary neurilemoma. A correlative cytological and histological study of 28 cases. Acta Pathol Microbiol Immunol Scand (A) 92: 91–101, 1984.

29. Delay D, Chamot L, Dragon V: Le cytodiagnostic par ponction-aspiration de metastases et recidives de cancers. Schweiz Med Wschr 106: 768–772, 1976.

30. Franzén S, Stenkvist B: Diagnosis of granular cell myoblastoma by fine-needle aspiration biopsy. Acta Pathol Microbiol Scand 72: 391–395, 1968.

31. Granberg I, Willems J S: Endometriosis of lung and pleura diagnosed by aspiration biopsy. Acta Cytol 21: 295–297, 1977.

32. Hajdu S I, Hajdu E O: Cytopathology of soft tissue and bone tumors. Monographs in clinical cytology. Wied G L (ed.), vol 12, Karger, Basel, 1989.

33. Kindblom L-G, Walaas L, Widehn S: Ultrastructural studies in the preoperative cytologic diagnosis of soft tissue tumors. Semin Diag Pathol 3: 317–344, 1985.

34. Koivuniemi A, Nickels J: Synovial sarcoma diagnosed by fine-needle aspiration biopsy. Acta Cytol 22: 515–518, 1978.

35. Krumerman M S: Leiomyosarcoma of the lung. Primary cytodiagnosis in two consecutive cases. Acta Cytol 21: 103–108, 1977.

36. Lindell M M Jr, Wallace S, deSantos L A, Bernardino M E: Diagnostic technique for the evaluation of the soft tissue sarcoma. Semin Oncol 8: 160–171, 1981.

37. Löwhagen T, Rubio C A: The cytology of the granular cell myoblastoma of the breast. Report of a case. Acta Cytol 21: 314–315, 1977.

38. Markhede G, Angervall L, Stener B: A multivariate analysis of the prognosis after surgical treatment of malignant soft-tissue tumours. Cancer 49: 1721–1733, 1982.

39. Mathews J B, Mason G I: Granular cell myoblastoma: an immunoperoxidase study using a variety of antisera to human carcinoembryonic antigen. Histopathology 7: 77–82, 1983.

40. Merck, Ch, Hagmar B: Myxofibrosarcoma. A correlative cytologic and histologic study of 13 cases examined by fine needle aspiration cytology. Acta Cytol 22: 137–144, 1980.

41. Nguyen G K: Cytopathologic aspects of leiomyoblastoma in fine needle aspiration biopsy. Report of two cases. Acta Cytol 27: 173–177, 1983.

42. Nickels J, Koivuniemi A: Cytology of malignant haemangiopericytoma. Acta Cytol 23: 119–125, 1979.

43. Nordgren H, Åkerman M: Electron microscopy of fine needle aspiration biopsy from soft tissue tumours. Acta Cytol 26: 179–188, 1982.

44. Ramzy I: Benign Schwannoma: demonstration of Verocay bodies using fine needle aspiration. Acta Cytol 21: 316–319, 1977.

45. Reif R M: The cytologic picture of proliferative myositis. Acta Cytol 26: 376–377, 1982.

46. Ryd W, Mugel S, Ayyash K: Ancient neurilemoma. A pitfall in the cytologic diagnosis of soft tissue tumors. Diagn Cytopath 2: 244–247, 1988.

47. Rydholm A, Berg N O, Dawidskiba S, Egund N, Idvall I, Pettersson H, Rööser B, Willén H, Åkerman M: Preoperative diagnosis of soft tissue tumors. Int Orthop (SICOT) 12: 109–114, 1988.

48. Rööser B, Herrlin K, Rydholm A, Åkerman M: Pseudomalignant myositis ossificans. Clinical, radiologic, and cytologic diagnosis. Acta Orthop Scand 60: 457–460, 1989.

49. Seidal T, Angervall L, Kindblom L-G: Rhabdomyosarcoma in patients of over 40 years of age. Definition and diagnosis. Acta Pathol Microbiol Immunol Scand (APMIS) 97: 236–248, 1989.

50. Seidal T, Mark K, Hagmar B, Angervall L: Alveolar rhabdomyosarcoma. A cytogenetic and correlated cytological and histological study. Acta Pathol Microbiol Immunol Scand (A) 90: 345–354, 1982.

51. Seidal T, Walaas L, Kindblom L-G, Angervall L: Cytology of embryonal rhabdomyosarcoma. A cytologic, light microscopic, electron microscopic and immunohistochemical study of seven cases. Diagn Cytopath 4: 292–300, 1988.

52. Shousha S, Lyssiotis T: Granular cell myoblastoma: positive staining for carcinoembryonic antigen. J Clin Pathol 32: 219–224, 1979.

53. Stener B: The management of soft tissue tumours. Int Orthop 1: 289–298, 1978.

54. Uehara H: Cytology of alveolar soft part sarcoma. Acta Cytol 22: 191–192, 1978.

55. Walaas L, Angervall L, Hagmar B, Säve-Söderberg J: A correlative cytologic and histologic study of malignant

11 *SUPPORTING TISSUES*

fibrous histiocytoma: An analysis of 40 cases examined by fine-needle aspiration cytology. Diagn Cytopath 2: 46–64, 1986.

56. Walaas L, Kindblom L-G: Lipomatous tumors. A correlative cytologic and histologic study of 27 tumors examined by fine needle aspiration cytology. Human Pathol 16: 6–18, 1985.

57. Westermark P, Stenqvist B: A new method for the diagnosis of systemic amyloidosis. Arch Int Med 132: 522–523, 1973.

58. Zbieranowski I, Bedard Y: Fine needle aspiration of Schwannomas: Value of electron microscopy and immunocytochemistry in the preoperative diagnosis. Acta Cytol 33: 381–385, 1985.

59. Zornoza J: Needle biopsy of metastases. Radiol Clin North Am 20: 569–590, 1982.

60. Zornoza J, Bernardino M E, Ordonez N G, Thomas J L, Cohen M A: Percutaneous needle biopsy of soft tissue tumours guided by ultrasound and computed tomography. Skeletal Radiol 9: 33–36, 1982.

Bone

61. Adler O, Rosenberger A: Fine needle aspiration biopsy of osteolytic metastatic lesions. Am J Roentgenol 133: 15–18, 1979.

62. Akthar M, Ashraf A, Sabbah R: Aspiration cytology of Ewing's sarcoma. Light and electron microscopic correlations. Cancer 56: 2051–2060, 1985.

63. Åkerman M, Berg N O, Persson B M: Fine needle aspiration biopsy in the evaluation of tumour-like lesions of bone. Acta Orthop Scand 47: 129–136, 1976.

64. Argawal P K, Wahal K M: Cytopathologic study of primary tumours of bones and joints. Acta Cytol 27: 23–27, 1983.

65. Armstrong P, Chalmers A, Green G, Irving J D: Needle aspiration biopsy of the spine in suspected disc infection. Br J Radiol 51: 333–337, 1978.

66. Batisser-Bielecka I: Cytopathologic diagnosis of an eosinophilic granuloma of bone by needle aspiration biopsy. Acta Cytol 33: 683–685, 1989.

67. Coley B L, Sharp G S, Ellis E B: Diagnosis of bone tumours by aspiration. Am J Surg 13: 215–224, 1931.

68. Dahl I, Åkerman M, Angervall L: Ewing's sarcoma of bone. A correlative cytological and histological study of 14 cases. Acta Pathol Microbiol Immunol Scand (A) 94: 363–369, 1986.

69. De Santos L A, Murray J A, Ayala A: The value of percutaneous needle biopsy in the management of primary bone tumours. Cancer 43: 735–744, 1979.

70. Finley J, Silverman, J, Dabbs D, West R, Dickens A, Feldman Ph, Frable W: Chordoma. Diagnosis by fine needle aspiration biopsy with histologic, immunocytochemical and ultrastructural confirmation. Diagn Cytopath 2: 330–337, 1986.

71. Franzén S, Stenkvist B: Cytologic diagnosis of eosinophilic granuloma — reticuloendotheliosis. Acta Pathol Microbiol Scand 72: 385–390, 1968.

72. Hajdu S I: Aspiration biopsy of primary malignant bone tumours. Front Radiat Ther Oncol 10: 73–81, 1975.

73. Katz R L, Silva E G, de Santos L, Lukeman J M: Diagnosis of eosinophilic granuloma of bone by cytology, histology, and electron microscopy of transcutaneous bone aspiration biopsy. J Bone Joint Surg 62: 1284–1290, 1980.

74. Kontozoglou T, Qizilbash A, Sianos J, Stead R: Chordoma: cytologic and immunocytochemical study of four cases. Diagn Cytopath 2: 55–61, 1986.

75. Lefer L G, Rosier R P: The cytology of chordoma. Acta Cytol 22: 51–53, 1978.

76. Lopez-Cardozo P: Atlas of clinical cytology. Leiden, 1978.

77. McLaughlin R E, Miller W R, Miller C W: Quadriparesis after needle aspiration of the cervical spine. J Bone Joint Surg 58: 1167–1168, 1976.

78. Olszewski W, Woyke S, Musiatowics B: Fine needle aspiration biopsy cytology of chondrosarcoma. Acta Cytol 27: 345–349, 1983.

79. Ottolenghi C E: Diagnosis of orthopedic lesions by aspiration biopsy. Results of 1061 punctures. J Bone Joint Surg 37: 443–464, 1955.

80. Ottolenghi C E: Aspiration biopsy of the spine. Technique for the thoracic spine and results of 28 biopsies in this region and overall results of 1050 of other spinal segments. J Bone Joint Surg 51: 1531–1544, 1969.

81. Sanerkin N G, Jeffree G M: Cytology of bone tumours. A colour atlas with text. John Wright & Sons, Bristol, 1980.

82. Schajowics F: Tumours and tumour-like lesions of bone and joints. Springer, New York, 1981.

83. Schajowics F, Derqui J C: Puncture biopsy in lesions of the locomotor system. A review of results in 4050 cases including 941 vertebral punctures. Cancer 21: 531–548, 1968.

84. Sneige N, Ayala A, Carrasco H, Murray J, Raymond A: Giant cell tumor of bone. A cytologic study of 24 cases. Diagn Cytopath 1: 111–117, 1985.

85. Stormby N, Åkerman M: Cytodiagnosis of bone lesions by means of fine needle aspiration biopsy. Acta Cytol 17: 166–172, 1973.

86. Walaas L, Kindblom L-G: Light and electron microscopic examinations of the fine needle aspirates in the preoperative diagnosis of osteogenic tumours. Diagn Cytopath 6: 27–38, 1990.

87. White V A, Fanning C V, Ayala A, Raymond A, Carrasco H, Murray J: Osteosarcoma and the role of fine-needle aspiration: a study of 51 cases. Cancer 62: 1238–1246, 1988.

88. Zornoza J (ed): Percutaneous needle biopsy. Williams & Wilkins, Baltimore, 1981.

89. Histiocytosis syndromes in children. The Writing Group of the Histiocyte Society. Lancet 1: 208–209, 1987.

INDEX

INDEX

INDEX

INDEX

INDEX

INDEX

INDEX